Edited by
Raju Francis and
D. Sakthi Kumar

Biomedical Applications of Polymeric Materials and Composites

Related Titles

Bagchi, D., Bagchi, M., Moriyama, H., Fereidoon, S. (eds.)

Bio-Nanotechnology – A Revolution in Food, Biomedical and Health Sciences

2013
Print ISBN: 978-0-470-67037-8
WOL obook PDF ISBN: 978-1-118-45191-5
eMobi ISBN: 978-1-118-45192-2
ePub ISBN: 978-1-118-45193-9
Adobe PDF ISBN: 978-1-118-45194-6

Smela, E.E., Carpi, F.F. (eds.)

Biomedical Applications of Electroactive PolymerActuators

2009
Print ISBN: 978-0-470-77305-5
Adobe PDF ISBN: 978-0-470-74468-0
ISBN: 978-0-470-74469-7

Narain, R. (ed.)

Chemistry of Bioconjugates
Synthesis, Characterization, and Biomedical Applications

2014
Print ISBN: 978-1-118-35914-3
WOL obook PDF ISBN: 978-1-118-77588-2
ePub ISBN: 978-1-118-77637-7
Adobe PDF ISBN: 978-1-118-77640-7

Kabasci, S. (ed.)

Bio-based Plastics – Materials and Applications

2014
Print ISBN: 978-1-119-99400-8
eMobi ISBN: 978-1-118-67662-2
ISBN: 978-1-118-67664-6
ePub ISBN: 978-1-118-67673-8
Adobe PDF ISBN: 978-1-118-67678-3

Kumar, C.S. (ed.)

Biofunctionalization of Nanomaterials

2015
Print ISBN: 978-3-527-31381-5

Taubert, A., Mano, J.F., Rodríguez-Cabello, J.C. (eds.)

Biomaterials Surface Science

2013
Print ISBN: 978-3-527-33031-7
ISBN: 978-3-527-64960-0
eMobi ISBN: 978-3-527-64961-7
ePub ISBN: 978-3-527-64962-4
Adobe PDF ISBN: 978-3-527-64963-1

Zhao, Y., Shen, Y. (eds.)

Biomedical Nanomaterials

2016
Print ISBN: 978-3-527-33798-9
WOL obook PDF ISBN: 978-3-527-69439-6
ePub ISBN: 978-3-527-69441-9
eMobi ISBN: 978-3-527-69442-6
Adobe PDF ISBN: 978-3-527-69443-3

Deng, T. (ed.)

Bioinspired Engineering of Thermal Materials

2016
Print ISBN: 978-3-527-33834-4
WOL obook PDF ISBN: 978-3-527-68759-6
ePub ISBN: 978-3-527-68761-9
eMobi ISBN: 978-3-527-68764-0
Adobe PDF ISBN: 978-3-527-68765-7

Pompe, W., Rödel, G., Weiss, H., Mertig, M.

Bio-Nanomaterials

Designing materials inspired by nature

2013
Print ISBN: 978-3-527-41015-6
ISBN: 978-3-527-65526-7
eMobi ISBN: 978-3-527-65527-4
ePub ISBN: 978-3-527-65528-1
Adobe PDF ISBN: 978-3-527-65529-8

Kargarzadeh, H., Ahmad, I., Thomas, S., Dufresne, A. (eds.)

Handbook of Cellulose Nanocomposites

2016
Print ISBN: 978-3-527-33866-5
WOL obook PDF ISBN: 978-3-527-68997-2
Adobe PDF ISBN: 978-3-527-68998-9
ePub ISBN: 978-3-527-68999-6
eMobi ISBN: 978-3-527-69004-6

Jawaid, M., Faruq, M. (eds.)

Nanocellulose and Nanohydrogel Matrices

Biotechnological and Biomedical Applications

2017
Print ISBN: 978-3-527-34172-6
Adobe PDF ISBN: 978-3-527-80382-8
WOL obook PDF ISBN: 978-3-527-80383-5
eMobi ISBN: 978-3-527-80384-2
ePub ISBN: 978-3-527-80385-9

Edited by Raju Francis and D. Sakthi Kumar

Biomedical Applications of Polymeric Materials and Composites

WILEY-VCH
Verlag GmbH & Co. KGaA

Editors

Prof. Raju Francis
Mahatma Gandhi University
School of Chemical Sciences
Priyadarsini Hills
686560 Kottayam
Kerala
India

Prof. D. Sakthi Kumar
Toyo University
Bio Nano Electronics Research Center
350-858 Kawagoe
Japan

Cover:
Getty Images, Medical Art Inc.

Library of Congress Card No.: applied for

British Library Cataloguing-in-Publication Data
A catalogue record for this book is available from the British Library.

Bibliographic information published by the Deutsche Nationalbibliothek
The Deutsche Nationalbibliothek lists this publication in the Deutsche Nationalbibliografie; detailed bibliographic data are available on the Internet at <http://dnb.d-nb.de>.

Print ISBN: 978-3-527-33836-8
ePDF ISBN: 978-3-527-69094-7
ePub ISBN: 978-3-527-69092-3
Mobi ISBN: 978-3-527-69093-0
oBook ISBN: 978-3-527-69091-6

Typesetting SPi Global, Chennai, India
Printing and Binding Markono Print Media Pte Ltd, Singapore

Printed on acid-free paper

Contents

List of Contributors

Surjith Alancherry
James Cook University
College of Science
Technology and Engineering
James Cook Drive
Townsville, QLD 4811
Australia

Solaiappan Ananthakumar
Council of Scientific and
Industrial Research-National
Institute for Interdisciplinary
Science and Technology
(CSIR-NIIST)
Functional Materials Section
Materials Science and
Technology Division (MSTD)
Thiruvananthapuram 695019
Kerala
India

Deepa K. Baby
Rajagiri School of Engineering
and Technology
Department of Basic science and
Humanities
Rajagiri Valley
Kakkanad, Kochi 682039
Kerala
India

Kateryna Bazaka
James Cook University
College of Science
Technology and Engineering
James Cook Drive
Townsville, QLD 4811
Australia

and

Queensland University of
Technology
Institute of Health and
Biomedical Innovation
Brisbane, QLD 4000
Australia

Brahatheeswaran Dhandayuthapani
Toyo University
BioNano Electronics Research Centre
Kawagoe
Saitama 3508585
Japan

and

Collaborative Research and Education Program
Nanoscale Research Facility
Indian Institute of Technology-Delhi
Hauz Khaz 110016
Delhi
India

Joby Eldho
R&D Deposition Materials
EMD Performance Materials
1429 Hilldale Avenue
Haverhill, MA 01832
USA

Harikrishna Erothu
Aston University
Chemical Engineering and Applied Chemistry
Aston Triangle
Birmingham
West Midlands B4 7ET
UK

Raju Francis
Mahatma Gandhi University
School of Chemical Sciences
Priyadarshini Hills
Kottayam 686560
Kerala
India

J. Mary Gladis
Indian Institute of Space Science and Technology
Department of Chemistry
Valiamala
Thiruvananthapuram 695547
India

Geethy P. Gopalan
Mahatma Gandhi University
School of Chemical Sciences
Priyadarshini Hills
Kottayam 686560
Kerala
India

Daniel S. Grant
James Cook University
College of Science, Technology and Engineering
James Cook Drive
Townsville, QLD 4811
Australia

Mohan V. Jacob
James Cook University
College of Science, Technology and Engineering
James Cook Drive
Townsville, QLD 4811
Australia

Nidhin Joy
Mahatma Gandhi University
School of Chemical Sciences
Priyadarshini Hills
Kottayam 686560
Kerala
India

Anitha C. Kumar
Acharya Nagarjuna University
Department of Chemistry
Nagarjuna Nagar
Guntur 522510
Andhra Pradesh
India

and

Aston University
Chemical Engineering and
Applied Chemistry
Aston Triangle
Birmingham
West Midlands B4 7ET
UK

Dasappan Sakthi kumar
Toyo University
BioNano Electronics Research
Centre
Kawagoe
Saitama 3508585
Japan

and

Collaborative Research and
Education Program
Nanoscale Research Facility,
Indian Institute of
Technology-Delhi
Hauz Khaz 110016
Delhi
India

Vazhayal Linsha
Council of Scientific and
Industrial Research-National
Institute for Interdisciplinary
Science and Technology
(CSIR-NIIST), Functional
Materials Section
Materials Science and
Technology Division (MSTD)
Thiruvananthapuram 695019
Kerala
India

Kallyadan Veettil Mahesh
Council of Scientific and
Industrial Research
National Institute for
Interdisciplinary Science and
Technology (CSIR-NIIST),
Functional Materials Section,
Materials Science and
Technology Division (MSTD)
Thiruvananthapuram 695019
Kerala
India

T.P.D. Rajan
Council of Scientific and
Industrial Research-National
Institute for Interdisciplinary
Science and Technology
(CSIR-NIIST), Materials Science
and Technology Division
Industrial Estate PO
Pappanamcode
Thiruvananthapuram 695018
India

Anjaly Sivadas
Mahatma Gandhi University
School of Chemical Sciences
Priyadarshini Hills
Kottayam 686560
Kerala
India

Preface

Natural and synthetic polymer materials and composites are extensively used as biomaterials for various biomedical applications such as tissue engineering, implantable devices, drug delivery, gene delivery, bioimaging, and so on. Advances in polymer chemistry have allowed the creation of a wide range of biomaterials based on polymers and composites for different biomedical applications according to the nature of their use. The versatility and ease of modification of the chemical, physical, surface, and biomimetic properties of polymers have made them very much dear to the researchers working in the biomedical field. Applications of biomaterials have led to the development of polymers that are biocompatible, biodegradable, and/or resorbable.

A variety of research results are published almost daily on polymers and composites by enhancing their properties as biomaterials to meet the ongoing and evolving challenges in the biomedical field. This book, *Biomedical Applications of Polymeric Materials and Composites,* is intended to update and provide detailed information to students, technicians, researchers, scientists, and teachers working in the biomedical field by taking the contents only from the very latest results and presenting an extensive summary of the various polymeric materials used in biomedical applications.

This book consists of 12 Chapters.

Chapter 1, "Biomaterials for biomedical applications," provides an introduction to the various biomaterials currently used in biomedical applications. Selection of the appropriate biomaterials plays a key role in the design and development of the biomedical product. Nowadays, the strategy for biomaterials to be used as biomedical devices is that they should be biocompatible and must elicit a desirable cellular response to harness control over cellular interactions during its usage. This chapter provides detailed information on the current approach for developing biomaterials that can create cellular response by including protein growth factors, anti-inflammatory drugs, gene delivery vectors, and other bioactive vectors. Polymers are generally known to be insulating materials; however, it has been discovered that some polymers can be conductors and semiconductors. Chapter 2, "Conducting polymers – An introduction," provides information on conducting polymers, as these polymers can be used for different applications in biomedical devices. Chapter 3, "Conducting Polymers: Biomedical Applications," details the importance of using conducting biopolymers in the biomedical field and provides information of various biopolymers that are used in this field.

Chapter 4, "Plasma-assisted fabrication and processing of biomaterials," provides information on low-temperature plasma-assisted methods to fabricate and modify the surface of biomaterials. Plasma is also used for sterilization and disease management. Chapter 5, "Smart electroactive polymers and composite materials," describes such materials. Upon application of an electric voltage, the shape of some polymeric materials can be modified, which can be used as actuators and sensors. Because of their similarities with some biological tissues based on the achievable stress and force, these polymers can be used as artificial muscles. Chapter 6, "Synthetic polymer hydrogels," provides information of some of the rapidly developing groups of materials that find applications in many fields such as pharmacy, medicine, and agriculture. Chapter 7, "Hydrophilic polymers," describes various natural, synthetic, and semisynthetic hydrophilic polymers. These types of polymers have the lion's share of applications in the field of biomaterials.

Chapter 8 describes the "Properties of stimuli-responsive polymers." These types of polymers are the most exciting and emerging class of materials, and have the ability to respond to external stimuli such as temperature, pH, ionic strength, light, and electric and magnetic fields. Since these materials can respond to external stimuli, they find many applications in the biomedical field. Chapter 9, "Stimuli-responsive polymers: Biomedical applications," provides details about various polymers that find applications in the biomedical field based on their stimuli-responsive properties. This interesting property has enabled the development of smart systems that are useful in bioimaging, sensing (diagnosis), controlled drug delivery, regenerative medicine (therapy), bioseparation, gating valves for transport, and microfluidics. Chapter 10, "Functionally engineered sol–gel inorganic gels and hybrid nanostructures for biomedical applications," describes nanostructured inorganic gels, mostly metal oxide gels and hybrid nanoarchitectures developed through sol–gel synthesis, and their various biomedical applications.

Chapter 11, "Relevance of Natural Degradable Polymers in the Biomedical field," highlights the importance of natural degradable polymers for biomedical applications. In modern medicine, natural degradable polymers have their own indisputable place, particularly in drug delivery applications, because they degrade after serving their specific roles. Natural degradable polymers alone cannot meet the demand for applications in the biomedical field. Therefore, with the help of modern chemistry, many biodegradable synthetic polymers have been developed with a wide range of applications such as sutures, implants, drug delivery vehicles, and so on. A variety of synthetic methods have allowed the development of many polymers that meet the functional demands and materials with the desired physical, chemical, biological, biochemical, and degradation properties. Chapter 12, "Synthetic biodegradable polymers for Medical and Clinical Applications," is included to describe the various synthetic degradable polymers that find interesting applications in the biomedical field.

We believe that this book provides in-depth discussions and details on the polymers and their composites that have applications in the biomedical field based on recent research results in this magnificent field. Throughout the book, we have focused on recent applications, with worked examples and case studies for training purposes, which will serve the purpose of this book, that is, to update students, technicians, researchers, scientists, and teachers who work in the biomedical field.

We express our sincere thanks and appreciation to the 20 scientists for contributing chapters to this book and their constant cooperation from submission of the first drafts to revision and final fine-tuning of their chapters commensurate with the reviews. We extend our appreciation to our respective host institutions, namely Mahatma Gandhi University, Kottayam, India, and Toyo University, Japan, for their encouragement and support.

Finally, we wish to extend our thanks to Wiley-VCH and all their staff involved in the publication and promotion of this book, which will hopefully be useful to those working in the biomedical field.

India
Japan
18 July 2016

Raju Francis
D. Sakthi Kumar

1
Biomaterials for Biomedical Applications

Brahatheeswaran Dhandayuthapani and Dasappan Sakthi kumar

1.1
Introduction

Biomaterials play numerous critical roles in biomedical applications. Historically, biomaterials were obtained from natural sources, such as purified collagen, gelatin, silk, or cotton. Advances in polymer chemistry supplemented these natural polymers with first-generation medical polymers. Currently, polymers are used in a wide range of biomedical applications, including applications in which the polymer remains in intimate contact with cells and tissues for prolonged periods. Although many of these polymer materials have been tested for various applications, it is widely recognized that the current range of biomaterials available will not be adequate for the vast range of applications in drug delivery, artificial organs, and tissue engineering technologies. To select appropriate materials for biomedical applications, it will help to understand the influence of these materials on viability, growth, and function of attached or adjacent cells. The selection of biomaterials plays a key role in the design and development of biomedical products. While the classical selection criterion for a safe, stable implant dictated choosing a passive, inert material, it is now deduced that any such device is capable of eliciting a cellular response [1, 2]. Therefore, it is now widely accepted that a biomaterial must interact with tissue to repair, rather than simply be a static replacement. Furthermore, biomaterials used directly in tissue repair or replacement applications (e.g., artificial skin) must be more than biocompatible; they must elicit a desirable cellular response. Consequently, a major focus of biomaterials for tissue engineering applications centers on harnessing control over cellular interactions with biomaterials, often including components to manipulate cellular response within the supporting biomaterial as a key design component. Specific examples of such components include protein growth factors, anti-inflammatory drugs, gene delivery vectors, and other bioactive factors to elicit the desired cellular response [3, 4].

Biomedical Applications of Polymeric Materials and Composites, First Edition.
Edited by Raju Francis and Sakthi Kumar.

It is important for the developer of biomedical products to have several biomaterial options available, because each application calls for a unique environment for cell–cell interactions. Examples of some such applications are as follows:

a) Support for new tissue growth (wherein cell–cell communication and cell availability to nutrients, growth factors, and pharmaceutically active agents must be maximized);
b) Prevention of cellular activity (where tissue growth, such as in surgically induced adhesions, is undesirable);
c) Guided tissue response (enhancing a particular cellular response while inhibiting others);
d) Enhancement of cell attachment and subsequent cellular activation (e.g., fibroblast attachment, proliferation, and production of extracellular matrix (ECM) for dermis repair);
e) Inhibition of cellular attachment and/or activation (e.g., platelet attachment to a vascular graft); and
f) Prevention of a biological response (e.g., blocking antibodies against homograft or xenograft cells used in organ replacement therapies).

The processability of biomaterials is a key step for developing biomedical applications. Nine potential biomedical applications areas have been identified [5]:

1) Membranes in extracorporeal applications such as oxygenators;
2) Bioactive membranes, for example, controlled release delivery systems and artificial cells;
3) Disposable equipment, for example, blood bags and disposable syringes;
4) Sutures and adhesives including biodegradable and nonbiodegradable materials;
5) Cardiovascular devices such as vascular grafts;
6) Reconstructive and orthopedic implants;
7) Ophthalmic devices such as corneas and contact lenses;
8) Dental restorative materials including dentures;
9) Degradable plastic commodity products.

This chapter surveys the various biomaterials that have been used or are under consideration for use in biomedical applications.

1.2 Polymers as Hydrogels in Cell Encapsulation and Soft Tissue Replacement

Hydrogels are one of the most promising classes of biomaterials for biomedical applications because they have good biocompatibility and a large amount of equilibrium water content [6]. Wichterle [7] achieved the following four crucial criteria with the design.

a) Preventing component release.
b) Creating a stable chemical and biochemical structure.

c) Having a high permeability for nutrients and waste.
d) Assuming physical characteristics similar to those of natural living tissue.

Hydrogels have water content and mechanical properties that are similar to those of human tissue and find use in many biomedical applications. The first biomedical use for synthetic hydrogels, which was established in 1954, was as an orbital implant. Wichterle designed soft contact lenses from hydrogels in 1961. Since then, hydrogel use for biomedical applications has included wound dressings, drug delivery systems, hemodialysis systems, artificial skin, and tissue engineering [8–10]. The structural similarity of hydrogels to that of the human ECM creates promising applications as a scaffold material for cell-based tissue engineering [10]. Hern and Hubbell [11] first modified PEGA with the adhesive peptide arginyl–glycyl–aspartic acid (RGD) to enhance cell adhesion and promote tissue spreading. In separate experiments, PEG methacrylate has been modified with phosphoester and RGD to enhance bone engineering [12, 13]. In addition, hyaluronic acid has been copolymerized with PEGDA+RGD to support cell attachment and proliferation as well as to improve cartilage repair [14, 15]. Poly(γ-benzyl L-glutamate) (PBLG) is one of the synthetic polypeptides that has attracted attention for use in drug delivery matrices [16]. Hydrogels developed by combining polyisobutylene (PIB) and hydrophilic polymer segments were used for coating Gore-Tex vascular grafts and showed good biocompatibility [17]. These hydrogels were also used as membrane carriers for insulin-producing porcine platelet implants [18]. Shu *et al.* [19] synthesized thiolated HA and then conjugated it to PEG for the benefit of *in situ* injection and cell encapsulation and proliferation. PEG and HA may be further modified by physical cross-linking of bioactive factors, which is one of the methods used to create biomimetic hydrogels. Growth factors remain active after encapsulation to enhance the proliferation and differentiation of encapsulated cells or to improve local tissue regeneration [20, 21]. Growth factors that have been entrapped in hydrogels include bone morphogenetic protein-2 (BMP-2), fibroblast growth factor, vascular endothelial growth factor (VEGF), insulin-like growth factor 1 (IGF-1), and transforming growth factor β (TGF-β), among others [21–25].

The examples in the following paragraph illustrate the effect of biomimetic hydrogels on three different tissues. Several groups have demonstrated *in vivo* secretion of cartilaginous matrix using chondrocytes encapsulated in hydrogels. The use of hydrogels to support chondrocyte growth and matrix production is well established. Current efforts focus on bringing hydrogels closer to clinical applications. Lee *et al.* [20] incorporated TGF-β1 into a chitosan scaffold in which chondrocytes were cultured. The chondrocytes cultured in scaffolds containing TGF-β1 exhibited significantly greater proliferation and GAG and type II collagen production than did chondrocytes cultured in control scaffolds lacking TGF-β1. Recently, thermoplastic biodegradable hydrogels have been designed for biomedical applications including drug delivery systems: polyisobutylene (PIB)-based materials as potential materials for soft tissue replacement, specifically for vascular grafts and breast implants [26] (Figure 1.1). Polyesters (PET),

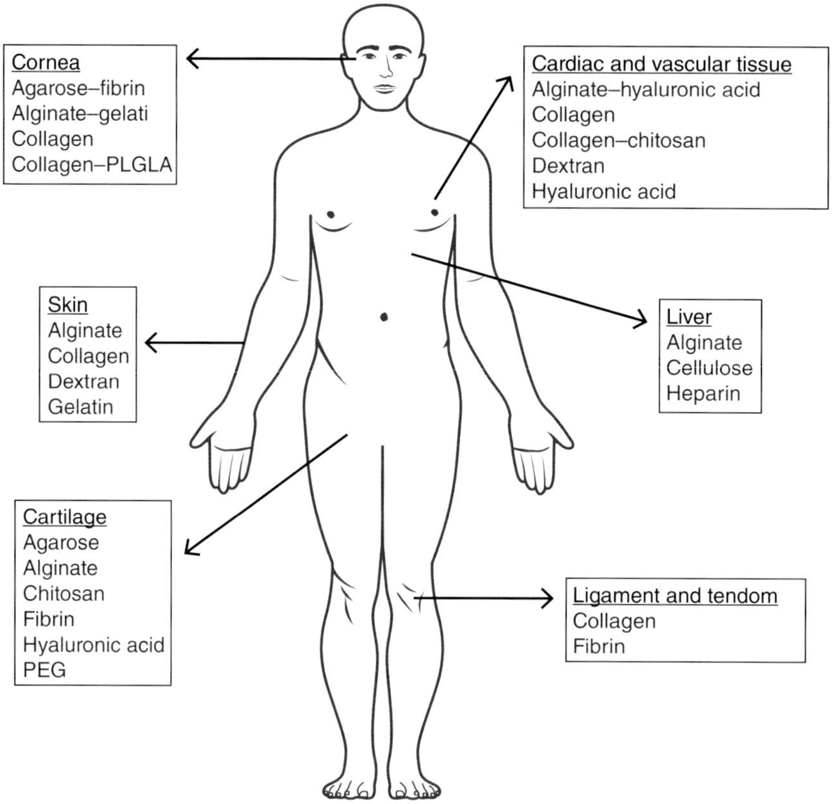

Figure 1.1 Polymer hydrogels used for tissue replacement.

fluoropolymers (PTFE), polypropylene (PP), polyurethanes (PU), and silicones have played a crucial role in the development of polymeric materials for soft tissue replacement [27]. This biomaterial represents a conceptually new soft biomaterial for potential biomedical application (Table 1.1).

1.3 Biomaterials for Drug Delivery Systems

A defining therapeutic feature of a biodegradable polymer used in modern drug delivery is facile degradation into oligomers or monomers with concomitant kinetically controlled drug release profiles. Polymeric delivery systems are mainly used to achieve either temporal or spatial control of drug delivery [28]. Essentially, polymeric vehicles enable drugs to be delivered over an extended period of time and to the local site of action. They are designed to enhance drug safety and efficacy, and to improve patient compliance. The use of polymers is designed to maintain therapeutic levels of the drug, reduce ide-effects, decrease the amount

Table 1.1 Natural and synthetic polymers commonly used in the synthesis of hydrogels [10].

Natural hydrogels	Synthetic polymers
Hyaluronic acid (HA)	Hydroxyethyl methacrylate (HEMA)
Chondroitin sulfate	Methoxyethyl methacrylate (MEMA)
Matrigel	*N*-Vinyl-2-pyrrolidone (NVP)
Alginate	*N*-Isopropyl Aam (NIPAAm)
Collagen	Acrylic Acid (AA)
Fibrin	Poly(ethylene glycol) acrylate (PEGA)
Chitosan	Poly(ethylene oxide) diacrylate (poly(ethylene glycol) diacrylate (PEGDA))
Silk	Poly(vinyl alcohol) (PVA)
Gelatin, Agarose, and Dextran	Poly(fumarates)

of drug molecule and the dosage frequency, and facilitate the delivery of drugs with short *in vivo* half-lives [29]. In polymer-based drug delivery, polyalkylcyanoacrylates (PACAs) have evolved diverse versatility as drug nanoparticle carriers for indomethacin [30], gangliosides [31], oligonucleotides [32], anti-epileptic medications including Ethosuximide [33], insulin [34], saquinavir [35], hemoglobin [36], and nucleoside analogs against human immunodeficiency virus (HIV) [37]. Translational research into poly(ethylene glycol) (PEG)–PACAs and actively targeted PACA systems [38, 39] have shown great promise for use *in vivo* such as the recently completed phase I and phase II studies of Doxorubicin Transdrug® for primary liver cancer.

Polyphosphazenes have been used for controlled release of naproxen [40–42], calcitonin [43], colchicines [44], (diamine) platinum [45], (dach) platinum (II) [46], insulin [47], other model proteins [48, 49], methylprednisolone [50, 51], methotrexate [52], tacrolimus [53], tempamine [54], and plasmid deoxyribonucleic acid [55]. Studies of blood biocompatibility *in vitro* with polyorganophosphazenes have shown no morphological changes or aggregation with platelets [56] and good biocompatibility after transplantation [57]. The first long-term biocompatibility *in vivo* study with polyphosphazene was reported in 2003 by Huang *et al.* [58] with a porcine coronary stent model, which showed no signs of either hyperplasia or proliferative response after 6 months. In the same family as polyphosphazenes, polyphosphoesters (PPEs) are inorganic polymers. To date, biocompatibility studies have been quite favorable, showing limited toxicity [59]. Numerous studies by Leong's group have used PPEs for block copolymer design including poly(2-aminoethyl propylene phosphate) (PPE-EA) for gene delivery [60–63] and PPE microspheres for nerve growth factor delivery. *In vivo* studies with the Paclimer delivery system, 10% w/w paclitaxel encapsulated in biodegradable polyphosphoester microspheres, with a single intratumoral or intraperitonel injection showed 80% release of the drug after 90 days in a human lung cancer xenograft model. This sustained release showed significant inhibition of nonsmall cell lung cancer nodules with three- to sixfold longer tumor doubling times compared with free paclitaxel and vehicle controls [64–66]. A recent translational canine study to evaluate dose escalation and neurotoxicity showed excellent results throughout the 120-day study with no evidence of systemic toxicity or gross morphological or physiological changes in the animals [67]. Polyesters represent perhaps the largest family of biodegradable polymers including aliphatic polyesters such as poly(glycolic acid) (PGA), poly(lactic acid) (PLA), poly(lactide-co-glycolide) (PLGA), polydioxanone, polyglyconate, polycaprolactone, and polyesteramide [68]. Several biodegradable polyesters, many of which are PGA derivatives, have also been used in nonviral gene delivery primarily to alleviate cytotoxicity such as poly[**α**-(4-aminobutyl)-L-glycolic acid] (PAGA) [69, 70], poly(D,L-lactic acid-co-glycolic acid) (PLGA) [71–73], PEG–PLGA–PEG [74] and poly(4-hydroxyl-1-proline esters) [75, 76]. PCL block copolymers have been used to deliver doxorubicin [77], cyclosporine A [78, 79], geldanamycin [80], rapamycin [81], 97 amphotericin B [82, 83], dihydrotestosterone [84], indomethacin [85, 86], and paclitaxel [87]. Polyorthoesters (POEs) were developed and reported by Heller *et al.*, nearly 40 years ago for use as implanted biomaterials and as drug delivery vehicles [88] (Figure 1.2).

Biodegradable polymers have truly revolutionized controlled drug delivery design and biomaterial applications for implants and tissue engineering. A biodegradable derivative of poly(ethylene glycol)-co-poly(L-lysine) (PEG–PLL) with grafted histidine residues has been synthesized for local gene therapy with transgene expression levels fourfold higher than PLL alone [89, 90]. With the help of biodegradable stents, clinicians can site-specifically control drug release to treat coronary artery disease through delivery of traditional small molecules

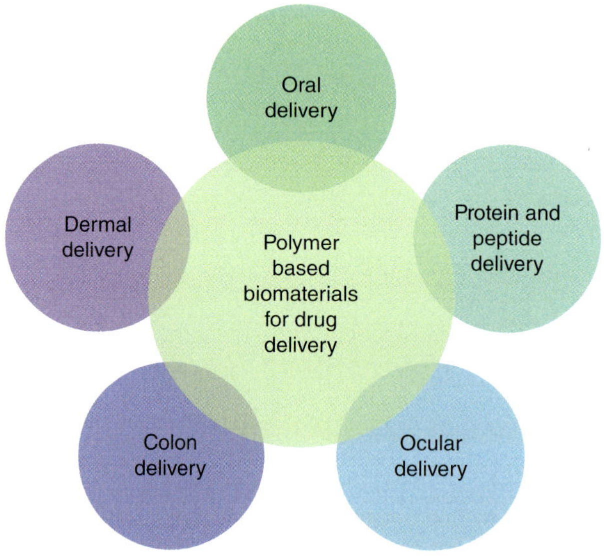

Figure 1.2 Biomaterials utilized for various drug delivery systems.

and, now, gene therapy [91, 92]. Biodegradable block copolymers and block copolypeptides have significantly endowed novel drug delivery systems with beneficial pharmacokinetic and biocompatible properties.

1.4 Biomaterials for Heart Valves and Arteries

Devices or natural tissues can be used to replace heart valves or arteries. These replacement materials are used when the natural heart valves or arteries fail to function properly, which can result in death or severe disability if left uncorrected. Such replacement materials help to restore the flow of blood that the body needs in order to function properly. Natural tissues are commonly used as replacement materials; alternatively, pyrolytic carbon mechanical valves are used to replace heart valves, while metal stents can be used to hold arteries open. However, there is interest in the development of polymers as replacement materials for heart valves and for use with stents. Heart valves are composed of connective tissue (collagen, elastin, and glycosaminoglycans [93], and open or close in response to pressure gradients and hemodynamics [94]. Flexible leaflet aortic replacement valves were developed in the 1960s [95]. There has been recent interest in developing polymeric valves from polyurethanes. Polyurethanes have good blood compatibility [96] and can be made into physiological shapes, forming valves that are flexible [97]. Synthetic poly(carbonate urethane) valves have been recently developed for both the aortic and the mitral positions [98]. *In vivo* results are promising, with tests being performed without anticoagulants in some cases, and show greater signs of durability than bioprostheses when tested in calves [99], or sheep [100].

Materials such as braided polyester, polybutester (a butylene terephthalate and poly(tetramethylene ether glycol) copolymer), polypropylene, PTFE, or e-PTFE can be used for replacement of mitral valves related repairs. However, during chordal replacement, the synthetic suture acts as a neochord. PTFE has been found to have material properties that are closer in nature to natural chordae than other materials such as braided polyester [101]. An alternative to synthetic chordae is the use of natural tissues, such as glutaraldehyde-tanned pericardial strips [102]. However, PTFE has been found to produce better clinical results than glutaraldehyde-tanned pericardial strips for chordal replacement [103]. Developments of new chordal replacement materials may further improve mitral valve repair in the long term. Tissue engineered synthetic chordae made from cultured fibroblast and smooth muscle cells have been reported, with added type I collagen [104, 105]. However, replacement synthetic chordae with properties closer in nature to real chordae may well provide benefits for mitral valve replacement (Figure 1.3).

Stents are usually composed of metal wires forming the outer boundaries of an open cylinder. The most widely used stents are made from stainless steel [106] and are relatively inert when in place. Stents have been very successful clinically and may well be used in over 50% of angioplasty procedures [107]. The placement of

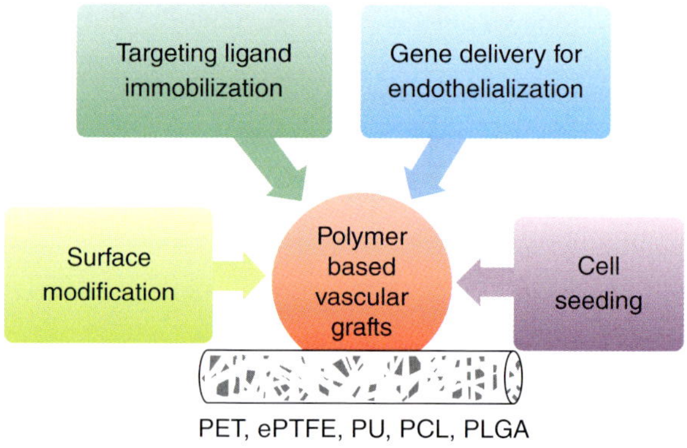

Figure 1.3 Polymers for artificial vascular grafts.

stents may damage the arterial endothelial layer [108], which may cause some of the problems associated with stents. Initially, stents were designed to be bioinert (by using materials such as stainless steel). However, coatings may be necessary to avoid restenosis. Polymer coatings, including natural polymers such as heparin (a polysaccharide), have been used on stents. Stents coated with resorbable polymers such as polycaprolactone and polyorthoester, and copolymers such as polyglycolic–polylactic acid, poly(hydroxybutyrate valerate), and poly(ethylene oxide)–poly(butylene terephthalate) have been compared *in vivo* as resorbable stent coatings [109]. Phosphorylcholine applied to the stents has the potential to prevent the stent from inducing the formation of a thrombus on its surface [110]. Currently, polymers within stents hold most promise as coatings used to control drug delivery or release from or near stents to reduce restenosis and thrombus formation.

Polymer fibers composed of polydioxanones (PDS) were first tested for use as monofilament biodegradable surgical sutures and the degradation profile was later found to be affected by gamma irradiation [111]. Katz *et al.* [112] reported biodegradable, poly(trimethylene carbonates) for monofilament surgical sutures currently marketed as Maxon. PLGA composed of LA–GA 10–90 has long-found utility as Vicryl (polyglactin 910), a biodegradable surgical suture licensed by Ethicon (Somerville, New Jersey) and, in 2002, Vicryl Plus became the first marketed suture designed to contain an antibacterial agent, Triclosan or 5-chloro-2-(2,4-dichlorophenoxy)phenol [113]. Lendlein and Langer reported a new thermoplastic elastomer based on PCL and poly(dioxanone), with both homopolymers having been used as suture materials [114]. Currently, much effort is being focused on using polyurethane (PU) in biomedical applications such as cardiac-assist pumps and blood bags, to chronic implants such as heart valves and vascular graft, hemodialysis bloodline sets, center venous catheters (CVCs), and intravenous (IV) bags [115, 116]. Lin *et al.*, demonstrated that water-soluble chitosan/heparin immobilized PU membranes effectively improved *in vitro* hemocompatibility and superior biocompatibility [117].

1.5 Biomaterials for Bone Repair

Bone is a metabolically active, highly vascularized tissue with a unique ability to regenerate without creating a scar [118]. Bone repair was proposed to be one of the first, major applications of tissue engineering [119]. The general concept of bone tissue engineering is based on the formation of a tissue engineering construct to encourage the regeneration of the damaged tissue [120]. The main physiological functions of the ECM include storage of the nutrients, growth factors, and cytokines as well as mechanical stabilization for anchorage-dependent cells [121]. In the context of bone tissue engineering, the scaffold should possess the following properties [122]:

a) biocompatibility,
b) bioresorbability/biodegradability,
c) open/interconnected porosity,
d) suitable topography and surface chemistry, and
e) appropriate mechanical properties.

To fulfill the above requirements, several different types of the materials have been proposed [123, 124]. Based on the origin, the scaffold materials may be divided into two main groups: (i) naturally derived materials such as collagen, glycosaminoglycans (GAGs), starch, chitosan, and alginates; and (ii) synthetic ones, including metals, ceramics, bioactive glasses, and polymers (listed in Table 1.2) [125–127]. In addition, the surface properties of the scaffold will influence cell adhesion and activity.

Table 1.2 Types of biomaterials used for preparation of scaffolds for bone tissue Engineering.

Polymer	3D architecture
Naturally derived materials	
Collagen	Fibrous, sponge, hydrogel
Starch	Porous
Chitosan	Sponge, fibers
Alginates	Hydrogel, sponge
Hyaluronic acid (HA)	Hydrogel
Polyhydroxyalkanotes (PHA)	Porous, hydrogel
Synthetic polymers	
Polyurethanes (PU)	Porous
Poly(-hydroxy acids) (i.e., PLLA, PGLA)	Porous
Poly(ε-caprolactone) (PCL)	Sponge, fibers
Poly(propylene fumarates) (PPF)	Hydrogel
Titanium	Mesh
Calcium phosphate	Porous

The current generation of synthetic bone substitutes is helping to overcome the problems associated with availability and donor-site morbidity. Alternatives to autografts and allograft preparations have included calcium-phosphates, bioactive glass, polymers, and many other composite materials [128–130]. Over the years, many materials have been described for application in bone repair (Table 1.3).

Organic and inorganic synthetic polymers have been used in a wide variety of biomedical applications. Other biodegradable polymers currently being studied for potential tissue engineering applications include polycaprolactone, polyanhydrides, and polyphosphazenes [131–133]. PMMA has also been widely used in dentistry. Other polymers such as polytetrafluoroethylene (PTFE) have also been used for augmentation and guided bone regeneration [134, 135]. Ceramics have also been widely used in orthopedic and dental applications [136] (Figure 1.4).

HA is biocompatible, and stimulates osseo-conduction [137, 138]. By recruiting osteoprogenitor cells and causing them to differentiate into osteoblast-like bone-forming cells, it is resorbed and replaced by bone at a slow rate [139]. Bioactive glasses are another class of interesting material as they elicit a specific biological response at the interface of the material, which results in the formation of a bond between tissues and the material [140]. Calcium phosphate (CaP)-based biomaterials have found many applications for bone substitution and repair. These materials show excellent *in vivo* biocompatibility, cell proliferation, and resorption [141].

Table 1.3 Types of biomaterials (polymers, ceramics, and composite) used for preparation of scaffolds for bone tissue Engineering.

Polymers	Ceramics	Composite/natural
Polylactic acid	Bioglass	Poly(D,L-lactide-co-glycolide) - bioactive glass
Polyglycolic acid	Sintered hydroxyapatite	Extracellular matrix (ECM)
Polycaprolactone	Glass-ceramic A–W	Hyaluronan-linear glycosaminoglycan (GAG)
Polyanhydrides	Hydroxyapatite (HA)-calcium phosphate-based ceramic	Demineralized bone matrix (DBM)
Polyphosphazenes	Collagraft – commercial graft. HA tricalcium phosphate ceramic fibrillar collagen	
Polymethylmethacrylate (PMMA)	Bioactive glass	
Polytetrafluoroethylene (PTFE)	Sol–gel-derived bioactive glass	

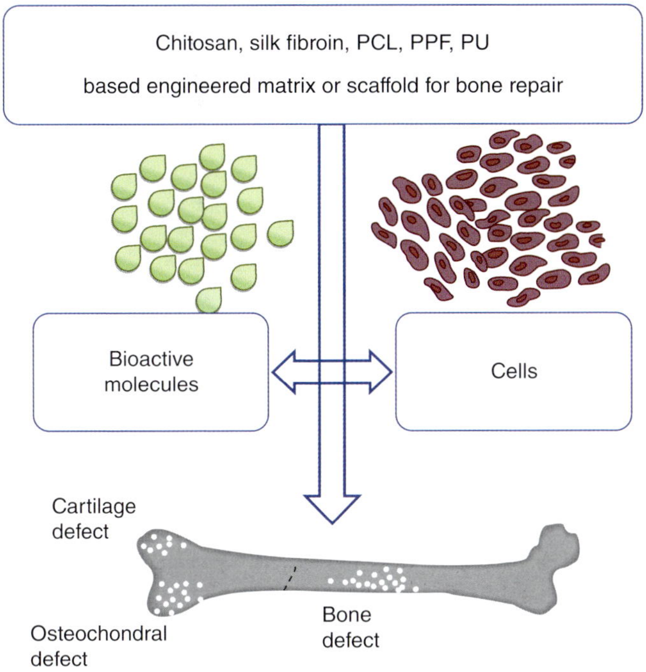

Figure 1.4 Polymer based matrix for bone repair.

1.6 Conclusion

In this chapter, a range of biomaterials from various polymers used for biomedical applications have been described. Biomaterials need to possess a number of key features to meet the stringent requirements of biomedical applications. The chosen biomaterial must provide a biocompatible and biodegradable matrix with interconnected pores to ensure that the body tolerates the conduit and also promotes nutrient and cellular diffusion. Furthermore, the material initially needs to provide mechanical stability and act as a template to guide three-dimensional tissue growth. There is great potential to produce replacement blood vessels and heart valves, which can be met with further advancements in tissue engineering. Developments in the area of cellular replacement tissues have led to replacement arteries and heart valves that can potentially allow host cell infiltration. Tissue engineering of an artery with an ECM made by cells in culture also led to a replacement artery with suitable properties for implantation. It is likely that there will be further advances with these technologies. Developments in polymeric material for use with stents in drug delivery systems, and to produce heart valves may allow further developments in replacement devices. While, at present, polymer stents have not proved to be successful, improvements in technology may allow their use in the future. The ultimate test for all new devices that are used to repair or replace arteries or heart valves is how well they perform clinically, and how they compare with existing devices. The development of these valves into successful clinical implants will ultimately depend on their long-term function, which can only be determined clinically. Furthermore, their long-term durability will also determine their clinical value and lead to complete optimization of their production; very useful techniques will be available that may help produce prominent cardiovascular replacement materials. Furthermore, just as it is true that no one material will satisfy all the design parameters required in all applications within the tissue engineering field, it is also true that a wide range of materials can be tailored for discrete applications, through the use of the most appropriate processing methodologies and processing parameters selected.

Abbreviations

AA	acrylic acid
BMP-2	bone morphogenetic protein-2
CVCs	center venous catheters
DBM	demineralized bone matrix
GAG	glycosaminoglycan
HA	hyaluronic acid
HEMA	hydroxyethyl methacrylate
IGF-1	insulin-like growth factor 1
IV	intravenous
MEMA	methoxyethyl methacrylate
NIPAAm	*N*-isopropyl Aam
NVP	*N*-vinyl-2-pyrrolidone
PACAs	polyalkylcyanoacrylates
PAGA	poly[**α**-(4-aminobutyl)-L-glycolic acid]
PCL	Polycaprolactone
PDS	polydioxanones
PEG	poly(ethylene glycol)
PEGA	poly(ethylene glycol) acrylate
PEGDA	poly(ethylene oxide) diacrylate (poly(ethylene glycol) diacrylate
PEG–PLL	poly(ethylene glycol)-co-poly(L-lysine)
PET	polyesters
PIB	polyisobutylene
PIB	polyisobutylene
PLA	poly(lactic acid)
PLGA	poly(D,L-lactic acid-co-glycolic acid)
PLGA	poly(lactide-co-glycolide)
PMMA	polymethylmethacrylate
POEs	polyorthoesters
PP	Polypropylene
PPE-EA	Poly(2-aminoethyl propylene phosphate)

PPF	poly(propylene fumarates)
PTFE	polytetrafluoroethylene
PTFE	fluoropolymers
PU	polyurethane
PVA	poly(vinyl alcohol)
TGF-β	transforming growth factor β
VEGF	vascular endothelial growth factor
CaP	calcium phosphate
ECM	extracellular matrix
PBLG	poly(γ-benzyl L-glutamate)
RGD	arginyl–glycyl–aspartic acid

References

1. Peppas, N.A. and Langer, R.L. (1994) New challenges in biomaterials. *Science*, **263**, 1715–1720.
2. Langer, R. and Tirrell, D.A. (2004) Designing materials for biology and medicine. *Nature*, **428**, 487–492.
3. Murphy, W.L. and Mooney, D.J. (1999) Controlled delivery of inductive proteins, plasmid DNA and cells from tissue-engineering matrices. *J. Periodontal. Res.*, **34**, 413–419.
4. Davies, N. (2004) in *Encyclopedia of Biomaterials and Biomedical Engineering* (eds G.E.B. Wnek and L. Gary), Marcel Dekker, New York, pp. 662–669.
5. Jones, A.J. and Denning, N.T. (1988) *Polymeric Biomaterials: Bio- and Ecocompatible Polymers, A Perspective for Australia*, Department of Industry, Technology and Commerce.
6. Park, H. and Park, K. (1996) in *Hydrogels in Bioapplications*, ACS Symposium Series, vol. 627 (eds R.M. Ottenbrite, S.J. Huang, and K. Park), American Chemical Society, Washington, DC, p. 1.
7. Wichterle, O. (1978) in *Soft Contact Lenses: Clinical and Applied Technology* (ed. M. Ruben), Baillière Tindall, London, pp. 3–5.
8. Levesque, S.G., Lim, R.M., and Shoichet, M.S. (2005) Macroporous interconnected dextran scaffolds of controlled porosity for tissue-engineering applications. *Biomaterials*, **26** (35), 7436–7446.
9. Li, Q., Wang, J., Shahani, S., Sun, D.D., Sharma, B., Elisseeff, J.H., and Leong, K.W. (2006) Biodegradable and photocrosslinkable polyphosphoester hydrogel. *Biomaterials*, **27** (7), 1027–1034.
10. Varghese, S. and Elisseeff, J.H. (2006) Hydrogels for musculoskeletal tissue engineering. *Adv. Polym. Sci.*, **203**, 95–144.
11. Hern, D.L. and Hubbell, J.A. (1998) Incorporation of adhesion peptides into nonadhesive hydrogels useful for tissue resurfacing. *J. Biomed. Mater. Res.*, **39** (2), 266–276.
12. Burdick, J.A., Mason, M.N., Hinman, A.D., Thorne, K., and Anseth, K.S. (2002) Delivery of osteoinductive growth factors from degradable PEG hydrogels influences osteoblast differentiation and mineralization. *J. Controlled Release*, **83** (1), 53–63.
13. Wang, D., Williams, C.G., Yang, F., Cher, N., Lee, H., and Elisseeff, J.H. (2005) Bioresponsive phophoester hydrogels for bone tissue engineering. *Tissue Eng.*, **11** (1–2), 201–213.
14. Park, Y.D., Tirelli, N., and Hubbell, J.A. (2003) Photopolymerized hyaluronic acidbased hydrogels and interpenetrating networks. *Biomaterials*, **24** (6), 893–900.
15. Shu, X.Z., Ghosh, K., Liu, Y., Palumbo, F.S., Luo, Y., Clark, R.A., and Prestwich, G.D. (2004) Attachment and spreading of fibroblasts on an RGD peptide-modified injectable hyaluronan

hydrogel. *J. Biomed. Mater. Res. Part A*, **68** (2), 365–375.

16. Cho, C.-S., Jeong, Y.-I., Kim, S.-H., Nah, J.-W., Kubota, M., and Komoto, T. (2000) Thermoplastic hydrogel based on hexablock copolymer composed of poly(**g**-benzyl l-glutamate) and poly(ethylene oxide). *Polymer*, **41**, 5185–5193.
17. Kennedy, J.P. (1994) Tailoring polymers for biological uses. *Chemtech*, **24**, 3.
18. Kennedy, J.P. (2000) *Designed Rubbery Biomaterials*, vol. 2, World Polymer Congress, IUPAC Macro 2000, Book of Abstracts, John Wiley & Sons, Ltd, London, p. 712.
19. Shu, X.Z., Liu, Y.C., Palumbo, F.S., Luo, Y., and Prestwich, G.D. (2004) In situ crosslinkable hyaluronan hydrogels for tissue engineering. *Biomaterials*, **25** (7–8), 1339–1348.
20. Lee, J.E., Kim, S.E., Kwon, I.C., Ahn, H.J., Cho, H., Lee, S.-H., Kim, H.J., Seong, S.C., and Lee, M.C. (2004) Effects of a chitosan scaffold containing TGF-beta1 encapsulated chitosan microspheres on in vitro chondrocyte culture. *Artif. Organs*, **28** (9), 829–839.
21. Burdick, J.A. and Anseth, K.S. (2002) Photoencapsulation of osteoblasts in injectable RGD-modified PEG hydrogels for bone tissue engineering. *Biomaterials*, **23** (22), 4315–4323.
22. Peters, M.C., Isenberg, B.C., Rowley, J.A., and Mooney, D.J. (1998) Release from alginate enhances the biological activity of vascular endothelial growth factor. *J. Biomater. Sci., Polym. Ed.*, **9** (12), 1267–1278.
23. Elisseeff, J., McIntosh, W., Fu, K., Blunk, B.T., and Langer, R. (2001) Controlled-release of IGF-I and TGF-beta1 in a photopolymerizing hydrogel for cartilage tissue engineering. *J. Orthop. Res.*, **19** (6), 1098–1104.
24. Lutolf, M.P., Weber, F.E., Schmoekel, H.G., Schense, J.C., Kohler, T., Muller, R., and Hubbell, J.A. (2003) Repair of bone defects using synthetic mimetics of collagenous extracellular matrices. *Nat. Biotechnol.*, **21** (5), 513–518.
25. Tabata, Y., Nagano, A., and Ikada, Y. (1999) Biodegradation of hydrogel carrier incorporating fibroblast growth factor. *Tissue Eng.*, **5** (2), 127–138.
26. Kennedy, J.P. and Richard, G.C. (1993) Polyisobutylene-toughened poly(methyl methacrylate). 1. Synthesis, characterization, and tensile properties of PMMA-l-PIB networks. *Macromolecules*, **26** (4), 567–571.
27. Bhowmick, A.K. and Stephens, H.L. (2001) *Handbook of Elastomers*, Marcel Dekker Inc., New York.
28. Ravin, H.A., Seligman, A.M., and Fine, J. (1952) Polyvinyl pyrrolidone as a plasma expander; studies on its excretion, distribution and metabolism. *J. Nucl. Med.*, **247** (24), 921–929.
29. Ammon, R. and Depner, E. (1957) Elimination and retention of various polyvinylpyrrolidone types in the body. *Z. Gesamte Exp. Med.*, **128** (6), 607–628.
30. Andrieu, V., Fessi, H., Dubrasquet, M., Devissaguet, J.P., Puisieux, F., and Benita, S. (1989) Pharmacokinetic evaluation of indomethacin nanocapsules. *Drug Des. Deliv.*, **4** (4), 295–302.
31. Polato, L., Benedetti, L.M., Callegaro, L., and Couvreur, P. (1994) In vitro evaluation of nanoparticle formulations containing gangliosides. *J. Drug Targeting*, **2** (1), 53–59.
32. Godard, G., Boutorine, A.S., Saison-Behmoaras, E., and Helene, C. (1995) Antisense effects of cholesterol-oligodeoxynucleotide conjugates associated with poly(alkylcyanoacrylate) nanoparticles. *Eur. J. Biochem.*, **232** (2), 404–410.
33. Fresta, M., Cavallaro, G., Giammona, G., Wehrli, E., and Puglisi, G. (1996) Preparation and characterization of polyethyl-2-cyanoacrylate nanocapsules containing antiepileptic drugs. *Biomaterials*, **17** (8), 751–758.
34. Aboubakar, M., Puisieux, F., Couvreur, P., Deyme, M., and Vauthier, C. (1999) Study of the mechanism of insulin encapsulation in poly(isobutylcyanoacrylate) nanocapsules obtained by interfacial polymerization. *J. Biomed. Mater. Res.*, **47** (4), 568–576.

35. Boudad, H., Legrand, P., Lebas, G., Cheron, M., Duchene, D., and Ponchel, G. (2001) Combined hydroxypropyl-beta-cyclodextrin and poly(alkylcyanoacrylate) nanoparticles intended for oral administration of saquinavir. *Int. J. Pharm.*, **218** (1–2), 113–124.
36. Chauvierre, C., Marden, M.C., Vauthier, C., Labarre, D., Couvreur, P., and Leclerc, L. (2004) Heparin coated poly(alkylcyanoacrylate) nanoparticles coupled to hemoglobin: a new oxygen carrier. *Biomaterials*, **25** (15), 3081–3086.
37. Hillaireau, H., Le Doan, T., and Couvreur, P. (2006) Polymer-based nanoparticles for the delivery of nucleoside analogues. *J. Nanosci. Nanotechnol.*, **6** (9–10), 2608–2617.
38. Stella, B., Arpicco, S., Peracchia, M.T., Desmaele, D., Hoebeke, J., Renoir, M., D'Angelo, J., Cattel, L., and Couvreur, P. (2000) Design of folic acid-conjugated nanoparticles for drug targeting. *J. Pharm. Sci.*, **89** (11), 1452–1464.
39. Peracchia, M.T., Fattal, E., Desmaele, D., Besnard, M., Noel, J.P., Gomis, J.M., Appel, M., d'Angelo, J., and Couvreur, P. (1999) Stealth PEGylated polycyanoacrylate nanoparticles for intravenous administration and splenic targeting. *J. Controlled Release*, **60** (1), 121–128.
40. Caliceti, P., Lora, S., Marsilio, F., and Veronese, F.M. (1995) Preparation and characterization of polyphosphazene-based controlled release systems for naproxen. *Farmaco*, **50** (12), 867–874.
41. Veronese, F.M., Marsilio, F., Lora, S., Caliceti, P., Passi, P., and Orsolini, P. (1999) Polyphosphazene membranes and microspheres in periodontal diseases and implant surgery. *Biomaterials*, **20** (1), 91–98.
42. Veronese, F.M., Marsilio, F., Caliceti, P., De Filippis, P., Giunchedi, P., and Lora, S. (1998) Polyorganophosphazene microspheres for drug release: polymer synthesis, microsphere preparation, in vitro and in vivo naproxen release. *J. Controlled Release*, **52** (3), 227–237.
43. Aldini, N.N., Caliceti, P., Lora, S., Fini, M., Giavaresi, G., Rocca, M., Torricelli, P., Giardino, R., and Veronese, F.M. (2001) Calcitonin release system in the treatment of experimental osteoporosis. Histomorphometric evaluation. *J. Orthop. Res.*, **19** (5), 955–961.
44. Ibim, S.M., el-Amin, S.F., Goad, M.E., Ambrosio, A.M., Allcock, H.R., and Laurencin, C.T. (1998) In vitro release of colchicine using poly(phosphazenes): the development of delivery systems for musculoskeletal use. *Pharm. Dev. Technol.*, **3** (1), 55–62.
45. Song, S.C. and Sohn, Y.S. (1998) Synthesis and hydrolytic properties of polyphosphazene/(diamine)platinum/saccharide conjugates. *J. Controlled Release*, **55** (2–3), 161–170.
46. Song, R., Joo Jun, Y., Ik Kim, J., Jin, C., and Sohn, Y.S. (2005) Synthesis, characterization and tumor selectivity of a polyphosphazene–platinum(II) conjugate. *J. Controlled Release*, **105** (1–2), 142–150.
47. Caliceti, P., Veronese, F.M., and Lora, S. (2000) Polyphosphazene microspheres for insulin delivery. *Int. J. Pharm.*, **211** (1–2), 57–65.
48. Andrianov, A.K., Marin, A., and Roberts, B.E. (2005) Polyphosphazene polyelectrolytes: a link between the formation of noncovalent complexes with antigenic proteins and immunostimulating activity. *Biomacromolecules*, **6** (3), 1375–1379.
49. Seong, J.Y., Jun, Y.J., Kim, B.M., Park, Y.M., and Sohn, Y.S. (2006) Synthesis and characterization of biocompatible poly(organophosphazenes) aiming for local delivery of protein drugs. *Int. J. Pharm.*, **314** (1), 90–96.
50. Huang, Y., Liu, X., Wang, L., Verbeken, E., Li, S., and De Scheerder, I. (2003) Local methylprednisolone delivery using a BiodivYsio phosphorylcholine-coated drug-delivery stent reduces inflammation and neointimal hyperplasia in a porcine coronary stent model. *Int. J. Cardiovasc. Intervent.*, **5** (3), 166–171.
51. Wang, L., Salu, K., Verbeken, E., Bosmans, J., Van de Werf, F., De Scheerder, I., and Huang, Y. (2005) Stent-mediated methylprednisolone

delivery reduces macrophage contents and in-stent neointimal formation. *Coron. Artery Dis.*, **16** (4), 237–243.
52. Huang, Y., Salu, K., Liu, X., Li, S., Wang, L., Verbeken, E., Bosmans, J., and De Scheerder, I. (2004) Methotrexate loaded SAE coated coronary stents reduce neointimal hyperplasia in a porcine coronary model. *Heart*, **90** (2), 195–199.
53. Huang, Y., Salu, K., Wang, L., Liu, X., Li, S., Lorenz, G., Wnendt, S., Verbeken, E., Bosmans, J., Van de Werf, F., and De Scheerder, I. (2005) Use of a tacrolimus-eluting stent to inhibit neointimal hyperplasia in a porcine coronary model. *J. Invasive Cardiol.*, **17** (3), 142–148.
54. Huang, Y., Wang, L., Li, S., Liu, X., Lee, K., Verbeken, E., van de Werf, F., and de Scheerder, I. (2006) Stent-based tempamine delivery on neointimal formation in a porcine coronary model. *Acute Card Care*, **8** (4), 210–216.
55. Luten, J., van Steenis, J.H., van Someren, R., Kemmink, J., Schuurmans-Nieuwenbroek, N.M., Koning, G.A., Crommelin, D.J., van Nostrum, C.F., and Hennink, W.E. (2003) Water-soluble biodegradable cationic polyphosphazenes for gene delivery. *J. Controlled Release*, **89** (3), 483–497.
56. Kawakami, H., Kanezaki, S., Sudo, M., Kanno, M., Nagaoka, S., and Kubota, S. (2002) Biodegradation and biocompatibility of polyorganophosphazene. *Artif. Organs*, **26** (10), 883–890.
57. Caliceti, P., Nicoli Aldini, N., Fini, M., Rocca, M., Gnudi, S., Lora, S., Giavaresi, G., Monfardini, C., Giardino, R., and Veronese, F.M. (1997) Bioabsorbable polyphosphazene matrices as systems for calcitonin controlled release. *Farmaco*, **52** (11), 697–702.
58. Huang, Y., Liu, X., Wang, L., Li, S., Verbeken, E., and De Scheerder, I. (2003) Long-term biocompatibility evaluation of a novel polymer-coated stent in a porcine coronary stent model. *Coron. Artery Dis.*, **14** (5), 401–408.
59. Wang, J., Zhang, P.C., Mao, H.Q., and Leong, K.W. (2002) Enhanced gene expression in mouse muscle by sustained release of plasmid DNA using PPE-EA as a carrier. *Gene Ther.*, **9** (18), 1254–1261.
60. Wang, J., Mao, H.Q., and Leong, K.W. (2001) A novel biodegradable gene carrier based on polyphosphoester. *J. Am. Chem. Soc.*, **123** (38), 9480–9481.
61. Huang, S.W., Wang, J., Zhang, P.C., Mao, H.Q., Zhuo, R.X., and Leong, K.W. (2004) Water soluble and nonionic polyphosphoester: synthesis, degradation, biocompatibility and enhancement of gene expression in mouse muscle. *Biomacromolecules*, **5** (2), 306–311.
62. Wen, J., Mao, H.Q., Li, W., Lin, K.Y., and Leong, K.W. (2004) Biodegradable polyphosphoester micelles for gene delivery. *J. Pharm. Sci.*, **93** (8), 2142–2157.
63. Mao, H.Q. and Leong, K.W. (2005) Design of polyphosphoester–DNA nanoparticles for non-viral gene delivery. *Adv. Genet.*, **53**, 275–306.
64. Xu, X., Yu, H., Gao, S., Ma, H.Q., Leong, K.W., and Wang, S. (2002) Polyphosphoester microspheres for sustained release of biologically active nerve growth factor. *Biomaterials*, **23** (17), 3765–3772.
65. Mao, H.Q., Shipanova-Kadiyaia, I., Zhao, Z., Dang, W., and Leong, K.W. (1999) *Encyclopedia of Controlled Drug Delivery*, John Wiley & Sons, Inc., New York.
66. Harper, E., Dang, W., Lapidus, R.G., and Garver, R.I.J. (1999) Enhanced efficacy of a novel controlled release paclitaxel formulation (Paclimer delivery system) for local-regional therapy of lung cancer tumor nodules in mice. *Clin. Cancer Res.*, **5** (12), 4242–4248.
67. Pradilla, G., Wang, P.P., Gabikian, P., Li, K., Magee, C.A., Walter, K.A., and Brem, H. (2006) Local intracerebral administration of paclitaxel with the paclimer delivery system: toxicity study in a canine model. *J. Neurooncol.*, **76** (2), 131–138.
68. Grigat, E., Koch, R., and Timmermann, R. (1998) BAK 1095 and BAK 2195: completely biodegradable synthetic

thermoplastics. *Polym. Degrad. Stab.*, **59** (1–3), 223–226.
69. Lim, Y., Kim, C., Kim, K., Kim, S.W., and Park, J. (2000) Development of a safe gene delivery system using biodegradable polymer, poly[**α**-(4-aminobutyl)-**l**-glycolic acid]. *J. Am. Chem. Soc.*, **122** (27), 6524–6525.
70. Lim, Y.B., Han, S.O., Kong, H.U., Lee, Y., Park, J.S., Jeong, B., and Kim, S.W. (2000) Biodegradable polyester, poly[**α**-(4-aminobutyl)-**l**-glycolic acid], as a nontoxic gene carrier. *Pharm. Res.*, **17** (7), 811–816.
71. Lim, Y.B., Kim, S.M., Suh, H., and Park, J.S. (2002) Biodegradable, endosome disruptive and cationic network-type polymer as a highly efficient and non-toxic gene delivery carrier. *Bioconjugate Chem.*, **13** (5), 952–957.
72. Panyam, J., Zhou, W.Z., Prabha, S., Sahoo, S.K., and Labhasetwar, V. (2002) Rapid endolysosomal escape of poly(**dl**-lactide-co-glycolide) nanoparticles: implications for drug and gene delivery. *FASEB J.*, **16** (10), 1217–1226.
73. Denis-Mize, K.S., Dupuis, M., MacKichan, M.L., Singh, M., Doe, B., O'Hagan, D., Ulmer, J.B., Donnelly, J.J., McDonald, D.M., and Ott, G. (2000) Plasmid DNA adsorbed onto cationic microparticles mediates target gene expression and antigen presentation by dendritic cells. *Gene Ther.*, **7** (24), 2105–2112.
74. Li, Z., Ning, W., Wang, J., Choi, A., Lee, P.Y., Tyagi, P., and Huang, L. (2003) Controlled gene delivery system based on thermosensitive biodegradable hydrogel. *Pharm. Res.*, **20** (6), 884–888.
75. Putnam, D. and Langer, R. (1999) Poly(4-hydroxy-**l**-proline ester): low-temperature polycondensation and plasmid DNA complexation. *Macromolecules*, **32** (11), 3658–3662.
76. Lim, Y., Choi, Y.H., and Park, J. (1999) A self-destroying polycationic polymer: biodegradable poly(4-hydroxy-**l**-proline ester). *J. Am. Chem. Soc.*, **121** (24), 5633–5639.
77. Chung, T.W., Liu, D.Z., Hsieh, J.H., Fan, X.C., Yang, J.D., and Chen, J.H. (2006) Characterizing poly(epsilon-caprolactone)-**β**-chitooligosaccharide-**β**-poly(ethylene glycol) (PCP) copolymer micelles for doxorubicin (DOX) delivery:effects of crosslinked of amine groups. *J. Nanosci. Nanotechnol.*, **6** (9–10), 2902–2911.
78. Aliabadi, H.M., Mahmud, A., Sharifabadi, A.D., and Lavasanifar, A. (2005) Micelles of methoxy poly(ethylene oxide)-**β**-poly(epsilon-caprolactone) as vehicles for the solubilization and controlled delivery of cyclosporine A. *J. Controlled Release*, **104** (2), 301–311.
79. Aliabadi, H.M., Brocks, D.R., and Lavasanifar, A. (2005) Polymeric micelles for the solubilization and delivery of cyclosporine A: pharmacokinetics and biodistribution. *Biomaterials*, **26** (35), 7251–7259.
80. Forrest, M.L., Zhao, A., Won, C.Y., Malick, A.W., and Kwon, G.S. (2006) Lipophilic prodrugs of Hsp90 inhibitor geldanamycin for nanoencapsulation in poly(ethylene glycol)-**β**-poly(epsilon-caprolactone) micelles. *J. Controlled Release*, **116** (2), 139–149.
81. Forrest, M.L., Won, C.Y., Malick, A.W., and Kwon, G.S. (2006) In vitro release of the mTOR inhibitor rapamycin from poly(ethylene glycol)-**β**-poly(epsiloncaprolactone) micelles. *J. Controlled Release*, **110** (2), 370–377.
82. Vandermeulen, G., Rouxhet, L., Arien, A., Brewster, M.E., and Preat, V. (2006) Encapsulation of amphotericin B in poly(ethylene glycol)-block-poly(epsiloncaprolactone-co-trimethylenecarbonate) polymeric micelles. *Int. J. Pharm.*, **309** (1–2), 234–240.
83. Vakil, R. and Kwon, G.S. (2006) Poly(ethylene glycol)-**β**-poly(epsilon-caprolactone) and PEG–phospholipid form stable mixed micelles in aqueous media. *Langmuir*, **22** (23), 9723–9729.
84. Allen, C., Han, J., Yu, Y., Maysinger, D., and Eisenberg, A. (2000) Polycaprolactone-bpoly(ethylene oxide) copolymer micelles as a delivery vehicle for dihydrotestosterone. *J. Controlled Release*, **63** (3), 275–286.

85. Kim, S.Y., Shin, I.G., Lee, Y.M., Cho, C.S., and Sung, Y.K. (1998) Methoxy poly(ethylene glycol) and epsilon-caprolactone amphiphilic block copolymeric micelle containing indomethacin. II. Micelle formation and drug release behaviours. *J. Controlled Release*, **51** (1), 13–22.
86. Shin, I.G., Kim, S.Y., Lee, Y.M., Cho, C.S., and Sung, Y.K. (1998) Methoxy poly(ethylene glycol)/epsilon-caprolactone amphiphilic block copolymeric micelle containing indomethacin. I. Preparation and characterization. *J. Controlled Release*, **51** (1), 1–11.
87. Cheon Lee, S., Kim, C., Chan Kwon, I., Chung, H., and Young Jeong, S. (2003) Polymeric micelles of poly(2-ethyl-2-oxazoline)-block-poly(epsilon-caprolactone) copolymer as a carrier for paclitaxel. *J. Controlled Release*, **89** (3), 437–446.
88. Choi, N.S. and Heller, J. (1979) Erodible agent releasing device comprising poly(ortho esters) and poly(ortho carbonates). US Patent 4,138,344, Alza Corporation.
89. Bikram, M., Lee, M., Chang, C.W., Janát-Amsbury, M.M., Kern, S.E., and Kim, S.W. (2005) Long-circulating DNA-complexed biodegradable multiblock copolymers for gene delivery: degradation profiles and evidence of dysopsonization. *J. Controlled Release*, **103** (1), 221–233.
90. Bikram, M., Ahn, C.H., Chae, S.Y., Lee, M.Y., Yockman, J.W., and Kim, S.W. (2004) Biodegradable poly(ethylene glycol)-co-poly(**l**-lysine)-γ-histidine multiblock copolymers for nonviral gene delivery. *Macromolecules*, **37** (5), 1903–1916.
91. Perin, E.C. (2005) Choosing a drug-eluting stent: a comparison between Cypher and Taxus. *Rev. Cardiovasc. Med.*, **6** (Suppl. 1), S13–S21.
92. Kohn, J. and Zeltinger, J. (2005) Degradable, drug-eluting stents: a new frontier for the treatment of coronary artery disease. *Expert Rev. Med. Devices*, **2** (6), 667–671.
93. Stevens, A. and Lowe, J. (1997) *Human Histology*, Mosby, London.
94. Caro, C.G., Pedley, T.J., Schroter, R.C., and Seed, W.A. (1978) *The Mechanics of the Circulation*, Oxford University Press, Oxford.
95. Roe, B.B., Kelly, P.B., Myers, J.L., and Moore, D.W. (1966) Tricuspid leaflet aortic valve prosthesis. *Circulation*, **33** (Suppl. I), I124–I130.
96. Zdrahala, R.J. and Zdrahala, I.J. (1999) Biomedical applications of polyurethanes: a review of past promises, present realities, and a vibrant future. *J. Biomater. Appl.*, **14** (1), 67–90.
97. Mackay, T.G., Wheatley, D.J., Bernacca, G.M., Fisher, A.C., and Hindle, C.S. (1996) New polyurethane heart valve prosthesis: design, manufacture and evaluation. *Biomaterials*, **17**, 1857–1863.
98. Daebritz, S.H., Fausten, B., Hermanns, B., Schroeder, J., Groetzner, J., Autschbach, R., Messmer, B.J., and Sachweh, J.S. (2004) Introduction of a flexible polymeric heart valve prosthesis with special design for the aortic position. *Eur. J. Cardiothorac. Surg.*, **25**, 946–952.
99. Daebritz, S.H., Sachweh, J.S., Hermanns, B., Fausten, B., Franke, A., Groetzner, J., Klosterhalfen, B., and Messmer, B.J. (2003) Introduction of a flexible polymeric heart valve prosthesis with special design for mitral position. *Circulation*, **108** (Suppl. II), II134–II139.
100. Wheatley, D.J., Raco, L., Bernacca, G.M., Sim, I., Belcher, P.R., and Boyd, J.S. (2000) Polyurethane: material for the next generation of heart valve prostheses? *Eur. J. Cardiothorac. Surg.*, **17**, 440–448.
101. Cochran, R.P. and Kunzelman, K.S. (1991) Comparison of viscoelastic properties of suture versus porcine mitral valve chordae tendineae. *J. Card. Surg.*, **6**, 508–513.
102. Ng, C.K., Nesser, J., Punzengruber, C., Pachinger, O., Auer, J., Franke, H., and Hartl, P. (2001) Valvuloplasty with glutaraldehyde-treated autologous pericardium in patients with complex mitral valve pathology. *Ann. Thorac. Surg.*, **71**, 78–85.

103. Kobayashi, Y., Nagata, S., Ohmori, F., Eishi, K., and Miyatake, K. (1996) Mitral valve dysfunction resulting from thickening and stiffening of artificial mitral valve chordae. *Circulation*, **94** (Suppl. II), II129–II132.
104. Shi, Y. and Vesely, I. (2003) Fabrication of tissue engineered mitral valve chordae using directed collagen gel shrinkage. *Tissue Eng.*, **9** (6), 1233–1242.
105. Shi, Y. and Vesely, I. (2004) Characterization of statically loaded tissue-engineered mitral valve chordae tendineae. *J. Biomed. Mater. Res. Part A*, **69**, 26–39.
106. Schoen, F.J. and Levy, R.J. (1999) Tissue heart valves: current challenges and future research perspectives. *J. Biomed. Mater. Res.*, **47**, 439–465.
107. Topol, E.J. and Serruys, P.W. (1998) Frontiers in interventional cardiology. *Circulation*, **98**, 1802–1820.
108. Padera, R.F. and Schoen, F.J. (2004) in *Biomaterials Science* (eds B.D. Ratner, A.S. Hoffman, F.J. Schoen, and J.E. Lemons), Elsevier, London, pp. 470–494.
109. Van der Giessen, W.J., Lincoff, A.M., Schwartz, R.S., van Beusekom, H.M.M., Serruys, P.W., Holmes, D.R., Ellis, S.G., and Topol, E.J. (1996) Marked inflamatory sequelae to implantation of biodegradable and nonbiodegradable polymers in porcine coronary arteries. *Circulation*, **94**, 1690–1697.
110. Whelan, D.M., van der Giessen, W.J., Krabbendam, S.C., van Vliet, E.A., Verdouw, P.D., Serruys, P.W., and van Beusekom, H.M.M. (2000) Biocompatibility of phosphorylcholine coated stents in normal porcine coronary arteries. *Heart*, **83**, 338–345.
111. Yang, K.K., Wang, X.L., and Wang, Y.Z. (2002) Poly(**p**-dioxanone) and its copolymers. *J. Macromol. Sci.*, **42** (3), 373–398.
112. Katz, A.R., Mukherjee, D.P., Kaganov, A.L., and Gordon, S. (1985) A new synthetic monofilament absorbable suture made from polytrimethylene carbonate. *Surg. Gynecol. Obstet.*, **161** (3), 213–222.
113. Miller, R.A., Brady, J.M., and Cutright, D.E. (1977) Degradation rates of oral resorbable implants (polylactates and polyglycolates): rate modifi cation with changes in PLA/PGA copolymer ratios. *J. Biomed. Mater. Res.*, **11** (5), 711–719.
114. Skarja, G.A. and Woodhouse, K.A. (2001) In vitro degradation and erosion of degradable, segmented polyurethanes containing an amino acid-based chain extender. *J. Biomater. Sci., Polym. Ed.*, **12**, 851–873.
115. Zhu, Y., Gao, C., He, T., and Shen, J. (2004) Endothelium regeneration on luminal surface of polyurethane vascular scaffold modified with diamine and covalently grafted with gelatin. *Biomaterials*, **25** (3), 423–430.
116. Yuan, Y., Ai, F., Zang, X., Zhuang, W., Shen, J., and Lin, S. (2004) Polyurethane vascular catheter surface grafted with zwitterionic sulfobetaine monomer activated by ozone. *Colloids Surf., B*, **35** (1), 1–5.
117. Lin, W.-C., Tseng, C.-H., and Yang, M.-C. (2005) In-vitro hemocompatibility evaluation of a thermoplastic polyurethane membrane with surface-immobilized water-soluble chitosan and heparin. *Macromol. Biosci.*, **5**, 1013–1021.
118. Sommerfeldt, D.W. and Rubin, C.T. (2001) Biology of bone and how it orchestrates the form and function of the skeleton. *Eur. Spine J.*, **10** (Suppl. 2), S86–S95.
119. Service, R.F. (2000) Tissue engineers build new bone, *Science*, **289** (5484), 1498–1500.
120. Hutmacher, D.W. and Garcia, A.J. (2005) Scaffold-based bone engineering by using genetically modified cells. *Gene*, **347** (1), 1–10.
121. Kneser, U., Schaefer, D.J., Polykandriotis, E., and Horch, R.E. (2006) Tissue engineering of bone: the reconstructive surgeon's point of view. *J. Cell. Mol. Med.*, **10** (1), 7–19.
122. Salgado, A.J., Coutinho, O.P., and Reis, R.L. (2004) Bone tissue engineering: state of the art and future trends. *Macromol. Biosci.*, **4**, 743–765.
123. Laurencin, C.T., Ambrosio, A.M., Borden, M.D., and Cooper, J.A. Jr.,

(1999) Tissue engineering: orthopedic applications. *Annu. Rev. Biomed. Eng.*, **1**, 19–46.

124. Vats, A., Tolley, N.S., Polak, J.M., and Gough, J.E. (2003) Scaffolds and biomaterials for tissue engineering: a review of clinical applications. *Clin. Otolaryngol. Allied Sci.*, **28**, 165–172.

125. Hutmacher, D.W. (2000) Scaffolds in tissue engineering bone and cartilage. *Biomaterials*, **21**, 2529–2543.

126. Lewandowska-Szumiel, M., Sikorski, K., Szummer, A., Lewandowski, Z., and Marczynski, W. (2007) Osteoblast response to the elastic strain of metallic support. *J. Biomech.*, **40**, 554–560.

127. Yang, Y. and El Haj, A.J. (2006) Biodegradable scaffolds – delivery systems for cell therapies. *Expert Opin. Biol. Ther.*, **6**, 485–498.

128. Burg, K.J., Porter, S., and Elam, J.F. (2000) Biomaterial developments for bone tissue engineering. *Biomaterials*, **21** (23), 2347–2359.

129. Hench, L.L. and Paschall, H.A. (1973) Direct chemical bond of bioactive glass- ceramic materials to bone and muscle. *J. Biomed. Mater. Res.*, **7**, 25–42.

130. Spector, M. (2006) Biomaterials-based tissue engineering and regenerative medicine solutions to musculoskeletal problems. *Swiss Med. Wkly.*, **136**, 293–301.

131. Gunatillake, P.A. and Adhikari, R. (2003) Biodegradable synthetic polymers for tissue engineering. *Eur. Cells Mater.*, **5**, 1–16.

132. Bass, E., Kuiper, J.H., Wood, M.A., Yang, Y., and El Haj, A.J. (2006) Micromechanical analysis of PLLA scaffolds for bone tissue engineering. *Eur. Cells Mater.*, **11** (3), 34.

133. Cohn, D. and Salomon, A.H. (2005) Designing biodegradable multiblock PCL/PLA thermoplastic elastomers. *Biomaterials*, **26**, 2297–2305.

134. Santhosh Kumar, T.R. and Krishnam, L.K. (2002) A stable matrix for generation of tissue engineered non thrombogenic vascular grafts. *Tissue Eng.*, **8** (5), 763–770.

135. Dahklin, C., Anderrsson, L., and Linde, A. (1991) Bone augmentation at fenestrated implants by an osteopromotive membrane technique. A controlled clinical study. *Clin. Oral Implants Res.*, **2** (4), 159–165.

136. Jarcho, M. (1981) Calcium phosphate ceramics as hard tissue prostheses. *Clin. Orthop. Relat. Res.*, **157**, 259–266.

137. Di Silvio, L., Dalby, M., and Bonfield, W. (1998) In vitro response of osteoblasts to hydroxyapatite reinforced polyethylene composites. *J. Mater. Sci. - Mater. Med.*, **9**, 845–848.

138. Schnettler, R., Alt, V., Dingeldein, E., Pfefferle, H.J., Kilian, O., Meyer, C., Heiss, C., and Wenisch, S. (2003) Bone ingrowth in _FGF-coated hydroxyapatite ceramic implants. *Biomaterials*, **24**, 4603–4608.

139. Kizuki, T., Ichinose, M.O.S., Nakamura, S., Hashimoto, K., Toda, Y., Yokogawa, Y., and Yamashita, K. (2006) Specific response of osteoblast-like cells on hydroxyapatite layer containing serum protein. *J. Mater. Sci. - Mater. Med.*, **17** (9), 859–867.

140. Hench, L.L., Splinter, R.J., Allen, W.C., and Greenlee, J.T.K. (1972) Bonding mechanisms at the interface of ceramic prosthetic materials. *J. Biomed. Mater. Res.*, **2** (1), 117–141.

141. Song, J., Saiz, E., and Bertozzi, C.R. (2003) A new approach to mineralization of biocompatible hydrogel scaffolds: an efficient process toward 3-dimensional bone like composites. *J. Am. Chem. Soc.*, **125**, 1236–1243.

2
Conducting Polymers: An Introduction

Nidhin Joy, Joby Eldho, and Raju Francis

2.1
Introduction

Polymers have been extensively used both as biomaterials, which are constituents of medical devices, and as constituents of drug delivery systems [1]. Many regulatory requirements must be met in order to use materials in the domain of human health [2]. For instance, sterility is mandatory concerning materials in direct contact with living tissues in the absence of a barrier such as intact skin. In addition, both polymers and devices have to be biocompatible, and their biocompatibility has to be evaluated by *in vitro* and *in vivo* tests [3, 4]. However, the regulations differ depending on whether the polymer is a constituent of a medical device or part of a medication. If a drug is included in a medical device for an auxiliary action, then the regulations for medical devices are applicable. If the main action is linked to the presence of the drug, then regulations for medications are applicable.

Polymers (plastics) are known to have good insulating properties and are among the most used materials in the modern world. However, it has been discovered that there are some polymers that have conducting properties. Polymer materials with metallic and semiconductor characteristics are called conducting polymers (CP), a combination of properties not exhibited by any other known material [5]. The most important component of a CP is the presence of conjugated double bonds along the backbone of the polymer. In conjugation, alternate single and double bonds exist between the carbon atoms.

Since the electrons in a conjugated system are only loosely bound, current flow may be possible. Every bond contains a localized "sigma" bond that forms a strong chemical bond. In addition, every double bond also contains a less strongly localized "pi" bond that is weaker [6, 7]. These enable the electrons to be delocalized over the whole polymer chain and so be shared by many atoms. This means that the delocalized electrons may move around the whole system. However, conjugation alone is not enough to make the polymer material conductive. Further, the polymer material needs to be doped for electron flow to occur. Doping is either the addition of electrons (reduction reaction) or the removal of electrons

Biomedical Applications of Polymeric Materials and Composites, First Edition.
Edited by Raju Francis and Sakthi Kumar.

(oxidation reaction) from the polymer. An oxidation doping (means removal of electrons) can be carried out using iodine. The iodine attracts an electron from the polymer from one of the bonds. Once doping is done, the electrons in the bonds are able to "jump" around the polymer chain. As the electrons move along the molecule, electric current flows. For better conductivity, the molecules must be well ordered and closely packed to limit the space "jumped" by the electrons. The conductivity of these polymers can be fine-tuned by chemical manipulation of the polymer backbone, by the nature of the dopant, by the degree of doping, and by blending with other polymers [8].

Polyacetylene, in view of possessing the simplest molecular framework, has attracted the most attention, especially of physicists, with an emphasis on understanding the mechanism of conduction. However, its insolubility, infusibility, and poor environmental stability have rendered it rather unattractive for technological applications. The technologically relevant front-runners belong to essentially four families: polyaniline (PANI), polypyrrole (PPy), polythiophenes (PT), and poly(para-phenylene vinylene) (PPV)

PANI is rather unique as it is the only polymer that can be doped by a protic acid and can exist in different forms depending upon the pH of the medium. While PANI is soluble in the neutral emeraldine form in highly polar aprotic solvents such as NMP, all other polymers are insoluble. However, as mentioned earlier, laterally substituted derivatives of the remaining three classes are soluble in pristine form and are solution processable. A typical example of a laterally substituted conjugated polymer that has been extensively investigated is P3-HT. PANI, PPy, and PT can be prepared by either chemical or electrochemical oxidation, the latter approach being often preferred as they result in polymeric films deposited on the anode surface, which can be removed to give free-standing films. The electrochemical method, in addition, may also be well suited for fabrication of microelectronic devices in which polymer films are directly deposited on to metal contacts. Although chemical oxidation yields powders, the reaction when performed in the presence of surfactants, in some cases, permits the preparation of emulsions, which upon drying form coherent films. In the case of the substituted derivatives, however, the chemical method is often preferred, as the resulting polymers are soluble and hence can be purified and solution processed.

PPV has also attracted a lot of attention in recent years, due to the availability of a synthetic route that gives a water-soluble polyelectrolyte precursor, which upon heating to about 200 °C under vacuum gives the wholly conjugated polymer. By virtue of this soluble precursor route, PPV films and fibers for a variety of applications are accessible.

CP have got wide applications in these fields, namely light-emitting diodes (LEDs), electrochromic displays, polymeric batteries, and so on [9]. They have also touched the biological field by taking its application in the field of biosensors [10–12]. Commonly used CP are shown in Table 2.1.

CP have also touched the arena of biomedical applications. One such application is the fabrication of a glucose biosensor. Such a device can not only sense the

Table 2.1 Various conducting polymers.

Structure	Maximum conductivity	Stability	Processability
Polyaniline 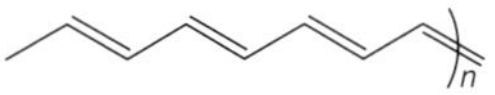	1.5×10^5	Reacts with air	Film not soluble or fusible
Polypyrrole 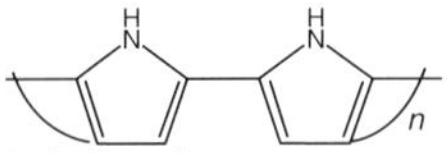	2000	Reasonably stable	Insoluble and infusible
Polythiophene 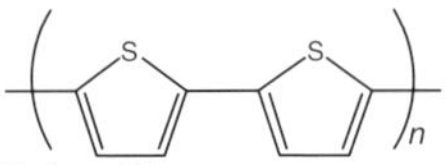	100	Stable	Insoluble and infusible
Polyaniline 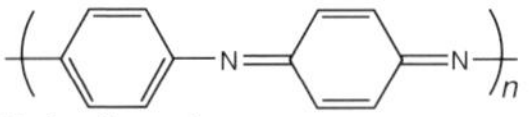	10	Stable	Soluble in neutral form
Polyphenylene 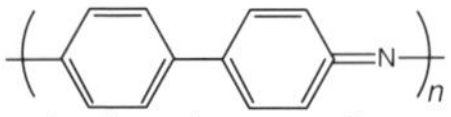	1000	Stable	Insoluble and infusible
Polyphenylene vinylene 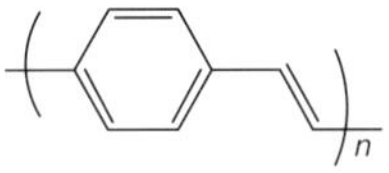	1000	Stable undoped form	Soluble precursor route available

presence of glucose but can also estimate its concentration. The principle involves immobilization of an enzyme and a suitable mediator on a conducting polymer matrix that is coated on to a suitable sensor chip. PPy- and PANI-based sensors have been fabricated, both of which are of the amperometric type (based on the measurement of the steady-state current at a fixed applied potential). One such sensor is based upon electrochemically polymerized PPy on an electrode from a solution that contains both glucose oxidase (a flavin-containing enzyme that oxidizes glucose) and ferrocene monocarboxylic acid (which is the electron transfer mediator that shuttles electrons from the redox center of the enzyme to the surface of the sensing electrode). In such a device, the amount of charge transferred (i.e., the current passed) is proportional to the concentration of glucose present in the solution. The specificity of the enzyme (which oxidizes only glucose) imparts to the device a very important characteristic, namely, its ability to sense glucose even in the presence of several other components (as would be the case in, say, blood or urine). Prototypes of such microamperometric glucose and galactose biosensors based on a silicon chip employing PPy have in fact been developed by several companies. These types of sensors are likely to soon find their way into analytical clinical laboratories for glucose estimation, for online supervision of diabetic patients, and so on.

2.2
Types of Conducting Polymers

Only emeraldine polymer exhibits conductivity. The emeraldine salt form which is the conducting form of the emeraldine polymer is formed when an emeraldine-based polymer is treated with acidic solution (either organic or inorganic protonic acids) with pH lower than 4. The insulator form of the same polymer is obtained if the polymer is treated with a solution with pH greater than 4 [13]. Common CP are poly(acetylene)s, poly (pyrrole)s, poly(thiophene)s, poly(terthiophene)s, poly(aniline)s, poly(fluorine)s, poly(3-alkylthiophene)s, polytetrathiafulvalenes, polynapthalenes, poly(-phenylene sulfide), poly(-phenylenevinylene)s, poly(3,4-ethylenedioxythiophene), polyparaphenylene, polyazulene, polyparaphenylene sulfide, polycarbazole, and polydiaminonaphthalene [14]. Among the various CP, PANI, polythiophene, and PPy are biocompatible and hence, cause minimal and reversible disturbance to the working environment and protect electrodes from fouling [15]. Nonetheless, only PANI and polypyrrole are most extensively used in biosensors for foodborne pathogen detection. Recently, conducting polymer nanocomposites that have improved properties have been fabricated to overcome the inherent limitations of pure CP. [16] Some of the most important CP and their synthetic techniques, properties, and applications are summarized and shown in Table 2.2.

The greater exposed surface area of conducting polymer nanocomposites/nanoparticles could greatly improve the diffusion. As a result of this, the basic characteristic of a biosensor, for example, low detection limit, gets enhanced. The oriented microstructure and the high surface area also facilitate high biomolecule loading, and, thereby, highly sensitive detection is possible. Besides, the relative stability is increased due to efficient bonding of biomolecule on the transducer surface, which increases reproducibility. These materials are particularly important due to their bridging role between the world of conducting polymers and nanoparticles [17]. The rewarding features of CP nanocomposites are also discussed in literature [18–23].

Pal and Alocilja have developed electrically active PANI-coated magnetic nanoparticle-based biosensor for the detection of *Bacillus anthracis* endospores in contaminated food samples. The 100 nm-diameter EAPM nanoparticles are synthesized from aniline (ANI) monomers coating the surface of gamma iron oxide cores. Experimental results show that the biosensor is able to discover *Bacillus anthracis* spores at concentrations as low as 4.2×10^2 spores/ml from the samples with a total detection time of 16 min. Nanocomposite of poly(anilineboronic acid), a self-doped PANI, with ss-DNA-wrapped single-walled carbon nanotubes(ss-DNA/SWNTs) to fabricate on a gold electrode by *in situ* electrochemical polymerization of 3-aminophenylboronic acid monomers in the presence of ss-DNA/SWNTs was used by Ma *et al.* [24]. The paper reported that the sensitivity increased by four orders of magnitude when nanocomposite

Table 2.2 Types of conducting polymers and their properties and applications.

Conducting polymer	Synthetic technique	Properties	Applications
Polypyrrole (PPy)	Electrochemical and chemical synthesis	High conductivity (up to 160 S cm^{-1}) when doped with iodine, opaque, brittle, amorphous material	Biosensors, antioxidants, drug delivery, bioactuators, neural prosthetics, cardiovascular applications
Polyaniline (PANI)	Electrochemical and chemical synthesis	Belongs to the semiflexible rod polymer family; requires simple doping/dedoping chemistry; high conductivity up to 100 S cm^{-1}	Biosensors, antioxidants, drug delivery, bioactuators, food industry, cardiovascular applications
Poly(3,4-diethylene-dioxythiophene) (PEDOT)	Electrochemical and chemical synthesis	High temperature stability; ability to suppress the so-called thermal runway of the capacitor transparent |conductor; high conductivity up to 210 S cm^{-1}	Biosensors, antioxidants, drug delivery, neural prosthetics
Polythiophenes (PT)	Electrochemical and chemical synthesis	Good electrical conductivity and optical property	Biosensors, food industry

was used to detect nanomolar concentrations of dopamine compared to the detection at an electrode modified with only poly(aniline boronic acid).

CPs are an exciting new class of electronic materials, which have attracted increasing interest since their discovery in 1977. They have many advantages, as compared to the non-CP, which are primarily due to their electronic and optic properties. In addition, they have been used in artificial muscles, fabrication of electronic device, solar energy conversion, rechargeable batteries, and sensors. Many scientists have been working on finding applications for the newly discovered CP, such as thin-film transistors [25], polymer LEDs [26], corrosion resistance [27], electromagnetic shielding [28], sensor technology [29], molecular electronics [30], supercapacitors [31], and electrochromic devices [32]. CP include PT, PPV, polycarbazole, PANI, and PPy.

CP are mainly of three types:

- Electron-conducting polymers
- Proton-conducting polymers
- Ion-conducting polymers

2.2.1
Poly(thiophene)

PT has received great scientific attention in the past 20 years. This is because of its interesting properties, such as good environmental and thermal stability, as well as by its wide application perspectives [33]. Numerous polyalkyl derivatives of thiophene have been synthesized so far by chemical and electrochemical approaches, resulting in CP with better solubility and higher capacitor behaviors [34].

CP have attracted attention to be used as electrochromic materials due to their inexpensive and potentially processable nature [35–37]. Thiophene-based polymers have received significant interest for their electrical properties, environmental stabilities, and a number of practical applications. For instance, these materials have been used as charge dissipation coatings in electron-beam lithography [38] and as active semiconducting material in organic thin-film transistors [39]. Recently, Shi and coworkers reported the preparation of PT films from a boron trifluoride–diethyl ether solution with thiophene monomer by electrochemical means so that the films possess tensile strength and are tougher and mechanically more durable than aluminum [40]. Thiophene-based polymers can also be used as potential materials for electrochromic devices [41]. An electrochromic material possesses the ability to reversibly change color by altering its redox state. For instance, poly(3-methylthiophene) (poly(3MTh)) is known to be blue in the oxidized state and red in the reduced state. Panero *et al.* have investigated the electrochromic devices by using poly(3MTh)-coated indium tin oxide glass electrodes and thus have obtained an optical contrast between the reduced and oxidized states of about 30% [42].

2.2.2
Poly(para-phenylene vinylene)

PPV is a conducting polymer of the rigid-rod polymer family with high levels of crystallinity. PPV is an important polymer in many electronic applications, such as LEDs and photovoltaic devices [43], which is due to its small optical bandgap and its bright yellow fluorescence. In addition, it can be easily doped to form electrically conductive materials. Therefore, its electronic and physical properties can be changed by the inclusion of functional groups. It is mostly synthesized via chemical routes, where a precursor is converted to PPV by thermal elimination of a leaving group. The deposition of PPV on to or inside polysilicon (PSi) could lead to the development of new functional hybrid devices. In literature, PPV and poly(2,5-dimethyl-para-phenylene vinylene) were prepared via the formation of a double bond by thermal elimination of an octylsulfinyl side group at 200 °C under vacuum [44]. Alves *et al.* have studied theoretical approaches of PPV and poly(p-phenylene) (PPP) [45]. PPV-based devices have drawbacks due to photodegradation. However, PPV and its derivatives find frequent application in research cells [46].

2.2.3 Poly(carbazole)

Carbazole(Cz) is a heterocyclic organic compound with active sides at the 3rd and 6th positions. The anodic polymerization of Cz [47], especially *N*-vinylcarbazole [48, 49], has been considered in relation to the polymer film electrodes. The interest in polycarbazoles is also stimulated by their possible applications in electrochromic display devices [50] and batteries [51]. Sarac *et al.* have synthesized and polymerized some ter-arenes based on *N*-ethylcarbazole and thiophene [52]. PVCz electroluminescence devices with better performance and modified configuration were also reported [53]. Electrocopolymerization of Cz with p-tolylsulfonylpyrrole (pTsp) was studied concerning two different types of electrodes, namely, CFMEs and platinum (Pt) button electrodes. Modified electrodes on the CFMEs are more suitable for decreasing the electrochemical potential values than the Pt button electrodes [54].

2.2.4 Polyaniline

The oxidized and reduced states of PANI films, including the effects of the dopants and electrolytes, have been extensively studied [55]. Sarac *et al.* [56] have studied aniline, which has been electropolymerized by the CV method on three different electrodes: Pt, glassy carbon, and CFME in acid aqueous solution (0.5 M H_2SO_4). Bhattacharya and De [57] have investigated PANI using gas sensors and corrosion protective coatings. The applicability of PANI as an ion-exchange resin and conducting polymer has attracted considerable scientific interest in recent decades due to its good combination of properties, such as diverse structure, thermal and radiation stability, low cost, ease of synthesis, and conducting properties. This resulted in its application to different fields, such as microelectronics, corrosion protection, sensors, and electrodes for batteries [58].

2.2.5 Polypyrrole

Among the various CP, PPy is more interesting due to its ease of synthesis, stability in the oxidized form, good redox properties, ability to give high electrical conductivity, commercial availability, water solubility, and useful electrical and optical properties [59–61]. So it has several applications, such as batteries, electrochemical biosensors, supercapacitors, conductive textiles and fabrics, EMI shielding, mechanical actuators, antistatic coatings, and drug delivery systems [42]. Its intrinsic properties are highly dependent on electropolymerization conditions [62].

Brajter-Toth and coworkers have proposed overoxidized PPy films as a substitute for Nafion films [63–65]. In its oxidized form, PPy is a positively charged conducting polymer [66]. Upon overoxidation, it loses its conductivity and charge [67]. The characterization of these films by X-ray photoelectron spectroscopy [68, 69] and Fourier transform infrared spectroscopy (FTIR) [70] reveals the overoxidation results on addition of carbonyl and carboxylic groups.

2.3 Synthesis of Conducting Polymers

CPs can be synthesized by different methods of chemical synthesis including step- or chain-growth polymerization. Condensation polymerization proceeds via the loss of small molecules, such as hydrochloric acid or water. Radical, cation, and anion polymerizations are all examples of addition polymerization [71]. The advantages and disadvantages of chemical and electrochemical polymerization methods are summarized in Table 2.3.

Electrochemical polymerization (Figure 2.1) occurs by applying an electrical current through electrodes placed into a solution containing the monomer of the polymer, the solvent, and the doping agent [72–75]. This method allows the deposition of a thin film of the polymer with well-controlled thickness (down to 20 nm) and morphology [71, 74, 76]. The electrical current causes the monomer to deposit and oxidize on the positively charged working electrode, forming insoluble polymer chains. Electrochemical polymerization allows the synthesis of the polymer only if its monomer can undergo oxidation in the presence of an electrical potential. All of the main conductive polymers currently in use (e.g., PPy, PANI, PEDOT) fulfill this criterion.

Table 2.3 Comparison of chemical and electrochemical polymerization methods used to prepare CPs.

Polymerization approach	Advantages	Disadvantages
Electrochemical polymerization	• Synthesis of thin film is possible • Doping is simultaneous • Ease of synthesis • Entrapment of molecules in CP	• Postcovalent modification of CP is difficult • Difficult to remove film from electrode surface
Chemical polymerization	• Postcovalent modification of bulk CP is possible. • More options to modify CP backbone covalently • Larger-scale production is possible	• Synthesis is more complicated • Cannot make thin films

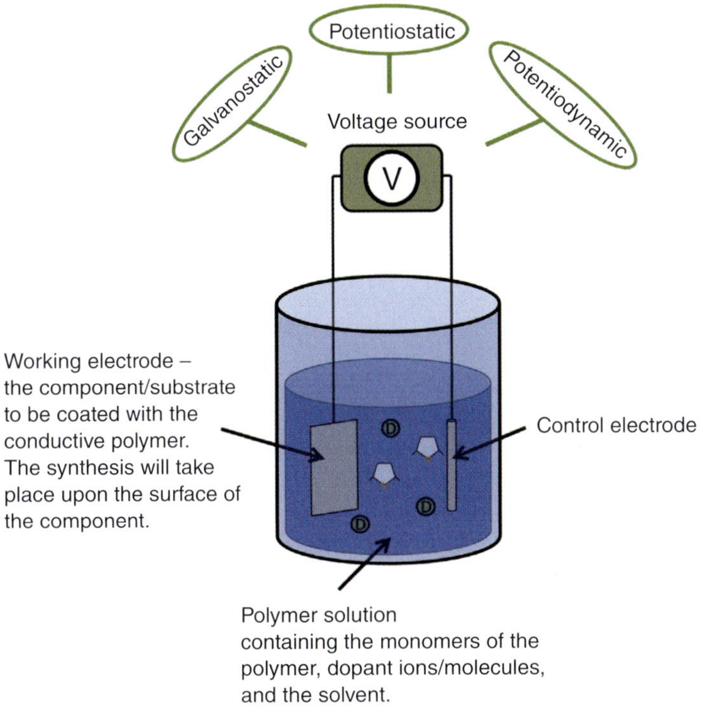

Figure 2.1 A schematic of the electrochemical synthesis setup [72].

2.4 Surface Functionalization of Conducting Polymers

2.4.1 Physical–Chemical Modifications

Both physical and chemical modifications are used for achieving the surface modification of the CP for incorporating biomolecules. Chemical modification has been extensively investigated using biomolecules as dopants or by immobilizing bioactive moieties on the surface of the material [77, 78]. Physical modification has been explored by increasing surface roughness using methods like creating microporous films using polystyrene sphere templates, fabricating composites of nanoparticles and polylactide, growing CPs within HG, blending with biomolecules to yield "fuzzy" structures, and so on.

2.4.2 Electrical Property Modification

Doping is the process of oxidizing (p-doping) or reducing (n-doping) a neutral polymer and providing a counterion or cation (i.e., dopant), respectively. Upon doping, a zero-charged CP system is produced owing to the close association of the counterions with the charged CP backbone. This process introduces charged polarons- (radical ions) or bipolarons- (dications or dianions) like charge carriers into the polymer. The attraction of electrons in one repeat unit to the nuclei in the neighboring units yields charge mobility along the chains as well as between the chains, often referred to as "electron hopping." Electrical conductivity was produced by this ordered movement of charge carriers along the conjugated CP backbone [71, 79]. Dopant concentration is the main factor that affects the electrochemical properties of the CP, that is, electrical conductivities can be varied by 15 magnitudes by changing dopant concentrations [80].

2.4.3
Mechanical Property Modification

As compared with those of a linear macromolecule, the tensile properties of CPs like polyacetylene and PPy have been accounted to be very unsatisfactory. In any case the tensile strength and moduli have been reported to increase as a consequence of annealing [81]. Moreover, the mechanical properties have additionally appeared to rely upon the strategy for the synthesis of CP [82]. The mechanical property of the CPs was influenced by the addition of dopant molecules. The expansion of dopants, for example, SbF5 and AsF5, has been reported to create a significant lessening in the modulus and quality of the material.

This may be because even if the addition of dopants causes an increment in the average cross-sectional area, no major contribution was accomplished toward the load-bearing capacity of the polymer, in this way lowering its modulus. Likewise, doping brought about embrittlement and scission, on account of the strong oxidizing capability of the dopants utilized. Sometimes doping diminishes the tensile modulus and attainable strain to around 1% in cases where the impact of doping is greater because of the lateral separation of the polymer chain required to accommodate the dopant molecule. Varying alkyl chain length is also a technique for the modification of mechanical properties.

Abbreviations

ANI	aniline
CP	conducting polymers
Cz	carbazole
EL	electroluminescence
GC	glassy carbon
LEDs	polymer light-emitting diodes
NMP	*N*-methyl pyrrolidone
P3-HT	poly(3-hexyl thiophene)
PANI	polyaniline
PEDOT	poly(3,4-diethylenedioxy thiophene)

PPP	poly(p-phenylene)
PPy	polypyrroles
PPV	poly(para-phenylene vinylene)
PT	polythiophenes
pTsp	p-tolylsulfonylpyrrole
PSi	polysilicon
PVCz	polyvinylcarbazole

References

1. Malliaras, G. (2013) Organic bioelectronics: a new era in organic electronics. *Biochim. Biophys. Acta*, **1830**, 4286–4287.
2. Higgins, M.J., Molino, P.J., Yue, Z., and Wallace, G.G. (2012) Organic conducting polymer–protein interactions. *Chem. Mater.*, **24**, 828–839.
3. Sayyar, S., Murray, E., Thompson, B.C., Gambhir, S., Officer, D.L., and Wallace, G.G. (2013) Covalently linked biocompatible graphene/polycaprolactone composites for tissue engineering. *Carbon*, **52**, 296–304.
4. Otero, T.F., Martinez, J.G., and Arias-Pardilla, J. (2012) Biomimetic electrochemistry from conducting polymers. A review: artificial muscles, smart membranes, smart drug delivery and computer/neuron interfaces. *Electrochim. Acta*, **84**, 112–128.
5. Fabbro, A., Bosi, S., Ballerini, L., and Prato, M. (2012) Carbon nanotubes: artificial nanomaterials to engineer single neurons and neuronal networks. *ACS Chem. Neurosci.*, **3**, 611–618.
6. Yoon, H., Hong, J.-Y., and Jang, J. (2007) Charge-transport behavior in shape-controlled poly(3,4- ethylenedioxythiophene) nanomaterials: intrinsic and extrinsic factors. *Small*, **3**, 1774–1783.
7. Yoon, H., Chang, M., and Jang, J. (2007) Formation of 1d poly(3,4-ethylenedioxythiophene) nanomaterials in reverse microemulsions and their application to chemical sensors. *Adv. Funct. Mater.*, **17**, 431–436.
8. Angelopoulos, M. (2001) Conducting polymers in microelectronics. *IBM J. Res. Dev.*, **45**, 57–75.
9. MacDiarmid, A.G., Yang, L.S., Huang, W.S., and Humphrey, B.D. (1987) Polyaniline: electrochemistry and application to rechargeable batteries. *Synth. Met.*, **18**, 393–398.
10. Bartlett, P.N. and Whitaker, R.G. (1988) Modified electrode surface in amperometric biosensors. *Med. Biol. Eng. Comput.*, **28**, 10–17.
11. He, P. and Dai, L. (2006) *BioMEMS and Biomedical Nanotechnology*, vol. 6, Springer, New York, pp. 171–201.
12. Balasubramanian, K. and Burghard, M. (2006) Biosensors based on carbon nanotubes. *Anal. Bioanal. Chem.*, **385**, 452–468.
13. Chiang, J.C. and Macdiarmid, A.G. (1986) Polyaniline-protonic acid doping of the emeraldine form to the metallic regime. *Synth. Met.*, **13**, 193–205.
14. Faridbod, F., Ganjali, M.R., Dinarvand, R., and Norouzi, P. (2008) Developments in the field of conducting and non-conducting polymer based potentiometric membrane sensors for ions over the past decade. *Sensors*, **8**, 2331–2412.
15. Geise, R.J., Adams, J.M., Barone, N.J., and Yacynych, A.M. (1991) Electropolymerized films to prevent interferences and electrode fouling in biosensors. *Biosens. Bioelectron.*, **6**, 151–160.
16. Fang, F.F., Choi, H.J., and Joo, J. (2008) Conducting polymer/clay nanocomposites and their applications. *J. Nanosci. Nanotechnol.*, **8**, 1559–1581.
17. Murugendrappa, M.V. and Prasad, M. (2007) Chemical synthesis, characterization, and direct-current conductivity

studies of polypyrrole/gamma-Fe O composites. *J. Appl. Polym. Sci.*, **103**, 2797–2801.

18. Malhotra, B.D., Chaubey, A., and Singh, S.P. (2006) Prospects of conducting polymers in biosensors. *Anal. Chim. Acta*, **578**, 59–74.
19. Teles, F.R.R. and Fonseca, L.R. (2008) Applications of polymers for biomolecule immobilization in electrochemical biosensors. *Mater. Sci. Eng., C*, **28**, 1530–1543.
20. Xiao, Y.H. and Li, C.M. (2008) Nanocomposites: from fabrications to electrochemical bioapplications. *Electroanalysis*, **20**, 648–662.
21. Galandova, J. and Labuda, J. (2009) Polymer interfaces used in electrochemical DNA- based biosensors. *Chem. Pap.*, **63**, 1–14.
22. Pal, S. and Alocilja, E.C. (2009) Electrically active polyaniline coated magnetic (EAPM) nanoparticle as novel transducer in biosensor for detection of Bacillus anthracis spores in food samples. *Biosens. Bioelectron.*, **24**, 1437–1444.
23. Ahuja, T.R. and Kumar, D. (2009) Recent progress in the development of nano-structured conducting polymers/nanocomposites for sensor applications. *Sens. Actuators, B*, **136**, 275–286.
24. Ma, Y.F., Ali, S.R., Dodoo, A.S., and He, H.X. (2006) Enhanced sensitivity for biosensors: multiple functions of DNA-wrapped single-walled carbon nanotubes in self-doped polyaniline nanocomposites. *J. Phys. Chem. B*, **110**, 16359–16365.
25. Halls, J.J.M., Walsh, C.A., Greenham, N.C., Marseglia, E.A., Friend, R.H., Moratti, S.C., and Holmes, A.B. (1995) Efficient photodiodes from interpenetrating polymer networks. *Nature*, **376**, 498–500.
26. Kraft, A., Grimsdale, A.C., and Holmes, A.B. (1998) Electroluminescent conjugated polymers-seeing polymers in a new light. *Angew. Chem. Int. Ed. Engl.*, **37**, 402–428.
27. Hepburn, A.R., Marshall, J.M., and Maud, J.M. (1991) Novel electrochromic films *via* anodic oxidation odcarbazolyl substituted polysilaxones. *Synth. Met.*, **43**, 2935–2938.
28. Dubois, J.C., Sagnes, O., and Henry, F. (1989) Polyheterocyclic conducting polymers and composites derivatives. *Synth. Met.*, **28**, C871–C878.
29. Roncali, J., Garreau, R., Delabouglise, D., Garnier, F., and Lemaire, M. (1989) Communications modification of the structure and electrochemical properties of poly(thiophene) by ether groups. *J. Chem. Soc., Chem. Commun.*, **11**, 679–781.
30. Bradley, D.D.C. (1991) Molecular electronics-aspects of the physics. *Chem. Br.*, **27**, 719–723.
31. Burke, A. (2000) Ultracapacitors: why, how, and where is the technology. *J. Power Sources*, **91**, 37–50.
32. Sonmez, G., Meng, H., Zhang, Q., and Wudl, F. (2003) A highly stable, new electrochromic polymer: Poly(1,4-bis(2,3(,)'4'ethylenedioxy)thienyl)-2-methoxy-5-2''ethylhexyloxybenzene. *Adv. Funct. Mater.*, **13**, 726–731.
33. Kutsche, C., Targove, J., and Haaland, P.J. (1993) Microlithographic patterning of polythiophene films. *J. Appl. Phys.*, **73**, 2602–2604.
34. Hotta, S., Rughooputh, D.D.V., Heeger, A.J., and Wudl, F. (1987) Spectroscopic studies of soluble poly(3-alkylthienylenes). *Macromolecules*, **20**, 212–215.
35. Mank, P.M.S., Mortimer, R.J., and Rossensky, D.R. (1995) *Electrochromism: Fundamental and Applications*, VCH Publishers, Weinheim and New York.
36. Gustafsson-Carlberg, J.C., Inganas, O., Andersson, M.R., Booth, C., Azens, A., and Granqvist, C.G. (1995) Tuning the bandgap for polymeric smart windows and displays. *Electrochim. Acta*, **40**, 2233–2235.
37. Havinga, E.E., Mutsaers, C.M.J., and Jenneskens, L.W. (1996) Absorption properties of alkoxy-substituted thienylene-vinylene oligomers as a function of the doping level. *Chem. Mater.*, **8**, 769–776.

38. Huang, W.S. (1994) Synthesizing and processing conducting polythiophene derivatives for charge dissipation in electron-beam lithography. *Polymer*, **35**, 4057–4064.
39. Dodabalapur, A., Torsi, L., and Katz, H.E. (1995) Organic transistors – 2-dimensional transport and improved electrical characteristics. *Science*, **268**, 270–271.
40. Shi, G.Q., Jin, S., Xue, G., and Li, C. (1995) A conducting polymer film stronger than aluminum. *Science*, **267**, 994–996.
41. Nawa, K., Imae, I., Shirota, Y., and Noman, N. (1995) Synthesis of a novel type of electrochemically doped vinyl polymer containing pendant terthiophene and its electrical and electrochromic properties. *Macromolecules*, **28**, 723–729.
42. Panero, S., Passerini, S., and Scrosati, B. (1993) Conducting polymers: new electrochromic materials for advanced optical devices. *Mol. Cryst. Liq. Cryst.*, **230**, 337–349.
43. Skothenn, T.A., Ronald, L.E., and Reynolds, J.R. (1997) *Handbook of Conducting Polymers*, 2nd edn, CRC Press, New York.
44. Kiebooms, R., Resel, R., Vanderzande, D., and Leising, G. (1999) Polymer LEDs based on N-alkylsulfinyl PPV precursor polymers. *MRS Proc.*, **558**, 409–413.
45. De Carvalho, L.C., Dos Santos, C.N., Alves, H.W.L., and Alves, J.L.A. (2003) Theoretical studies of poly(para-phenylene vinylene) (PPV) and poly(para-phenylene) (PPP). *Microelectron. J.*, **34**, 623–625.
46. Sariciftci, N.S., Braun, D., Zhang, C., Srdanov, V.I., Heeger, A.J., Stucky, G., and Wudl, F. (1993) Semiconducting polymer-buckminsterfullerene heterojunctions – diodes, photodiodes, and photovoltaic cells. *Appl. Phys. Lett.*, **62**, 585–587.
47. Saraswathi, R., Hillman, A.R., and Martin, S.J. (1999) Mechanical resonance effects in electroactive polycarbazole films. *J. Electroanal. Chem.*, **460**, 267–272.
48. Skompska, M. and Peter, L.M. (1995) Electrodeposition and electrochemical properties of poly(n-vinylcarbazole) films on platinum electrodes. *J. Electroanal. Chem.*, **383**, 43–52.
49. Skompska, M. and Hillman, A.R. (1997) Electrochemical quartz crystal microbalance studies of the electrodeposition and subsequent crosslinking of poly(N-vinylcarbazole) films. *J. Electroanal. Chem.*, **433**, 127–134.
50. Monk, P.M.S., Mortimer, R.J., and Rosseinsky, D.R. (1995) *Electrochromism Fundamentals and Applications*, VCH Verlagsgesellschaft, Weinheim.
51. Kakuta, T., Shirota, Y., and Makowa, H. (1985) A rechargeable battery using electrochemically doped poly(N-vinylcarbazole). *J. Chem. Soc., Chem. Commun.*, **9**, 553–554.
52. Sezer, E., Van Hooren, M., Sarac, A.S., and Hallensleben, M.L. (1999) Synthesis and electrochemical polymerization of ter-arenes based on N-ethyl carbazole and thiophene. *J. Polym. Sci., Part A: Polym. Chem.*, **37**, 379–381.
53. Bruetting, W., Berleb, S., Egerer, G., Schwoerer, M., Wehrmann, R., and Elschner, A. (1997) Full colour electroluminescence using dye dispersed polymer blends. *Synth. Met.*, **91**, 325–327.
54. Sarac, A.S., Ates, M., Parlak, E.A., and Turcu, E.F. (2007) Characterization of micrometer-sized thin films of electrocoated carbazole with p-tolylsulfonylpyrrole on carbon fiber microelectrodes. *J. Electrochem. Soc.*, **154**, 283–291.
55. Grzeszcuk, M. and Poks, P. (1999) Double layer and redox capacitances of polyaniline electrodes in aqueous trichloroacetic acid. *J. Electrochem. Soc.*, **146**, 642–647.
56. Sarac, A.S., Ates, M., and Kilic, B. (2008) Electrochemical impedance spectroscopic study of polyaniline on platinum, glassy carbon and carbon fiber microelectrodes. *Int. J. Electrochem. Sci.*, **3**, 777–786.
57. Bhattacharya, A. and De, A. (1996) Conducting composites of polypyrrole and polyaniline – A review. *Prog. Solid State Chem.*, **24**, 141–181.

58. Syed, A.A. and Dinesan, M.K. (1991) Polyaniline – a novel polymeric material -review. *Talanta*, **38**, 815–837.
59. Wise, D.L., Wirek, G.E., Trantolo, D.J., Cooper, T.M., and Gresser, D. (1998) *Electrical and Optical Polymer Systems*, Marcel Dekker, New York.
60. Rodriguez, J., Grande, H.J., and Otero, T.F. (1997) *Handbook of Organic Conductive Molecules and Polymers*, John Wiley & Sons, Inc., New York.
61. Simonet, J. and Rault-Berthelot, J. (1991) Electrochemistry – a technique to form, to modify and to characterize organic conducting polymers. *Prog. Solid State Chem.*, **21**, 1–48.
62. Gupta, N. and Santhanam, K.S.V. (1993) Electron-transfer chemiluminescence of buckminsterfullerene radical-anion and thianthrenecation. *Curr. Sci.*, **65**, 75–77.
63. Witkowski, A., Freund, M.S., and Brajter-Toth, A. (1991) Effect of electrode substrate on the morphology and selectivity of overoxidized polypyrrole films. *Anal. Chem.*, **63**, 622–626.
64. Hsueh, C. and Brajter-Toth, A. (1994) Electrochemical preparation and analytical applications of ultrathin overoxidized polypyrrole films. *Anal. Chem.*, **66**, 2458–2464.
65. Freund, M., Bodalbhai, L., and Brajter-Toth, A. (1991) Anion-excluding polypyrrole films. *Talanta*, **38**, 95–99.
66. Diaz, A. and Castillo, J.I. (1980) A polymer electrode with variable conductivity-polypyrrole. *J. Chem. Soc., Chem. Commun.*, **9**, 397–398.
67. Beck, F., Braun, P., and Oberst, M. (1987) Organic electrochemistry in the solid state-overoxidation of polypyrrole. *Ber. Bunsen Ges. Phys. Chem.*, **91**, 967–974.
68. Ge, H., Qi, G., Kang, E., and Neoh, K.G. (1994) Study of overoxidized polypyrrole using X-ray photoelectron spectroscop. *Polymer*, **35**, 504–508.
69. Palmisano, F., Malitesta, C., Centonze, D., and Zambonin, P.G. (1995) Correlation between permselectivity and chemical-structure of overoxidized polypyrrrole membranes used in electroproduced enzyme biosensors. *Anal. Chem.*, **67**, 2207–2211.
70. Christensen, P.A. and Hamnett, A. (1991) Insitu spectroscopic investigations of the growth, electrochemical cycling and overoxidation of polypyrrole in aqueous-solution. *Electrochim. Acta*, **36**, 1263–1286.
71. Guimard, N.K., Gomez, N., and Schmidt, C.E. (2007) Conducting polymers in biomedical engineering. *Prog. Polym. Sci.*, **32**, 876–921.
72. Balint, R., Cassidy, N.J., and Cartmell, S.H. (2014) Conductive polymers: towards a smart biomaterial for tissue engineering. *Acta Biomater.*, **10**, 2341–2353.
73. Martins, N.C.T., Moura e Silva, T., Montemora, M.F., Fernandes, J.C.S., and Ferreira, M.G.S. (2008) Electrodeposition and characterization of polypyrrole films on aluminium alloy 6061-T6. *Electrochim. Acta*, **53**, 4754–4763.
74. Herrasti, P., Díaz, L., Ocón, P., Ibáñez, A., and Fatas, E. (2004) Electrochemical and mechanical properties of polypyrrole coatings on steel. *Electrochim. Acta*, **49**, 3693–3699.
75. Choi, S. and Park, S. (2002) Electrochemistry of conductive polymers. XXVI. Effects of electrolytes and growth methods on polyaniline morphology. *J. Electrochem. Soc.*, **149**, 26–34.
76. Wallace, G.G., Smyth, M., and Zhao, H. (1999) Conducting electroactive polymer-based biosensors. *Trends Anal. Chem.*, **18**, 245–251.
77. Cui, X., Wiler, J., Dzaman, M., Altschuler, R.A., and Martin, D.C. (2003) In vivo studies of polypyrrole/peptide coated neural probes. *Biomaterials*, **24**, 777–787.
78. Zhong, Y.H., Yu, X.J., Gilbert, R., and Bellamkonda, R.V. (2001) Stabilizing electrode-host interfaces: a tissue engineering approach. *J. Rehabil. Res. Dev.*, **38**, 627–632.
79. Guimard, N.K., Sessler, J.L., and Schmidt, C.E. (2007) Design of a novel electrically conducting biocompatible polymer with degradable linkages for biomedical applications. *Mater. Res. Soc. Symp. Proc.*, **950**, 99–104.

80. Malhotra, B.D. and Singhal, R. (2003) Conducting polymer based biomolecular electronic devices. *Pramana*, **61**, 331–343.
81. Machado, J.M., Masse, M.A., and Karasz, F.E. (1989) Anisotropic mechanical properties of uniaxially oriented electrically conducting poly(p-phenylenevinylene). *Polymer*, **30**, 1992–1996.
82. Diaz, A.F. and Hall, B. (1983) Mechanical properties of electrochemically prepared polypyrrole films. *IBM J. Res. Dev.*, **27**, 342–347.

3
Conducting Polymers: Biomedical Applications

Nidhin Joy, Geethy P. Gopalan, Joby Eldho, and Raju Francis

3.1
Applications

Conducting polymers (CPs) are organic polymers that may either have metallic conductivity or be semiconductors and can conduct electricity. The biggest advantage of CPs is their processability, mainly by dispersion. Bioapplications of CPs are attractive because of their inherent biocompatibility and unique optical and electrical transduction mechanisms [1–3]. CPs consisting of conjugated π-electron systems also offer advantages of having enhanced chemical and physical properties [4, 5]. These features make CPs attractive for many biomedical applications. There are various extraordinary qualities of CPs that make them appropriate for integration with living systems:

1) Mixed conduction of both electronic and ionic charge carriers is advantageous for communication with biological systems that depend mostly on ionic fluxes.
2) CPs form ideal interfaces with electrolyte solutions that lack native oxides and dangling bonds.
3) CPs are easily fabricated by chemical and electrochemical polymerization.
4) CP structure is readily modified by synthetic variables, and can be deposited on substrates via electrochemical deposition or drop casting methods.
5) Conducting polymeric framework has "soft" mechanical properties almost similar to those of the majority of biological tissues and, therefore, there is very low mechanical mismatch in implanted devices.
6) Their biocompatibility enables various biomedical applications.
7) The solution processing of CPs facilitates easy fabrication and unique form factors. Solution processability becomes important when designing flexible devices or inexpensive single-use sensors. These characteristics provide a new solution for interfacing electronics with biology and biodiagnostics.

The application of CPs at the interface with biology is an energizing new pattern in organic electronics research [6–8]. The coupling of organic electronic

Biomedical Applications of Polymeric Materials and Composites, First Edition.
Edited by Raju Francis and Sakthi Kumar.

devices (such as electrodes and transistors) with biological systems, in an effort to bridge the biotic/abiotic interface, is included in the early field of organic bioelectronics.

Recently, CP nanomaterials have shown outstanding chemical and physical properties compared with those of ceramic and metal nanomaterials. Thus, significant efforts have been made to fabricate CPs that enable various biomedical applications, such as high-performance biosensing and cellular interfacing. Although sensing or measuring devices based on CP nanomaterials have shown excellent electrical and physical properties, their limitations, such as the minimum detectable level, cytotoxicity assessments, and reliable synthesis methods, remain challenges to realizing high-performance biomedical geometries.

CP nanomaterials are promising candidates that have shown excellent performance in biomedical applications [9–16]. Nanoscale CPs exhibit outstanding properties compared with their bulk counterparts. In addition, they possess unique properties associated with high surface-to-volume ratios, such as highly sensitive sensing and low impedance with cells. Studies have provided information on the effects of interfacing CP nanomaterials in biological systems: (i) charge transfer via CP nanomaterial arrays, (ii) immobilization of CP nanomaterials and biomaterials, (iii) cell adhesion properties on CP nanomaterials, and (iv) the cytotoxicity of size and shape-controlled CP nanomaterials.

Cytotoxicity assessments are essential for the purpose of using CP nanomaterials for biomedical applications; however, they have generally been neglected. Only a few papers have been published concerning the cytotoxicity of CP nanomaterials. Although CPs are generally known as safe materials, the unique physicochemical properties of CP nanomaterials can induce adverse biological effects on living cells [17]. The surface area of nanomaterials increases exponentially with decreasing size, resulting in increased uptake and interaction with biological tissues. Thus, systematic toxicity evaluations of CP nanomaterials are important for understanding the toxicological issues associated with nanomaterials and providing toxicological information with relevance to biomedical applications. The investigation of neuronal development and outgrowth has received considerable attention from biomedical engineers over the past few decades [18–20]. Several research groups have exploited CP nanomaterials to improve the properties of neural interfaces as well as methods in tissue engineering [21, 22]. Such CP nanomaterials were substituted for metal electrodes because of their enhanced charge-transfer characteristics, leading to high cell adhesion in biological assays [19]. Because neuronal stimulation and monitoring are required for many clinical diagnostics and remedies, the unique electrical properties of CP nanomaterials may provide advantages for therapeutic and other purposes [23, 24]. In addition, the electronic properties of CP nanomaterials can be modified according to the charge transport required for electrical cellular interfacing. CPs nanomaterials can be subjected to large strains and have high strength even though they are lightweight, and they can be applied at body temperature and can circulate through the body [25–27]. Moreover, CP nanomaterials can be actuated or tuned with existing technologies. Therefore, CP

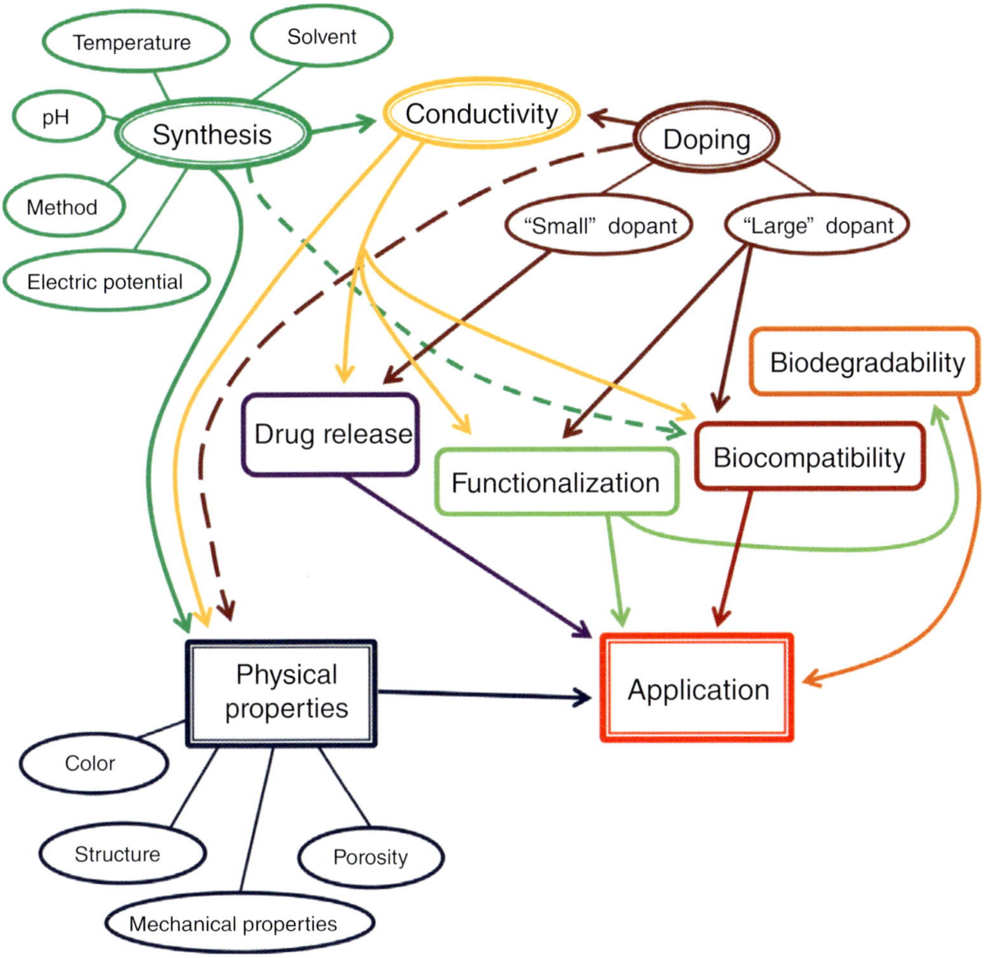

Figure 3.1 Everything is connected in the world of conductive polymers [28]. (Balint http://www.sciencedirect.com/science/article/pii/S1742706114000671. Used under CC-BY 3.0 license http://creativecommons.org/licenses/by/3.0/.)

nanomaterials have advantages in drug delivery systems, that is, the process of releasing a pharmaceutical compound at specifically targeted points in the living body; researches have made considerable efforts in the field of CP nanomaterials to take advantage of their properties that could control the administration of a therapy through physiological or chemical triggers. In this chapter, we provide general information on CP nanomaterials and their biomedical applications focusing especially on cellular interfacing and biosensing (Figure 3.1) [28].

In the field of bioelectronics emerged a champion material called poly(3,4-ethylenedioxythiophene)/polystyrene sulfonate (PEDOT/PSS). The p-conjugation gives PEDOT its semiconducting properties, while the PSS acts as a p-type dopant and raises the room temperature electrical conductivity to high levels

(100 S cm^{-1}, even up to 1000 S cm^{-1} with proper optimization). Polarons present on the PEDOT chain balances the fixed negative charges on the PSS chain, resulting in an enhanced electronic conductivity.

Also the use of CPs in extracting polar compounds has several advantages: the inherent and unusual multifunctionality of these compounds resulted in high extraction efficiency (e.g., ion-exchange properties, $\pi-\pi$ interactions, hydrogen bonding, acid-base properties, polar functional groups, and electroactivity) [29, 30] and switchable ion-exchange behavior [31]. Conductive polypyrrole (PPy) hollow fibers were fabricated by electrospinning and *in situ* polymerization over electrospun polycaprolactone (PCL) fibers [32]. These fibers were used for the solid-phase extraction of two important neuroendocrine markers of behavioral disorders, namely, 5-hydroxyindole-3-acetic acid and homovanillic acid from human plasma, with a successful recovery of 90.7% and 92.4%, respectively.

3.1.1 Drug Delivery

A drug delivery system is designed to deliver medicine at specifically targeted places in the living body. The medicine can be transported by carriers such as NPs and biomolecules [33, 34]. Polymeric microspheres and hydrogel-type compounds have been investigated before for their ability to target specific points and reduce drug toxicity. Moreover, controlled release and active targeting delivery systems are required. CP nanomaterials are biocompatible and can be activated by low voltages or light. The application of CP nanomaterials for drug delivery has currently not been explored in depth but is promising. The Martin group developed PEDOT NTs having well-defined internal and external surface textures, which showed controlled release of dexamethasone (DEX) by external electrical stimulation [35]. The PEDOT NTs lowered the impedance between the tissue and recording site by growing the surface area for ionic-to-electronic charge transfer. To produce the PEDOT NT delivery system, biodegradable PLLA or poly(lactic-co-glycolic acid)(PLGA) was first electrospun onto the electrode, followed by electrochemical deposition of PEDOT on the electrospun NFs. Then, the drug was loaded into the NFs after the fiber templates were removed. The neural probes consisting of PEDOT NTs enabled the electrical stimulation or signal recording of neurons. This methodology opens new pathways for the controlled release of drugs and biomolecules through electrical stimulation. PEDOT:PSS NPs were developed as an organic photothermal agent, activated by strong near-infrared (IR) absorbance, for the photothermal treatment of cancer [36]. Layer-by-layer coating with charged PEDOT:PSS polymers, followed by grafting with branched PEG, resulted in PEDOT:PSS–PEG NPs that were highly stable in the physiological environment and possessed "stealth-like" behavior after intravenous injection, with a long blood circulation half-life. As a photothermal agent, PEDOT:PSS–PEG NPs were used for *in vivo* cancer treatment and demonstrated excellent therapeutic efficacy in a mouse tumor model under near-IR irradiation at a low laser power density. Carbonized PPy NPs for drug delivery were prepared by pyrolysis of PPy NPs [37]. The final NPs displayed uniform sizes, large micropore volumes, and high surface areas. Magnetic phases formed during pyrolysis were useful for selective NP separation. Hydrophobic medicines, such as ibuprofen, were incorporated into the carbonized PPy NPs by surface adsorption and pore filling, and further plasma modification enhanced drug sustainability via surface covalent coupling. Drug-loaded NPs demonstrated sustained release properties. The carbonized PPy NPs also showed low toxicity and were readily incorporated into cells.

The applications of drug delivery systems are targeting cell clusters rather than the individual cells [38]. The utilization of CPs in the areas of bioanalytical sciences is of immense interest since their biocompatibility opens up the possibility of using them in "*in vivo*" biosensor applications for continuous monitoring of drugs or metabolites in biological fluids or as a means of opening up the field to a variety of new analytes [39–41]. Soluble CP polyaniline (PANI) grafted to lignin, poly(aniline sulfonic acid), and PPy are effective scavengers of the stable 1,1-diphenyl-2-picrylhydrazyl(DPPH) free radical. This property might be especially advantageous in tissues suffering from oxidative stress due to its attractive ability to lower the excessive levels of reactive radical species. This free radical-reducing ability of CPs is matched by efficient scavenging of DPPH radicals, with two and four radicals scavenged per aniline or pyrrole monomer unit during the 30 min test period. This shows that CPs can act as effective antioxidants when present in biological media [42, 43]. Various vitamins and polyphenol free radical-scavenging antioxidants in beverages, fruits, and vegetables are of great interest. These antioxidants have the ability to protect against diseases like cardiovascular diseases and cancer [44, 45]. Controlled drug release can also be facilitated using a change in CP redox state to increase permeation of dexamethasone (drug) [46, 47]. Electrical stimulation of CPs has been used to release a number of therapeutic proteins and drugs like nerve growth factor (NGF), heparin, and DEX. A fast release of heparin from the HG immobilized onto PPy films has been observed when PPy was electrically stimulated. Another study showed the utilization of PEDOT nanotubes polymerized on top of electrospun PLGA nanofibers for the potential release of the drug DEX. Here, PEDOT was integrated around the DEX-loaded PLGA nanofibers. DEX molecules remained inside the PEDOT nanotubes when the PLGA fibers degraded. The volume of the PEDOT nanotube changes upon electrical stimulation owing to the expulsion of anions [35]. Although the CPs possess immense potential in drug delivery applications, they have certain disadvantages that are attributed to the initial burst release of the drug and the hydrophobic nature of the polymer, which limits their application. Nevertheless, the drug delivery systems are of immense scientific interest and give hope for the treatment of cancer and also for minimum invasive techniques for several neural and cardiovascular applications.

Uniform pore-sized nanoporous membranes are used for achieving pulsatile release of drugs based on electric stimulus [44, 48]. Fluorescein isothiocyanate-labeled bovine serum albumin as a model protein drug was used for demonstrating successful release of pulsatile drug. This device could be used for intermittent and fast drug delivery (therapeutic methods of hormone-related diseases as well as chronic diseases). The main goal is the use of biodegradable polymers that could eliminate surgery for removing the implant.

Cellulose-PPy composite film was also used as a self-powered drug delivery system. This was constructed by electrochemical deposition of drug-contained PPy film on the inner and outer surfaces of a porous cellulose film. The amount of the drug released and the release rate were effectively controlled by adjusting the thickness and type of the active metal, respectively. The authors expected that this system could be used for *in vivo* applications because cellulose film is biodegradable, and the system was flexible and lightweight [27].

Abidian *et al.* reported a new method for the preparation of CP nanotubes that can be used for precise controlled drug release [35]. The fabrication process involved electrospinning of a biodegradable polymer (e.g., PLGA), into which a drug (e.g., DEX) was incorporated. Subsequently, a CP (e.g., PEDOT) was electrochemically deposited around the drug-loaded electrospun nanofibers. The proposed method seems to provide a useful means for creating low impedance, biologically active polymer coatings, which can facilitate integration of electronic active devices with living tissues. Highly localized stimulation of neurite outgrowth and guidance for neural tissue regeneration and spatially and temporally controlled drug delivery for ablation of specific cell populations are the other interesting biomedical applications of these electrically active polymer nanotubes.

Drug delivery systems based on CPs are of immense scientific interest for cancer treatment and also for the development of minimally invasive techniques (neural and cardiovascular applications). Significant burst release effect and a great hydrophobic nature of polymeric chains limit their applications.

3.1.1.1 **Release and Diffusion**

Niamlang and Sirivat [49] investigated the Dapp of SA (as a model drug) doped into PPV, as well as the mechanism of its release from PPV blended with PAAm hydrogel. They compared it with the release of SA from PAAm hydrogel loaded with SA. Measurements were carried out both in the presence and in the absence of an external electric field of 0.1 V, which was applied either to the anode or to cathode terminals. For the first 3 h, SA was not released from the SA-doped PPV, without electric stimulation. Afterward it started to diffuse through the PPV/PAAm blend until equilibrium concentration was reached. When the electric field was applied to the anodic terminal, SA was initially not released by SA-doped PPV, because ionic interaction between conductive polymer and SA counter ions prevented it. On the other hand, when the potential was applied to the cathode, the release was very pronounced and increased with the increase in the strength of the electric field. The release of SA loaded into PAAm hydrogel was also affected by the applied current. However, Dapp of SA diffusing from PAAm hydrogel was smaller by one order of magnitude than Dapp of SA released by SA-PPV. Chansai *et al.* [50] prepared PAA hydrogel, cross-linked by EGDMA. Various degree of cross-linking was obtained by changing the proportion of EGDMA. Cross-linked PAA hydrogels were blended with PPy doped with SSA (as a model drug). Diffusion of SSA through the PAA hydrogels was compared with their diffusion through the matrices of the conductive blends. When the degree of cross-linking was decreased and the strength of the applied electric field was increased, the diffusion coefficients increased. Investigators concluded that PPy promotes transport of SSA through PPA matrix, and its rate of release can be controlled by adjustment of the appropriate parameters. Cho *et al.* [51] investigated mesoporous silica nanoparticles (100 nm in diameter) loaded with NGF and imbedded into PPy film. This system was able to control the release of NGF, which induced specific cellular response in the PC12 cells targeted by it. Their spreading, adhesion, and proliferation were significantly increased. These effects were strongly enhanced by electric stimulation of the PPy film. Luo and Cui [52] investigated the electrically controlled drug release from the sponge like nanostructured PPy film. It was found that the drug can be loaded not only into the bulk of PPy but also onto its nanoholes. The choice of molecules that can be loaded into the holes is not limited rigorously by their size or charge. Such system allows the simultaneous release of two kinds of drugs, which may be required for a given treatment, for example, for simultaneous delivery of enzyme and its cofactor. Wadhwa *et al.* [53] electrochemically controlled release of DEX from PPy-coated electrode. 0.5 $\mu g\,cm^{-2}$ of DEX was released during each cycle of cyclic voltammetry (CV). A total of 16 $\mu g\,cm^{-2}$ of DEX could thus be released after 30 CV cycles. *In vitro* studies of murine glial cells showed that the number of reactive astrocytes could thus be reduced without any toxic side effects. Authors believe that this kind of system can also be used for local delivery of other drugs and agents for treatment of injuries and disorders. Abidjan *et al.* [35] prepared conductive nanotubes coated on neural electrodes by electrospinning the biodegradable poly (L-lactic acid) (PLA) as a template in which DEX was incorporated. This step was followed by an electrochemical deposition of PPy or PRDOT doped with saline solution. DEX could be released after biodegradation or dissolution in chloroform of PLA. Alternatively, the core of the polymer could be removed by soaking it in CH_2Cl_2, and the conductive tubes (containing DEX inside it) could be deposited on the tips of the microelectrodes. DEX could be delivered by activating the microelectrodes.

Stevenson *et al.* [54] investigated polyterthiophene (PTT) as an electrostimulated material for the release of DEX. Disodium phosphate of DEX can be released from PTT at therapeutically relevant levels. Sirivisoot *et al.* [55] released DEX and/or penicillin/streptomycin (P/S) in a controlled fashion, from PPy immobilized on an anodized nanotubular titanium (MWNT-Ti). Pyrrole monomers were oxidized by P/S or by DEX (incorporated as anionic dopants). CV was used to stimulate the release of drugs from PPy. Results of CV showed that 80% of drugs could be released on demand by applying five cycles of voltage sweep at a scan rate of 0.1 $V\,s^{-1}$. This investigation indicated that controlled release of these drugs improved bone implants. They enhanced adhesion of osteoblasts and inhibited fibroblast (scar-tissue cells) formation. Stauffer *et al.* [56] modulated local neural activity by controlled drug release from PPy coated on recording microelectrodes. However, without an external reservoir, the number of molecules that can be thus released was quite limited. These investigators attempted to increase drug load, to attain identical release at each pulse applied, and to increase its efficiency, by creating a nanostructure polymer film. They attempted to optimize stimulation drug release, and conditions of polymer synthesis, in order to attain maximal, identical release at each pulse applied. Moreover, electroactive polymers, other than PPy, could also be used for the electrochemically controlled release of various agents. Kang, Borgens, and Cho deposited PPy electrochemically on colloidal polystyrene arrays, which served as a template for the formation of a well-ordered porous PPy doped with NGF and sodium salt of poly(styrene sulfonate) (NaPSS). They deposited, under constant cathodic potential of 0.9 V aqueous mixture of 0.1 M pyrrole, 0.1 M NaPSS and 100 μg ml^{-1} of NGF. The resulting porous film of doped PPy was dried and stored in vacuum. The PPY-NGF-doped film was incubated at 37 °C in PBS solution, and 0.1 V potential applied for 2 h in order to release NGF. The release profile of NGF doped into the open structure porous PPy increased dramatically in comparison with NGF doped onto a flat PPy sheets, especially when it was stimulated electrically. Cell adhesion, metabolic activity, and neurite extension of cells cultured on the porous PPy were superior to those which were cultured on flat PPy sheets. Cho and Borgens prepared biotin-doped porous PPY. 9 mM of biotin, and 0.01 M NaDBS were used instead of NGF and NaPSS, and the applied potential was 0.7 V and not 0.9 V. When the biotin-doped PPy was exposed to a suspension of gold–streptavidin (Au–Sa), it absorbed gold particles as a result of the biotin–streptavidin interaction. The absorbed Au–Sa nanoparticles can be released in a controlled fashion by applying negative–positive potentials ranging from 1 to 2 V. When +2 V potential was used, all the nanoparticles were released within 60 s. This experiment demonstrated that biotin doping combined with biotin–streptavidin interactions can be used for controlled release of many important biological substances. Shepherd and Wallace [57] achieved autonomously controlled drug release due to galvanic coupling between an electrode (I) immersed in PBS solution at pH = 7.2 and biodegradable Mg alloy attached to it (which dissolves during the release of a drug to form Mg^{2+}ions) and electrode (II) connected to it, enveloped by a film of conductive polymer doped with a drug to be released and immersed in an identical PBS solution. The rate of drug release may be adjusted by changing the thickness and/or porosity of the coating method of preparation or the type of the conducing polymer. Majumdar *et al.* [58] applied a mathematical framework of the dynamics and performance involved in the molecular drug release of a given drug from an ECP, in order to calculate parameters of its release. A huge set of simulations varying in operational parameters and design were considered. Authors believe that the system developed by them will enable optimization of a wide range of therapeutic applications of ECPs for controlled drug release and delivery.

3.1.1.2 **Targeting and Delivery**

Wuang *et al.* [59] synthesized nanoparticles of PPy with Fe_3O_4 encapsulated in them by emulsion polymerization (with PVA as surfactant). The size (80–100 nm) and shape of the PPy-Fe_3O_4 nanoparticles were well defined. Their magnetization values were >20 emu g^{-1} and electric conductivity was about 1 S cm^{-1}. At Fe_3O_4

content of 28%, they were well dispersed and did not show any significant toxicity. Surfactant's functional groups allowed immobilization of folic acid or other biomolecules. Folic acid bonded to them targeted efficiently MCT-7 human breast cancer cells, as a result of the receptor-induced endocytosis and possibly also some nonspecific binding. It is hoped that these nanoparticles will serve as cancer cell-targeting agents and as intracellular seeds in cancer treatment therapy. George *et al.* [60] proposed to attach drugs to be delivered to biotin molecules, which were attached as dopants to PPy. In this way, they circumvented problems related to the choice of dopant and were not limited by the molecular weight of the drug. They investigated neurite outgrowth from PC12 cells cultured on PPy doped with biotin to which NGF molecules were attached through streptavidin links. Stimulation of PP by the 3 V potential was applied at 24 °C across BPS solution. Abidian *et al.* [35] reported that DEX loaded into PLGA tubes surrounded by PEDOT could be delivered at a given moment by electric pulse, which caused contraction of PEDOT surrounding PLGA containing DEX and pushed part of the drug into the surrounding solution or blood.

Micro- and nanostructured materials, often characterized by a significant amount of surfaces and interfaces, have been attracting intensive interest because of their demonstrated or anticipated unique properties compared with conventional materials. As an important type of carrier for foreign species, micro- and nanocontainers are common in nature, for example, the vesicles in living cells. A vesicle is a small, intracellular, membrane-enclosed container that stores or transports substances within a cell. In recent years, laboratorially available micro- and nanocontainers have been obtained with the advancement of nanotechnology resulting from scientific exploration of nature. CPCs, in particular, have aroused great attention because of their special inherent properties. Noticeably, the biggest advantage of nanostructured CPs is that their structure and properties can be adjusted reversibly by the doping/dedoping process. Therefore, CPs have been widely studied as actuators in aqueous solution. The polymer matrix expands and contracts with the flux of counter ions during the electrochemically controlled reversible doping and dedoping. So far, various structures of conductive-polymer containers have been produced by chemical or electrochemical approaches, including porous films, hollow spheres, tube like structures, and so on. Numerous novel methods have been introduced to fabricate CPCs. Among them, hard templates, soft templates, and nanofabrication are usual and typical routes. Meanwhile, the formation mechanisms of these CPCs have been investigated based on the comprehensive understanding of their chemical, electrical, and mechanical properties.

CPCs are considered to be competitive potential candidates for applications in encapsulation, drug delivery, and controlled release. A great deal of such examples is available in recent reports, reviews, and books. However, there are seldom systematic summaries, including the methods, corresponding mechanisms, and applications of these containers. Because of their significant possibilities for the future, the current state of knowledge concerning the aspects mentioned earlier is reviewed in this chapter with a systematic perspective.

Current drug delivery methods pose specific problems that scientists are endeavoring to address. For example, many drug potencies and therapeutic effects are limited or reduced because the drugs partially degrade before they reach the target in the body. Further, injectable medications could be made more cheaply and administered more easily if they were dosed orally [61]. However, this improvement cannot take place until methods are developed for the safe delivery of drugs through specific areas of the body or through an area where healthy bone and tissue are badly affected. The goal of all drug delivery systems is to transport medications intact to specifically targeted parts of the body through a medium that can control the release of the drugs by means of either a physiological or a chemical trigger. To achieve this, researchers have put enormous effort into the fields of micro- and nanotechnology. During the past decades, polymeric microspheres, polymer micelles, and hydrogel-type materials have all been proven to be effective in enhancing drug targeting specificity, lowering systemic drug toxicity, improving treatment absorption rates, and providing protection for pharmaceuticals against biochemical degradation.

So far, many sophisticated and potent drugs have been developed. However, conventional dosage forms such as oral delivery and injection have been found to be unsuitable for many of these new protein- and DNA-based drugs. Since they fail to target a specific area, these delivery routes often require frequent administration of drugs in high dosages. Consequently, the body experiences a rapid release of the drug, which renders these dosage forms unsuitable for many of the new drugs, because their toxicity requires observation for concentration spikes. Therefore, the blood concentrations and target areas of these drugs must be carefully controlled. Furthermore, since the efficacy of many new and traditional drugs is strongly influenced by their temporal administration, it is necessary to deliver drugs at a controlled rate. For example, many therapeutic agents are most effective when delivered in a pulsatile release profile. For these reasons, new cost-effective technologies for controlled drug delivery are demanded for the administration of the new drugs. Progress has been made in recent years following advances in nanotechnology, by way of microparticles, biocapsules, microneedles, and micropumps. The ideal drug delivery system that can self-regulate the delivery rate in response to the patient's physiological condition to obtain the optimal therapeutic effect is yet to be attained.

The reasons why CPs are the ideal materials for biomedical actuators and relevant applications have been summarized by Smela [62]. These lightweight materials have large strain and high strength. They are able to work at room or body temperature and in body fluids, and they only require low voltages for actuation. Many CPs are also biocompatible and suitable for processing by microfabrication with existing technology. CPs have been chosen as the material for micropump drug delivery systems. Experiments were conducted to choose the polymer or polymer composites most suitable for the application. Numerous articles have indicated that PPy is a good candidate because of its *in vivo* stability and biocompatibility. Different micropump designs were also modeled by computer simulation. CPs possess reversible electrochemical responses, where they expand upon oxidation and contract on reduction. The volume change originates from the insertion or expulsion of counter ions from an electrolyte for charge balancing, together with the movement of solvent molecules. When conducting electroactive polymers expand, they generate force and movement in a particular direction. This electrochemically controlled actuation has been investigated for a wide range of applications, including artificial muscles, microrobotics, and microfluidics. Electrochemical switching of an electronically conducting polymer is accompanied by charge compensation through ion flux into or out of a membrane formed from such a polymer, which can be made to work as an ion gate. PPy functions very well as an ion-gate membrane, which is positively charged in its oxidized state and is neutral in its reduced state. The ion-gate membrane can be used to control the delivery of drugs, which can be accumulated in the membrane, for example, during oxidation, and then released by electrochemically controlled reduction of the membrane.

PPy is particularly suitable for this purpose because the monomer is nontoxic, and the electrochemical synthesis of the polymer membrane can be performed in aqueous solution. Glutamate and dopamine (DA) can be released from a PPy membrane using potential control. Pyo has shown that controlled release of adenosine 5′-triphosphate (ATP) can be achieved using the same polymer membrane [63]. Hepel and Mahdavi have used a composite PPy film as an ion-gate membrane for the potential controlled release of a cationic drug, chlorpromazine [64]. The electrochemical synthesis conditions have a great influence on the redox properties of the PPy membrane, and these determine the ion-gate function of the membrane. In a recent study, efforts were made toward the electrochemical polymerization of PPy conductive polymer in order to find the optimum conditions for producing a PPy membrane that could exchange anions [65]. Furthermore, Iseki *et al.* evaluated the efficiency of a PPy membrane as a device for drug delivery using model compounds, which in aqueous solution produces anions with therapeutic activity. The selected anions were salicylate, nicoside, and naproxen. These anions have an aromatic structure and are of medium size [66]. The delivery of anions from the membrane was studied by using an electrochemical quartz crystal microbalance (EQCM), as well as high-pressure liquid chromatography (HPLC) as an analytical tool. In a report by D.G. Shchukin, the release and reloading cycles of a PPy microcontainer system were visualized by fluorescence microscopy, employing FITC-labeled dextran as a probe. The initial dextran-loaded PPy microcontainer electrode demonstrated a high uptake yield in solution without applied potential bias. Changing to a reductive potential resulted in the release of the encapsulated material. Further, hollow polyelectrolyte capsules could be reloaded with new portions of FITC-dextran at a positive potential bias. Twenty minutes of incubation at an oxidative potential was sufficient to reload the capsules inside the PPy microcontainer electrode. The incubation time or release time could be reduced by increasing the potential bias (Figure 3.2) [66].

Martin *et al.* demonstrated that PEDOT nanotubes can precisely release individual drugs and bioactive molecules at desired points in time by using electrical stimulation [35]. By applying a positive voltage, electrons were injected into the

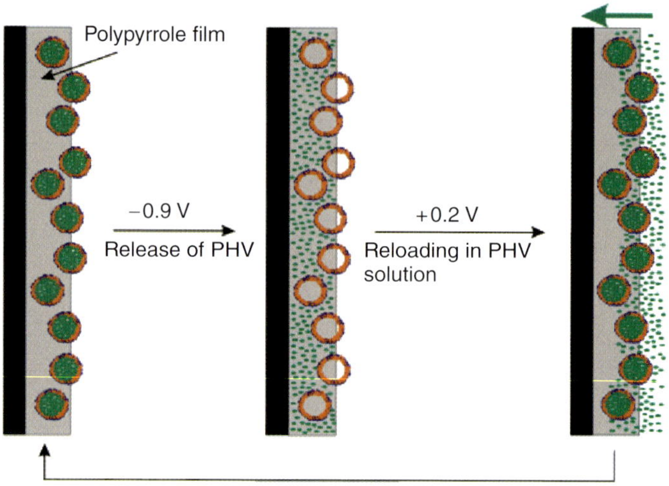

Figure 3.2 Schematic representation of functioning of polypyrrole microcontainer electrochemical system. (Shchukin 2006 [67]. Reproduced with permission from American Chemical Society.)

chains, and then positive charges in the polymer chains were compensated. To maintain overall charge neutrality, counter ions were expelled toward the solution, and the nanotubes contracted. PEDOT contraction then produced a mechanical force creating pressure within the nanotubes. Expulsion of PLGA degradation products and DEX occurs either through the ends or through openings or cracks on the surface of the PEDOT nanotubes as a result of hydrodynamic force inside the nanotubes. This research provided a general method capable of facilitating the integration of electronically active devices into living tissues.

Encapsulation, drug delivery, and controlled release are the main goal of scientists in preparing CPCs. Considering their special structures and unique properties, CPCs could also be applied to other aspects. For example, because of their high specific area, CP microcontainers are considered to be good candidates for sensing applications. Dai *et al.* found that the response current for PPy microcontainers is roughly double that of the corresponding PPy film when using them to detect glucose [68]. Furthermore, CPCs are capable of serving as a catalyst support due to their hollow structures and high surface-to-volume ratios. Despite their potential applications in other fields, encapsulation of certain foreign species and delivery and release of contents continue to be the focus of research.

The ability to nanostructure CPs allows biological signaling factors to be incorporated into these materials, through a variety of routes [69]. It is perceived that electrochemical reduction of oxidatively doped CPs allows the release of microscopic doses of biological inclusions to supply tissues with appropriate biological cues in a controlled manner [44]. Biological release profiles can also be controlled either through polymer composition or structure or through the application of electrical potentials, which releases charged biomolecules via ionic flux [70]. Such bioactive CPs can be designed for targeted cell responses. This functionality has been predominantly exploited in the field of neuroprostheses to promote neural cell growth toward microelectrodes and is hypothesized to aid in the survival and rescue of degenerative cells [71, 72]. The provision of cell adherence proteins and growth factors within CPs have significantly improved *in vivo* cell interactions with electrodes, but wider applications of bioactive CPs have not been thoroughly investigated. It is hypothesized that bioactive CPs could find applications in the prevention of infection and reduction of inflammation through the provision of antibiotics, anti-inflammatories, and other appropriate drug formulations.

The utility of incorporating CPs into biomaterials to take electrical stimulation on tissue regeneration such as nerve, skeletal, or other living tissues has been explored by researchers. For example, biocompatible PANI and its derivatives have both H9c2 cardiac myoblasts, and PC12 pheochromocytoma cells can adhere, grow, and differentiate well [73, 74]. PPy enhanced the effect of NGF in inducing neuronal differentiation of PC12 cells with electric stimulation. Polyvinylidine difluoride (PVDF) and poled polytetrafluoro ethylene (PTFE) promote enhanced neurite outgrowth *in vitro* and nerve regeneration *in vivo* as a consequence of either transient or static surface charges in the material [75].

Electrospinning and spin coating are the two methods for NF synthesis. These fibers are noticing for drug gene/cell delivery, wound dressings, artificial blood vessels, and substrates for tissue regeneration, immobilization of enzymes, and catalyst systems, because they have interconnected porous networks. Nonwoven mats of electrospun NFs can copy the extracellular matrices (ECM) since their construction becomes similar that of the collagen structure of the ECM (a 3D system of collagen NFs 50–500 nm in distance across). What's more, electrospun synthetic materials can offer several advantages for tissue regeneration: correct and controllable topography (e.g., nanoscale size, 3D porosity, and alignment), encapsulation and local sustained release of drugs, and surface functionalization. Electrospun NF mats can likewise be utilized for the development of complex nanosensory systems to identify biomolecules (e.g., glucose recognition) in less than nanomolar concentrations [76].

3.1.2 Electrode Coating

The most common biomedical applications for which CPs have been explored are implantable bioelectrodes for stimulating or recording from tissues. Typical neuroprosthetic implant electrodes are fabricated from platinum, gold, or alloys of these metals and iridium oxide. Despite recent advances in surface modification to increase the available surface area of conventional electrodes, their minimal interaction with neural tissue limits their capacity to provide optimal stimulation of and recording from neural cells [10]. The provision of a conductive polymer coating has the potential to surmount these limitations by providing a softer interface with a high surface area for delivering higher charge densities with lower thresholds.

Bioelectrodes are used extensively in the area of biological–machine systems integration (BMSI), particularly in relation to neural interfacing. The primary purpose of the BMSI is to provide neural interfaces for both sensory (recording) and actuation (neurostimulation purposes). The majority of recent advances in BMSI for manipulation and locomotion are in the domain of neural and rehabilitation engineering, the motivation being to improve the quality of life of the severely paralyzed or those suffering from profound losses to various sense organs.

Cellulose paper can be viewed as a smart material that can be utilized as a sensor and an actuator [77, 78]. The material has clear advantages with respect to lightweight, dryness, biodegradability, biocompatibility, low cost, large deformation, low actuation voltage, and low power consumption. Cellulose paper can be electrically activated due to the combination of ion migration and piezoelectric effect which originates from its crystal structure. The performance of cellulose can be enhanced by coating the paper with conductive polymers, for example, PPy and PANI [79, 80]. The ion migration effect can be improved by nanocoating the cellulose film with PPy and ionic fluids (e.g., 1-butyl- 3-methylimidazolium tetra fluoroborate) [81]. This hybrid nanocomposite showed durable bending actuation in ambient and temperature conditions. Results seem promising for creating cellulose-based paper actuators for ultralightweight devices and biomedical applications.

Cochlear implant, bionic eye, and deep brain stimulators are examples of stimulating devices. In the case of the last device, direct electrical stimulation of cortical and deep brain structures has been carried out for many years to control epileptic seizures and symptoms associated with degenerative neurological disorders such as Parkinson's disease. Replacing loss of motor control through functional electrical stimulation (FES) of nerve fibers and muscle is another example. While these prostheses are utilized to electrically bring out reactions in specific neural tissue through controlled stimulation paradigms, in many cases they are also required to perform recording functions that output information relating to characteristics of the neural – tissue interface – typically the interfacial impedance. Existing neural recording devices are typically more research based, with intensive investigation underway in the areas of brain–computer interfacing and nerve interfacing for prosthetic control purposes. Cochlear implant is a commercially available device that has for several decades restored hearing percepts to patients suffering from sensorineural deafness. This device communicates with the neural tissue via a flexible electrode array inserted in the cochlea. While the electrodes are fabricated from platinum and provide an effective long-term stimulation platform, it is hypothesized that CP electrodes could reduce implant power consumption and improve signal fidelity by increasing the electroactive surface area. This would benefit patients by allowing more complex signal modulation resulting in an improved dynamic range. The psychophysical outcome of such technology would be clearer hearing percepts of sounds, which are currently poor due to high background noise, such as music and speech in crowded environments [82]. In addition, the modification of CPs to incorporate biofunctional molecules might be used both to reduce tissue damage resulting from implantation and rescue or aid in the survival of diseased neural cells [83]. The vision prosthesis, also known as the bionic eye, is a stimulating device currently under development. Several groups around the world [84–86] are designing implants to restore perception of sight to blind patients by bypassing the degenerative photoreceptor tissue and electrically stimulating the remaining functional cells. Such devices are designed to aid patients blinded by degenerative diseases of the retina such as age-related macular degeneration (AMD) and retinitis pigmentosa (RP) [87]. In both these diseases the photoreceptor layer regresses, but a number of cell types within the retina, such as the retinal ganglion cells (RGCs), remain functional and can be electrically stimulated by electrodes placed in close apposition to the target cells [88, 89]. One of the major technological barriers in developing such a device is the construction of the high-density electrode array. CPs can potentially offer one alternative to allow small electrodes to be constructed with appropriate characteristics for long-term charge delivery.

In stimulating electrode applications, the current density supplied by the electrode and the current threshold required for cell activation are integral in determining the quality of the delivered signal. As the size of the electrodes is reduced to increase the number of discrete stimulation points (or resolution), the current density inversely increases. This is a major limitation for conventional platinum electrodes as the typical charge-carrying capacity of this metal is $6\,mC\,cm^{-2}$ [90], and the safe charge injection limit is $250\,mC\,cm^{-2}$, above which hydrolysis of the platinum can result in the evolution of toxic chemical species that can cause adverse tissue reactions [91]. Conventional CPs have been reported as carrying charge densities of up to approximately $200\,mC\,cm^{-2}$ [92, 93]. It has been proposed that CP coatings can provide significantly higher charge-carrying surface areas available per geometric electrode area.

CPs have also found application in neural recording and sensing of many organ systems in the body, with particular emphasis in the brain (cortical) interfacing to provide the so-called brain–computer interfaces (BCIs). Other applications include improving biosignal detection in diagnostics and mapping approaches for corrective surgery. Studies have shown that the distance between the recording electrodes and neural tissue has a significant influence on the signal to noise ratio (SNR) [94, 95]. The application of a CP coating provides closer apposition between the recording electrode and neural tissue, resulting in improved signal detection with less noise. An improved SNR can potentially be used to distinguish previously unattainable signals, leading to better diagnostics and improved surgical outcomes through more accurate localization and mapping [96].

3.1.3
Biological Sensors

Conversion of a biological response into an electrical signal is done by a biosensor, which is an analytical device. It consists of two main components: a bioreceptor or biorecognition element, which recognizes the target analyte, and a transducer, for converting the recognition event into a measurable electrical signal. A bioreceptor can be a tissue, microorganisms, organelles, cells, enzymes, antibodies, nucleic acids, and biomimic, and the transduction may be optical, electrochemical, thermometric, piezoelectric, magnetic, and piezoelectricor combinations of one or more of the previous techniques.

A biosensor is a device having a biological sensing element either intimately connected to or integrated within a transducer. The aim is to produce a digital electronic signal, which is proportional to the concentration of a specific biochemical or enzyme. CP conductivity is sensitive to chemical agents, and this allows them to be structured for use as biosensors, with the conductivity being proportional to the detected biochemical. The ability to alter the CP molecular structure and morphology makes them a superior choice for biosensors that are easily tailored to enhance the sensitivity and selectivity of a device to specific biochemicals [97].

Amperometric biosensors based on CPs with incorporated enzymes such as glucose oxidase (GOx), alcohol dehydrogenase, glutamate oxidase, and peroxidase [98–101] have found application in both biomedical and food industries. The most common CP-based biosensor is used in the detection of glucose in diabetic patients. In this CP-based biosensor, GOx is immobilized on the surface of either (PPy) or (PEDOT). The GOx enzyme catalyzes the conversion of glucose to D-gluconolactone, and the electron release from the oxidation reaction alters the current passing through the CP in proportion to the concentration of converted glucose in solution.

The bioreceptor recognizes the target analyte, and the corresponding biological responses are then converted into equivalent electrical signals by the transducer. The amplifier in the biosensor responds to the small input signal from the transducer and delivers a large output signal. The amplified signal is then processed by the signal processor where it can later be stored, displayed, and analyzed. In medicine, security, food, process industries, defense, environment, and so on, biosensors are used.

Some of the attractive features of CPs for biosensor applications include:

- Availability of varied range of monomer types.
- Availability of synthetic analogs of monomers.
- Composites can be prepared combining CPs with non-CPs or with nonpolymer materials such as carbon, carbon nanotubes (CNTs), metals, and so on.
- It can be prepared both electrochemically and chemically.
- It can be prepared in a range of soluble and insoluble forms.
- It has unique electrical, electronic, magnetic, and optical properties.
- Compliance with micro- and nanoscale fabrication.
- Compatibility with a diverse range of fabrication techniques such as electrochemical, optical, mass-based, and so on.
- Biomaterials such as enzymes, antibodies, whole cells, and nucleic acids can be incorporated into the polymer matrix.
- Strong biomolecular interactions.
- Low detection limits.
- Enhanced sensitivity.

- Reversible responses at ambient temperatures.
- Cost effectiveness.

CPs have tremendous technological potential for the development of sensors. They are inexpensive, can be miniaturized, and can be easily fabricated as compared with other miniaturized sensors. The primary output of these sensors is electrical in nature and hence easier to integrate into a single chip for further signal processing, which may lead to the development of "multiple sensors" or "sensor arrays" (Figure 3.3).

Even though many CP-based biosensors for foodborne pathogen detection have been reported in recent years, only very few applications in food samples have been reported to date. Among other CPs, PANI and PPy were most extensively reported and PPy was found to be a better choice for DNA biosensors. Foodborne pathogen detection based on electrochemical detection is preferred to optical detection. To fabricate a CP-based biosensor, it is important not only to consider the properties of CPs but also to focus on the method of immobilization that plays a vital role. For the fabrication of biosensors and many other nanoelectronic devices, CPs combine with nanomaterials/NPs as a composite shows enhanced sensitivity and very low detection limit.

Biosensor is a device that has a biological sensing element either connected to or integrated within a transducer. The purpose is to produce a digital electronic signal, proportional to the concentration of a specific chemical or a set of chemicals [102]. The biochemical transducer or biocomponent imparts selectivity or specificity to the biosensor. A transducer transforms the biochemical signal into an electronic signal. A suitable transducing system can be fitted in a sensor assembly depending on the nature of the biochemical interaction with the species of interest [103, 104]. Biocomponents that can function as biochemical transducers are tissues, yeast, bacteria, antibodies/antigens, liposomes, organelles,

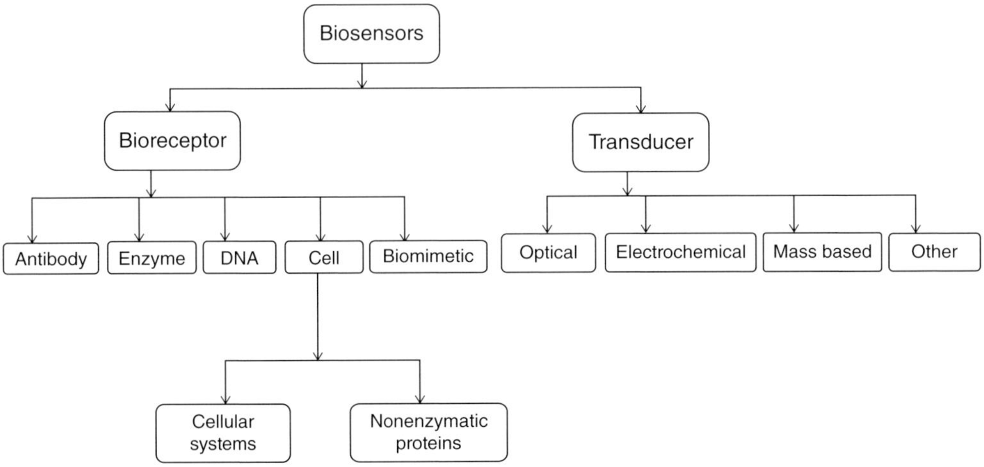

Figure 3.3 Biosensors classification.

enzymes, and so on [105, 106]. Within a biosensor, the recognition of the biomolecule incorporated possesses a level of selectivity, but it can be affected by extreme conditions, such as temperature, pH, and ionic strength [107]. Most of the biological molecules, such as enzymes, receptors, antibodies, cells, and so on, have a very short lifetime in solution phase. However, they can be fixed in a suitable matrix. The immobilization of the biological component against the environmental conditions results in decreased enzyme activity [108, 109]. The activity of immobilized molecules depends on the surface area, porosity, and the hydrophilic character of the immobilizing matrix. These are the bound reaction conditions and the methodology chosen for the immobilization process. CPs have attracted much interest as suitable matrices of biomolecules that can be utilized to improve stability, speed, and sensitivity and can, therefore, be useful in medical diagnostics [110, 111]. In order to obtain a long operational life of the biomolecules, or enzyme in an analytic device, the technique of the enzyme immobilization onto the transducer is key to developing a good biosensor. Enzymes can be immobilized onto the transducer by using such methods as adsorption, covalent attachment, cross-linking, and entrapment. As for the adsorption method, it uses the hydrophilic or hydrophobic properties of the material, such as ion- exchange resin [112] and nylon [113], to construct the enzyme electrode. The method of covalent attachment uses the functional group in the biomolecules, such as $-NH_2$, $-COOH$, and $-SH$, for binding with transducer chemically [114]. Covalent attachment, based on ethyldimethylaminopropylcarbodiimide (EDC) and *N*-hydroxysuccinimide (NHS) coupling chemistry, has been used to improve the stability of the desired biomolecules onto CPs [102]. Cosnier *et al.* reported the electropolymerization of a dicarbazole monomer functionalized with NHS group. The immobilization of both polyphenol oxidase (PPO) and thionine, which is a redox dye, has been carried out [115]. p-Aminophenol (*p*-AP) has been widely used as a raw chemical material and an important intermediate in various fields, such as medicine, petroleum industry, and photography, and in the preparation of sulfur and azo dyes, rubber, feeding stuff, and others. As a result, large amounts of *p*-AP may enter the environment as a pollutant [116]. Sarac *et al.* have demonstrated that by using thin film, electrocoated poly[*N*-vinylcarbazole-co-vinylbenzene sulfonic acid] (p[NVCzVBSA]), poly[carbazole-comethylthiophene] (p[CzMeTh]), and polycarbazole(PCz) carbon fiber microelectrodes can be used for the detection of some biologically important species, such as *p*-AP. These modified carbon fiber electrodes are found to be effective systems to determine *p*-AP. Thin film coated p[NVCzVBSA] is the most suitable modified electrode for the detection of p-AP [117].

Developing high-performance biosensor is of great interest in the fields of national security, food safety testing, and environmental monitoring [102, 118, 119]. Thus, the preparation of well-controlled nanomaterials having sensitive and selective analyte detection is an important and challenging goal. The following issues require further consideration for high-performance biosensor design: (i) an enlarged surface area for enhanced interactions with analytes and (ii) chemical functionalization for selective responses [120–122]. Based on these considerations, various carbon-based nanomaterials including graphene and CNTs and metal- or ceramic-based nanomaterials, have been shown to control sensing in devices. Numerous studies on carbon nanomaterial-based biosensors have been performed to advance the development of next-generation biosensors [123–126]. Although carbon-based biosensors offer advantages in biosensing applications, intrinsic shortcomings still remain due to their inert surfaces. CP nanomaterials can be used in miniaturized biosensors that enable a cost-efficient, portable, and high-density design [127, 128]. In particular, functionalized CP nanomaterials exhibit improved sensing performance via the immobilization process [41, 129–131]. The modification is readily achieved by grafting functional groups onto the polymer backbone, leading to a stability in the liquid state compared to noncovalent bonding. CP nanomaterials will open up novel biosensor applications and likely play an expanding role in future biosensor technology.

For example, PANI-CSA-Ni composite nanowire was successfully synthesized using camphor sulfonic acid (CSA) as a dopant as well as a surfactant. In this process, CSA-ANI micelles act as soft template facilitating the formation of PANI nanowire. The use of PANI-CSA-Ni composite nanowire as sensing material was also investigated. It was observed that PANI-CSA-Ni nanowire composite shows nearly four-order decreases in AC impedance in the presence of cigarette smoke. Therefore, such material has potential for use in cigarette smoke detection [132] (Figure 3.4).

DA is a monoamine neurotransmitter of both the central and the peripheral nervous systems. It plays an important role in neural immune communication [133]. In order to achieve simultaneous voltammetric measurement of DA and ascorbic acid (AA), Ciszewski and Milczarek have investigated different polymer

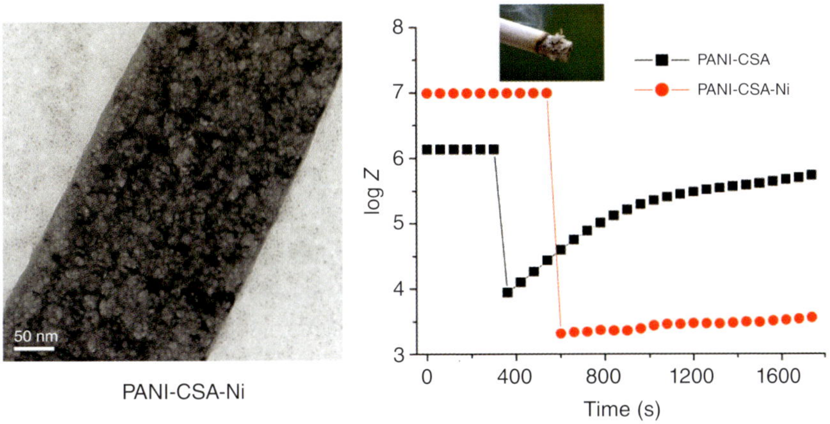

Figure 3.4 TEM and log impedance (*Z*) versus time plot of the PANI-CSA-Ni nanowire (red line) after exposure to cigarette smoke and log impedance response with time of PANI-CSA (black line) in the presence of cigarette smoke. (Chowdhury 2011 [132]. Reproduced with permission from American Chemical Society.)

coatings [134] and introduced new carbon electrode materials [135]. The voltammetric resolution obtained is good, but some of the approaches either show a less favorable detection capability with the conventionally sized electrodes, used in all of these studies [136], or require a nonphysiological pH of the medium [137]. Despite these great achievements, it seems that further efforts are necessary in order to introduce a suitable voltammetric microprobe for simple, selective, and reliable simultaneous measurement of DA and AA at their physiological concentrations. Modified PCz/carbon fiber microelectrode (CFME) is studied for biosensor applications to detect DA concentration by Sarac and coworkers. Results show that the electrodes have a reversible and stable behavior over the 68 days of testing for DA (100 μM) in buffer solution. A detection limit for PCz thin films is obtained as low as 0.1 μM using CV. Hence, this sensor can be considered to be a promising sensor for DA detection [138]. Polymer films of *N*-vinylcarbazole (*N*-VCz) have been electrocoated on CFME. Their responses to DA have been studied in different solutions [139]. Organophosphates (OPs) have been used as pesticides in modern agriculture given their low tenacity and high insecticidal activity [140]. Yet, due to their long-term accumulation in the environment, OP pollutions have caused serious public concern from the perspective of food safety and human health [141, 142]. Many analytic methods, containing gas chromatography [143], liquid chromatography [144], ultraviolet spectroscopy [145], and others, have been developed to assess OP disclosures. Although these methods could quantitatively provide an accurate evaluation of the health risk of integrated OP disclosures, they still suffer from some intrinsic disadvantages either of low detection specificity and sensitivity or of expensive analysis settings that entails well-trained personnel and inconvenience for field applications. Hence, simple, sensitive, selective, and field-deployable tools are still highly desired for the biomonitoring and diagnostic evaluation of OP disclosures.

Amperometric acetylcholinesterase (AChE) biosensors demonstrate a promising alternative to traditional methods owing to their good selectivity, sensitivity, rapid response, and miniature size. AChE biosensors have shown satisfactory results for pesticides analysis [146], where the enzymatic activity is employed as an indicator of quantitative measurement of insecticides [45]. Du *et al.* reported immobilized AChE on (PPy) and PANI copolymer doped with multiwalled carbon nanotubes (MWCNTs). The synthesized PANI–PPy–MWCNT copolymer presents a porous and homogeneous morphology, which provides an ideal size to entrap enzyme molecules. Because of the biocompatible microenvironment offered by the copolymer network, the obtained composite is designed for AChE attachment, arising from a stable AChE biosensor for screening of OP disclosure [147].

Biosensors use the ability of triiodide to oxidize polyacetylene to measure glucose concentration. Glucose is oxidized with oxygen with the help of GOx. This produces hydrogen peroxide, which oxidizes iodide ions to form triiodide ions. Hence, conductivity is proportional to the glucose concentration [148].

PANI is one of the most extensively studied CPs because of its simple synthesis [149] and doping/dedoping chemistry [150], low cost, high conductivity, and excellent environmental stability. PANI has wide applicability in rechargeable batteries [151], erasable optical information storage [152], shielding of electromagnetic interference [153], microwave- and radar-absorbing materials [154], sensors [155], indicators [156], catalysts [157], electronic and bioelectronic components [158], membranes [159], electrochemical capacitors [160], electrochromic devices [161], nonlinear optical [162] and light-emitting devices [163], electromechanical actuators [164], and antistatic [165] and anticorrosion coatings [166]. Its electromagnetic and optical properties depend mostly on its oxidation state and degree of protonation [167]. The green emeraldine salt form of PANI is conducting. The preparation of bulk quantities of conducting granular PANI is usually performed by the oxidative polymerization of aniline with ammonium peroxydisulfate (APS) in an acidic aqueous solution (initial pH <2.0). Colloidal PANI nanoparticles are prepared by dispersion polymerization of aniline in the presence of various colloidal stabilizers [168, 169]. The average size of colloidal PANI nanoparticles decreases with increasing stabilizer/aniline ratio. PANI colloids often have nonspherical (rice grain, needle like, etc.) core–shell morphology. The colloidal nanoparticle core most likely has a composite nature, that is, it is composed of both the PANI and the incorporated stabilizer, while the shell is formed by the stabilizer.

Nowadays, conducting PANI nanostructures are the focus of intense research owing to their significantly enhanced dispersibility and processability and substantially improved performance in many applications, as compared with granular and colloidal PANI [170–175]. The continuously growing interest in the study of zero-dimensional (0-D) (solid nanospheres), one-dimensional (1D) (NFs (nanowires), nanorods (nanosticks), nanoneedles, rice-like nanostructures, nanotubes), two-dimensional (2D) (nanoribbons (nanobelts), nanosheets (nanoplates, nanoflakes, nanodisks, leaf like nanostructures), nanorings (cyclic nanostructures), net like nanostructures), and three-dimensional (3D) PANI nanostructures (hollow nanospheres, dendritic, and polyhedral nanoparticles, flower like, rhizoid-like, brain-like, urchin-like, and star like nanostructures, etc.) has dramatically increased in recent years. The major focus of research has been the preparation, characterization, processing, and application of PANI nanofibers (PANI-NFs) and nanotubes (PANI-NTs). PANI-NFs are 1-D PANI nanoobjects of cylindrical profile with diameters 100 nm, without a discernible internal cavity, while PANI-NTs are 1-D PANI nanoobjects with an internal cavity. PANI nanowires (conducting or semiconducting doped PANI-NFs) and PANI nanorods (short and straight PANI-NFs) are also referred.

Extensive research in the broad field of preparation and characterization of nanostructured composite PANI materials, containing PANI nanostructures and micro-/submicro-/nanoparticles of various metals, oxides, organic/bioorganic compounds, and biological materials, has developed intensively with the aim to design nanomaterials with unique physicochemical properties and applicability. Therefore, the objective of this review is not only to provide insight into the recent developments regarding preparation, characterization, processing, and application of pure PANI nanostructures but also to give comprehensive information about composite materials that contain PANI nanostructures. It should be noted that the PANI nanocomposites prepared by the formation of PANI thin solid films on the surface of other nanostructured materials (nanofibers and nanotubes of various inorganic, organic, and biological materials, for example, CNTs, nanorods of tobacco mosaic virus, etc.) are not the subject of this review.

Progress in the development of nanostructured PANI for sensor applications has recently been reviewed [3, 23, 24, 176]. Films of PANI-NFs possess much faster gas-phase PANI nanostructures doping/dedoping times compared with conventionally cast films [177]. The NF films show essentially no thickness dependence in their performance. This is consistent with the porous nature of the NFs films, which enables gas molecules to diffuse in and out of the fibers rapidly. This also leads to a much greater doping or dedoping over short times for the NFs films. The better performance in both sensitivity and time response of PANI-NF film relative to its conventional bulk counterpart is caused by higher effective surface area and shorter penetration depth for target molecules. Using an interfacial polymerization method for the synthesis of PANI-NFs, Kaner's group has developed NF sensors (Figure 3.5) and compared them with conventional PANI sensors [22, 101, 178].

The changes in electrical resistance were monitored as a function of time as the thin films of PANI-NFs were exposed to the various gases. Five different response mechanisms were explored: acid doping (HCl), base dedoping (ammonia), reduction (hydrazine), swelling (chloroform), and polymer chain conformational changes (methanol). In all cases, the PANI-NFs performed better than conventional thin films. PANI-NF composites with metal salts can be used as a chemical sensor for hydrogen sulfide [179] and arsine [180]. Hydrogen sensors, based on conductivity changes in PANI-NFs [181, 182], have been reported. A controlled multipotential process was used to deposit PANI-NF arrays on a lithium niobate substrate with gold finger paired electrodes to form a surface acoustic wave device (hydrogen sensor) [183]. The lithium niobate surface acoustic wave transducer coated first with aluminum nitride and then with PANI-NFs by rapid mixing chemical oxidative method, in the presence of CSA,

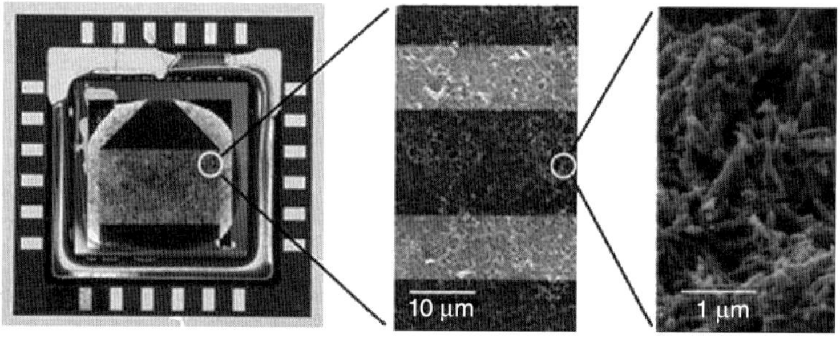

Figure 3.5 PANI-NF sensors. (Virji 2004 [170]. Reproduced with permission from American Chemical Society.)

has demonstrated a large and reproducible response to different concentrations of the hydrogen gas, making it an ideal candidate for hydrogen sensing at room temperature [184]. PANI-NFs deposited on lithium tantalate surface acoustic wave transducers [185] and Au and Pt electrodes [186] have also been used as hydrogen gas sensors. The great sensitivity of the Pt/PANI-NF sensor can be used to detect hydrogen at a concentration of 10 ppm [40]. Chemical gas sensors for nitrogen dioxide detection, using PANI-NFs synthesized by an interfacial polymerization method [187] and a plasma-induced polymerization technique [188], have been reported. Composites of PANI-NFs, synthesized using a rapid mixing method, with amines have recently been presented as novel materials for phosgene detection [189]. Chemiresistor sensors with nanofibrous PANI films as a sensitive layer, prepared by chemical oxidative polymerization of aniline on Si substrates, which were surface modified by amino-silane self-assembled monolayers, showed sensitivity to very low concentration (0.5 ppm) of ammonia gas [190]. Ultrafast sensor responses to ammonia gas of the dispersed PANI-CSA nanorods [191] and patterned PANI nanobowl monolayers containing Au nanoparticles [192] have recently been demonstrated. The gas response of the PANI-NTs to a series of chemical vapors such as ammonia, hydrazine, and triethylamine was studied [193, 194]. The results indicated that the PANI-NTs show superior performance as chemical sensors. Electrospun-isolated PANI-CSA NF sensors of various aliphatic alcohol vapors have been proven to be comparable to or faster than those prepared from PANI-NF mats [195]. An electrochemical method for the detection of ultratrace amount of 2,4,6-trinitrotoluene with synthetic copolypeptide-doped PANI-NFs has recently been reported [196]. PANI-NFs, prepared through the *in situ* oxidative polymerization method, were used for the detection of aromatic organic compounds [197].

Good biocompatibility of PANI-NFs enables them to become a simple and effective platform for the integration of proteins/enzymes and electrodes, which can provide analytical access to a large group of enzymes for a variety of bioelectrochemical applications. The (GOx)-PANI-NFs/glassy carbon [198] and (GOx)-PANI-NFs/carbon cloth [199] electrodes have displayed desirable features in electrocatalytic oxidation of glucose. An amperometric glucose biosensor prepared by self-assembly of GOx and dendrimer-encapsulated Pt nanoparticles on PANI-NFs has been described [200]. The unique sandwich-like layer structure showed excellent response performance to glucose and provided a favorable microenvironment to keep the bioactivity of GOx and to prevent enzyme leakage. A sensitive glucose biosensor based on a composite of conducting PANI-NFs and Au NPs, which shows excellent reproducibility and good operational stability, was also reported [201]. An amperometric glucose biosensor with good electrocatalytic activity toward oxidation of glucose and exhibited rapid response, low detection limit, useful linear range, high sensitivity, and biological affinity, as well as good stability and repeatability, was developed by electrochemically entrapping GOx on the inner wall of highly ordered PANI-NTs, which were synthesized using an AAO membrane as a template [202]. CSA-doped PANI/PS NFs, prepared using the electrospinning technique, have been used for sensing

H_2O_2 and glucose [203]. Sensitive H_2O_2 biosensors using HRP immobilized in PS nanoparticle/cauliflower like nanostructured PANI [204], Au–Pt alloy nanoparticle/PANI-NT/chitosan nanocomposite membranes [205], and processable PANI-NF/chitosan film [206] have been fabricated. Cholesterol biosensors based on cholesterol oxidase covalently immobilized onto electrophoretically deposited PANI film, derived from a PANI-NF colloidal suspension, have been reported [207]. A lipase/glutaraldehyde/PANI-NT/indium tin oxide (ITO) bioelectrode has recently been used to estimate triglycerides in serum samples using an impedimetric technique [208].

Sensitive electrochemical DNA biosensors based both on electrochemically fabricated PANI-NFs and methylene blue [209] and on the synergistic effect between PANI-NFs and MWCNTs in chitosan film have been successfully prepared [210]. Highly sensitive electrochemical impedance spectroscopic detection of DNA hybridization based on Aunano–CNT/PANI-NFs films has recently been reported [211]. PANI-NTs doped by poly(methyl vinyl ether-alt-maleic acid) were used to construct a simple electrochemical oligonucleotide sensor, where oligonucleotide probes were covalently grafted onto residual carboxylic acid functionalities on the nanotubes [212–214]. The potential pulse amperometry technique was used to obtain a direct and fast electrochemical readout. An ultrasensitive electrochemical DNA biosensor using a conducting PANI-NT array as the signal-enhancement element has also been presented [215]. A PANI-NT array with a highly organized structure was fabricated with a well-controlled nanoscale dimension on a graphite electrode using a thin nanoporous layer as a template, and 21 mer oligonucleotide probes were immobilized on these PANI-NTs. In comparison with Au nanoparticle or CNT-based DNA biosensors, this PANI-NT array-based DNA biosensor could achieve similar sensitivity without catalytic enhancement, purification, or end-opening processing. The electrochemical results showed that the conducting PANI-NTs array had a signal-enhancement capability, allowing the DNA biosensor to readily detect the target oligonucleotide at concentrations as low as 1.0×10^{-15}. In addition, this biosensor demonstrated good capability of differentiating the perfect matched target oligonucleotide from one-nucleotide mismatched oligonucleotides, even at a concentration of 4×10^{-14} M. This detection specificity indicates that this biosensor could be applied to single-nucleotide polymorphism analysis and single-mutation detection. Au nanoparticle/PANI-NT membranes on a glassy carbon electrode were constructed for the electrochemical sensing of the immobilization and hybridization of DNA [216]. The synergistic effect of the two kinds of nanomaterials, Au nanoparticles and PANI-NTs, dramatically enhanced the sensitivity for DNA hybridization recognition. The detection limit was 3.1×10^{-13} M. The biosensor also had good selectivity, stability, and reproducibility.

A nanogapped microelectrode-based PANI-NF biosensor array was fabricated for ultrasensitive electrical detection of microribonucleic acids (miRNAs) [217]. Deposition of conducting PANI-NFs was carried out by an enzyme-catalyzed method, where the electrostatic interaction between anionic phosphate groups in miRNA and cationic aniline molecules was exploited to guide the formation of the PANI-NFs on the hybridized target miRNA. The conductance of the deposited PANI-NFs was correlated directly with the amount of the hybridized miRNA, with a detection limit of 5.0×10^{-15} M.

A fast and sensitive continuous-flow nanobiodetector for detecting micro-organism cells in a flowing liquid, based on PANI-NFs fabricated as a freestanding nanonetwork in a microgap between two Au electrodes, was recently developed [218]. A direct-charge transfer biosensor, using antibodies as the sensing element and conducting PANI-NFs as the molecular electrical transducer, was developed for the detection of the foodborne pathogen *Bacillus cereus* [219]. A new type of nanobiodetector based on a limited number of PANI-NFs has recently been designed and tested against bacteria *Klebsiella pneumoniae, Pseudomonas aeruginosa, Escherichia coli,* and *Enterococcus faecalis* [220]. The cells' "defects" accumulated in PANI-NFs lead to an abrupt change in their electrical conductivity above a threshold density (the percolation limit). The device works like an "on–off" switch with nearly linear response above a threshold number of cells in the suspension examined. Nanostructured ultrathin films of self-assembled PANI-NFs cast onto interdigital microelectrodes have been used as efficient sensoactive layers in taste sensors for quality assessment of orange juices [221]. Unique highly carbonized PANI-NTs as a new thermally stable nanomaterial for nanosensors and nanodevices with a wide range of possible applications, comparable with CNTs, have been prepared [222].

Cell-based sensors, used for monitoring barrier tissue integrity in situ with high sensitivity and temporal resolution, result from the direct integration of barrier tissue with an organic electrochemical transistor (OECT) [223]. Barrier tissue comprises tightly packed layers of epithelial cells, such as the gastrointestinal (GI) tract and the blood-brain barrier. These cell layers allow the passage of ions, water, and nutrients but help to block the passage of toxins and pathogens. The ability of barrier tissue to impose this extremely controlled transport arises from the presence of protein complexes at the neighboring cell border, including the adherens junction (AJ) and the tight junction (TJ) [224]. So, disruptions in barrier tissue integrity are often indicative of the presence of toxins and pathogens. Here we use Caco-2 cell grown on a permeable membrane *in vitro* model for the GI tract, characterized by localized junctional proteins, low permeability to tracer molecules, and high transepithelial electrical resistance (TER) [225]. The sensor presented here follows OECT mechanism which consists of a CP (PEDOT : PSS) channel in contact with an electrolyte (cell culture medium) [226]. A gate electrode (Ag/AgCl) is immersed in the electrolyte, and either side of the transistor channel connects with the source and drain used for measuring the drain current (ID). On applying positive gate voltage (VG), cations from the electrolyte drift into the PEDOT : PSS channel and decrease the drain current (ID) due to dedoping the CP. The changes in the barrier tissue integrity affect the ID transient response. The OECT barrier tissue sensor was used to monitor the effect of a specific calcium chelator such as ethylene glycol-bis(2-aminoethylether)-*N, N, N′,N′*-tetraacetic acid (EGTA), on barrier tissue integrity. The junctional protein complexes are dynamic in nature, such as changes in the extracellular environment affect their assembly and function. Some junctional proteins are internalized in lower extracellular calcium level [227]. EGTA has effectively modified extracellular environment, leading to an increase in paracellular diffusion across tissue barrier [228]. Negligible changes in the response of the OECT were observed, when 100 mM EGTA was introduced to the basolateral side of the barrier tissue layer; it indicated no disruption of barrier properties. The sensitivity of the OECT sensor is equal to or greater than traditional end point characterization techniques including immunofluorescence staining of junctional proteins, permeability assays, and electrical impedance spectroscopy and benefits from an extremely high temporal resolution. This device fabrication and operation opens up new possibilities for creative solutions for large-scale diagnostic screening and *in vitro* model development.

3.1.4
Bioactuators

Bioactuators are used to create mechanical force, which in turn can be utilized as artificial muscles. The phenomenon of change in the volume of the CP scaffold upon electrical stimulation is the working principle for the construction of bioactuators. In artificial muscle applications, two layers of CPs are placed between nonconductive materials (triple-layer arrangement) [229, 230]. Oxidation and reductions occur when current is applied. The oxidized film expands owing to the inflow of dopant ions, whereas the reduced film expels the dopant ions and in the process shrinks [62].

The combined effect of simultaneous expansion and contraction is translated into a mechanical force that bends the polymer, which mimics the impact of muscles in biological systems [231]. CP actuators have numerous elements that make them perfect candidates for artificial muscles, including the fact that they (i) can be electrically controlled; (ii) possess high strength; (iii) have a large strain which is favorable for linear, volumetric, or bending actuators; (iv) require low voltage for actuation; (v) work at room/body temperature; (vi) can be positioned continuously between minimum and maximum values; (vii) can be readily microfabricated and are lightweight; and (viii) can operate in body fluids. PPy, PANI, and PPy–PANI composites and composites of these polymers with CNT have the ability to function as actuators. Of these materials, PPy-PANI shows strong mechanical property due to the high work per cycle [232, 233].

Electrochemical actuators are based on the expansion and contraction that tests a polymer in an electrolyte solution as an outcome of the change in electronic charge [234–236]. This is produced by the exchange of ions being the extension and contraction effect dependent on the size and number of counterions that enter or exit the polymer [231]. Bioactive drug-doped CPs used in actuators, for example, microfluidic pumps [47, 237], could lead to a controlled local release. For example, the treatment of the inflammatory response of neural prosthetic devices requires the release of anti-inflammatory drugs at wanted focuses in time [238].

3.1.5 Tissue Engineering Applications

CPs have recently received much attention as being advantageous substrates for tissue engineering scaffolds, because they can induce electrical stimuli for various cell types, including neurons, osteoblasts, fibroblasts, and skeletal myoblasts [239–243]. Because the orientation and diameter of NFs present unique topographical features that affect the behaviors of many cell types, CP NFs with well-controlled topographical features could be valuable as scaffold materials for translating model studies in tissue engineering [244–247]. The general CP properties desired for tissue engineering applications include conductivity, redox stability, reversible oxidation, hydrophobicity, biocompatibility, 3D geometry, and surface topography. One of the most promising CPs is PPy, which can be prepared by simple processes (*in situ* chemical oxidation or by VDP on a substrate) followed by oxidant treatment [248]. PPy NFs have shown attractive characteristics such as biocompatibility, facile modulation of adhesion, and differentiation of cell types as well as the ability to release and entrap biomolecules in bioapplications [46]. However, PPy performed poorly in a tissue engineering scaffold under mechanical forces because of its brittle backbone. Therefore, composites based on PPy have been constructed to overcome this limitation [43]. For example, PPy-coated PLGA, prepared by nano thick deposition, was used for conducting nanoscaffolds with high surface areas, interconnecting pores, and nanofibrous topographies [249].

CPs are broadly utilized as a part of tissue engineering applications because of their ability to subject cells to electrical stimulation. [250]. Little evidence of cytotoxicity was seen after long-term exposure to current [251]. Abidian *et al.* [252] demonstrated the biocompatibility of PPy and electrical conductivity of PEDOT, in film and nanotube morphology, by culturing neuronal cells using an *in vitro* dorsal root ganglion (DRG) model. CP in electrochemical synthesis allows direct deposition of a polymer on the electrode surface while simultaneously trapping the protein molecules [253]. Different approaches have been analyzed to overcome the drawback of CPs (hydrophobicity), which include the use of monomers that contain both redox centers and hydrophilic chain blends with polyelectrolytes and CP–HG composites.

In vitro cell culture using PC12 cells and embryonic hippocampal neurons demonstrated biocompatible cellular interactions, suitable for neuronal applications. In addition, the low electrical potential, $10\,\mathrm{mV\,cm^{-1}}$, facilitated neurite outgrowth on the aligned PPy-PLGA NFs. Xie and colleagues developed conductive PCL-PPy and polylactate (PLA)-PPy core–sheath NFs that facilitated neurite growth and extension [254]. The conductive core–sheath NFs were prepared by combining electrospinning with aqueous polymerization. The maximum length of neurites can be achieved by the synergistic effects of aligned conductive NFs: 1.83-fold (random NFs) and 1.47-fold (aligned NFs). PPy-polyurethane (PU) nanocomposites were also designed for tissue engineering scaffolds for C2C12 myoblast cells [255]. The scaffolds were prepared by chemical polymerization in a PU emulsion mixture with drop wise addition of an oxidant. The PPy–PU nanocomposites exhibited nontoxic, conductive, and elastomeric properties, resulting in cellular growth and subsequent cell differentiation. The dopant placed in the CPs can affect their cytocompatibility and the delivery of biomolecules [256]. Among various dopants, the smallest dopants (para toluene sulfonate and dodecylbenzenesulfonate) showed best biocompatibility with the neural tissue culture. As a result, electrochemically synthesized PPy/para toluene sulfonate enhanced the auditory nerve matrix, with release of neurotrophin. PEDOT-COOH nanodots (NDs) were prepared as a nanoplatform for enhanced cell capturing, synthesized by electropolymerization on ITO-coated glass [257]. The NDs were modified with the EpCAM antibody, a tumor cell-binding antibody. The enlarged cell-capturing efficacy resulted in the synergistic effects of ligand–receptor reactions and structural and mechanical matching between tumor cells and PEDOT-COOH NDs. The NDs have inherent advantages of facile fabrication, functional groups, and matching mechanical properties. PANI-NF-collagen composite films were introduced as an electronically conductive and biocompatible scaffold for mammalian cell culture [258]. The conductivity was related to the weight ratio of PANI-NFs. In addition, a PANI-coated Pt electrode was used to evaluate the biochemical mechanisms of tissue damage, in terms of both phospholipid peroxidation and protein denaturation under electrical stimulation.136 PANI was deposited onto the Pt electrode by *in situ* polymerization. PANI-NFs exhibited valuable properties, including inactivity against lipid peroxidation, increased protein adsorption, good stability, and anticorrosive effects.

It is well known that melanins are naturally occurring pigments which exhibit unique electrical properties [259]. This initiated their use as scaffolds for tissue engineering applications because of being biodegradable and semiconducting biomaterials. Here, melanin thin films with little concern for potential cytotoxicity were produced by the spin coating technique from dimethyl sulfoxide as the solvent. Melanin thin films increased Schwann cell growth and neurite extension compared with collagen films *in vitro*. In addition, melanin implants were significantly resorbed after 8 weeks. Recently Rachocki *et al.* have developed new biodegradable proton-conducting carbohydrate polymer films based on alginic acid (constituted by nearly 61% of mannuronic and 39% of guluronic acid) and benzimidazole [260].

An electroactive silsequioxane precursor containing an aniline trimer (i.e., N-(4-aminophenyl)-N′-(4′-(3-triethoxysilyl-propylureido)phenyl-1,4-quinonenedii mine) (ATQD)) could be a promising biomaterial for tissue engineering; it was reported by Wei *et al.* [261]. Self-assembled monolayers of ATQD on glass substrates were covalently modified with an adhesive oligopeptide, cyclic Arg-Gly-Asp (RGD) (Figure 3.6).

Measurement by atomic force microscopy gave the mean height of the monolayer coating on the surfaces as ~3 nm. The bioderivatized electroactive scaffold material, ATQD-RGD, supported adhesion and rapid growth of PC12 neuronal-like cells. Significantly, electroactive surfaces triggered spontaneous neuritogenesis in PC12 cells, in the absence of neurotrophic growth factors, such

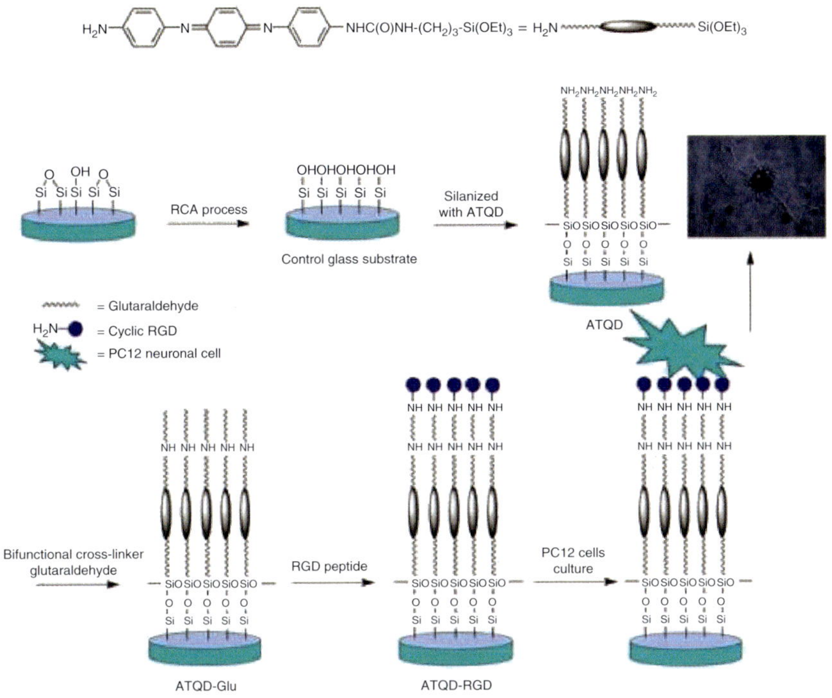

Figure 3.6 Scheme of self-assembled monolayers of ATQD-RGD. (Guo 2007 [261]. Reproduced with permission from American Chemical Society.)

as NGF. Therefore, covalent grafting of bioactive molecules, such as adhesion peptides, appears to be the best strategy to improve the biocompatibility of conventionally nonbiocompatible materials and consequently may permit to overcome the apparently poor cell biocompatibility of PANI.

Electrically conducting biomaterials have gained great attention in various biomedical studies especially to influence cell and tissue responses. Aufan *et al.* developed a simple method to create wrinkle topographies of conductive (wPPy) on soft polydimethylsiloxane surfaces via a swelling–deswelling process during and after PPy polymerization and by varying the thickness of the PPy top layers [262]. *In vitro* cell culture studies on NIH 3T3 fibroblasts and PC12 neuronal cells indicated that the conductive wrinkle topographies promote cell adhesion and neurite outgrowth of PC12 cells. wPPy-on-PDMS materials offer a novel design strategy for biomaterials for potential tissue engineering scaffold applications (Figure 3.7).

3.1.5.1 **Neural Applications**

Neural probe applications require materials with hydrophobicity, high surface area, and cell specificity for detection of neuron signals. Typical neuroprosthetic implants are usually fabricated from gold, platinum, or alloys of these metals and

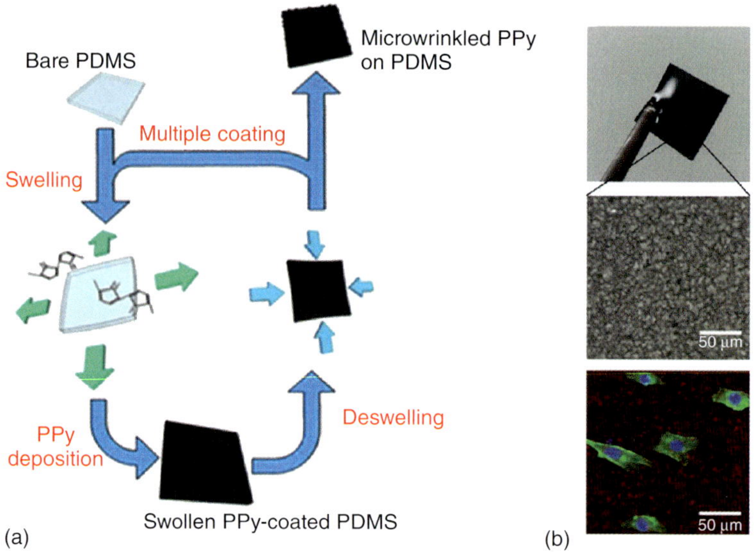

Figure 3.7 Conductive wrinkle topographies on PDMS. (a) Schematic diagram of wPPy formation. (b) Images of PPy wrinkle-coated PDMS for cell culture applications: a photograph of the wPPy-on-PDMS (top), its optical microscopic image (middle), and a fluorescent image of NIH3T3 cells grown on the wPPy substrate (bottom). (Aufan 2015 [262]. Reproduced with permission from American Chemical Society.)

iridium oxide, but the minimal interaction of these materials with neural tissue limits their ability to provide optimal stimulation and recording from neural cells. Neuroprostheses are utilized to electrically evoke responses in specific neural tissue through controlled stimulation paradigms, and they are also used for recording functions that output information on the status of the neural tissue interface. To maintain signal quality and activation of neural cells, neural interface has contact between the excitable tissue and the electrode. The effect of biological inclusions on polymer properties and their performance in neural prosthetics require a greater understanding of the CP film characteristics for long-term performance.

Kang *et al.* reported electrically conductive, porous PPy surfaces and demonstrated their use as an interactive substrate for neuronal growth. NGF-loaded porous CPs were initially prepared by electrochemical deposition of a mixture of pyrrole monomers and NGF into 2D or 3D particle arrays followed by subsequent removal of a sacrificial template. A four-point probe study demonstrated remarkable electrical activities despite the presence of voids. In addition, the effects of these surfaces on cellular behaviors using PC12 cells both in the presence and absence of electrical stimulation suggest that the surface topography as well as an applied electrical field can play a crucial role in determining further cell responses. Indeed, surface-induced preferential regulation leads to enhanced cellular viability and neurite extension (Figure 3.8) [263].

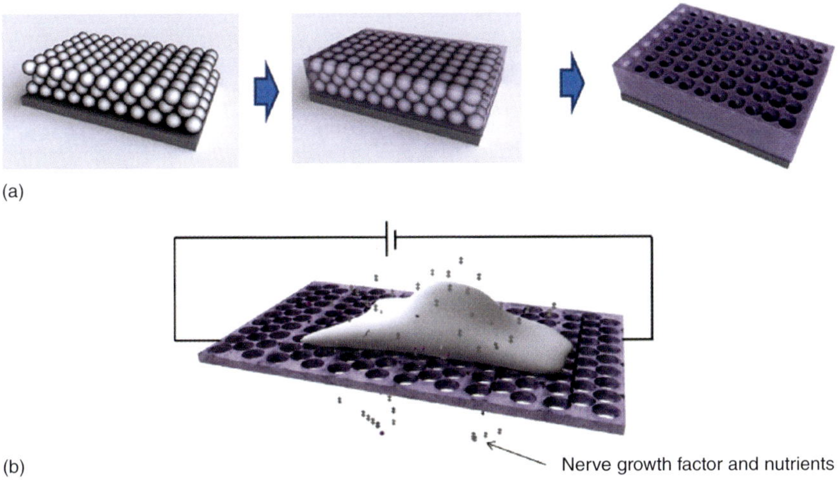

Figure 3.8 (a) The preparation of NGF-doped porous polypyrrole surfaces and (b) cellular interaction with a porous surface in the presence of electrical stimulation. (Kang 2011 [263]. Reproduced with permission from American Chemical Society.)

Nerve grafts or conduits guide the repair of injured neural tissue. Neural repair in the central nervous system, as in the case of spinal injury, as well as peripheral nerve damage associated with trauma, often results in uncontrolled growth of neural tissue. The result is that no effective conduction path is obtained, and both movement and sensory response can be lost in the body portion distal to the injury. CPs have potential application in nerve-graft technology, where an electroactive path is desirable for guiding tissue growth to bridge the gap in a damaged neural conduction path. CPs can be patterned to form channels along which neural cells extend, and the preferential adherence of cells to CPs may limit uncontrolled growth that could lead to cross talk and poor reconstruction of the damaged nerve. Currently, CPs are not frequently used because most are nonbiodegradable, but recent developments of novel composite CPs consisting of degradable block copolymers indicate that these materials will potentially provide superior scaffolds for nerve repair [264, 265].

The use of mixed heteroaromatic conductive segments of pyrrole and thiophene with flexible aliphatic chains via degradable ester linkages for making a novel biodegradable CP has recently been developed for biomedical applications. The authors specifically claimed its utility for peripheral nerve regeneration as well as spinal cord regeneration, wound healing, bone repair, and muscle tissue stimulation [266].

For nerve regeneration applications, electrically conductive polymer composites (PCLF-PPy) composed of polycaprolactone fumarate (PCLF) [267] and PPy have been developed [268]. This is possible because PCLF is a derivative of PCL that can be easily processed into complex 3D structures and exhibits biocompatibility, good mechanical properties, and tunable degradation rates that make it a future promising base material for application as nerve guidance conduits [269]. *In vitro* studies on PC12 neuronal-like cells and DRG explants showed that PCLF-PPy materials synthesized with naphthalene-2-sulfonic acid sodium salt or dodecylbenzene sulfonic acid sodium salt supported cell attachment, neurite extension, and proliferation and will be promising materials for future studies involving electrical stimulation.

For nerve regeneration applications, two novel biodegradable block copolymers of PPy with PCL and poly(ethyl cyanoacrylate) (PECA) were examined, that is, PPy-PCL and PPy-PECA copolymer [270]. The new conducting degradable biomaterials had good biocompatibility and support proliferation and growth of PC12 neuronal-like cells *in vitro* and neurons *in vivo*.

Scaffolds comprising conductive core–sheath NFs have been synthesized via *in situ* polymerization of pyrrole on electrospun PCL or PLA NFs [254]. Since PPy constitutes a thin coating on biodegradable NFs, the amount of PPy occupied in a nerve conduit could be significantly reduced for *in vivo* applications. The synergistic effect of topographic cue and electrical stimulation on axonal regeneration from cultured neuronal populations was examined and could consequently provide potential applications in neural tissue engineering.

Silk fibroin (SF) NF-based scaffolds prepared by electrospinning have been studied in detail for their widespread applications in biomedicine (e.g., tissue engineering in blood vessels, skin, bone, and cartilage) [271]. SF is highly biocompatible and is able to carry out appropriate cellular activity without evoking rejection, inflammation, or immune activation in the host [272]. Fibers of fibroin meshes have also been thin coated with PPy by chemical polymerization [273]. New materials were also established to support the adherence and proliferation of adult human mesenchymal stem cells (ahMSCs) or human fibroblasts (hFb).

Because of their low solubility and fast crystallization that easily blocks the nozzle, it is known that electrospinning of semi-CPs have been rarely carried out. Among the semi-CPs, poly(3-hexylthiophene) (P3HT) has been considered the best candidate since it has very high field effect mobilities (i.e., 0.1 $cm^2 V s^{-1}$ can be attained) [274]. A mixture of PLGA and poly(3-hexylthiophene) (PHT) was electrospun into 2D random (196 nm) and 3D axially aligned NFs (80–200 nm). Aligned PLGA-PHT NFs had a significant influence on the adhesion and proliferation of Schwann cells as indicated by *in vitro* cell studies. The new electrically conducting axially aligned NFs gave both electrical and structural cues and could be seriously used as scaffolds for neural regeneration [275].

3.1.5.2 Cardiovascular Applications

The complexity of the electrical conduction pathways is of great interest in the field of cardiac tissue engineering. The cardiac cells make the proper intercellular connections and matrix architecture so as to enable the electrical impulses to be transmitted in the appropriate direction at normal speed [276]. Further, the contraction of the cardiac muscle is driven by the waves of electrical impulses generated, which induces the mechanical stretch in the native heart. Any impairment in the electrical signal conducting pathway leads to cardiovascular diseases [277].

Li *et al.* showed the potential for using PANI as an electroactive polymer in the culture of excitable cells for cardiac and/or neuronal tissue engineering applications [278]. Different approaches of covalently attaching oligopeptides to PANI and electrospinning PANI–gelatin blend NF scaffold were examined as potential candidates for cardiac tissue engineering applications using H9c2 myoblast cells. In addition, a PPy–heparin composite was observed to be a good substrate for endothelial cell growth, and a PPy–hyaluronic acid (HA) composite seemed to promote vascularization. Also, PPy doped with erythrocytes can be used for the detection of blood rhesus factor via the rhesus factor antigens present on the cell surface [279]. Compared with unmodified one, erythrocyte-containing PPy bound more antibody, as proved by ELISA [280]. Tryptophan and oligopeptide (YIGSR)-modified PANI as well as PANI–collagen complexes showed that H9c2 cardiac cell viability was preserved, and that biocompatibility was improved using these modified CP scaffolds [281]. The mechanical properties of the CP construct play a vital role in cardiac applications. Attempts have been made to enhance the mechanical properties of CPs by making composites or blends and doping with large molecules that possess the desired mechanical properties to mimic the native myocardium.

One of the major challenges of cardiac tissue engineering is to generate a bioactive substrate with suitable chemical, biological, and conductive properties that could mimic the ECM both structurally and functionally, particularly to reconstruct infarct myocardium. Scaffolds constituted by PPy/PCL/gelatin NFs were obtained by electrospinning of different concentrations of PPy to PCL/gelatin solution [282]. The most balanced properties of conductivity, mechanical properties, and biodegradability and matching the requirements for regeneration of cardiac tissue were exhibited by conductive NFs containing 15% PPy. In addition, the scaffold promoted cell attachment, proliferation, interaction, and expression of cardiac-specific proteins.

3.1.5.3 Applications in Brain Recording

Electronic devices that interface with living tissue have become a necessity in clinics to improve findings and medications. One such illustration is electrocorticography (ECoG) electrode arrays, which are progressively utilized for functional mapping of cognitive processes before certain types of brain surgery (e.g., surgery for tumors), for diagnostic purposes (epilepsy) [283], and for brain-machine interfaces, an assistive innovation for people with serious motor disabilities [284]. High-quality electrical contacts are formed by complying with these electrode and curvilinear shape of the brain. Thin sheets of polymeric materials with metal electrodes are customarily utilized for this purpose [285]. Scientists prepared ECoG arrays with CPs electrodes utilizing microfabrication methods [286]. The arrays consisted of a parylene substrate, parylene insulation, and gold contact pads and interconnects. PEDOT:PSS film was deposited in appropriate holes in the insulation layer which defines the electrodes. The electrode arrays had adequate mechanical strength to be self-supporting and to be manipulated by a surgeon. The recordings were done after the addition of bicuculline (GABAA receptor antagonist) that enables the genesis of sharp-wave events which mimic epileptic spikes, and data were validated against a commercial implantable electrode. [287]. The PEDOT:PSS electrodes were found to outperform conventional metal electrodes, which highlight the significance of incorporating CP in a highly conformable electrode array format.

3.1.5.4 Applications in Scaffolds

Composite materials are currently used as a temporary substrate to trigger tissue generation by specific electrochemical signals as well as by continuous mechanical triggering until the regeneration processes are finished. Initial works giving novel conductive material well suited as biocompatible scaffolds for tissue engineering signals the development of PANi–gelatin blend NFs [278]. Many PANi and poly(D,L-lactide) (PDLA) compositions at different weight percentages were successfully electrospun from 1,1,1,3,3,3-hexafluoroisopropanol solutions, and their conductivity and biocompatibility were evaluated [288]. Even though the usefulness of polymer blend as the primary component of a biomedical device has limited use due to polymer degradation and shrinkage, it is found to be useful as biocompatible coatings on medical devices like sensors.

The use of composites from the blending of CPs and biocompatible polymers is strongly emerging as a promising strategy for the reappearance of myocardium due to their specific conductive and biological recognition properties. These findings are able to guarantee a more efficient electroactive stimulation of cells. Composite substrates made of synthesized polyaniline (sPANI) doped with CSA and PCL electrospun fibers were examined as scaffolds for cardiac tissue regeneration [289]. In particular, conductibility tests indicated that sPANI short fibers enabled a more efficient transfer of electric signals due to the spatial organization of the percolative network of electroactive needlelike phases. Based on this information, sPANI/PCL electrospun membranes have been optimized to mimic the morphological and functional features of the cardiac muscle ECM. Biological assays (i.e., evaluation of cell survival rate and immune staining of sarcomeric α-actinin of cardiomyocites-like cells) indicated that conductive signals offered by PANI needles promoted the cardiogenic differentiation of human mesenchymal stem cells into cardiomyocite-like cells. These preliminary results exhibited that the development of electroactive biodegradable substrates opens the path to another era of synthetic patches for the support of the regeneration of damaged myocardium.

Nanofibrous blends of HCl-doped poly(aniline-co-3-aminobenzoic acid) (3ABAPANI) copolymer and PLA were created by electrospinning solutions of the polymers, in varying proportions, in a DMF/THF mixture [290]. The nanofibrous electrospun 3ABAPANI-PLA blends gave improved cell growth, potent antimicrobial capability against Staphylococcus aureus and electrical conductivity. This new class of nanofibrous blends can potentially be utilized as tissue engineering scaffolds and new generation of functional wound dressings that may take out deficiencies of currently available antimicrobial dressings.

Combination of temperature-responsive CPs together with CNTs has excellent smart matrix with outstanding cell viability and proliferation. Electrospun microfabric scaffolds of poly(*N*-isopropylacrylamide) (PNIPAM)–CNT–PANI show excellent cell proliferation and viability that was attributed to the balanced hydrophilic functions, conductance, and mechanical strength provided by the PNIPAM, PANI, and MWNTs, respectively [291]. A temperature-dependent cell detachment behavior was observed by varying incubation at below LCST of PNIPAM. Thermoresponsive poly(NIPAM-co-methacrylic acid) in 3D conducting smart tissue scaffolds is also reported [292].

To support 3D cell culture *in vitro*, a novel fluffy-PPy scaffold composed of discrete hollow PPy fibers with interconnected pores of ~100 μm has been developed [293]. Cardiomyocytes as model cells were observed to enter into the interior of the fluffy-PPy scaffold smoothly with no extra help to achieve the 3D cell culture after only three days. Cell proliferation was found to be higher than that cultured on traditional electrospun mesh-PPy scaffolds. Results demonstrated that the 3D cell culture in fluffy fibrous scaffolds could enhance cells' survival *in vitro* compared with traditional 2D cell culture on electrospun fibrous meshes.

Advanced platforms for cell culturing and tissue engineering need polymer structures with controlled dimensions. The nature of polymeric structure and tissue to be repaired are some real worries that should be considered. Muscle is a suitable tissue to develop proper functional nano- and microstructured cell culture platforms since it includes a characteristic "bundled tubular" structure and cell systems that respond to electrical stimulation. Consequently, biosynthetic platforms support *ex vivo* growth of partially differentiated muscle cells in an aligned linear orientation that is consistent with the structural requirements of muscle tissue [294, 295]. In this platform, PLA/PLGA fibers are spatially aligned on a PPy-conducting substrate. Long multinucleated myotubes could be formed from differentiation of adherent myoblasts, which aligns longitudinally to the fiber axis to form linear cell-seeded biosynthetic fiber constructs. The capacity to remove the muscle cell-seeded polymer fibers when required gives the way to utilize the biodegradable fibers as linear muscle-seeded scaffold components suitable for *in vivo* implantation into muscle. Moreover, the conducting substrate with fibers placed provided the potential to develop electrical stimulation paradigms for optimizing the *ex vivo* growth and synchronization of muscle cells on the biodegradable fibers prior to implantation into damaged muscle tissue.

The designed scaffold also suggested to control axonal growth and Schwann cell migration. In addition, improved neurite outgrowth and Schwann cell migration were accomplished after direct electrical stimulation through the conductive polymer layer [296].

3.2 Conclusions

CPs have electrical and optical properties similar to those of metals and inorganic semiconductors, but they also possess attractive properties similar to those of common polymers. In most of the applications, CPs possess either a doped conducting state or a neutral semiconducting state. During the past decade, numerous applications such as biosensors, artificial muscles, coatings for neuroprosthetics, and drug delivery systems were proposed in this field – all of them showed the biomedical applications of CPs. However, their nondegradability has led to great attention being directed toward the recently developed degradable and electrically conductive polymers (DECPs). In many of the reported studies, biocompatibility testing has been limited to *in vitro* screening, and any further advancement of these materials requires appropriate functional animal studies before they can be used in clinical applications. It is clear that CPs are promising materials to fulfill material requirements in medical implants, in particular implants used in neural stimulation and sensing. Tissue engineering is another area where these materials may find applications, mainly as substrates for regeneration of tissues where electrical conductivity can enhance cell growth. However, the area is full of unresolved technological challenges motivating researchers to conduct further research and development work.

Abbreviations

AA	ascorbic acid
AChE	amperometric acetylcholinesterase
ATP	adenine triphenyl phosphate
BMSI	biological–machine systems integration
CNT	carbon nanotube
CP	conducting polymer
CPCs	conducting-polymer containers
CSA	camphor sulfonic acid
Dapp	apparent diffusion coefficients
DP	dopamine
DPPH	1,1-diphenyl-2-picrylhydrazyl
DRG	dorsal root ganglia
ECM	extracellular matrices
ECoG	electrocorticography
EGDMA	ethylene glycol dimethacrylate
EQCM	electrochemical quartz crystal microbalance
GOx	glucose oxidase
HA	hyaluronic acid
MDL	minimum detectable level
miRNAs	micro ribonucleic acids
MWCNT	multiwalled carbon nanotubes

NF	nanofibers
NGF	nerve growth factor
NHS	*N*-hydroxysuccinimide
N-VCz	*N*-vinylcarbazole
OECT	electrochemical transistor
OPs	organophosphates
PAAm	polyacrylamide
p-AP	p-aminophenol
PANI	polyaniline
PCL	polycaprolactone
PCLF	polycaprolactone fumarate
PCz	polycarbazole
PECA	poly(ethyl cyanoacrylate)
PDLA	poly(D,L-lactide)
PEDOT	poly(3,4-ethylenedioxythiophene)
PEDOT:PSS	poly(3,4-ethylenedioxythiophene):polystyrene sulfonate
PEG	polyethylene glycol
PHT	poly(3-hexylthiophene)
PLA	polylactic acid
PLGA	poly(lactic-co-glycolic acid)
PNIPAM	poly(*N*-isopropylacrylamide)
p[NVCzVBSA]	poly[*N*-vinylcarbazole-co-vinylbenzene sulfonic acid
PPO	polyphenol oxidase
PPV	poly(p-phenylene vinylidene)
PPy NPs	polypyrrole nanoparticles
RP	retinitis pigmentosa
SA	salicylic acid
SF	silk fibroin
SNR	signal to noise ratio
SSA	5-sulfosalicylicylic acid
sPANI	synthesized polyaniline

References

1. Yoon, H. and Jang, J. (2009) Conducting-polymer nanomaterials for high-performance sensor applications: issues and challenges. *Adv. Funct. Mater.*, **19**, 1567–1576.
2. Yoon, H., Choi, M., Lee, K., and Jang, J. (2008) Versatile strategies for fabricating polymer nanomaterials with controlled size and morphology. *Macromol. Res.*, **16**, 85–102.
3. Jang, J. (2006) Conducting polymer nanomaterials and their applications. *Adv. Polym. Sci.*, **199**, 189–260.
4. Yoon, H., Hong, J.-Y., and Jang, J. (2007) Charge-transport behavior in shape-controlled poly(3,4-ethylenedioxythiophene) nanomaterials: intrinsic and extrinsic factors. *Small*, **3**, 1774–1783.
5. Yoon, H., Chang, M., and Jang, J. (2007) Formation of 1d poly(3,4-ethylenedioxythiophene) nanomaterials in reverse microemulsions and their application to chemical sensors. *Adv. Funct. Mater.*, **17**, 431–436.

6. Malliaras, G. (2013) Organic bioelectronics: a new era in organic electronics. *Biochim. Biophys. Acta*, **1830**, 4286–4287.
7. Owens, R.M. and Malliaras, G.G. (2010) Organic electronics at the interface with biology. *MRS Bull.*, **35**, 449–456.
8. Berggren, M. and Richter-Dahlfors, A. (2007) Organic bioelectronics. *Adv. Mater.*, **19**, 3201–3213.
9. Guimard, N.K., Gomez, N., and Schmidt, C.E. (2007) Conducting polymers in biomedical engineering. *Prog. Polym. Sci.*, **32**, 876–921.
10. Green, R.A., Lovell, N.H., Wallace, G.G., and Poole-Warren, L.A. (2008) Conducting polymers for neural interfaces: challenges in developing an effective long-term implant. *Biomaterials*, **29**, 3393–3399.
11. Bendrea, A.-D., Cianga, L., and Cianga, I. (2011) Review paper: progress in the field of conducting polymers for tissue engineering applications. *J. Biomater. Appl.*, **26**, 3–84.
12. Higgins, M.J., Molino, P.J., Yue, Z., and Wallace, G.G. (2012) Organic conducting polymer–protein interactions. *Chem. Mater.*, **24**, 828–839.
13. Svennersten, K., Larsson, K.C., Berggren, M., and Richter-Dahlfors, A. (2011) Organic bioelectronics in nanomedicine. *Biochim. Biophys. Acta, Gen. Subj.*, **1810**, 276–285.
14. Sayyar, S., Murray, E., Thompson, B.C., Gambhir, S., Officer, D.L., and Wallace, G.G. (2013) Covalently linked biocompatible graphene/polycaprolactone composites for tissue engineering. *Carbon*, **52**, 296–304.
15. Otero, T.F., Martinez, J.G., and Arias-Pardilla, J. (2012) Biomimetic electrochemistry from conducting polymers. A review: artificial muscles, smart membranes, smart drug delivery and computer/neuron interfaces. *Electrochim. Acta*, **84**, 112–128.
16. Oh, J.K., Drumright, R., Siegwart, D.J., and Matyjaszewski, K. (2008) The development of microgels/nanogels for drug delivery applications. *Prog. Polym. Sci.*, **33**, 448–477.
17. Nel, A., Xia, T., Mädler, L., and Li, N. (2006) Toxic potential of materials at the nanolevel. *Science*, **311**, 622–627.
18. Han, D. and Cheung, K.C. (2011) Biodegradable cell-seeded nanofiber scaffolds for neural repair. *Polymers*, **3**, 1684–1733.
19. Fabbro, A., Bosi, S., Ballerini, L., and Prato, M. (2012) Carbon nanotubes: artificial nanomaterials to engineer single neurons and neuronal networks. *ACS Chem. Neurosci.*, **3**, 611–618.
20. Hou, S.T., Jiang, S.X., Smith, R.A., and Kwang, W.J. (2008) Permissive and repulsive cues and signalling pathways of axonal outgrowth and regeneration. *Int. Rev. Cell Mol. Biol.*, **267**, 125–181.
21. Lu, Y., Li, T., Zhao, X., Li, M., Cao, Y., Yang, H., and Duan, Y.Y. (2010) Electrodeposited polypyrrole/carbon nanotubes composite films electrodes for neural interfaces. *Biomaterials*, **31**, 5169–5181.
22. Lee, J.Y. and Schmidt, C.E. (2010) Pyrrole–hyaluronic acid conjugates for decreasing cell binding to metals and conducting polymers. *Acta Biomater.*, **6**, 4396–4404.
23. Thompson, B.C., Richardson, R.T., Moulton, S.E., Evans, A.J., O'Leary, S., Clark, G.M., and Wallace, G.G. (2010) Conducting polymers, dual neurotrophins and pulsed electrical stimulation: dramatic effects on neurite outgrowth. *J. Controlled Release*, **141**, 161–167.
24. Gelmi, A., Higgins, M.J., and Wallace, G.G. (2010) Physical surface and electromechanical properties of doped polypyrrole biomaterials. *Biomaterials*, **31**, 1974–1983.
25. Svirskis, D., Travas-Sejdic, J., Rodgers, A., and Garg, S. (2010) Electrochemically controlled drug delivery based on intrinsically conducting polymers. *J. Controlled Release*, **146**, 6–15.
26. Jiang, S., Sun, Y., Cui, X., Huang, X., He, Y., Ji, S., Shi, W., and Ge, D. (2013) Enhanced drug loading capacity of polypyrrole nanowire network for controlled drug release. *Synth. Met.*, **163**, 19–23.
27. Ge, D., Ru, X., Hong, S., Jiang, S., Tu, J., Wang, J., Zhang, A., Ji, S., Linkov, V.,

Ren, B., and Shi, W. (2010) Coating metals on cellulose–polypyrrole composites: a new route to self-powered drug delivery system. *Electrochem. Commun.*, **12**, 1367–1370.
28. Balint, R., Cassidy, N.J., and Cartmell, S.H. (2014) Conductive polymers: towards a smart biomaterial for tissue engineering. *Acta Biomater.*, **10**, 2341–2353.
29. Mohammadi, A., Ameli, A., and Alizadeh, N. (2009) Headspace solid-phase microextraction using a dodecylsulfate-doped polypyrrole film coupled to ion mobility spectrometry for the simultaneous determination of atrazine and ametryn in soil and water samples. *Talanta*, **78**, 1107–1114.
30. Li, X., Zhong, M., and Chen, J. (2008) Electrodeposited polyaniline as a fiber coating for solid-phase microextraction of organochlorine pesticides from water. *J. Sep. Sci.*, **31**, 2839–2845.
31. Li, M., Wei, Z., and Jiang, L. (2008) Polypyrrole nanofiber arrays synthesized by a biphasic electrochemical strategy. *J. Mater. Sci.*, **18**, 2276–2280.
32. Tian, T., Deng, J., Xie, Z., Zhao, Y., Feng, Z., Kang, X., and Gu, Z. (2012) Polypyrrole hollow fiber for solid phase extraction. *Analyst*, **137**, 1846–1852.
33. Zhang, X.Q., Xu, X., Bertrand, N., Pridgen, E., Swami, A., and Farokhzad, O.C. (2012) Interactions of nanomaterials and biological systems: implications to personalized nanomedicine. *Adv. Drug Delivery Rev.*, **64**, 1363–1384.
34. Shim, M.S. and Kwon, Y.J. (2012) Stimuli-responsive polymers and nanomaterials for gene delivery and imaging applications. *Adv. Drug Delivery Rev.*, **64**, 1046–1059.
35. Abidian, M.R., Kim, D.H., and Martin, D.C. (2006) Conducting-polymer nanotubes for controlled drug release. *Adv. Mater.*, **18** (4), 405–409.
36. Cheng, L., Yang, K., Chen, Q., and Liu, Z. (2012) Organic stealth nanoparticles for highly effective *in vivo* near-infrared photothermal therapy of cancer. *ACS Nano*, **6**, 5605–5613.
37. Oh, W.K., Yoon, H., and Jang, J. (2010) Size control of magnetic carbon nanoparticles for drug delivery. *Biomaterials*, **31**, 1342–1348.
38. Venugopal, J., Molamma, P., Choon, A.T., Deepika, G., Giri Dev, V.R., and Ramakrishna, S. (2009) Continuous nanostructures for the controlled release of drugs. *Curr. Pharm. Des.*, **15**, 1799–1808.
39. Adeloju, S.B. and Wallace, G.G. (1996) Conducting polymers and the bioanalytical sciences: new tools for biomolecular communication a review. *Analyst*, **121**, 699–703.
40. Harwood, G.W.J. and Pouton, C.W. (1996) Amperometric enzyme biosensors for the analysis of drug and metabolites. *Adv. Drug Delivery Rev.*, **18**, 163–191.
41. Ahuja, T., Mir, I.A., and Kumar, D. (2007) Biomolecular immobilization on conducting polymers for biosensing applications. *Biomaterials*, **28**, 791–805.
42. Gizdavic-Nikolaidis, M., Travas-Sejdic, J., Graham-Bowmaker, A., Ralph Cooney, P., Thompson, C., and Kilmartin, P.A. (2004) The antioxidant activity of conducting polymers in biomedical applications. *Curr. Appl. Phys.*, **4**, 347–350.
43. Gizdavic-Nikolaidis, M., Travas-Sejdic, J., Graham Bowmaker, A., Ralph Cooney, P., and Kilmartin, P.A. (2004) Conducting polymers as free radical scavengers. *Synth. Met.*, **140**, 225–232.
44. Li, Y., Neoh, K.G., Cen, L., and Kang, E.T. (2005) Controlled release of heparin from polypyrrole–poly(vinyl alcohol) assembly by electrical stimulation. *J. Biomed. Mater. Res. Part A*, **73A** (2), 171–181.
45. Li, Y., Neoh, K.G., Cen, L., and Kang, E.T. (2005) Porous and electrically conductive polypyrrole–poly(vinyl alcohol) composite and its applications as a biomaterial. *Langmuir*, **21**, 10702–10709.
46. Stassen, I., Sloboda, T., and Hambitzer, G. (1995) Membrane with controllable permeability for drugs. *Synth. Met.*, **71**, 2243–2244.

47. Pernaut, J.M. and Reynolds, J.R. (2000) Use of conducting electroactive polymers for drug delivery and sensing of bioactive molecules. A redox chemistry approach. *J. Phys. Chem. B*, **104**, 4080–4090.
48. Yang, S.Y., Yang, J.A., Kim, E.S., Jeon, G., Oh, E.J., Choi, K.Y., Hahn, S.K., and Kim, J.K. (2010) Single-file diffusion of protein drugs through cylindrical nanochannels. *ACS Nano*, **4**, 3817–3822.
49. Niamlang, S. and Sirivat, A. (2009) Electrically controlled release of salicylic acid from poly(p-phenylene vinylene)/polyacrylamide hydrogels. *Int. J. Pharm.*, **371**, 126–133.
50. Chansai, P., Sirivat, A., Niamlang, S., Chotpattananont, D., and Viravaidya-Pasuwat, K. (2009) Controlled transdermal iontophoresis of sulfosalicylic acid from polypyrrole/poly(acrylic acid) hydrogel. *Int. J. Pharm.*, **381**, 25–33.
51. Cho, Y., Shi, R., Ivanisevic, A., and Ben Borgens, R. (2009) A mesoporous silica nanosphere-based drug delivery system using an electrically conducting polymer. *Nanotechnology*, **20**, 275102–275114.
52. Luo, X. and Cui, X.T. (2009) Sponge-like nanostructured conducting polymers for electrically controlled drug release. *Electrochem. Commun.*, **11**, 1956–1959.
53. Wadhwa, R., Lagenaur, C.F., and Cui, X.T. (2006) Electrochemically controlled release of dexamethasone from conducting polymer polypyrrole coated electrode. *J. Controlled Release*, **110**, 531–541.
54. Stevenson, G., Moulton, S.E., Innis, P.G., Gordon, G., and Wallace, G.G. (2010) Polyterthiophene as an electrostimulated controlled drug release material of therapeutic levels of dexamethasone. *Synth. Met.*, **160**, 1107–1114.
55. Sirivisoot, S., Pareta, R., and Webster, T.J. (2011) Electrically controlled drug release from nanostructured polypyrrole coated on titanium. *Nanotechnology*, **22**, 085101.
56. Stauffer, W.R., Lau, P.-M., Bi, Q.-B., and Cui, X.T. (2011) Rapid modulation of local neural activity by controlled drug release from polymer-coated recording microelectrodes. *J. Neural Eng.*, **8**, 044001–044008.
57. Shepherd, L. and Wallace, G.G. (2008) Galvanic coupling conducting polymers to biodegradable Mg initiates autonomously powered drug release. *J. Mater. Chem.*, **18**, 3608–3613.
58. Majumdar, S., Kargupta, K., Ganguly, S., and Ray, P. (2011) Studies on the performance of conducting polymer based molecular release system. *Polym. Eng. Sci.*, **51**, 2001–2012.
59. Wuang, S.C., Neoh, K.G., Kang, E.-T., Pack, D.W., and Leck, D.E. (2007) Synthesis and functionalization of polypyrrole-Fe_3O_4 nanoparticles for applications in biomedicine. *J. Mater. Chem.*, **17**, 3354–3362.
60. George, P.M., LaVan, D.A., Burdick, J.A., Chen, C.-Y., Liang, E., and Langer, R. (2006) Electrically controlled drug delivery from biotin-doped conductive polypyrrole. *Adv. Mater.*, **18**, 577–581.
61. Geetha, S., Rao, C.R.K., Vijayan, M., and Trivedi, D.C. (2006) Biosensing and drug delivery by polypyrrole. *Anal. Chim. Acta*, **568** (1–2), 119–125.
62. Smela, E. (2003) Conjugated polymer actuators for biomedical applications. *Adv. Mater.*, **15** (6), 481–494.
63. Pyo, M. (1994) Controlled-release of biological molecules from conducting polymer-modified electrodes – the potential-dependent release of adenosine 5′-triphosphate from poly(pyrrole adenosine 5′-triphosphate) films. *J. Electroanal. Chem.*, **368** (1–2), 329–332.
64. Hepel, M. and Mahdavi, F. (1997) Application of the electrochemical quartz crystal microbalance for electrochemically controlled binding and release of chlorpromazine from conductive polymer matrix. *Microchem. J.*, **56** (1), 54–64.
65. Kontturi, K., Murtomaki, L., Pentti, P., and Sundholm, G. (1998) Preparation and properties of a pyrrole-based ion-gate membrane as studied by the EQCM. *Synth. Met.*, **92** (2), 179–185.
66. Iseki, M. (1993) Effect of cations on the electrochemical-behavior of

p-toluenesulfonate-doped polypyrrole in various aqueous-solutions. *J. Electroanal. Chem.*, **358** (1–2), 221–233.
67. Shchukin, D.G., Köhler, K., and Möhwald, H. (2006) Microcontainers with electrochemically reversible permeability. *J. Am. Chem. Soc.*, **128** (14), 4560–4561.
68. Bajpai, V., He, P.G., and Dai, L.M. (2004) Conducting-polymer microcontainers: controlled syntheses and potential applications. *Adv. Funct. Mater.*, **14** (2), 145–151.
69. Green, R.A., Lovell, N.H., and Poole-Warren, L.A. (2010) Impact of co-incorporating laminin-peptide dopants and neurotrophic growth factors on conducting polymer properties. *Acta Biomater.*, **6**, 63–71.
70. Isaksson, J., Kjall, P., Nilsson, D., Robinson, N., Berggren, M., and Richter-Dahlfors, A. (2007) Electronic control of Ca2+ signalling in neuronal cells using an organic electronic ion pump. *Nat. Mater.*, **6** (9), 673–679.
71. Richardson, R.T., Thompson, B., Moulton, S., Newbold, C., Lum, M.G., Cameron, A., Wallace, G., Kapsa, R., Clark, G., and O'Leary, S. (2007) The effect of polypyrrole with incorporated neurotrophin-3 on the promotion of neurite outgrowth from auditory neurons. *Biomaterials*, **28** (3), 513–523.
72. Thompson, B.C., Moulton, S.E., Ding, J., Richardson, R., Cameron, A., O'Leary, S., Wallace, G.G., and Clark, G.M. (2006) Optimising the incorporation and release of a neurotrophic factor using conducting polypyrrole. *J. Controlled Release*, **116** (3), 285–294.
73. Wei, Y., Lelkes, P.I., MacDiarmid, A.G., Guterman, E., Cheng, S., and Palouian, K. (2004) *Contemporary Topics in Advanced Polymer Science and Technology*, (eds Q. Zhou and S.Z.D. Cheng), Peking University Press, Beijing, pp. 430–436.
74. Bidez, P., Li, S., MacDiarmid, A.G., Venancio, E.C., Wei, Y., and Lelkes, P.I. (2006) Polyaniline, an electroactive polymer, supports adhesion and proliferation of cardiac myoblasts. *J. Biomater. Sci., Polym. Ed.*, **17**, 199–212.
75. Kotwal, A. and Schmidt, C.E. (2001) Electrical stimulation alters protein adsorption and nerve cell interactions with electrically conducting biomaterials. *Biomaterials*, **22**, 1055–1064.
76. Tiwari, A., Terada, D., Yoshikawa, C., and Kobayashi, H. (2010) An enzyme-free highly glucose-specific assay using self-assembled aminobenzene boronic acid upon polyelectrolytes electrospun nanofibers-mat. *Talanta*, **82**, 1725–1732.
77. Kim, J. and Seo, Y.B. (2002) Electro-active paper actuators. *Smart Mater. Struct.*, **11**, 355–360.
78. Kim, J., Yun, S., and Ounaies, Z. (2006) Discovery of cellulose as a smart material. *Macromolecules*, **39**, 4202–4206.
79. Kim, J., Deshpande, S.D., Yun, S., and Li, Q. (2006) A comparative study of conductive polypyrrole and polyaniline coatings on electro-active papers. *Polym. J.*, **38**, 659–668.
80. Kim, J., Yun, S., and Deshpande, S.D. (2007) Synthesis, characterization and actuation behavior of polyaniline-cellophane based electro-active paper actuator. *Polym. Int.*, **56**, 1530–1536.
81. Kim, J., Yun, S., Mahadeva, S.K., Yun, K., Yang, S.Y., and Maniruzzaman, M. (2010) Paper actuators made with cellulose and hybrid materials. *Sensors*, **10**, 1473–1485.
82. Huang, C.Q. and Shepherd, R.K. (1999) Reduction in excitability of the auditory nerve following electrical stimulation at high stimulus rates IV Effects of stimulus intensity. *Hear. Res.*, **132** (1–2), 60–68.
83. Richardson, R.T., Wise, A.K., Thompson, B.C., Flynn, B.O., Atkinson, P.J., Fretwell, N.J., Fallon, J.B., Wallace, G.G., Shepherd, R.K., Clark, G.M., and O'Leary, S.J. (2009) Polypyrrole-coated electrodes for the delivery of charge and neurotrophins to cochlear neurons. *Biomaterials*, **30**, 2614–2624.
84. Weiland, J. and Humayan, M. (2003) Past, present and future of artificial vision. *Artif. Organs*, **27**, 961–962.
85. Zrenner, E. (2002) Will retinal implants restore vision? *Science*, **295**, 1022–1025.

86. Lovell, N.H., Hallum, L.E., Chen, S., Dokos, S., Byrnes-Preston, P., Green, R.A., Poole-Warren, L.A., Lehmann, T., and Suaning, G.J. (2007) Advances in retinal neuroprosthetics, in *Handbook of Neural Engineering* (ed. M. Akay), Wiley-Blackwell, London.
87. Humayun, M.S. (1999) Pattern electrical stimulation of the human retina. *Vision Res.*, **39** (15), 2569–2576.
88. Humayun, M.S., Prince, M., De Juan, E. Jr.,, Barron, Y., Moskowitz, M., Klock, I.B., and Milam, A.H. (1999) Morphometric analysis of the extramacular retina from postmortem eyes with retinitis pigmentosa. *Invest. Ophthalmol. Vis. Sci.*, **40** (1), 143–148.
89. Humayun, M.S., De Juan, E. Jr.,, Dagnelie, G., Greenberg, R.J., Propst, R.H., and Phillips, D.H. (1996) Visual perception elicited by electrical stimulation of retina in blind humans. *Arch. Ophthalmol.*, **114** (1), 40–46.
90. Kim, D.R., Abidian, M., and Martin, D.C. (2004) Synthesis and characterization of conducting polymers grown in hydrogels for neural applications. *Mater. Res. Soc. Symp. Proc.*, **1**, 1–6.
91. Rose, T.L. and Robblee, L.S. (1990) Electrical stimulation with Pt electrodes VIII Electrochemically safe charge injection limits with 0 2 mspulses. *IEEE Trans. Biomed. Eng.*, **37** (11), 1118–1120.
92. Green, R.A. (2009) Conducting polymers for neural interfaces: impact of physicochemical properties on biological performance. PhD thesis. Graduate School of Biomedical Engineering, University of New South Wales.
93. Green, R.A., Lovell, N.H., and Poole-Warren, L.A. (2009) Cell attachment functionality of bioactive conducting polymers for neural interfaces. *Biomaterials*, **30** (22), 3637–3644.
94. Cui, X., Wiler, J., Dzaman, M., Altschuler, R.A., and Martin, D.C. (2003) *In vivo* studies of polypyrrole/peptide coated neural probes. *Biomaterials*, **24** (5), 777–787.
95. Kim, D.H., Richardson-Burns, S.M., Hendricks, J.L., Sequera, C., and Martin, D.C. (2006) Effect of immobilized nerve growth factor on conductive polymers: electrical properties and cellular response. *Adv. Funct. Mater.*, **17** (1), 1–8.
96. Snellings, A., Anderson, D.J., and Aldridge, J.W. (2003) Use of multichannel recording electrodes and independent component analysis for target localization in deep brain structures. Proceedings of the 1st International IEEE EMBS Conference on Neural Engineering, Capri Island, Italy, pp. 305–308.
97. Liu, J., Agarwal, M., and Varahramyan, K. (2008) Glucose sensor based on organic thin film transistor using glucose oxidase and conducting polymer. *Sens. Actuators, B*, **135** (1), 195–199.
98. Gao, M., Dai, L., and Wallace, G.G. (2003) Glucose sensor based on glucose-oxidase-containing polypyrrole/aligned carbon nanotube coaxial nanowire electrodes. *Synth. Met.*, **137**, 1393–1394.
99. Vernitskaya, T.V. and Efimov, O.N. (1997) Polypyrrole: a conducting polymer; its synthesis, properties and applications. *Russ. Chem. Rev.*, **66** (5), 443–457.
100. Wang, J. and Musameh, M. (2005) Carbon-nanotubes doped polypyrrole glucose biosensor. *Anal. Chim. Acta*, **539**, 209–213.
101. Huang, J., Virji, S., Weiller, B.H., and Kaner, R.B. (2004) Nanostructured polyaniline sensors. *Chem. Eur. J.*, **10**, 1314–1319.
102. Gerard, M., Chaubey, A., and Malhotra, B.D. (2002) Application of conducting polymers to biosensors. *Biosens. Bioelectron.*, **17**, 345–359.
103. Svorc, J., Miertus, S., Katrlik, J., and Stredansk, M. (1997) Composite transducer for amperometric biosensors. The glucose sensor. *Anal. Chem.*, **69**, 2086–2089.
104. Urban, G., Jachimowicz, A., Kohl, F., Kuttner, H., Olcaytug, F., Kamper, H., Pittner, F., Mann-Buxbaum, E., Schalkhammer, T., Prohaska, O., and Schonauer, M. (1990) High resolution thin film temperature sensor arrays for

medical applications. *Sens. Actuators, A*, **21**, 650–654.

105. Sadik, O. and Wallace, G.G. (1993) Pulsed amperometric detection of proteins using antibody containing conducting polymers. *Anal. Chim. Acta*, **279**, 209–212.

106. Foulds, N.C. and Lowe, C.R. (1988) Immobilization of glucose oxidase in ferrocene modified pyrrole polymers. *Anal. Chem.*, **60** (22), 2473–2478.

107. Karyakin, A.A., Vuki, M., Lukachova, L.V., Karyakina, E.E., Orlov, A.V., Karpachova, G.P., and Wang, J. (1999) Processable polyaniline as an advanced potentiometric pH transducers. *Anal. Chem.*, **71**, 2534–2540.

108. Hammerle, M., Schuhmann, W., and Schmidt, H.L. (1992) Amperometricpolypyrrole enzyme electrodes: effect of permeability and enzyme location. *Sens. Actuators, B*, **6**, 106–112.

109. Evtugyn, G.A., Budnikov, H.C., and Nikolskaya, E.B. (1998) Sensitivity and selectivity of electrochemical enzyme sensors for inhibitor determination. *Talanta*, **46**, 465–484.

110. Adeloju, S.B. and Wallace, G.G. (1996) Conducting polymers and the bioanalytical sciences: new tools for biomolecular communications- a review. *Analyst*, **21**, 699–703.

111. Sung, W.J. and Bae, Y.H. (2000) A glucose oxidase electrode based on electropolymerized conducting polymer with polyanion-enzyme conjugated dopant. *Anal. Chem.*, **72**, 2177–2181.

112. Zhujun, Z. and Seitz, W.R. (1986) Optical sensor for oxygen based on immobilized hemoglobin. *Anal. Chem.*, **58**, 220–222.

113. Gamati, S., Luong, J.H.T., and Mulchandani, A. (1991) A microbial biosensor for trimethylamine using pseudomonas a aminovorans cells. *Biosens. Bioelectron.*, **6**, 125–131.

114. Cass, A.E.G., Davis, G., Francis, G.D., Hill, H.A.O., Aston, W.J., Higgins, I.J., Plotkin, E.V., Scott, L.D.L., and Turner, A.P.F. (1984) Ferrocenemediated enzyme electrode for amperometric determination of glucose. *Anal. Chem.*, **56**, 667–671.

115. Cosnier, S., Fologea, D., Szunerits, S., and Marks, R.S. (2000) Poly (dicarbazole-N-hydroxysuccinimide) film: a new polymer for the reagent less grafting of enzymes and redox mediators. *Electrochem. Commun.*, **2**, 827–831.

116. Filik, H., Hayvalı, M., Kılıc, E., Apak, R., Aksua, D., Yanaza, Z., and Cengel, T. (2008) Development of an optical fibre reflectance sensor for p-aminophenol detection based on immobilised bis-8-hydroxyquinoline. *Talanta*, **77**, 103–109.

117. Jamal, M., Sarac, A.S., and Magner, E. (2003) Conductive copolymermodified carbon fibre microelectrodes: electrode characterization and electrochemical detection of p-aminophenol. *Sens. Actuators, B*, **97**, 57–66.

118. Ramanavičius, A., Ramanavičienė, A., and Malinauskas, A. (2006) Electrochemical sensors based on conducting polymer-polypyrrole. *Electrochim. Acta*, **51**, 6025–6037.

119. Bartlett, P. and Birkin, P. (1993) The application of conducting polymers in biosensors. *Synth. Met.*, **61**, 15–21.

120. Song, H.S., Kwon, O.S., Lee, S.H., Park, S.J., Kim, U.K., Jang, J., and Park, T.H. (2012) Human taste receptor-functionalized field effect transistor as a human-like nanobioelectronic tongue. *Nano Lett.*, **13**, 172–178.

121. Park, S.J., Kwon, O.S., Lee, S.H., Song, H.S., Park, T.H., and Jang, J. (2012) Ultrasensitive flexible graphene based FET-type bioelectronic nose. *Nano Lett.*, **12**, 5082–5090.

122. Yoon, H., Lee, S.H., Kwon, O.S., Song, H.S., Oh, E.H., Park, T.H., and Jang, J. (2009) Polypyrrole nanotubes conjugated with human olfactory receptors: high-performance transducers for FET type bioelectronic noses. *Angew. Chem. Int. Ed.*, **48**, 2755–2758.

123. He, P. and Dai, L. (2006) *BioMEMS and Biomedical Nanotechnology*, vol. **6**, Springer, New York, pp. 171–201.

124. Balasubramanian, K. and Burghard, M. (2006) Biosensors based on carbon nanotubes. *Anal. Bioanal. Chem.*, **385**, 452–468.

125. Sotiropoulou, S. and Chaniotakis, N.A. (2003) Carbon nanotube array-based biosensor. *Anal. Bioanal. Chem.*, **375**, 103–105.
126. Sinha, N., Ma, J., and Yeow, J.T.W. (2006) Carbon nanotube-based sensors. *J. Nanosci. Nanotechnol.*, **6**, 573–590.
127. Contractor, A., Sureshkumar, T.N., Narayanan, R., Sukeerthi, S., Lal, R., and Srinivasa, R. (1994) Conducting polymer-based biosensors. *Electrochim. Acta*, **39**, 1321–1324.
128. Wallace, G., Smyth, M., and Zhao, H. (1999) Conducting electroactive polymer-based biosensors. *TrAC, Trends Anal. Chem.*, **18**, 245–251.
129. Elkaoutit, M., Naggar, A.H., Naranjo-Rodriguez, I., Dominguez, M., and De Cisneros, J.L.H.-H. (2009) Electrochemical AFM investigation of horseradish peroxidase enzyme electro-immobilization with polypyrrole conducting polymer. *Synth. Met.*, **159**, 541–545.
130. Ekiz, F., Rende, E., Timur, S., and Toppare, L. (2012) A novel functional conducting polymer: synthesis and application to biomolecule immobilization. *J. Mater. Chem.*, **22**, 22517–22525.
131. Yousef Elahi, M., Bathaie, S.Z., Kazemi, S.H., and Mousavi, M.F. (2011) DNA immobilization on a polypyrrole nanofiber modified electrode and its interaction with salicylic acid/aspirin. *Anal. Biochem.*, **411**, 176–184.
132. Chowdhury, D. (2011) Ni-coated polyaniline nanowire as chemical sensing material for cigarette smoke. *J. Phys. Chem. C*, **115**, 13554–13559.
133. Zhan, D., Mao, S., Zhao, Q., Chen, Z., Hu, H., Jing, P., Zhang, M., Zhu, Z., and Shao, Y. (2004) Electrochemical investigation of dopamine at the water/1, 2-dichloroethane interface. *Anal. Chem.*, **76**, 4128–4136.
134. Ciszewski, A. and Milczarek, G. (1999) Polyeugenol-modified platinum electrode for selective detection of dopamine in the presence of ascorbic acid. *Anal. Chem.*, **71** (5), 1055–1061.
135. Miyazaki, K., Matsumoto, G., Yamada, M., Yasui, S., and Kaneko, H. (1999) Simultaneous voltammetric measurement of nitrite ion, dopamine, serotonin with ascorbic acid on the GRC electrode. *Electrochim. Acta*, **44** (21–22), 3809–3820.
136. Erdogdu, G., Mark, H.B., and Karagoezler, E. (1996) Voltammetric resolution of ascorbic acid and dopamine at conducting polymer electrodes. *Anal. Lett.*, **29** (2), 221–231.
137. Sun, Y., Ye, B., Zhang, W., and Zhou, X. (1998) Simultaneous determination of dopamine and ascorbic acid at poly(neutral red) modified electrodes. *Anal. Chim. Acta*, **363** (1), 75–80.
138. Ates, M., Sarac, A.S., Turhan, C.M., and Ayaz, N.E. (2009) Polycarbazole modified carbon fiber microelectrode: surface characterization and dopamine sensor. *Fiber Polym.*, **10** (1), 46–52.
139. Sarac, A.S., Dogru, E., Ates, M., and Parlak, E.A. (2006) Electrochemical synthesis of N-methylpyrrole and N-methylcarbazole copolymer on carbon fiber microelectrodes, and their characterization. *Turk. J. Chem.*, **30**, 401.
140. Young, S., Balluz, L., and Malilay, J. (2004) Natural and technologic hazardous material releases during and after natural disasters: a review. *Sci. Total Environ.*, **322** (1–3), 3–20.
141. Wang, H., Wang, J., Choi, D., Tang, Z.W., Wu, H., and Lin, Y.H. (2009) EQCM immunoassay for phosphorylated acetylcholinesterase as a biomarker for organophosphate exposures based on selective zirconia adsorption and enzyme-catalytic precipitation. *Biosens. Bioelectron.*, **24** (8), 2377–2383.
142. Scott, G., Fulton, M., Moore, D., Wirth, E., Chandler, G., Key, P., Daugomah, J., Strozier, E., Devane, J., Clark, J., Lewis, M., Finley, D., Ellenberg, W., and Karnaky, K. (1999) Assessment of risk reduction strategies for the management of agricultural nonpoint source pesticide runoff in estuarine ecosystems. *Toxicol. Ind. Health*, **15** (1–2), 200–213.
143. Frenich, A.G., Gonzalez-Rodrıguez, M.J., Arrebola, F.J., and Martınez Vidal, J.L. (2005) Potentiality of gas chromatography-triple quadrupole-mass spectrometry in vanguard and

rearguard methods of pesticide residues in vegetables. *Anal. Chem.*, **77** (14), 4640–4648.

144. Cappielo, A., Famiglini, G., Palma, P., and Mangani, F. (2002) Trace level determination of organophosphorus pesticides in water with the new direct-electron ionization LC/MS interface. *Anal. Chem.*, **74** (14), 3547–3554.

145. Ganzera, M., Aberham, A., and Stuppner, H. (2006) Development and validation of an HPLC/UV/MS method for simultaneous determination of 18 preservatives in grapefruit seed extract. *J. Agric. Food Chem.*, **54** (11), 3768–3772.

146. Du, D., Chen, S.Z., Cai, J., and Song, D. (2007) Comparison of drug sensitivity using acetylcholinesterase biosensor based on nanoparticleschitosan sol–gel composite. *J. Electroanal. Chem.*, **611** (1–2), 60–66.

147. Du, D., Ye, X., Cai, J., Liu, J., and Zhang, A. (2010) Acetylcholinesterase biosensor design based on carbon nanotube-encapsulated polypyrrole and polyaniline copolymer for amperometric detection of organophosphates. *Biosens. Bioelectron.*, **25**, 2503–2508.

148. Reynolds, J.R., Baker, C.K., Jolly, C.A., Poropatic, P.A., and Ruiz, J.P. (1989) *Conductive Polymers and Plastics* (ed. J.M, Margolis), Chapman & Hall, New York, pp. 1–40.

149. Stejskal, J. and Gilbert, R.G. (2002) Polyaniline, preparation of a conducting polymer. *Pure Appl. Chem.*, **74**, 857–867.

150. Chiang, J.C. and MacDiarmid, A.G. (1986) 'Polyaniline': protonic acid doping of the emeraldine form to the metallic regime. *Synth. Met.*, **13**, 193–205.

151. MacDiarmid, A.G., Yang, L.S., Huang, W.S., and Humphrey, B.D. (1987) Polyaniline: electrochemistry and application to rechargeable batteries. *Synth. Met.*, **18**, 393–398.

152. McCall, R.P., Ginder, J.M., Leng, J.M., Coplin, K.A., Ye, H.J., Epstein, A.J., Asturias, G.E., Manohar, S.K., Masters, J.G., Scherr, E.M., Sun, Y., and MacDiarmid, A.G. (1991) Photoinduced absorption and erasable optical information storage in polyanilines. *Synth. Met.*, **41**, 1329–1332.

153. Trivedi, D.C. and Dhawan, S.K. (1993) Shielding of electromagnetic interference using polyaniline. *Synth. Met.*, **59**, 267–272.

154. Makeiff, D.A. and Huber, T. (2006) Microwave absorption by polyaniline–carbon nanotube composites. *Synth. Met.*, **156**, 497–505.

155. Dutta, D., Sarma, T.K., Chowdhury, D., and Chattopadhyay, A. (2005) A polyaniline-containing filter paper that acts as a sensor, acid, base, and endpoint indicator and also filters acids and bases. *J. Colloid Interface Sci.*, **283**, 153–159.

156. Drelinkiewicz, A., Waksmundzka-Góra, A., Sobczak, J.W., and Stejskal, J. (2007) Hydrogenation of 2-ethyl-9, 10-anthraquinone on Pd-polyaniline(SiO_2) composite catalyst: the effect of humidity. *Appl. Catal., A*, **333**, 219–228.

157. Zhao, C., Xing, S., Yu, Y., Zhang, W., and Wang, C. (2007) A novel all-plastic diode based upon pure polyaniline material. *Microelectron. J.*, **38**, 316–320.

158. Willner, I., Willner, B., and Katz, E. (2007) Biomolecule–nanoparticle hybrid systems for bioelectronic applications. *Bioelectrochemistry*, **70**, 2–11.

159. Blinova, N.V., Stejskal, J., Trchová, M., Ćirić-Marjanović, G., and Sapurina, I. (2007) Polymerization of aniline on polyaniline membranes. *J. Phys. Chem. B*, **111**, 2440–2448.

160. Sun, L.-J., Liu, X.-X., Lau, K.K.-T., Chen, L., and Gu, W.-M. (2008) Electrodeposited hybrid films of polyaniline and manganese oxide in nanofibrous structures for electrochemical supercapacitor. *Electrochim. Acta*, **53**, 3036–3042.

161. Bessière, A., Duhamel, C., Badot, J.-C., Lucas, V., and Certiat, M.-C. (2004) Study and optimization of a flexible electrochromic device based on polyaniline. *Electrochim. Acta*, **49**, 2051–2055.

162. Halvorson, C., Cao, Y., Moses, D., and Heeger, A.J. (1993) Third order nonlinear optical susceptibility of polyaniline. *Synth. Met.*, **57**, 3941–3944.

163. Wang, H.L., MacDiarmid, A.G., Wang, Y.Z., Gebier, D.D., and Epstein, A.J. (1996) Application of polyaniline (emeraldine base, EB) in polymer light-emitting devices. *Synth. Met.*, **78**, 33–37.
164. Kaneto, K., Kaneko, M., Min, Y., and MacDiarmid, A.G. (1995) 'Artificial muscle': electromechanical actuators using polyaniline films. *Synth. Met.*, **71**, 2211–2212.
165. Soto-Oviedo, M.A., Araújo, O.A., Faez, R., Rezende, M.C., and De Paoli, M.-A. (2006) Antistatic coating and electromagnetic shielding properties of a hybrid material based on polyaniline/organoclaynanocomposite and EPDM rubber. *Synth. Met.*, **156**, 1249–1255.
166. Kalendová, A., Veselý, D., and Stejskal, J. (2008) Organic coatings containing polyaniline and inorganic pigments as corrosion inhibitors. *Prog. Org. Coat.*, **62**, 105–116.
167. Stejskal, J., Kratochvíl, P., and Jenkins, A.D. (1996) The formation of polyaniline and the nature of its structures. *Polymer*, **37**, 367–369.
168. Armes, S.P. (1998) Colloidal dispersions of conducting polymers, in *Handbook of Conducting Polymers*, 2nd edn (eds T.A. Skotheim, R.L. Elsenbaumer, and J.R. Reynolds), Marcel Dekker, New York.
169. Stejskal, J. (2001) Colloidal dispersions of conducting polymers. *J. Polym. Mater.*, **18**, 225–258.
170. Virji, S., Huang, J., Kaner, R.B., and Weiller, B.H. (2004) Polyaniline nanofiber gas sensors: examination of response mechanisms. *Nano Lett.*, **4** (3), 491–496.
171. Huang, J. (2006) Syntheses and applications of conducting polymer polyaniline nanofibers. *Pure Appl. Chem.*, **78**, 15–28.
172. Zhang, D. and Wang, Y. (2006) Synthesis and applications of one-dimensional nano-structured polyaniline: an overview. *Mater. Sci. Eng., B*, **134**, 9–19.
173. Bhadra, S., Khastgir, D., Singha, N.K., and Lee, J.H. (2009) Progress in preparation, processing and applications of polyaniline. *Prog. Polym. Sci.*, **34**, 783–810.
174. Wan, M. (2009) Some issues related to polyaniline micro-/nanostructures. *Macromol. Rapid Commun.*, **30**, 963–975.
175. Liu, P. and Zhang, L. (2009) Hollow nanostructured polyaniline: preparation, properties and applications. *Crit. Rev. Solid State Mater. Sci.*, **34**, 75–87.
176. Rajesh , Ahuja, T., and Kumar, D. (2009) Recent progress in the development of nano-structured conducting polymers/nanocomposites for sensor applications. *Sens. Actuators, B*, **136**, 275–286.
177. Huang, J., Virji, S., Weiller, B.H., and Kaner, R.B. (2003) Polyanilinenanofibers: facile synthesis and chemical sensors. *J. Am. Chem. Soc.*, **125**, 314–315.
178. Li, D., Huang, J., and Kaner, R.B. (2009) Polyaniline nanofibers: a unique polymer nanostructure for versatile applications. *Acc. Chem. Res.*, **42**, 135–145.
179. Virji, S., Fowler, J.D., Baker, C.O., Huang, J., Kaner, R.B., and Weiller, B.H. (2005) Polyaniline nanofiber composites with metal salts: chemical sensors for hydrogen sulfide. *Small*, **1**, 624–627.
180. Virji, S., Kojima, R., Fowler, J.D., Kaner, R.B., and Weiller, B.H. (2009) Polyaniline nanofiber-metal salt composite materials for arsine detection. *Chem. Mater.*, **21**, 3056–3061.
181. Virji, S., Kaner, R.B., and Weiller, B.H. (2006) Hydrogen sensors based on conductivity changes inn polyaniline nanofibers. *J. Phys. Chem. B*, **110**, 22266–22270.
182. Sadek, A.Z., Wlodarski, W., Kalantar-Zadeh, K., Baker, C., and Kaner, R.B. (2007) Doped and dedoped polyaniline nanofiber based conductometric hydrogen gas sensors. *Sens. Actuators, A*, **139**, 53–57.
183. Yu, X., Li, Y., and Kalantar-zadeh, K. (2009) Synthesis and electrochemical properties of template-based polyaniline nanowires and template-free nanofibril arrays: two potential

nanostructures for gas sensors. *Sens. Actuators, B*, **136**, 1–7.

184. Atashbar, M.Z., Sadek, A.Z., Wlodarski, W., Sriram, S., Bhaskaran, M., Cheng, C.J., Kaner, R.B., and Kalantar-zadeh, K. (2009) Layered SAW gas sensor based on CSA synthesized polyaniline nanofiber on AlN on 64YX LiNbO3for H_2 sensing. *Sens. Actuators, B*, **138**, 85–89.
185. Arsat, R., Yu, X.F., Li, Y.X., Wlodarski, W., and Kalantar-zadeh, K. (2009) Hydrogen gas sensor based on highly ordered polyaniline nanofibers. *Sens. Actuators, B*, **137**, 529–532.
186. Fowler, J.D., Virji, S., Kaner, R.B., and Weiller, B.H. (2009) Hydrogen detection by polyaniline nanofibers on gold and platinum electrodes. *J. Phys. Chem. C*, **113**, 6444–6449.
187. Yan, X.B., Han, Z.J., Yang, Y., and Tay, B.K. (2007) NO2gas sensing with polyaniline nanofibers synthesized by a facile aqueous/organic interfacial polymerization. *Sens. Actuators, B*, **123**, 107–113.
188. Tiwari, A., Kumar, R., Prabaharan, M., Pandey, R.R., Kumari, P., Chaturvedi, A., and Mishra, A.K. (2010) Nanofibrous polyaniline thin film prepared by plasma induced polymerization technique for detection of NO_2gas. *Polym. Adv. Technol.*, **21** (9), 615–620.
189. Virji, S., Kojima, R., Fowler, J.D., Villanueva, J.G., Kaner, R.B., and Weiller, B.H. (2009) Polyaniline nanofiber composites with amines: novel materials for phosgene detection. *Nano Res.*, **2**, 135–142.
190. Sutar, D.S., Padma, N., Aswal, D.K., Deshpande, S.K., Gupta, S.K., and Yakhmi, J.V. (2007) Preparation of nanofibrous polyaniline films and their application as ammonia gas sensor. *Sens. Actuators, B*, **128**, 286–292.
191. Manigandan, S., Jain, A., Majumder, S., Ganguly, S., and Kargupta, K. (2008) Formation of nanorods and nanoparticles of polyaniline using Langmuir Blodgett technique: performance study for ammonia sensor. *Sens. Actuators, B*, **133**, 187–194.
192. Jiang, S., Chen, J., Tang, J., Jin, E., Kong, L., Zhang, W., and Wang, C. (2009) Au nanoparticlesfunctionalized two dimensional patterned conducting PANI nanobowl monolayer for gas sensor. *Sens. Actuators, B*, **140**, 520–524.
193. Gao, Y., Li, X., Gong, J., Fan, B., Su, Z., and Qu, L. (2008) Polyaniline nanotubes prepared using fiber mats membrane as the template and their gas-response behavior. *J. Phys. Chem. C*, **112**, 8215–8222.
194. Gao, Y., Yao, S., Gong, J., and Qu, L. (2007) Preparation of polyaniline nanotubes via 'thin glass tubes template' approach and its gas response. *Macromol. Rapid Commun.*, **28**, 286–291.
195. Pinto, N.J., Ramos, I., Rojas, R., Wang, P.-C., and Johnson, A.T. Jr., (2008) Electric response of isolated electrospun polyaniline nanofibers to vapors of aliphatic alcohols. *Sens. Actuators, B*, **129**, 621–627.
196. Wang, F., Wang, W., Liu, B., Wang, Z., and Zhang, Z. (2009) Copolypeptide-doped polyaniline nanofibers for electrochemical detection of ultratrace trinitrotoluene. *Talanta*, **79**, 376–382.
197. Li, W., Hoa, N.D., Cho, Y., Kim, D., and Kim, J.-S. (2009) Nanofibers of conducting polyaniline for aromatic organic compound sensor. *Sens. Actuators, B*, **143**, 132–138.
198. Zhao, M., Wu, X., and Cai, C. (2009) Polyaniline nanofibers: synthesis, characterization, and application to direct electron transfer of glucose oxidase. *J. Phys. Chem. C*, **113**, 4987–4996.
199. Horng, Y.Y., Hsu, Y.K., Ganguly, A., Chen, C.C., Chen, L.-C., and Chen, K.-H. (2009) Direct-growth of polyaniline nanowires for enzyme-immobilization and glucose detection. *Electrochem. Commun.*, **11**, 850–853.
200. Xu, L., Zhu, Y., Tang, L., Yang, X., and Li, C. (2008) Dendrimer-encapsulated Pt nanoparticles/polyaniline nanofibers for glucose detection. *J. Appl. Polym. Sci.*, **109**, 1802–1807.
201. Xian, Y., Hu, Y., Liu, F., Xian, Y., Wang, H., and Jin, L. (2006) Glucose biosensor based on Au nanoparticles–conductive polyaniline nanocomposite. *Biosens. Bioelectron.*, **21**, 1996–2000.

202. Wang, Z., Liu, S., Wu, P., and Cai, C. (2009) Detection of glucose based on direct electron transfer reaction of glucose oxidase immobilized on highly ordered polyaniline nanotubes. *Anal. Chem.*, **81**, 1638–1645.

203. Aussawasathien, D., Dong, J.-H., and Dai, L. (2005) Electrospun polymer nanofiber sensors. *Synth. Met.*, **154**, 37–40.

204. Luo, X., Vidal, G.D., Killard, A.J., Morrin, A., and Smyth, M.R. (2007) Nanocauliflowers: a nanostructured polyaniline-modified screen-printed electrode with a self-assembled polystyrene template and its application in an amperometric enzyme biosensor. *Electroanalysis*, **19**, 876–883.

205. Wang, X., Yang, T., Feng, Y., Jiao, K., and Li, G. (2009) A novel hydrogen peroxide biosensor based on the synergistic effect of gold-platinum alloy nanoparticles/polyaniline nanotube/chitosan nanocomposite membrane. *Electroanalysis*, **21**, 819–825.

206. Du, Z., Li, C., Li, L., Zhang, M., Xu, S., and Wang, T. (2009) Simple fabrication of a sensitive hydrogen peroxide biosensor using enzymes immobilized in processable polyaniline nanofibers/chitosan film. *Mater. Sci. Eng., C*, **29**, 1794–1797.

207. Dhand, C., Singh, S.P., Arya, S.K., Datta, M., and Malhotra, B.D. (2007) Cholesterol biosensor based on electrophoretically deposited conducting polymer film derived from nano-structured polyaniline colloidal suspension. *Anal. Chim. Acta*, **602**, 244–251.

208. Dhand, C., Solanki, P.R., Sood, K.N., Datta, M., and Malhotra, B.D. (2009) Polyaniline nanotubes for impedimetric triglyceride detection. *Electrochem. Commun.*, **11**, 1482–1486.

209. Zhu, N., Chang, Z., He, P., and Fang, Y. (2006) Electrochemically fabricated polyaniline nanowire-modified electrode for voltammetric detection of DNA hybridization. *Electrochim. Acta*, **51**, 3758–3762.

210. Yang, T., Zhou, N., Zhang, Y., Zhang, W., Jiao, K., and Li, G. (2009) Synergistically improved sensitivity for the detection of specific DNA sequences using polyaniline nanofibers and multiwalled carbon nanotubes composites. *Biosens. Bioelectron.*, **24**, 2165–2170.

211. Zhou, N., Yang, T., Jiang, C., Du, M., and Jiao, K. (2009) Highly sensitive electrochemical impedance spectroscopic detection of DNA hybridization based on Aunano–CNT/PANnano films. *Talanta*, **77**, 1021–1026.

212. Peng, H., Zhang, L., Kilmartin, P.A., Zujovic, Z., Soeller, C., and Travas-Sejdic, J. (2009) Quantum dots and nanostructured conducting polymers for biosensing applications. *Int. J. Nanotechnol.*, **6**, 418–430.

213. Zhang, L., Peng, H., Kilmartin, P.A., Soeller, C., and Travas-Sejdic, J. (2007) Polymeric acid doped polyaniline nanotubes for oligonucleotide sensors. *Electroanalysis*, **19**, 870–875.

214. Peng, H., Zhang, L., Soeller, C., and Travas-Sejdic, J. (2009) Conducting polymers for electrochemical DNA sensing. *Biomaterials*, **30**, 2132–2148.

215. Chang, H., Yuan, Y., Shi, N., and Guan, Y. (2007) Electrochemical DNA biosensor based on conducting polyaniline nanotube array. *Anal. Chem.*, **79**, 5111–5115.

216. Feng, Y., Yang, T., Zhang, W., Jiang, C., and Jiao, K. (2008) Enhanced sensitivity for deoxyribonucleic acid electrochemical impedance sensor: gold nanoparticle/polyaniline nanotube membranes. *Anal. Chim. Acta*, **616**, 144–151.

217. Fan, Y., Chen, X., Trigg, A.D., Tung, C.-H., Kong, J., and Gao, Z. (2007) Detection of microRNAs using target-guided formation of conducting polymer nanowires in nanogaps. *J. Am. Chem. Soc.*, **129**, 5437–5443.

218. Langer, K., Barczyński, P., Baksalary, K., Filipiak, M., Golczak, S., and Langer, J.J. (2007) A fast and sensitive continuous flow nanobiodetector based on polyaniline nanofibrils. *Microchim. Acta*, **159**, 201–206.

219. Pal, S., Alocilja, E.C., and Downes, F.P. (2007) Nanowire labeled direct-charge

transfer biosensor for detecting Bacillus species. *Biosens. Bioelectron.*, **22**, 2329–2336.

220. Langer, J.J., Langer, K., Barczyński, P., Warchoł, J., and Bartkowiak, K.H. (2009) New 'ON-OFF'-type nanobiodetector. *Biosens. Bioelectron.*, **24**, 2947–2949.
221. Medeiros, E.S., Gregório, R., Martinez, R.A., and Mattoso, L.H.C. (2009) A taste sensor array based on polyaniline nanofibers for orange juice quality assessment. *Sens. Lett.*, **7**, 24–30.
222. Langer, J.J. and Golczak, S. (2007) Highly carbonized polyaniline micro- and nanotubes. *Polym. Degrad. Stab.*, **92**, 330–334.
223. Jimison, L.H. *et al.* (2012) Measurement of barrier tissue integrity with an organic electrochemical transistor. *Adv. Mater.*, **24**, 5919–5923.
224. Farquhar, M.G. and Palade, G.E. (1963) Junctional complexes in various epithelia. *J. Cell Biol.*, **17**, 375–412.
225. Artursson, P., Palm, K., and Luthman, K. (2001) Caco-2 monolayers in experimental and theoretical predictions of drug transport. *Adv. Drug Delivery Rev.*, **46**, 27–43.
226. Bernards, D.A. and Malliaras, G.G. (2007) Steady-state and transient behavior of organic electrochemical transistors. *Adv. Funct. Mater.*, **17**, 3538–3544.
227. Ivanov, A.I., Nusrat, A., and Parkos, C.A. (2004) Endocytosis of epithelial apical junctional proteins by a clathrin-mediated pathway into a unique storage compartment. *Mol. Biol. Cell*, **15**, 176–188.
228. Knipp, G.T., Ho, N.F.H., Barsuhn, C.L., and Borchardt, R.T. (1997) Paracellular diffusion in Caco- 2 cell monolayers: effect of perturbation on the transport of hydrophilic compounds that vary in charge and size. *J. Pharm. Sci.*, **86**, 1105–1110.
229. Otero, T.F. and Sansihena, J.M. (1997) Bilayer dimensions and movement in artificial muscles. *Bioelectrochem. Bioenerg.*, **42**, 117–122.
230. Otero, T.F. and Cortes, M.T. (2003) A sensing muscle. *Sens. Actuators, B*, **96**, 152–156.
231. Gandhi, M.R., Murray, P., Spinks, G.M., and Wallace, G.G. (1995) Mechanism of electromechanical actuation in polypyrrole. *Synth. Met.*, **73**, 247–256.
232. Spinks, G.M., Campbell, T.E., and Wallace, G.G. (2005) Force generation from polypyrroleactuators. *Smart Mater. Struct.*, **14**, 406–412.
233. Spinks, G.M., Xi, B., Troung, V.T., and Wallace, G.G. (2005) Actuation behavior of layered composites of polyaniline, carbon nanotubes and polypyrrole. *Synth. Met.*, **151**, 85–91.
234. Baughman, R.H., Shacklette, R.L., Elsenbaumer, R.L., Plichta, E.J., and Becht, C. (1990) in *Conjugated Polymeric Materials: Opportunities in Electronics, Optoelectronics, and Molecular Electronics*, NATO ASI Series E, vol. **182** (eds J.L. Brédas and R.R. Chance), Applied Science, Mons, pp. 559–582.
235. Pei, Q.B. and Inganläs, O. (1992) Conjugated polymers and the bending cantilever method: electrical muscles and smart devices. *Adv. Mater.*, **4**, 277–278.
236. Otero, T.F. and Cortes, M.T. (2003) Artificial muscles with tactile sensitivity. *Adv. Mater.*, **15**, 279–282.
237. Adeloju, S.B., Shaw, S.J., and Wallace, G.G. (1997) Pulsed-amperometric detection of urea in blood samples on a conducting polypyrrole-urease biosensor. *Anal. Chim. Acta*, **341**, 155–160.
238. Reinhard, C.S., Radomsky, M.L., Saltzman, W.M., Hilton, J., and Brem, H. (1683) Polymeric controlled release of dexamethasone in normal rat brain. *J. Controlled Release*, **1991**, 331–339.
239. Subramanian, A., Krishnan, U., and Sethuraman, S. (2009) Development of biomaterial scaffold for nerve tissue engineering: biomaterial mediated neural regeneration. *J. Biomed. Sci.*, **16**, 108–118.
240. Ravichandran, R., Sundarrajan, S., Venugopal, J.R., Mukherjee, S., and Ramakrishna, S. (2010) Applications of conducting polymers and their issues in biomedical engineering. *J. R. Soc. Interface*, **7**, S559–S579.

241. Prabhakaran, M.P., Ghasemi-Mobarakeh, L., and Ramakrishna, S. (2011) Electrospun composite nanofibers for tissue regeneration. *J. Nanosci. Nanotechnol.*, **11**, 3039–3057.
242. Mawad, D., Stewart, E., Officer, D.L., Romeo, T., Wagner, P., Wagner, K., and Wallace, G.G. (2012) A single component conducting polymer hydrogel as a scaffold for tissue engineering. *Adv. Funct. Mater.*, **22**, 2692–2699.
243. Ateh, D.D., Navsaria, H.A., and Vadgama, P. (2006) Polypyrrole-based conducting polymers and interactions with biological tissues. *J. R. Soc. Interface*, **3**, 741–752.
244. Perez-Madrigal, M.M., Armelin, E., Del Valle, L.J., Estrany, F., and Aleman, C. (2012) Bioactive and electroactive response of flexible polythiophene:polyester nanomembranes for tissue engineering. *Polym. Chem.*, **3**, 979–991.
245. Lu, Y., Li, Y., Pan, J., Wei, P., Liu, N., Wu, B., Cheng, J., Lu, C., and Wang, L. (2012) Poly(3,4-ethylenedioxythiophene)/poly(styrenesulfonate)-poly(vinyl alcohol)/poly(acrylic acid) interpenetrating polymer networks for improving optrode-neural tissue interface in optogenetics. *Biomaterials*, **33**, 378–394.
246. Collins, G., Federici, J., Imura, Y., and Catalani, L.H. (2012) Charge generation, charge transport, and residual charge in the electrospinning of polymers: a review of issues and complications. *J. Appl. Phys.*, **111**, 044701–044718.
247. Armelin, E., Gomes, A.L., Perez-Madrigal, M.M., Puiggali, J., Franco, L., Valle, L.J.D., Rodriguez-Galan, A., Campos, J.S.D.C., Ferrer-Anglada, N., and Aleman, C. (2012) Biodegradable freestanding nanomembranes of conducting polymer: polyester blends as bioactive platforms for tissue engineering. *J. Mater. Chem.*, **22**, 585–594.
248. Jang, J. and Oh, J.H. (2004) A facile synthesis of polypyrrole nanotubes using a template-mediated vapour deposition polymerization and the conversion to carbon nanotubes. *Chem. Commun.*, **10** (7), 882–883.
249. Lee, J.Y., Bashur, C.A., Goldstein, A.S., and Schmidt, C.E. (2009) Polypyrrole-coated electrospun PLGA nanofibers for neural tissue applications. *Biomaterials*, **30**, 4325–4335.
250. Schmidt, C.E., Shastri, V.R., Vacanti, J.P., and Langer, R. (1997) Stimulation of neurite outgrowth using an electrically conducting polymer. *Proc. Natl. Acad. Sci. U.S.A.*, **94**, 8948–8953.
251. Williams, R.L. and Doherty, P.J. (1994) A preliminary assessment of poly (pyrrole) in nerve guide studies. *J. Mater. Sci. Mater. Med.*, **5**, 429–433.
252. Abidian, M.R., Corey, J.M., Kipke, D.R., and Martin, D.C. (2010) Conducting-polymer nanotubes improve electrical properties, mechanical adhesion, neural attachment, and neurite outgrowth of neural electrodes. *Small*, **6**, 421–429.
253. Bartlett, P.N. and Whitaker, R.G. (1988) Modified electrode surface in amperometricbiosensors. *Med. Biol. Eng. Comput.*, **28**, 10–17.
254. Xie, J., Macewan, M.R., Willerth, S.M., Li, X., Moran, D.W., Sakiyama-Elbert, S.E., and Xia, Y. (2009) Conductive core-sheath nanofibers and their potential application in neural tissue engineering. *Adv. Funct. Mater.*, **19**, 2312–2318.
255. Broda, C.R., Lee, J.Y., Sirivisoot, S., Schmidt, C.E., and Harrison, B.S. (2011) A chemically polymerized electrically conducting composite of polypyrrole nanoparticles and polyurethane for tissue engineering. *J. Biomed. Mater. Res. Part A*, **98A**, 509–516.
256. Thompson, B.C., Moulton, S.E., Richardson, R.T., and Wallace, G.G. (2011) Effect of the dopant anion in polypyrrole on nerve growth and release of a neurotrophic protein. *Biomaterials*, **32**, 3822–3831.
257. Sekine, J., Luo, S.C., Wang, S., Zhu, B., Tseng, H.R., and Yu, H.H. (2011) Functionalized conducting polymer nanodots for enhanced cell capturing: the synergistic effect of capture agents

and nanostructures. *Adv. Mater.*, **23**, 4788–4792.

258. Kim, H.S., Hobbs, H.L., Wang, L., Rutten, M.J., and Wamser, C.C. (2009) Biocompatible composites of polyaniline nanofibers and collagen. *Synth. Met.*, **159**, 1313–1318.

259. Bettinger, C.J., Bruggeman, J.P., Misra, A., Borenstein, J.P., and Langer, R. (2009) Biocompatibility of biodegradable semiconducting melanin films for nerve tissue engineering. *Biomaterials*, **30**, 3050–3057.

260. Rachocki, A., Pogorzelec-Glaser, K., Pawlaczyk, C., and Tritt-Goc, J. (2011) Morphology, molecular dynamics and electric conductivity of carbohydrate polymer filmbased on alginic acid and benzimidazole. *Carbohydr. Res.*, **346**, 2718–2726.

261. Guo, Y., Li, M.Y., Mylonakis, A., Han, J.J., MacDiarmid, A.G., Chen, X.S., Lelkes, P.I., and Wei, Y. (2007) Electroactive oligoaniline-containing self-assembled monolayers for tissue engineering applications. *Biomacromolecules*, **8**, 3025–3034.

262. Aufan, M.R., Sumi, Y., Kim, S., and Lee, J.Y. (2015) Facile synthesis of conductive polypyrrole wrinkle topographies on polydimethylsiloxane via a swelling–deswelling process and their potential uses in tissue engineering. *ACS Appl. Mater. Interfaces*, **7**, 23454–23463.

263. Kang, G., Borgens, R.B., and Cho, Y. (2011) Well-ordered porous conductive polypyrrole as a new platformfor neural interfaces. *Langmuir*, **27**, 6179–6184.

264. De Ruiter, G.C.W., Malessy, M.J.A., Yaszemski, M.J., Windebank, A.J., and Spinner, R.J. (2009) Designing ideal conduits for peripheral nerve repair. *J. Neurosurg.*, **26**, 1–9.

265. Huang, L., Hu, J., Lang, L., Wang, X., Zhang, P., Jing, X., Wang, X., Chen, X., Lelkes, P.I., Macdiarmid, A.G., and Wei, Y. (2007) Synthesis and characterization of electroactive and biodegradable ABA block copolymer of polylactide and aniline pentamer. *Biomaterials*, **28**, 1741–1751.

266. Schmidt, C.E. and Rivers, T.J. (2004) Biodegradable, electrically conducting polymer for tissue engineering applications. US Patent 6, 696, 575.

267. Wang, S., Lu, L., Gruetzmacher, J.A., Currier, B.L., and Yaszemski, M.J. (2006) Synthesis and characterizations of biodegradable and crosslinkable poly(epsilon-caprolactonefumarate), poly(ethylene glycol fumarate), and their amphiphilic copolymer. *Biomaterials*, **27**, 832–841.

268. Runge, M.B., Dadsetan, M., Baltrusaitis, J., Knight, A.M., Ruesink, T., Lazcano, E., Lu, L., Windebank, A.J., and Yaszemsk, M.J. (2010) The development of electrically conductive polycaprolactone fumarate-polypyrrole composite materials for nerve regeneration. *Biomaterials*, **31**, 5916–5926.

269. Abbari, E., Wang, S., Lu, L., Gruetzmacher, J.A., Ameenuddin, S., Hefferan, T.E., Currier, B.L., Windebank, A.J., and Yaszemski, M.J. (2005) Synthesis, material properties, and biocompatibilityof a novel self-cross-linkable poly(caprolactone fumarate) as an injectable tissue engineering scaffold. *Biomacromolecules*, **6**, 2503–2511.

270. Durgam, H., Sapp, S., Deister, C., Khaing, Z., Chang, E., Luebben, S., and Schmidt, C.E. (2010) Novel degradable copolymers of polypyrrole support cell proliferation and enhance neurite out-growth with electrical stimulation. *J. Biomater. Sci., Polym. Ed.*, **21**, 1265–1282.

271. Wang, Y.Z., Kim, H.J., Vunjak-Novakovic, G., and Kaplan, D.L. (2006) Stem cell-based tissue engineering with silk biomaterials. *Biomaterials*, **27**, 6064–6082.

272. Yang, Y., Chen, X., Ding, F., Zhang, P., Liu, J., and Gu, X. (2007) Biocompatibility evaluation of silk fibroin with peripheral nerve tissues and cells *in vitro*. *Biomaterials*, **28**, 1643–1652.

273. Aznar-Cervantes, S., Roca, M.I., Martinez, J.G., Meseguer-Olmo, L., Cenis, J.L., Moraleda, J.M., and Otero, T.F. (2012) Fabrication of conductive electrospun silk fibroin scaffolds by

coating with polypyrrole for biomedical applications. *Biochemistry*, **85**, 36–43.
274. Sirringhaus, H., Brown, P.J., Friend, R.H., Nielsen, M.M., Bechgaard, K., Langeveld-Voss, B.M.W., Spiering, A.J.H., Janssen, R.A.J., and Meijer, E.W. (2000) Microstructure–mobility correlation in self-organised, conjugated polymer field-effect transistors. *Synth. Met.*, **111–112**, 129–132.
275. Subramanian, A., Krishnan, U.M., and Sethuraman, S. (2012) Axially aligned electrically conducting biodegradable nanofibers for neural regeneration. *J. Mater. Sci. - Mater. Med.*, **23**, 1797–1809.
276. Zimmermann, W.H., Fink, C., Kralish, D., Remmers, U., Weil, J., and Eschenhagen, T. (2000) Three-dimensional engineered heart tissue from neonatal rat cardiac myocytes. *Biotechnol. Bioeng.*, **68**, 106–114.
277. Zimmermann, W.H. *et al.* (2002) Cardiac grafting of engineered heart tissue in syngenic rats. *Circulation*, **106**, I151–I157.
278. Li, M., Guo, Y., Wei, Y., MacDiarmid, A.G., and Lelkes, P.I. (2006) Electrospinning polyaniline-contained gelatin nanofibers for tissue engineering applications. *Biomaterials*, **27**, 2705–2715.
279. Campbell, T.E., Hodgson, A.J., and Wallace, G.G. (1999) Incorporation of erythrocytes into polypyrrole to form the basis of a biosensor to screen for Rhesus (D) blood groups and rhesus (D) antibodies. *Electroanalysis*, **11**, 215–222.
280. Richardson-Burns, S.M., Hendricks, J.L., Brian, F., Povlich, L.K., Dong-Hwan, K., and Martin, D.C. (2007) Polymerization of the conducting polymer poly (3, 4- ethylenedioxythiophene) (PEDOT) around living neural cells. *Biomaterials*, **28**, 1539–1552.
281. Meng-yan, L. *et al.* (2007) Electroactive and nanostructured polymers as scaffold materials for neuonal and cardiac tissue engineering. *Chin. J. Polym. Sci.*, **25**, 331–339.
282. Kai, D., Prabhakaran, M.P., Jin, G., and Ramakrishna, S. (2011) Polypyrrole-contained electrospun conductive nanofibrous membranes for cardiac tissue engineering. *J. Biomed. Mater. Res. Part A*, **99**, 376–385.
283. Kuruvilla, A. and Flink, R. (2003) Intraoperative electrocorticography in epilepsy surgery: useful or not? *Seizure*, **12**, 577–584.
284. Schalk, G., McFarland, D.J., Hinterberger, T., Birbaumer, N., and Wolpaw, J.R. (2004) BCI2000: a general-purpose, brain-computer interface (BCI) system. *IEEE Trans. Biomed. Eng.*, **51**, 1034–1043.
285. Kim, D.H. *et al.* (2010) Dissolvable films of silk fibroin for ultrathin conformal bio-integrated electronics. *Nat. Mater.*, **9**, 511–517.
286. Khodagholy, D. *et al.* (2011) Highly conformable conducting polymer electrodes for *in vivo* recordings. *Adv. Mater.*, **23**, 268–272.
287. Chagnac-Amitai, Y. and Connors, B.W. (1989) Horizontal spread of synchronized activity in neocortex and its control by GABA-mediated inhibition. *J. Neurophysiol.*, **61**, 747–758.
288. McKeon, K.D., Lewis, A., and Freeman, J. (2010) Electrospunpoly(D, L-Lactide) and polyaniline scaffold characterization. *J. Appl. Polym. Sci.*, **115**, 1566–1572.
289. Borriello, A., Guarino, V., Schiavo, L., Alvarez-Perez, M.A., and Ambrosio, L. (2011) Optimizing PANi doped electroactive substrates as patches for the regeneration of cardiac muscle. *Mater. Sci. Eng., C*, **22**, 1053–1062.
290. Gizdavic-Nikolaidis, M., Ray, S., Bennett, J.R., Easteal, A.J., and Cooney, R.P. (2010) Electrospun functionalized polyaniline copolymer-based nanofibers with potential application in tissue engineering. *Macromol. Biosci.*, **10**, 1424–1431.
291. Tiwari, A., Sharma, Y., Hattori, S., Terada, D., Sharma, A.K., Turner, A.P.F., and Kobayashi, H. (2013) Influence of poly(N-isopropylacrylamide)-CNT-polyaniline three dimensional electrospun microfabric scaffolds on cell growth and viability. *Biopolymers*, **99**, 334–341.
292. Sharma, Y., Tiwari, A., Hattori, S., Terada, D., Sharma, A.K., Ramalingan,

M., and Kobayashi, H. (2012) Fabrication of conducting electrospun nanofibers scaffold for three-dimensional cells culture. *Int. J. Biol. Macromol.*, **51**, 627–631.

293. Jin, L., Wang, T., Feng, Z.-Q., Zhu, M., Leach, M.K., Naim, Y.I., and Jiang, Q. (2012) Fabrication and characterization of a novel polypyrrole fibrous scaffold designed for 3D cell culture. *J. Mater. Chem.*, **22**, 18321–18326.

294. Razal, J., Kita, M., Quigley, A.F., Kennedy, E., Moulton, S.E., Kapsa, R.M.I., Clark, G.M., and Wallace, G.G. (2009) Wet-spun biodegradable fibers on conducting platforms: novel architectures for muscle regeneration. *Adv. Funct. Mater.*, **19**, 3381–3388.

295. Quigley, A.F., Razal, J.M., Thompson, B.C., Moulton, S.E., Kita, M., Kennedy, E.L., Clark, G.M., Wallace, G.G., and Lapsa, R.M.I. (2009) A conducting-polymer platform with biodegradable fibers for stimulation and guidance of axonal growth. *Adv. Mater.*, **21**, 4393–4397.

296. Yu, M., Huang, Y., Ballweg, J., Shin, H., Huang, M., Savage, D.E., Lagally, M.G., Dent, E.W., Blick, R.H., and Williams, J.C. (2011) Semiconductor nanomembrane tubes: three-dimensional confinement for controlled neurite outgrowth. *ACS Nano*, **5**, 2447–2457.

4
Plasma-Assisted Fabrication and Processing of Biomaterials

Kateryna Bazaka, Daniel S. Grant, Surjith Alancherry, and Mohan V. Jacob

4.1
Introduction

Plasma creates a highly reactive chemical environment that can be used to selectively induce specific biological responses, fabricate materials with a wide range of physico-chemical, mechanical, and biological properties, and modify surfaces in a highly controlled manner. In this chapter, we will first briefly review how plasma is used for sterilization and disease management. We will then focus on the use of plasma environments for surface functionalization and fabrication of carbon-based structures, from soft polymers to amorphous carbons and carbon nanotubes.

The suitability of materials for use within a biological environment is a function of both their mechanical characteristics and their surface properties [1–3]. Historically, major emphasis has been placed on selecting materials with the most favorable mechanical properties and chemical inertness. However, as our understanding of the interplay between living cells and abiotic surfaces grows, current practices have progressed beyond merely favoring inert surfaces, to employing techniques that enable the controlled development of surface morphology and chemistry [4–9]. As a result, the typical approach for the development of devices that are to be exposed to some biological medium is to select materials possessing the requisite bulk mechanical properties (e.g., strength, density, wear resistance, machinability), and to then employ surface modification techniques to control interactions between the material's surface and constituent components of the biological medium [10].

Surface characteristics such as roughness, specific chemistry, hydrophilicity, surface charge, surface energy, and surface reactivity play a significant role in mediating biocompatibility factors relating to protein adsorption, cell adhesion, immunological responses, and surface-tissue integration [11, 12]. There exists a wide range of methods that can be employed to modify a surface, including self-assembly, imprinting, pulsed laser processing, chemical etching, mechanical polishing, and many others. The selection of a specific technique is dependent

Biomedical Applications of Polymeric Materials and Composites, First Edition.
Edited by Raju Francis and Sakthi Kumar.

on the type of the material being processed (e.g., metallic, ceramic, or polymeric), and the desired outcome (e.g., altering surface chemistry, topography, or hardness).

It must be noted that while most surface-modification techniques aim to alter surface chemistry as the dominant factor in regulating interactions between a material's surface and the biological medium in which it exists, other factors such as surface architecture and roughness should also be considered when engineering a surface for biotechnology applications [13]. Furthermore, consideration must be given to the surface properties of the biological bodies that the material is expected to interact with, and the environmental conditions (e.g., pH, biomolecule concentration, and presence or absence of micro-organisms) of the application site where the interaction is to occur [6, 14, 15].

The process of introducing atoms or molecules with known chemical behavior (i.e., functional groups) to the surface of a given material is known as surface functionalization, and, given the inherently inert nature of many presently used biomaterials, is of particular importance in biotechnology applications [10]. These inert surfaces elicit nonspecific protein adhesion immediately upon exposure to a biological system, and in the case of medical implants, this nonspecific protein adhesion often induces foreign body reactions such as prolonged inflammation at the surface–medium interface, and the formation of collagenous fibrous tissue that encapsulates the device [4, 16].

The principal role of surface functionalization in biotechnology is to effect selective immobilization of biogenic substances (e.g., proteins, peptides, and polysaccharides) at the material's surface [14]. This immobilization is often best achieved via covalent bonding, which presents several advantages over other less stable immobilization mechanisms such as electrostatic interactions and ligand–receptor pairing. Advantages include an extended half-life of attached biogenic substances, and a capacity to inhibit both their metabolism and migration, all of which permit continued bioactivity of in-dwelling implants [10].

Selective immobilization of biogenic substances ultimately regulates interactions between the material's surface and the biological medium, with many far-reaching implications of technological significance. From a medical perspective, it prospectively permits surface engineering that can bring about a moderated foreign-body response, and selectivity in cell adhesion and proliferation (including an ability to inhibit bacterial adhesion and subsequent biofilm development and tissue overgrowth) [17]. This ability to control the interplay between material surfaces and biological mediums has led to the adoption of surface functionalization techniques in a number of fields, including: drug delivery, biosensors, medical implants and instruments, and industrial environments (where it has been employed to control bacterial adhesion and subsequent biofilm formation that promotes bioinduced corrosion of piping and other metal work) [4, 18, 19].

The desirability of specific surface-functionalization techniques employed to achieve selective biogenic substance immobilization may be assessed on two fronts. First, and most importantly for the performance of the device in question, factors relating to the process outputs must be considered. This includes an analysis of variations in bulk material properties (which are typically sought to be kept to a minimum), as well as the selectivity, amount, and distribution of attached functional groups. If a number of techniques can be employed to achieve comparably equivalent functionalization performance, then practical factors relating to the process itself must be taken into consideration. To this end, elements relating to technique cost, material wastage, environmental effects, reproducibility, and production rates must be analyzed [20, 21].

In this chapter, we will focus on plasma-enabled processing as a highly versatile tool for selective modification of a wide range of implantable materials, including temperature-sensitive polymeric materials and living tissues. By varying processing conditions, a wide range of outcomes can be attained, including highly controlled micro- and nanostructuring of the surface (e.g., via etching and deposition), alterations to surface chemistry, including homogenous and heterogeneous functionalization with functional chemistries and surface chemical gradients (e.g., via surface activation), and enhancing mechanical properties of the surface layer (via cross-linking). Furthermore, plasma-enhanced fabrication enables controlled synthesis of a wide range of nanomaterials that can be either directly grown on the surface of the material or deposited on the catalyst support and then used in material fabrication (bulk and surface).

4.1.1 Plasma in Medicine

Plasma-assisted technologies have found numerous applications in medicine, materials science, and biotechnology. In medicine, thermal plasmas have long been used to cut, ablate, and cauterize tissues by means of heating. On the other hand, low-temperature, nonequilibrium plasmas produce minimum heating, and thus can be applied to materials and tissues to induce a highly specific response. Clinically, low-temperature plasma can be used for sterilization and decontamination, wound healing, blood coagulation, and cancer treatment.

4.1.2 Plasma Sterilization

Low-temperature plasma can be used to effectively kill pathogens residing on surfaces of medically relevant materials and devices, in liquids, and on living tissues. Furthermore, plasma can be used to clean the surface of proteins, pyrogens, peptides, and other microorganism-related biomolecules without damaging the substrate. It can also be used to effectively deactivate and remove bacterial spores, making it highly suited for decontamination and sterilization of biomaterial surfaces [22, 23]. Exposing pure water to a carrier gas in an electrical discharge produces an acidic solution, a so-called plasma acid, which can be used for biological decontamination for several days. The pH of such a solution can be controlled by changing the carrier gas; for example, using the gliding arc plasmatron, solutions with a lower pH were obtained with air as the carrier gas than with oxygen [24].

Resistive barrier discharge plasmas have been demonstrated to be effective on *Escherichia coli*, *Pseudomonas fluorescens* (5RL), methicillin-resistant *Staphylococcus aureus*, spores, and bacteriophages [25]. In addition to medically relevant bacteria, atmospheric pressure plasma was demonstrated to rapidly and completely eradicate biofilms of four biofouling marine bacterial species on polystyrene and stainless steel surfaces [26]. The kill rate and physical removal of biofilms were controlled by regulating the process parameters, such as air flow [25].

In terms of plasma device set up, low-pressure systems, for example, a double inductively coupled plasma or a very high frequency capacitively coupled plasma, are best used for laboratory inactivation of spores and germs, whereas atmospheric-pressure plasmas, for example, dielectric barrier discharge, are better suited for wound and skin sterilization [27]. Wavelength-dependent photo sterilization efficiency is observed for double inductively coupled plasma, where irradiation below 235 nm effectively kills *Aspergillus brasiliensis* spores, whereas irradiation between 235 and 300 nm is required for deactivation of *Bacillus atrophaeus* spores [27].

Treatment of bleeding rat wounds contaminated with high concentrations of *S. aureus* for 1 min resulted in a 3-log reduction in bacteria cell numbers [28]. In humans, treatment of wounds using MicroPlaSter alpha and MicroPlaSter beta plasma devices resulted in a significant reduction in bacterial load, regardless of the species of bacteria [29]. Treatment was safe, with no side-effects observed in the treated patients. Similar results were reported for the decontamination of fingertips of healthy volunteers as a means of hands hygiene [30]. Although in this study dielectric barrier discharge plasma was shown to be more effective at reducing the bacterial load than low-temperature atmospheric pressure plasma jets, both types of plasma treatments were effective and well tolerated by the patients. Histology and electron microscopy examination of healthy *ex vivo* human skin samples subjected to plasma treatment using FlatPlaSter 2.0 and MiniFlatPlaSter showed the treatment to be tolerable up to 2 min, with no DNA damage [31].

The antimicrobial activity of plasma is closely associated with reactive oxygen species (ROS) and reactive nitrogen species (RNS) that are generated in medically relevant plasmas [32]. These species play a key role in oxidation–reduction biochemistry, a critical process in the biology of aerobic organisms. ROS and RNS are also intimately involved in the immune reactions, with recent findings pointing to their key role in the antimicrobial and antiparasite activity of medical agents [32]. Indeed, recent reports have suggested that classic antibiotics kill bacteria by stimulating the formation of ROS [33, 34] although this finding remains a subject of debate [35, 36]. In addition to ROS, RNS and other reactive species, neutral species, electric fields, charges, and photons generated in nonequilibrium plasmas also contribute to the antimicrobial activities of these plasmas [32, 37].

The process of plasma-induced killing of bacteria is not fully elucidated [38]. Bacterial cells, as well as cells of most living organisms, are coated by a liquid film. Therefore, it is likely that plasma species may interact with this film before they reach the surface of the cell itself. Computational studies have shown that

ROS, such as OH, HO_2, and H_2O_2 can travel deep into the liquid layer and reach the bioorganism. At the same time, O, OH, and HO_2 radicals can react with water molecules through hydrogen-abstraction reactions (H-reaction), whereas no H-abstraction reaction occurs for H_2O_2 [39]. Furthermore, it is important to consider that a wound is not a homogenous environment, but rather a morphologically complex surface, potentially complete with dirt, oil, blood, and other contaminants [40, 41]. These complexities may affect the depth of penetration, and thereby the effectiveness of the reactive species generated in the plasma.

4.1.3
Plasma Treatment of Cells

In addition to wound sterilization, low-temperature (at or below physiological level) plasmas can be used to suppress inflammation and encourage healing [42, 43]. Tissue-tolerable plasma has been investigated for treatment of inflammatory diseases, such as psoriasis, where plasma treatment was also found to temporarily reduce the bacterial colonization on skin lesions [44]. Plasma treatment of inflamed tissues in ulcerative colitis disease suppressed the progression of the disease while no damage to colon tissues was observed [45].

Immune system cells, such as monocytes and $CD4^+$, $CD8^+$, B, NK, NKT, T_H17, and $\gamma\delta$ T cells, regulate immune responses and modulate inflammation in all types of tissues. Plasma treatment of these cells for 5–60 s resulted in a notably reduced cell viability that varied with the cell type, with lymphocyte-type cells showing significantly lower survival rates compared to monocytes [46]. It is likely that different types of immune cells possess inherently different coping mechanisms to mitigate plasma cytotoxicity.

Exposure of primary human immune cells to plasma induces oxidative stress, significantly oxidizing glutathione and thus changing cellular redox balance [47]. This change leads to mitochondrial oxidation and reduced mitochondrial membrane potential, thus inducing apoptosis [47].

Depending on the dose, plasma treatment of eukaryotic cells can induce either proliferation or apoptosis, with the effect attributed to the extent of formation of intracellular ROS within the cell. Plasma-generated active neutral species may induce the formation of organic peroxides in cell medium, thus facilitating DNA damage, replication arrest, or formation of single-stranded DNA breaks [48]. However, plasma was not found to lead to the formation of bulky adducts/thymine dimers. Exposure of blood samples to the plasma jet for 40–80 s yielded significant incremental differences in micronuclei, IL-1β, and TNF-α, whereas shorter exposure times (i.e., 20 s) did not lead to these changes [49].

Given that different cell types respond differently to plasma-generated species and radiation, selective biomanipulation of cells can be achieved. In addition to affecting cell proliferation, plasma treatment can be used to control local cell adhesion without inducing necrosis. Similarly, plasmas can be used for displacement of cells from the substrate by inducing apoptosis [48, 50]. Atmospheric plasmas alter cell migration rates as a function of plasma treatment time and localization of the treatment zone [51]. Cancer cells can be selectively targeted [52, 53]. For instance, treatment of glioblastoma brain tumor cells and normal astrocytes with plasma-activated medium resulted in selective killing of glioblastoma cells, manifested by morphological changes and reduced size consistent with apoptosis. The killing mechanism involved plasma-induced downregulation of expression of AKT kinase, the survival signals in cancers. Such selectivity in a co-culture may be used for safe anticancer therapy [54–56]. Plasma treatment of prostate cancer primary cells derived from patient tumor tissue exacted irreversible DNA damage [57].

The mechanisms of plasma effects on healthy cells need to be elucidated further. On exposing human keratinocyte cells to atmospheric pressure argon plasma induced changes of charges of several cell proteins, yet no fragmentation, degradation, or complexation of cell proteins was observed [58]. At the mRNA levels, such plasma treatment prompted an upregulation of vascular endothelial growth factor-a, heparin-binding epidermal growth factor, granulocyte macrophage colony-stimulating factor, prostaglandin-endoperoxide synthase 2 and interleukin-6 [59], promoting the synthesis and secretion of corresponding proteins. The release of these cytokines and growth factors may stimulate resolution of chronic wounds.

Plasma treatment of amino acids in aqueous solution resulted in hydroxylation and nitration of aromatic rings in tyrosine, phenylalanine, and tryptophan; sulfonation and disulfide linkage formation of thiol groups in cysteine; sulfoxidation of methionine; and amidation and ring opening of five-membered rings in histidine and proline [60]. Plasma treatment was also found to preferentially decrease sulfur-containing and aromatic amino acids. Plasma interactions with L-alanine caused the decrease in the $-CH_3$ bond, $>C(NH_2)COOH$ bond, and $-COOH$ bond peaks of the main component [61]. Degradation increased with ion energy and dose, and photon energy, with energy over 6 eV sufficient to degrade this amino acid. In terms of the relative importance of different plasma-generated effects, argon plasma ions were found to be the most significant, followed by UV photons, and metastable radicals [62]. Results from the treatment with $Ar-O_2$ plasma suggest that surface etching dominates the chemical degradation process [62].

4.1.4 Plasma-Assisted Surface Modification

From a biomaterials perspective, plasma-assisted techniques are widely used for the long-lasting, highly controlled modification of a variety of medically relevant surfaces [63–65]. Over the past two decades, plasma-assisted nanoscale synthesis and modification has developed into a sophisticated highly flexible process for the fabrication of a broad selection of pure and hybrid nanoscale objects spanning across a vast number of materials systems and length scales [66]. In terms of energy, material efficiency, and degree of organization, plasmas are equal or even superior to commonly used thermal, wet chemistry, or laser-assisted processing methods [66]. The plasma environment can be tailored to facilitate one-step synthesis of functional materials from natural precursors [67–73].

Numerous advantageous properties can be attributed to the use of plasma-assisted functionalization of biomaterial surfaces, as achieved via either plasma treatment or plasma polymerization. First and foremost, the ability to change plasma species energy and density by easily varying process parameters affords the surface engineer ample opportunity to develop new functionalization-related surface environments [74]. Importantly, this breadth of choice is also accompanied by a high degree of reproducibility in the achieved functional group type and coverage when a given system operates under identical conditions [75].

Plasma-assisted functionalization processes exhibit low substrate dependence and can, as such, be applied to virtually all materials commonly employed in biotechnology applications, including polymers such as poly(methyl methacrylate) (PMMA), polyurethane (PU), polytetrafluoroethylene (PTFE), polypropylene (PP), and poly(ethylene terephthalate) (PET) [10]. Vitally, only the top few nanometers of these materials are subjected to modification, and as such the polymers retain their bulk physical properties [76]. This process is also line-of-sight independent, and can as such accommodate the functionalization of three-dimensional geometries [77, 78]. This feature can be coupled with the fact that the process is highly scalable, and as such lends itself to the functionalization of micro- or nano-scaled artifacts, allowing it to cater to the prominent trend of miniaturizing the detail of biotechnology devices [5, 79].

The application of masking techniques to the substrate during either the plasma treatment or plasma polymerization process can facilitate spatial patterning of surface functionalities (i.e., form well-defined regions of functional groups, or conversely an absence of functional groups) [79, 80], or the formation of functional group gradients [81–83]. This surface patterning ability has been exploited by researchers such as Leclair *et al.* in order to micropattern glass substrates using plasma-deposited fluoropolymer thin films, resulting in single-cell positioning and neural circuit arrangements, as depicted in Figures 4.1 and 4.2 [84]. Gradients of a specific chemical moiety or several chemical groups across the surface can

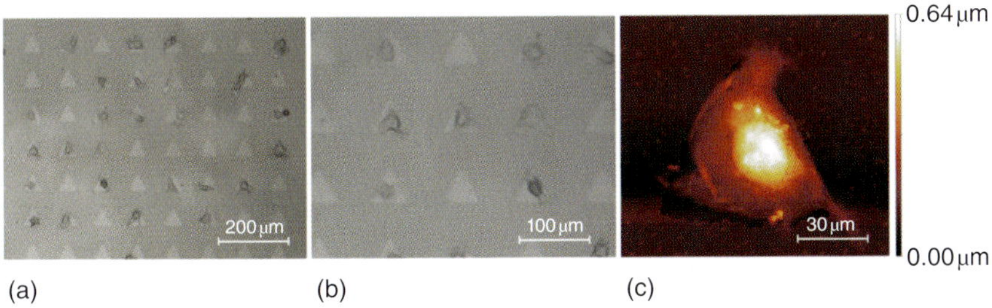

Figure 4.1 (a, b) Optical images of myoblast cells cultured on the single-cell patterning substrates. (c) AFM image of a single cell adopting the triangular shape of the pattern feature. (Leclair 2011 [84]. Reproduced with permission of Elsevier.)

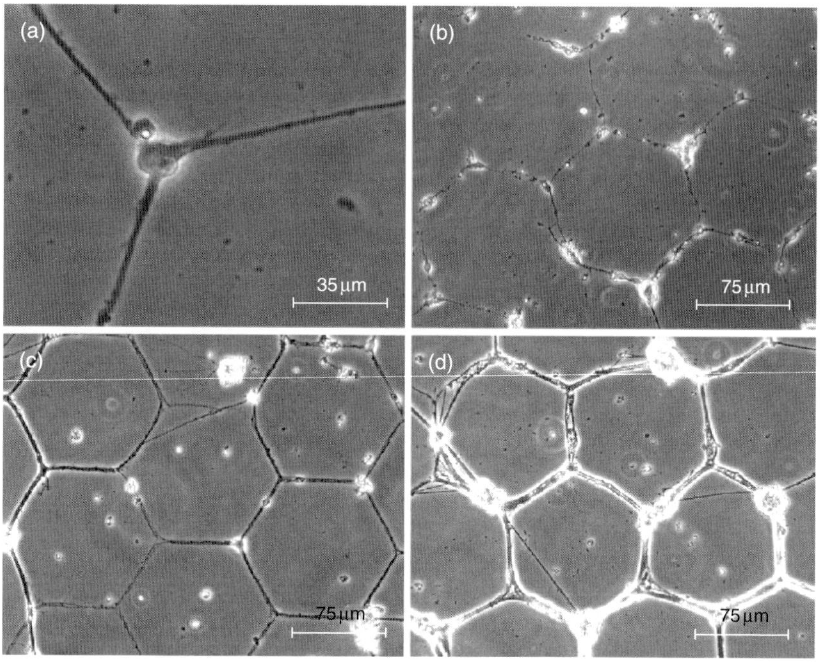

Figure 4.2 Optical images of live neurons cultured on the hexagonal grid pattern, after incubation times of (a, b) 4 days, (c) 7 days, and (d) 21 days. (Leclair 2011 [84]. Reproduced with permission of Elsevier.)

be employed to study cell–surface interactions, yielding a large number of data points per sample [85]. In a similar manner, morphological gradients can be employed to study the response of cells to various surface topographies.

Specific surface topographies can be achieved in a two-step process, where chemical functionalization is followed by time-dependent immersion of the substrate into a nanoparticle solution, where nanoparticles preferentially bind to the deposited chemistry [86]. The material is then coated with a thin polymer layer, resulting in a surface that displays a nanoparticle density gradient, yet is chemically homogeneous. The final coating step can be omitted, and instead biomolecules with a preferential attachment for the nanoparticles can be used to create a biomolecule gradient. Given that protein fouling is observed on most biomaterial surfaces, understanding the relationship between biomolecule density and cells can provide further insights into cell–surface dynamics.

Single-cell patterning achieved using plasma lithography technology (Figure 4.1a,b) may facilitate the controlled study of cell, cell-to-cell, and cell–material interactions, free from the interference generated by the bulk presence of cells [87–89]. Moreover, the demonstrated ability to moderate cell shape and spreading area (Figure 4.1c) also lends the process a prospective capacity for influencing cell migration [90, 91], differentiation [92], and proliferation [93].

By taking advantage of the cell's preferential adhesion to the glass substrate over that of the fluoropolymer thin film, the researchers were able to successfully fabricate live two-dimensional neural circuits cultured on patterned samples. These networks were strongly characterized by cell nuclei adhesion at the nodal locus' connecting glass channels (Figure 4.2a,b), and by subsequent neurite alignment and growth along the glass channels (Figure 4.2c,d). This plasma polymerization process used to fabricate neural networks with controlled morphology has numerous prospective applications, including that of neuron-based biosensors, which may be achieved by monitoring variations in neuron electrical activity in response to chemical influences in the culture environment [84].

Beyond patterning, the benefits associated with plasma techniques for accomplishing surface functionalization also extend to a preclusion of the need for certain biomaterial surface-cleaning and preparation techniques, which may by their very nature introduce contaminants onto the surface. This includes contaminants such as silicon and aluminum from grit blasting media, processing fluids (e.g., etchants and cleaning solvents), and residues from sterilization procedures (e.g., autoclaving or ethylene oxide) [94]. It also obviates the need to use other avenues for achieving surface functionalization, including the use of wet chemicals or photochemical treatment. These alternative techniques can be subject to a number of limitations, including high substrate dependence, difficulties in reproducibility, the production of hazardous chemical waste, and prospectively low functionalization yield and specificity [95–98].

Finally, it must be noted that plasma-based methods for achieving surface functionalization also impose a number of constraints upon the selection of bulk materials suitable for the process. The functionalization process is often (though by no means exclusively) undertaken at low pressure, and as such the polymeric material may need to exhibit stability while under vacuum at (or slightly above) room temperature [77, 78]. The vast majority of polymeric materials employed in biotechnology are more than capable of satisfying these process requirements.

4.1.5 Plasma Functionalization

Plasma treatment involves the use of nonpolymerizing gases (with frequently used gases including Ar, O_2, H_2, N_2, and NH_3) to produce a plasma state consisting of neutral atoms and molecules, positively and negatively charged atoms and molecules, electrons, and photons [99]. The plasma can be subjected to several modes of classification based upon its working pressure (e.g., low or high/atmospheric pressure), the method of transferring energy from the electric field to the plasma species (e.g., DC, RF capacitively coupled, and microwave discharge), and its thermal state (i.e., thermal equilibrium or nonequilibrium plasma).

Plasma treatment makes use of careful selection of the process gas and conditions to achieve controlled changes in surface chemistry and topology [100].

It can be applied to polymeric materials in order to enhance their cytocompatibility, hemocompatibility, and antibacterial properties. This enhancement is accomplished (notwithstanding the effects of nanostructuring) by the controlled introduction of specific functional groups (such as carboxyl, amine, and hydroxyl groups) onto the polymer's surface [14].

Surface functionalization is achieved by bombardment of the polymeric substrate with energetic species present within the plasma. Bombardment leads to the removal of contaminant surface species, the cleavage of covalent bonds on the substrate surface, and the subsequent development of unsaturations and free radicals. These surface free radicals establish covalent bonds with active plasma species and subsequently facilitate the adhesion of functional groups at the surface [101]. The specificity of these functional groups (i.e., the number of a specific type of functional group per 100 C atoms) can be controlled to some extent via intelligent selection of the process gas [100]. For example, oxygen or hydroxyl group functionalization can be achieved using O_2, H_2O, O_2/O_3, and O_2/H_2O_2 gases [102–104] amine groups can be introduced using N_2, N_2/H_2, and NH_3 gases [105, 106] and carboxyl groups such as COOH can be introduced using CO_2 [105, 107].

There exists an extensive compilation of publications exploring the interplay between plasma treated polymeric materials and cell interaction [17]. One representative example of these publications is the study conducted by Švorčík *et al.* [108] into the *in vitro* cytocompatibility of Ar plasma treated polyethylene [17]. This study focussed, in part, on the effects of Ar plasma treatment on polyethylene (PE), as determined by its influence on the adhesion and proliferation of rat vascular smooth muscle cells (VSMC), and mouse embryonic NIH 3T3 fibroblasts.

Here, the plasma treated PE exhibited markedly greater cell population density, attributable in part to plasma-induced surface oxidation, which promoted surface wettability and the subsequent uptake of adhesion supporting biomolecules. A comparison of the growth rates for both VSMC and NH 3T3 fibroblasts on pristine and plasma treated PE surfaces (Figure 4.3) clearly demonstrates superior cell

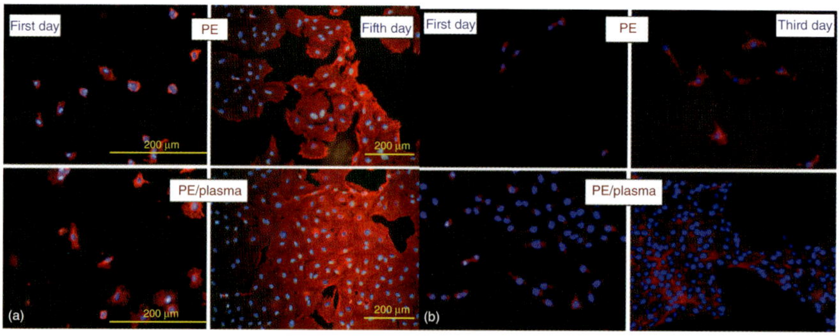

Figure 4.3 VSMC adhered (first day) and grown (fifth day) on pristine and plasma treated PE (a), and 3T3 adhered (first day) and grown (third day) on pristine and plasma treated PE (b). (Jacobs 2012 [17]. Reproduced with permission of Elsevier.)

adhesion and spreading on the plasma treated surfaces, leading to an enhanced state of proliferation for the cell types under consideration.

Plasma treatment may find preferential employment over plasma polymerization in situations where it would be inappropriate to apply a polymeric layer to the substrate, or when a higher degree of nonspecific hetero-functionalization of the surface is sought. In qualifying this latter point, it bears mentioning that while it is possible to use plasma treatment to produce highly homo-functionalized surfaces, doing so may require additional chemical reduction of the functional groups formed by the plasma [109].

4.1.6 Plasma-Enabled Synthesis of Polymers

Plasma polymerization differs from plasma treatment in that its process gas makes use of monomeric units containing specific functional groups, leading to the production of a functionalized polymer coating over the bulk substrate material. This method of surface functionalization finds preferential use over plasma treatment when a high degree of mono-functionalization is sought, or when a nonpolymeric substrate material (e.g., metal or ceramic) is to be used.

The properties of the polymer coating depend on the processing parameters, including fabrication power, pressure, properties of the monomer and carrier gas, flow rates, temperature of the substrate, and many others [110]. For protective coatings, highly cross-linked polymers are used. These coatings are fabricated at higher input power, resulting in a high degree of fragmentation and a significant loss of original chemical functionality. Where surface functionality is to be retained, low-temperature low-power plasmas are used. However, these conditions also result in coatings with inferior mechanical properties, stability, and adhesion to substrate, which may undermine the clinical usefulness of these coatings [111].

Selectivity of the functional groups to be retained in the plasma-deposited polymeric layer can be achieved via careful selection of the monomeric unit (e.g., allyl alcohol for OH groups, acrylic acid for COOH groups, and allylamine for NH_2 groups) [112]. At low power, the chemical structure of the monomer, such as the presence of unsaturation, is particularly important [113]. Polymerization of unsaturated monomers results in coatings with lower hardness, and higher solubility, and density compared to films produced from saturated monomers. The retention of the selected functional groups can then be accomplished by exercising control over a number of plasma parameters, with special emphasis on the plasma energy density, as indicated by the Yasuda factor: $\mathrm{YF} = W/MF$, where W = wattage in $\mathrm{J\,s^{-1}}$, M = monomer molecular weight in $\mathrm{kg\,mol^{-1}}$, and F = monomer flow rate in $\mathrm{mol\,s^{-1}}$ [114].

While retention of monomer functional groups during plasma polymerization is easier to achieve than retention of the entire monomer structure, it still stands that lowering the input power (i.e., operating at a lower Yasuda factor) suppresses monomer fragmentation [115], and leads to an increased retention of monomer functional groups within the deposited polymer layer [116, 117]. However, caution must be exercised when using a low energy density plasma, as it also leads to increased retention or entrapment of complete monomer and oligomer units throughout the deposited polymer layer. These entrapped species may, subsequently, lower the thermal stability of the deposited polymer layer as they evaporate at temperatures below 100 °C [116].

A complementary method for increasing functional group retention involves operating at a higher process pressure, resulting in a reduction in the electron mean-free-path and a subsequent decrease in electron temperature. In turn, this lower electron temperature leads to a decrease in monomer fragmentation, and an increase in the number of intact monomer units incorporated into the deposited layer. The extent of functional group retention may be prospectively calculated as $\varphi = [c_{\mathrm{fg}}\ M]_n \times c_{\mathrm{fg}}\ M$, where M = monomer molecular weight in kg mol^{-1}, n = number of monomer units, and c_{fg} = concentration of functional groups per monomer unit [116]. Efforts to limit the residence time of the monomer within the plasma and to avoid ionic bombardment may also lead to further preservation of the monomer structure within the plasma-polymerized film [118].

In addition to direct incorporation of functional groups at the surface during the plasma *on* state, polymer surfaces may also be functionalized by plasma-induced chemical radical graft polymerization. In this process, an inert gas (e.g., Ar or He) is used in the plasma *on* state to activate the surface as per the case for plasma treatment. Thereafter, the activated surface is exposed to unsaturated monomeric units, which subsequently graft to free radical sites at the surface [21]. This can be accomplished using any process that exposes the post-plasma activated surface to the monomer, or by processes employing on–off cycles (such as pulsed plasma techniques) [119].

The efficacy of plasma-induced grafting has been comprehensively demonstrated on a number of polymeric substrate materials [109, 120, 121]. Furthermore, the technique has the capacity to immobilize a variety of biogenic molecules and other functional structures [63, 122], and to enhance the properties of the biomaterial for a specific application [123]. For example, proteins, such as streptavidin can be covalently linked to aldehyde functionalities without losing their binding ability, or nonspecifically adsorbed to ethanol functionalities, leading to protein denaturation [124]. Xia *et al.* used surface modification of poly(L-lactic acid) (PLLA) to promote endothelialization [125]. In this study, PLLA was subjected to a three-step plasma process, consisting of (i) surface activation via Ar plasma treatment, (ii) carboxylic group surface functionalization via acrylic acid (AA) graft polymerization, and (iii) biomolecule immobilization via covalent bonding between the surface carboxylic groups and amine groups present on the selected biomolecules (viz., gelatin and chitosan). Human umbilical vein endothelial cells (HUVECs) were then grown on the pristine and surface-modified PLLA surfaces.

The effectiveness of this plasma-induced grafting process is demonstrated in Figure 4.4 by the preferential focal-adhesion and spreading of the endothelial

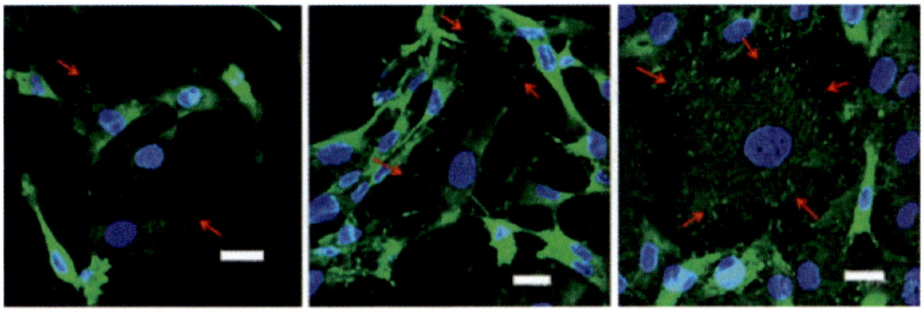

(a) (b) (c)

Figure 4.4 Surface dependent focal adhesion formation (denoted by arrows). Cells were seeded on (a) PLLA, (b) PLLA-gAA-chitosan, and (c) PLLA-gAA-gelatin at a seeding density of 10^4 cell cm^{-2} and cultured for 12 h. Scale = 20 μm. (Xia 2010 [125]. Reproduced with permission of Springer.)

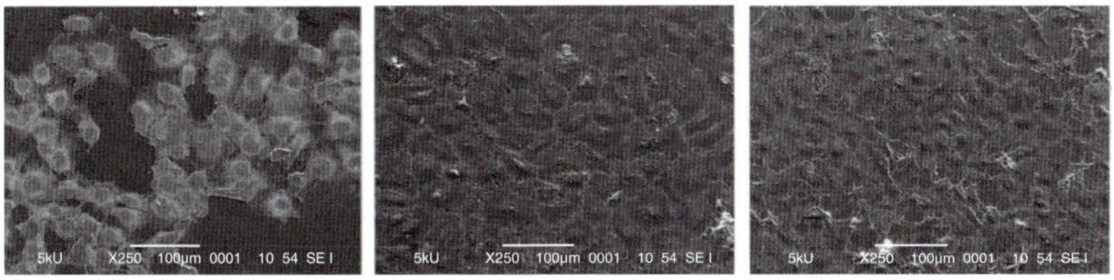

(a) (b) (c)

Figure 4.5 Cell morphology observed on (a) PLLA, (b) PLLA-gAA-gelatin, and (c) PLLA-gAA-chitosan by SEM at day 7. Complete endothelialization was observed on both modified PLLA substrates, but not on PLLA substrate. Scale = 100 μm. (Xia 2010 [125]. Reproduced with permission of Springer.)

cells on the PLLA samples with plasma grafting assisted immobilization of gelatin (b) and chitosan (c) biomolecules. These enhanced cell attributes (relative to those exhibited by the pristine PLLA surface) are then further complemented by the complete endothelialization of the plasma grafted surfaces, as presented in Figure 4.5.

Improved surface endothelialization achieved by plasma-based techniques such as those presented here may find prospective applications in blood-contacting devices, effectively masking the underlying polymeric biomaterial from platelets and fibrinogen present within the blood, and subsequently circumventing immunogenic complications [126, 127].

4.1.7 Plasma-Enhanced Fabrication of Amorphous and Graphene-Like Carbon

4.1.7.1 Plasma Polymerized Diamond-Like Carbon (DLC) Films

Diamond-like carbon (DLC) is a group of metastable carbon materials with a significant fraction of sp^3 carbon–carbon bonds. They exist as amorphous carbon (a-C) and hydrogenated amorphous carbon (a-C:H). The amorphous carbon is characterized by high sp^3 content (between 40% and 80%) whereas the hydrogenated form comprises predominantly sp^2 bonded carbon together with 20–30% hydrogen [128]. For decades, DLC has been considered as a technologically important material due to its outstanding properties such as extreme hardness, high chemical inertness, high wear and corrosion resistance, low coefficient of friction, transparency to IR light, and good biocompatibility. The properties of DLC thin films are highly dependent on the ratio of sp^3/sp^2 carbon bonds in their structure. In turn, the sp^3/sp^2 ratio is very sensitive to the deposition process and parameters.

DLC films can be prepared using a range of techniques, including plasma-enhanced chemical vapor deposition (PECVD), ion beam deposition, filtered cathodic vacuum arc, plasma immersion ion implantation, magnetron sputtering, ion beam sputtering, pulsed laser deposition, and mass selected ion beam deposition. Of these, plasma-based methods have gained considerable research attention in recent years [129–134]. A comparative experimental analysis of PECVD of a-C:H films using methane and acetylene as precursor gases showed that deposition rate, surface roughness, hardness, mass density, and hydrogen content were affected by both the choice of the precursor and deposition parameters.

4.1.7.2 DLC films as Hemocompatible Coatings

Hemocompatibilty is an essential prerequisite for implants, especially those that are in direct contact with blood such as prosthetic heart valves, blood pumps, stents, and other blood contacting devices. One of the major challenges faced by these implants is thrombus formation on the device's surface arising from the adsorption of plasma proteins and subsequent platelet adhesion when the device comes into contact with blood. The process of thrombus formation is closely related to the ratio of adsorbed albumin to fibrinogen (plasma proteins) on the implant surface. It is better to have a higher albumin to fibrinogen ratio as fibrinogen accelerates platelet adhesion whereas albumin prevents it. A number of *in vitro* and *in vivo* studies have confirmed the blood biocompatibility of DLC films [132, 135–137]. In general, the hemocompatibility of DLC films depends on wettability, surface composition, surface roughness, and surface charge [138]. Hasebe *et al.* studied the platelet adhesion and activation characteristics of PECVD DLC and fluorinated DLC (F-DLC) [139]. It was found that nano-order surface roughness (below 100 nm) had no obvious effect on nonthrombogenic properties of these films. Moreover, F-DLC has shown lower platelet adhesion than DLC for every grade of roughness.

Several studies have reported the improvement of hemocompatibility of DLC films by incorporating other elements [140–142]. Being amorphous in nature, the DLC structure is flexible to accommodate the doping element and shows properties dependent on the nature of the dopant and level of doping (Figure 4.6). It is observed that the doping element (X) preferentially substitutes sp^2 (C=C) hybridized carbon forming C–X bonds by keeping the sp^3 hybridized carbon

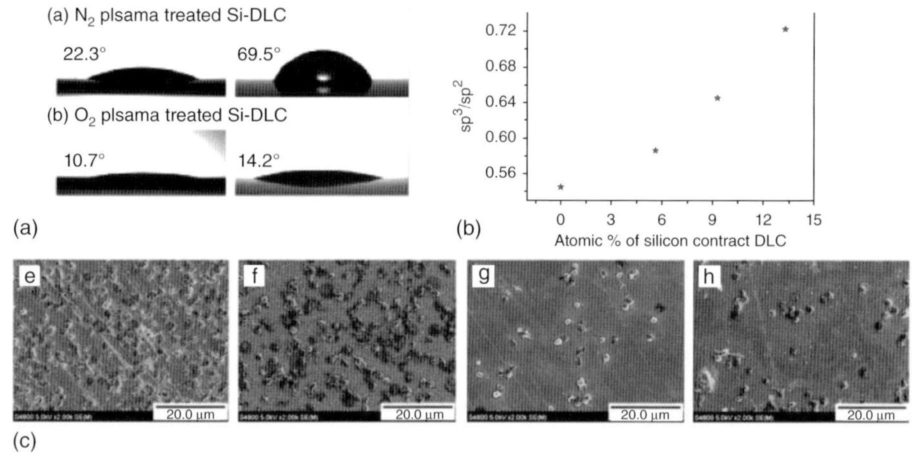

Figure 4.6 (A) Optical microscopic images of DI water droplets showing the difference of oxygen and nitrogen plasma treatment on maintaining the hydrophilic nature of Si-DLC surface. The oxygen treated surfaces exhibit prolonged wettability by showing consistent wetting angle measured for a period of 20 days, whereas nitrogen treated surface lost its hydrophilic nature. (Orlanda 2010 [143]. American Chemical Society.) (B) Variation of sp^3/sp^2 ratio with respect to silicon doping concentration in DLC film. (Ahmed 2013 [144]. Reproduced with permission of Elsevier.) (C) SEM images showing platelet adhesion on substrates coated with TIN, A-Si and F-DLC coatings. The adhered platelets are significantly reduced in F-DLC films (g and h) compared to others. (Chou 2013 [145]. Reproduced with permission of Elsevier.)

relatively unaltered. This will change the sp^3/sp^2 ratio, which in turn affects the properties of the film [144]. A detailed description of the various studies to enhance the blood biocompatibility of DLC films by doping with different elements is available in these review articles and references therein [141, 142, 146]. Recently, Ahmed *et al.* [147] prepared DLC and Si-DLC through radio frequency PECVD using acetylene as a source gas and tetramethylsilane as a dopant source. On comparing the adsorption of human serum albumin (HSA) on these films, the authors observed an increased adsorption of HSA on Si-DLC. In addition, the amount of HSA adsorbed on Si-DLC increased with the Si content. The sp^3/sp^2 ratio also increased with increase in Si concentration. Another couple of studies by the same authors about glycine adsorption on PECVD-deposited silicon and fluorine doped DLC film revealed that silicon and fluorine concentration could control the glycine adsorption rate on DLC surfaces. The DLC films with lower concentrations of silicon and fluorine, had a higher adsorption rate than films having higher concentration of these elements [148].

Chou *et al.* conducted hemolysis ratio and platelet covered area studies of fluorinated DLC films coated on titanium alloy through radio frequency PECVD. They showed that a higher concentration of fluorine in DLC films is not favorable to maintain hemocompatibility [145]. Ohgoe *et al.* [149] observed reduced hemolysis and improved hemolytic performance for fluorine doped DLC coatings prepared from C_6F_5H precursor gas. The fluorinated DLC dominated undoped DLC as well as bare surface (SU 304) by exhibiting a low friction coefficient and reduced surface energy, which resulted in improved hemolytic performance. Recently, Shiba *et al.* reported the hemocompatibility studies of radio frequency plasma polymerized DLC films on four different polymers to ascertain the applicability of microchannels for blood analyzing devices. The authors obtained a satisfactory result for DLC coated polydimethylsiloxane and cyclic olefin polymers [150].

Apart from doping, surface treatment of DLC films with appropriate plasma also enhances the blood compatibility [143, 151]. The plasma used for surface treatment has significant influence in deciding the end properties of DLC films. Plasma can modify the surface bonds, hydrophilicity, and surface charge of the DLC surface. Roy *et al.* reported the protein adsorption and blood coagulation time of Si-DLC films surface treated with O_2, N_2, and CF_4 plasma [151]. It was found that the plasma affects the polar component of surface energy and makes the surface hydrophilic or hydrophobic depending on the nature of the plasma used. Hydrophilic Si-DLC surfaces with reduced platelet adhesion and improved blood coagulation time were obtained for oxygen and nitrogen plasma surface treatment. On the other hand, CF_4 plasma made the surface hydrophobic with low hemocompatibility. The hydrophilicity of the surface is an important factor governing platelet adhesion as well as prolonged wettability. Yi *et al.* showed that long-lasting hydrophilic Si-DLC could be made by precisely controlling the Si concentration in the DLC film and subsequent oxygen surface treatment [152]. They prepared Si-DLC films with different Si concentrations (0–3.25 at.%) through radio frequency PECVD using benzene and a mixture of benzene and silane as the precursor gases. The Si-DLC films with Si concentration from 0.66 to 2.42 at.% maintained their hydrophilic nature up to 20 days and were suggested for applications like biocoatings for contact lenses where long-lasting wettability is needed.

4.1.7.3 DLC Films as Antibacterial Coatings

Bacterial adhesion, proliferation, and biofilm formation are another major concern for implantable devices, with the majority of implant failure and surgical removal occurring due to implant-associated infections and inflammation. DLC films have been considered as promising antibacterial coatings for implantable devices. The decisive parameters that control bacterial adhesion on DLC films are the structure, chemical bonds, surface roughness, surface charge, hydrophilicity, and hydrogen content. Marciano *et al.* reported the bactericidal properties of PECVD DLC films from a methane gas precursor [153]. The antibacterial property of 22% hydrogen containing films was evaluated against *E. coli*, *P. aeruginosa*, *Salmonella typhimurium*, and *S. aureus*. The antibacterial activity ranged from 25% to 55% depending on the bacterial species (Figure 4.7). The antibacterial effect of DLC films was attributed to the rupture of cell membranes from the direct contact of bacteria with nanocarbon aggregates on the DLC film.

Though DLC films exhibit antibacterial properties, the majority of the reported studies deal with doped DLC films since even better properties could be achieved

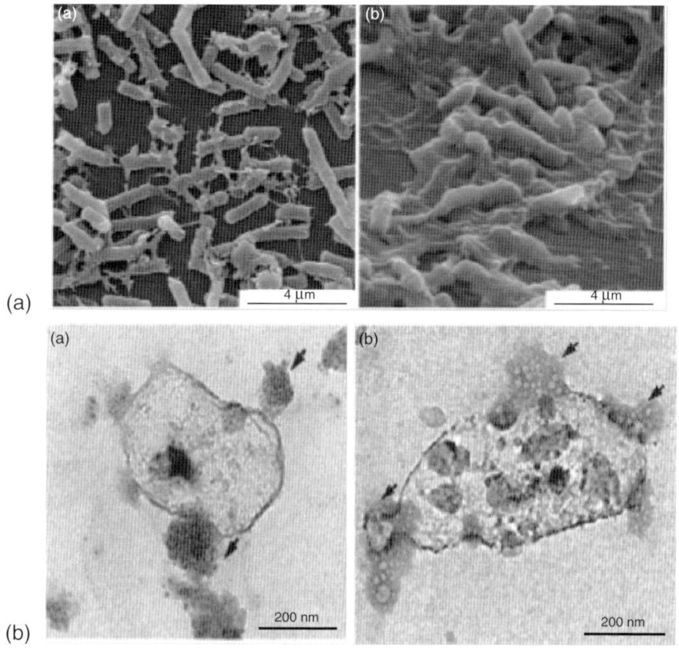

Figure 4.7 (A) The SEM images showing the antibacterial activity of DLC film against bacterium *E. coli* and *P. aeruginosa*. The bacterium tends to lose its shape with cytoplasmic projections indicating the rupturing of cell wall when bacteria come in contact with DLC films. (Marciano 2011 [153]. Reproduced with permission of Elsevier.) (B) The TEM images describing the antibacterial activity of Cu embedded nanostructured DLC film against bacterium *S. aureus* and *E. coli*. The cytoplasm leakage is clearly visible (arrow marked region) due to destruction of cell walls by Cu diffusion. The inset picture represents the adhered bacterium *S. aureus* (round morphology) and *E. coli* (tubular morphology) on glass substrate for the same incubation time. (Lee 2013 [154]. Reproduced with permission of Taylor and Francis.)

through doping. The activity of bacterium *Klebsiella pneumonia* on silicon and fluorine incorporated DLC films prepared through radio frequency PECVD on stainless steel substrates was reported by Ren *et al.* [155]. The F-DLC with 39.2% fluorine and Si-DLC with 19.2% silicon reduced the bacterial adhesion by 68% compared to the undoped film. The doped DLC films were characterized by low surface energy and low interaction energy between bacteria and film surface, which accounts for the better antibacterial properties.

Staphylococcal biofilm formation on DLC and F-DLC coated ultrahigh molecular weight polyethylene (UHMWPE) was investigated by Del-Prado *et al.* [156]. A marginal decrease in biofilm thickness and bacterial coverage was obtained for DLC-coated UHMWPE compared to the uncoated sample. A species-specific effect is also observed, with *S. aureus* being affected mainly by F-DLC, whereas *S. epidermidis* was affected by DLC coatings. An antibacterial nanostructured a-C:H/Cu composite was prepared by Lee *et al.* through a combined radio frequency

PECVD and magnetron sputtering system [154]. The a-C:H/Cu composite containing more than 27.8 at.% Cu displayed excellent antibacterial performance (>99.9%) against *S. aureus* and *E. coli* after incubation for 24 h. The authors also showed that the incorporated Cu particles could diffuse into the bacterial cell by destroying the cell wall and cell membrane and causing bacterial apoptosis. Similarly, Lan *et al.* [157] reported that silver containing DLC films were effective against *E. coli*. It was noticed that even the lowest Ag/C ratio (0.07) resulted in an activity of 93%, which increased to 98% upon increasing the Ag/C ratio to 0.25%. In this case, Ag^+ ions kill the bacteria by diffusing into the cytoplasm of the cell.

4.1.7.4 DLC Films as Corrosion Resistant and Low Wear Coatings

The use of orthopedic implants shows a dramatic increase every year. Unfortunately, surgical removal and replacement also increases. The major problems associated with orthopedic implants are implant-associated infections and loosening of joints due to wear and corrosion [142]. The mechanism of wear is complex, and is mainly related to the type of materials involved in joints, geometry, and implant surroundings. Metals, alloys, polymers, and ceramics have been used to fabricate different parts of prosthesis. These artificial joints are expected to be dynamic in the presence of body fluids containing corrosive elements, subjected to wear and tear and corrosion. The wear rates of metal/ceramic-on-polymer (UHMWPE), metal-on-metal, and ceramic-on-ceramic implants are estimated in the 5–30, 1–3, and 0.05 $mm^3\ year^{-1}$range respectively [142]. The debris particles released out of these joints may be cytotoxic and can cause inflammation of tissue surrounding the implant, which leads to device removal and replacement.

Since DLC coatings possess high hardness, wear resistance, chemical inertness, and a low friction coefficient, they are considered as an excellent material to engineer the surface properties of artificial joint components to overcome the aforementioned problems [142, 146, 158, 159]. One of the major advantages of DLC films in biological applications are their noncytotoxic nature. For instance, it was reported that delaminated DLC debris particles did not induce any inflammation or toxic reactions on bone marrow cell cultures, demonstrating excellent cell compatibility [146]. Another study, by Wang *et al.* [160] showed that ammonia surface treated radio frequency plasma polymerized DLC displayed better cytocompatibility to mouse MC3T3-E1 pre-osteoblasts than the untreated DLC films. As explained earlier, the DLC surface becomes hydrophilic by forming amine-terminated bonds after surface modification.

Mechanically, the DLC films showed hardness up to 90 GPa and extreme resilience. However, tribological behavior of DLC films depends on intrinsic as well as extrinsic factors. The friction values reported for DLC films span a range of 0.001–0.7 and normalized wear rate values as low as $10^{-11}\ mm^3\ N^{-1}\ m^{-1}$ [161]. It is postulated that the tribological performance of implant surfaces benefits from protein adsorption, whereby a protein layer acts as a natural lubricating layer to reduce wear rate [162, 163]. It is worth noting that DLC as well as alloyed DLC films act as good host surfaces to proteins and, therefore, serve as an ideal material for orthopedic implant coatings. Liu *et al.* [162] reported that the corrosion resistance and wear rate of DLC coated CoCrMo alloy was improved by adsorption of protein when subjected to bovine calf serum. As discussed in the previous section, doping of DLC could control the protein adsorption as it changes the surface characteristics. Another study by Escudeiro *et al.* [163] observed that incorporation of zirconium ion into DLC film enhances the protein adsorption characteristics and showed better wear properties. The surface was characterized by the reduced surface energy.

The tribological performance of DLC coatings for orthopedic replacements is usually analyzed *in vitro* using pin on disc tests, hip simulators, or spine and knee simulator analysis. Liu *et al.* [162] studied the tribocorrosion behavior of filtered cathodic vacuum arc derived DLC, coated on CaCrMo alloy in a simulated biological environment (i.e., in the presence of 50 vol% bovine calf serum and 0.9% NaCl solution) by using a ball-on-disk reciprocating tribometer and three electrode electrochemical cell. The testing was performed at 1 N normal load, 0.5 Hz sliding frequency, 6 mm stroke length, and with an estimated contact pressure of 800 MPa. Under sliding conditions, the DLC coated alloy showed better corrosion resistance, smaller friction force, and a lower wear rate than the bare alloy. A pin-on-disc simulation test with an applied normal force of 1 N, linear speed 20 cm s^{-1}, and 10 000 cycles performed by Escudeiro *et al.* [163] on zirconium incorporated DLC films revealed that Zr-DLC films exhibited a significant reduction in the wear rate of the titanium alloy counter-body. On comparing the corrosion, tribological performance, and impact fatigue behavior of plasma derived DLC and TIN coatings on 316L stainless steel, Wang *et al.* [164] observed that DLC has no impact fatigue after 10^4 cycles, with 700 N impact and 700 N static loads, whereas TIN showed impact fatigue under these conditions (Figure 4.8). In addition, DLC coatings exhibited stable tribological behavior under a simulated body environment, with an average coefficient of friction of ~0.35 measured using a pin-on-disc experimental set-up. Moreover, DLC coatings exhibited a higher corrosion resistance by showing highest polarization corrosion resistance R_p (1543 kΩ cm^2) and lower corrosion current I_{corr} (0.055 μA cm^{-2}) than TIN and bare stainless steel.

Though a number of wear studies have been reported using the above-mentioned simulations, the results are incomparable due to inconsistencies in choosing experimental parameters such as load, contact pressure, number of cycles, speed, testing environment, and counter-surface [142]. Only a handful of literature is available that describes the simulations as per ASTM or ISO standard procedures. Recently, Thorwarth *et al.* [165] reported a simplified spinal simulation with reference to ASTM-F 2423-05 performed on radio frequency PECVD DLC layers on biomedical $CoCr_{28}Mo_6$ alloy. It is worth mentioning that DLC coated CCM articulations detected little or no noticeable wear after 101 million cycles of testing. Franta *et al.* [166] studied the tribocorrosion behavior of DLC coated and uncoated titanium alloy using a hinge-type knee prosthesis wear test according to the ISO standard for knee joint prosthesis. Interestingly, the coated implant did not show any contact damage and exhibited good tribological performance with significant improvement in implant lifetime. A hinge-type knee

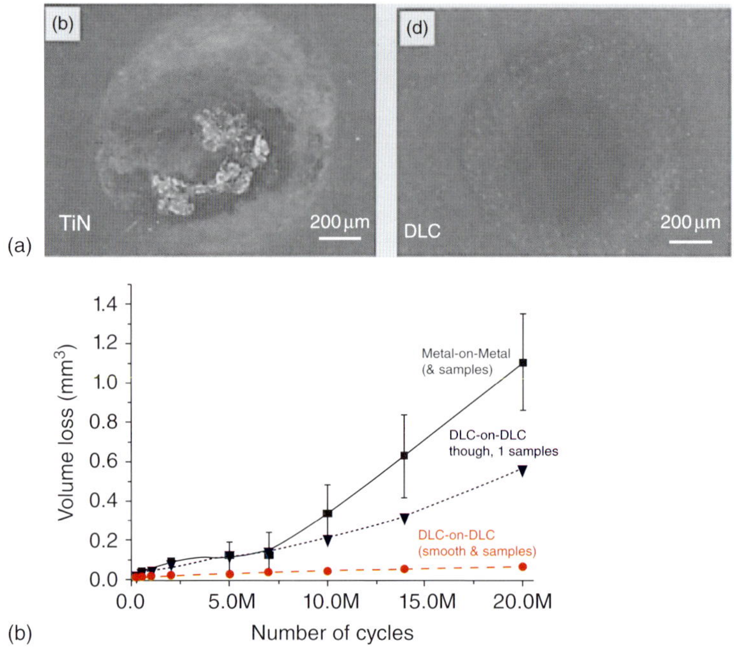

Figure 4.8 (A) The SEM micrographs showing the stability of DLC films over TIN coatings for 10^4 cycles of impact fatigue test. The DLC film does not show cohesive or adhesive failure during the course of the experiment. (Wang 2010 [164]. Reproduced with permission of Elsevier.) (B) Wear volume produced by metal-on-metal and DLC-on-DLC pairs with respect to number of test runtime. The smooth DLC pairs exhibit significantly reduced wear volume compared to MoM pairs. (Thorwarth 2014 [165]. Reproduced with permission of Elsevier.)

simulator with loading conforming to ISO 14 243, and in the presence of sodium chloride solution, reported an increase in the service life of the DLC/PEEK articulating system by up to 2 million cycles.

The DLC films are usually characterized by high residual stress. This high internal compressive stress, together with the coefficient of thermal expansion mismatch with the substrate, leads to DLC film/substrate interfacial cracking and delamination. In addition, the residual stress is found to increase with DLC film thickness, preventing the implant surfaces with thick DLC coatings from being used. Hence, providing better adhesion between DLC and the substrate, especially on metal substrate, is one of the major goals for attaining long-lasting coatings on articulating surfaces. One way of meeting this requirement is by introducing suitable interlayers between the DLC and substrate material. In general, layers of Ti, Si, Cr, Cr-CrN, Ta, Nb, and functionally graded layers (Me, MeN, MeNC, or Me/MeC where Me corresponds to metallic ion) are used as adhesion promoting layers [142, 163]. Interlayer stability and high cycle simulator performance of a DLC coating with Ta interlayer was reported by Thorwarth *et al.* [165]. The authors found that an amorphous/α tantalum interlayer gave excellent adhesion for a DLC layer to CCM alloy with little or no noticeable wear rate after 101 million cycles. In addition, overloading and third body (cortical bone chips) wear did not show any kind of coating failure, local defects or defect propagation, and projected them as potential candidates for coatings on metal-on-metal articulations. Another approach is by forming multilayer structures. Xu *et al.* [167] effectively reduced the internal stress of DLC films by fabricating alternating DLC layers rich in sp^2 (soft DLC) and sp^3 (hard DLC) through the filtered cathodic vacuum arc method. It was proposed that soft DLC is susceptible to plastic deformation and effectively relieves the stress produced by hard DLC. Further, lowest compressive stress was observed for low bilayer thickness (35 nm for each layer) due to an increase in the number of layers as well as the interface region. In addition, these multilayer structures exhibit better wear properties than single-layer DLC films. Recently, Sahoo *et al.* [168] reported that DLC/Cr multilayers displayed enhanced adhesion and modulus properties. Although interlayers provides better adhesion *in vitro*, the long-term stability of these interlayers still remains a challenge for researchers.

4.1.7.5 **Efficacy of DLC Films Tested *in vivo***

Though DLC films show exceptional properties *in vitro*, the *in vivo* results are contradictory. The major problem encountered is the longevity of the devices in real body systems. As far as DLC coated orthopedic devices are concerned, delamination of DLC coatings from the articulating surfaces and reduced lifetime are the prime reasons for device failure. In addition, localized defects and pin holes created in the coating allow the diffusion of body fluids containing corrosive elements into the interstitials, which could corrode the adhesion-promoting interlayer and further enhance the delamination. As this process is very slow implant failure usually occurrs after a few years of operation.

Very little literature is available on *in vivo* and explant studies of DLC coated orthopedic implants. Taeger *et al.* compared the survivorship of DLC coated femoral heads and alumina oxide heads articulating with polyethylene in total hip arthroplasty (THA) in a medical follow-up study [169]. After an average period of 9 years, excessive failure of DLC coated heads was noticed with a fourfold increase in the number of patients undergoing revision surgery due to aseptic loosening compared to THA having alumina femoral heads. Further, the DLC film was found to delaminate from the head and failed *in vivo* for longevity. Another *ex vivo* case study conducted by Joyce with metal-on-metal metatarsophalangeal (MTP) prosthesis also addressed the delamination of DLC coatings and failure of the implant in real practice [170].

Hauert *et al.* analyzed the stability of Si-based adhesive interlayers of DLC coated metallic metatarsophalangeal (MTP) prosthesis explanted after 4 years [171]. It appeared that DLC coatings were partly or fully delaminated from the components. The study also revealed that the key reason for delamination is the corrosive nature of the Si interlayer that was provided to increase the adhesion between the DLC and alloy. Furthermore, on a separate crevice experiment the authors proved the instability of Si against body fluids. Similarly, the *in vivo* studies of DLC coated blood contacting devices did not perform as well as expected. Mikhalovska *et al.* reported significantly increased neointima around DLC coated stents compared to TiO or ZrO coated stents assessed 8 weeks after stenting inside white rabbits [172]. There are other medical follow-up studies that have shown both satisfactory and nonsatisfactory results. The various *in vivo* studies on DLC coated stents and heart valves are summarized in the review article by Hauert *et al.* [142]. It is important to mention that *in vivo* studies have failed to reproduce the excellent properties observed for this material *in vitro*.

4.1.7.6 **Plasma-Enhanced Synthesis of Graphene and Carbon Nanoparticles**

Nonequilibrium and kinetics-driven phenomena of low-temperature plasma can be used for the catalyst-free energy-efficient production of self-organized nanosolids from conventional precursors, for example, methane. While the dissociation of carbon is purely thermal in the case of conventional thermal CVD, the plasma environment enables electron- and ion-assisted dissociation that complements plasma heating effects to promote faster monomer break-down. Ionic and radical species recombine on the surface of the carbon nanoparticle, inducing highly localized heating that removes the need for general substrate heating. A lower substrate temperature not only reduces the energy cost of synthesis, but also minimizes the evaporation and desorption of carbon units from the surface of the substrate. Plasma-generated reactive hydrogen species prolong particle catalytic activity, while the electric field enables surface organization and alignment of the formed particle. The unique chemistry of plasma can be used to convert raw carbon sources such as foodstuff, raw materials, and waste materials into carbon nanoparticles and graphene layers [173, 174]. The plasma environment can be used to functionalize carbon nanotubes during or post synthesis, enabling their use in a variety of biosensing applications.

Graphene-based materials have a wide range of potential applications in medicine and biotechnology [8, 175]. As films, graphene-based nanomaterials inhibit the growth of *E. coli*, via a combination of membrane and oxidation stress, while showing minimal cytotoxicity [176–178]. Graphene oxide was demonstrated to have the highest antibacterial activity, sequentially followed by reduced graphene oxide, graphite, and graphite oxide. Highly organized surface nanostructures, such as arrays of vertically aligned CNTs with a length gradient [179], can be used for a variety of biomedical application, including cell-surface studies and highly controlled cell attachment. NIH-3T3 fibroblast cells, grown on supported thin films of graphene and carbon nanotubes, displayed good growth rate and gene transfection efficiency up to 250% more than that of cells grown on a cover glass [180]. Graphene was found to be a suitable biocompatible scaffold for proliferation of human mesenchymal stem cells, accelerating their specific differentiation into bone cells with a rate comparable to that achieved by common growth factors [181]. Graphene has also been shown to enhance neurite numbers, average neurite length, and expression of growth-associate protein-43 compared with tissue culture polystyrene substrates, suggesting its use for neural interfacing [182].

Carbon nanotubes can be added to bulk biomaterials to improve their mechanical properties for tissue engineering and implant applications [183]. A film produced by casting a solution containing few-layered graphene sheets (0.1 – 0.3 wt%) dispersed in chitosan/acetic acid had an elastic modulus 200% higher than that of pure chitosan film [184]. There was no significant difference in the biocompatibility between the pure and graphene-enhanced chitosan, with L929 cells adhering well to both surfaces. Plasma can be used for fabrication of carbon nanodots from a range of highly purified and raw resources, including chicken eggs [185], simple carbohydrates [186], amino acids, and polymers. These quantum dots have bright luminescence, resistance to photobleaching, aqueous stability, and low cytotoxicity superior to most other dyes commonly used in biomedical applications. They are often used in highly sensitive cellular imaging, where their photostability facilitates extended high-resolution imaging with multiple passes. They are equally useful for real-time tracking of biomolecules and cells over prolonged periods of time. For visualization, the dots may be linked to a biomolecule, such as an antibody, peptide, nucleic acid fragment, and so on, that targets a specific biomarker on the cells to be visualized. This allows for imaging of specific tissues, such as tumors. Individual cells can also be labeled and thus tracked to observe their real-time behavior.

4.2 Conclusion

Plasmas have a plethora of applications in the areas of medicine and biotechnology. In medicine, thermal effects of plasma have long been exploited for tissue ablation and cauterization. Current research mainly focuses on the nonthermal effects of plasmas, specifically their ability to induce specific biological responses or chemical modification via plasma-generated reactive and neutral species and irradiation. Because of their low temperature, nonthermal plasmas have minimal deleterious effects on the surrounding healthy tissues, yet allow for prompt decontamination from pathogenic microorganisms and removal of dead tissue. It can potentially suppress inflammation and promote tissue healing.

The same reactive species can be effectively used to transform a wide range of organic and inorganic precursors into thin polymer films with tunable properties and good substrate adhesion. Furthermore, plasma effects can be successfully used for highly controlled surface modification, with the ability to even process most temperature-sensitive biomaterials without changing their bulk properties.

Plasmas that generate higher temperatures can be used to fabricate a broad range of carbon nanomaterials, including ordered carbons (e.g., graphene sheets, nanotubes and nanoparticles), carbon quantum dots, and amorphous carbons. These materials can be deposited directly onto biomaterials to modify the surface profile, particularly to improve chemical stability and prevent wear as well as to enhance blood- and tissue-compatibility and promote specific cell/tissue responses. These carbon nanostructures can also be used to change the bulk properties of biomaterials, often to improve the mechanical and biological properties of the resultant structure. Carbon nanomaterials have promising drug delivery, sensing, and bioimaging applications.

References

1. Qi, L., Li, N., Huang, R., Song, Q., Wang, L., Zhang, Q., Su, R., Kong, T., Tang, M., and Cheng, G. (2013) The effects of topographical patterns and sizes on neural stem cell behaviour. *PLoS One*, **8**, e59022.
2. Zheng, W., Zhang, W., and Jiang, X. (2013) Precise control of cell adhesion by combination of surface chemistry and soft lithography. *Adv. Healthc. Mater.*, **2** (1), 95–108.
3. Valamehr, B., Jonas, S.J., Polleux, J., Qiao, R., Guo, S., Gschweng, E.H., Stiles, B., Kam, K., Luo, T.-J.M., Witte, O.N., Liu, X., Dunn, B., and Wu, H. (2008) Hydrophobic surfaces for enhanced differentiation of embryonic stem cell-derived embryoid bodies. *Proc. Natl. Acad. Sci. U.S.A.*, **105** (38), 14459–14464.
4. Ratner, B.D. and Bryant, S.J. (2004) Biomaterials: where we have been and where we are going. *Annu. Rev. Biomed. Eng.*, **6** (1), 41–75.
5. Chu, P.K., Chen, J.Y., Wang, L.P., and Huang, N. (2002) Plasma-surface modification of biomaterials. *Mater. Sci. Eng., R*, **36** (5-6), 143–206.
6. Williams, D.F. (2008) On the mechanisms of biocompatibility. *Biomaterials*, **29** (20), 2941–2953.
7. Bazaka, O. and Bazaka, K. (2014) Surface modification of biomaterials for biofilm control, in *Biomaterials and Medical Device-Associated Infections* (eds E., Ivanova and R., Crawford), Woodhead Publishing, p. 103.
8. Bazaka, O. and Bazaka, K. (2015) in *Antibacterial Surfaces* (eds E. Ivanova and R. Crawford), Springer International Publishing, pp. 113–147.
9. Bazaka, K., Jacob, M.V., Chrzanowski, W., and Ostrikov, K. (2015) Antibacterial surfaces: natural agents, mechanisms of action, and plasma surface modification, *RSC Adv.*, **5** (60), 48739–48759.
10. Goddard, J.M. and Hotchkiss, J.H. (2007) Polymer surface modification for the attachment of bioactive compounds. *Prog. Polym. Sci.*, **32** (7), 698–725.
11. Junkar, I., Cvelbar, U., and Lehocky, M. (2011) Plasma treatment of biomedical materials. *Mater. Technol.*, **45** (3), 221–226.
12. Deng, X. and Lahann, J. (2014) Orthogonal surface functionalization through bioactive vapour-based polymer coatings. *J. Appl. Polym. Sci.*, **131** (14), 40315.
13. Crawford, R.J., Webb, H.K., Truong, V.K., Hasan, J., and Ivanova, E.P. (2012) Surface topographical factors influencing bacterial attachment. *Adv. Colloid Interface Sci.*, **179–182**, 142–149.
14. Desmet, T., Morent, R., De Geyter, N., Leys, C., Schacht, E., and Dubruel, P. (2009) Nonthermal plasma technology as a versatile strategy for polymeric biomaterials surface modification: a review. *Biomacromolecules*, **10** (9), 2351–2378.
15. Montanaro, L., Campoccia, D., and Arciola, C.R. (2007) Advancements in molecular epidermiology of implant infections and future perspectives. *Biomaterials*, **28** (34), 5155–5168.
16. Anderson, J.M. (2001) Biological responses to materials. *Annu. Rev. Mater. Res.*, **31** (1), 81–110.
17. Jacobs, T., Morent, R., De Geyter, N., and Dubrual, P. (2012) Plasma surface modification of biomedical polymers: influence on cell-material interaction. *Plasma Chem. Plasma Process.*, **32** (5), 1039–1073.

18. Hoa, X.D., Kirk, A.G., and Tabrizian, M. (2007) Toward integrated and sensitive surface plasmon resonance biosensors: a review of recent progress. *Biosens. Bioelectron.*, **23** (2), 151–160.
19. Slowing, I., Trewyn, B.G., and Lin, V.S.-Y. (2006) Effect of surface functionalization of MCM-41-type mesoporous silica nanoparticles on the endocytosis by human cancer cells. *J. Am. Chem. Soc.*, **128** (46), 14792–14793.
20. Sioshansi, P. and Tobin, E.J. (1996) Surface treatment of biomaterials by ion beam processes. *Surf. Coat. Technol.*, **83** (1–3), 175–182.
21. Siow, K.S., Britcher, L., Kumar, S., and Griesser, H.J. (2006) Plasma methods for the generation of chemically reactive surfaces for biomolecule immobilization and cell colonization – a review. *Plasma Processes Polym.*, **3** (6-7), 392–418.
22. Pavlovich, M.J., Chen, Z., Sakiyama, Y., Clark, D.S., and Graves, D.B. (2013) Effect of discharge parameters and surface characteristics on ambient-gas plasma disinfection. *Plasma Processes Polym.*, **10** (1), 69–76.
23. Rossi, F., Kylián, O., Rauscher, H., Hasiwa, M., and Gilliland, D. (2009) Low pressure plasma discharges for the sterilization and decontamination of surfaces. *New J. Phys.*, **11** (11), 115017.
24. Robinson, R.D., Gutsol, K., Rabinovich, A., and Fridman, A.A. (2012) Plasma acid production in a gliding arc plasmatron. *Plasma Med.*, **2** (4), 249–258.
25. Balasundaram, A., Alexeff, I., and Sawhney, R.S. (2011) Design of experiment-based testing of air, charged ions, and hydrogen peroxide in a direct current steady-state plasma sterilizer. *Plasma Med.*, **1** (3–4), 179–189.
26. Alkawareek, M.Y., Gorman, S.P., Graham, W.G., and Gilmore, B.F. (2014) Eradication of marine biofilms by atmospheric pressure non-thermal plasma: a potential approach to control biofouling? *Int. Biodeterior. Biodegrad.*, **86**, Part A, 14–18.
27. Awakowicz, P., Baldus, S., Stapelmann, K., Engelhardt, M., Bibinov, N., and Denis, B. (2012) Optical emission spectroscopy as a tool for characterization of technical plasmas in medical applications. *Plasma Med.*, **2** (1–3), 151–168.
28. Dobrynin, D., Wasko, K., Friedman, G., Fridman, A.A., and Fridman, G. (2011) Cold plasma sterilization of open wounds: live rat model. *Plasma Med.*, **1** (2), 109–114.
29. Isbary, G., Heinlin, J., Shimizu, T., Zimmermann, J.L., Morfill, G., Schmidt, H.U., Monetti, R., Steffes, B., Bunk, W., Li, Y., Klaempfl, T., Karrer, S., Landthaler, M., and Stolz, W. (2012) Successful and safe use of 2 min cold atmospheric argon plasma in chronic wounds: results of a randomized controlled trial. *Br. J. Dermatol.*, **167** (2), 404–410.
30. Daeschlein, G., Scholz, S., Ahmed, R., von Woedtke, T., Haase, H., Niggemeier, M., Kindel, E., Brandenburg, R., Weltmann, K.D., and Juenger, M. (2012) Skin decontamination by low-temperature atmospheric pressure plasma jet and dielectric barrier discharge plasma. *J. Hosp. Infect.*, **81** (3), 177–183.
31. Isbary, G., Köritzer, J., Mitra, A., Li, Y.F., Shimizu, T., Schroeder, J., Schlegel, J., Morfill, G.E., Stolz, W., and Zimmermann, J.L. (2013) Ex vivo human skin experiments for the evaluation of safety of new cold atmospheric plasma devices. *Clin. Plasma Med.*, **1** (1), 36–44.
32. Graves, D.B. (2012) The emerging role of reactive oxygen and nitrogen species in redox biology and some implications for plasma applications to medicine and biology. *J. Phys. D: Appl. Phys.*, **45** (26), 263001.
33. Kohanski, M.A., Dwyer, D.J., Hayete, B., Lawrence, C.A., and Collins, J.J. (2007) A common mechanism of cellular death induced by bactericidal antibiotics. *Cell*, **130** (5), 797–810.
34. Dwyer, D.J., Kohanski, M.A., and Collins, J.J. (2009) Role of reactive oxygen species in antibiotic action and resistance. *Curr. Opin. Microbiol.*, **12** (5), 482–489.
35. Liu, Y. and Imlay, J.A. (2013) Cell death from antibiotics without the

involvement of reactive oxygen species. *Science*, **339** (6124), 1210–1213.

36. Keren, I., Wu, Y., Inocencio, J., Mulcahy, L.R., and Lewis, K. (2013) Killing by bactericidal antibiotics does not depend on reactive oxygen species. *Science*, **339** (6124), 1213–1216.
37. Laroussi, M. (2002) Nonthermal decontamination of biological media by atmospheric-pressure plasmas: review, analysis, and prospects. *IEEE Trans. Plasma Sci.*, **30** (4), 1409–1415.
38. Neyts, E.C., Yusupov, M., Verlackt, C.C., and Bogaerts, A. (2014) Computer simulations of plasma–biomolecule and plasma–tissue interactions for a better insight in plasma medicine. *J. Phys. D: Appl. Phys.*, **47** (29), 293001.
39. Yusupov, M., Neyts, E.C., Simon, P., Berdiyorov, G., Snoeckx, R., van Duin, A.C.T., and Bogaerts, A. (2014) Reactive molecular dynamics simulations of oxygen species in a liquid water layer of interest for plasma medicine. *J. Phys. D: Appl. Phys.*, **47** (2), 025205.
40. Dobrynin, D., Fridman, G., Friedman, G., and Fridman, A. (2012) in *Plasma for Bio-Decontamination, Medicine and Food Security*, NATO Science for Peace and Security Series A: Chemistry and Biology (eds Z. Machala, K. Hensel, and Y. Akishev), Springer Netherlands, 299, p. 293.
41. Dobrynin, D., Fridman, G., Friedman, G., and Fridman, A.A. (2012) Deep penetration into tissues of reactive oxygen species generated in floating-electrode dielectric barrier discharge (FE-DBD): an *in vitro* agarose gel model mimicking an open wound. *Plasma Med.*, **2** (1–3), 71–83.
42. Sladek, R.E.J., Stoffels, E., Walraven, R., Tielbeek, P.J.A., and Koolhoven, R.A. (2004) Plasma treatment of dental cavities: a feasibility study. *IEEE Trans. Plasma Sci.*, **32** (4), 1540–1543.
43. Nosenko, T., Shimizu, T., and Morfill, G.E. (2009) Designing plasmas for chronic wound disinfection. *New J. Phys.*, **11** (11), 115013.
44. Klebes, M., Lademann, J., Philipp, S., Ulrich, C., Patzelt, A., Ulmer, M., Kluschke, F., Kramer, A., Weltmann, K.D., Sterry, W., and Lange-Asschenfeldt, B. (2014) Effects of tissue-tolerable plasma on psoriasis vulgaris treatment compared to conventional local treatment: a pilot study. *Clin. Plasma Med.*, **2** (1), 22–27.
45. Chakravarthy, K., Dobrynin, D., Fridman, G., Friedman, G., Murthy, S., and Fridman, A.A. (2011) Cold spark discharge plasma treatment of inflammatory bowel disease in an animal model of ulcerative colitis. *Plasma Med.*, **1** (1), 3–19.
46. Bekeschus, S., Kolata, J., Muller, A., Kramer, A., Weltmann, K.-D., Broker, B., and Masur, K. (2013) Differential viability of eight human blood mononuclear cell subpopulations after plasma treatment. *Plasma Med.*, **3** (1–2), 1–13.
47. Bekeschus, S., von Woedtke, T., Kramer, A., Weltmann, K.-D., and Masur, K. (2013) Cold physical plasma treatment alters redox balance in human immune cells. *Plasma Med.*, **3** (4), 267–278.
48. Kalghatgi, S., Kelly, C.M., Cerchar, E., Torabi, B., Alekseev, O., Fridman, A., Friedman, G., and Azizkhan-Clifford, J. (2011) Effects of non-thermal plasma on mammalian cells. *PLoS One*, **6** (1), e16270.
49. Ahmed, M.M., El-Aragi, G.M., Elhadary, A.M.A., and Montaser, S.A. (2012) Cytogenetic and immunological effects on human blood cultures resulting from cold pulsed atmospheric pressure plasma Jet exposure. *Plasma Med.*, **2** (4), 191–205.
50. Kieft, I.E., Kurdi, M., and Stoffels, E. (2006) Reattachment and apoptosis after plasma-needle treatment of cultured cells. *IEEE Trans. Plasma Sci.*, **34** (4), 1331–1336.
51. Volotskova, O., Shashurin, A., Stepp, M.A., Pal-Ghosh, S., and Keidar, M. (2011) Plasma-controlled cell migration: localization of cold plasma-cell interaction region. *Plasma Med.*, **1** (1), 85–92.
52. Ishaq, M., Bazaka, K., and Ostrikov, K. (2015) Intracellular effects of atmospheric-pressure plasmas on

melanoma cancer cells. *Phys. Plasmas*, **22** (12), 122003.
53. Ishaq, M., Bazaka, K., and Ostrikov, K. (2015) Pro-apoptotic NOXA is implicated in atmospheric-pressure plasma-induced melanoma cell death. *J. Phys. D: Appl. Phys.*, **48** (46), 464002.
54. Keidar, M., Walk, R., Shashurin, A., Srinivasan, P., Sandler, A., Dasgupta, S., Ravi, R., Guerrero-Preston, R., and Trink, B. (2011) Cold plasma selectivity and the possibility of a paradigm shift in cancer therapy. *Br. J. Cancer*, **105** (9), 1295–1301.
55. Vandamme, M., Robert, E., Lerondel, S., Sarron, V., Ries, D., Dozias, S., Sobilo, J., Gosset, D., Kieda, C., Legrain, B., Pouvesle, J.-M., and Pape, A.L. (2012) ROS implication in a new antitumor strategy based on non-thermal plasma. *Int. J. Cancer*, **130** (9), 2185–2194.
56. Ishaq, M., Evans, M., and Ostrikov, K. (2013) Effect of atmospheric gas plasmas on cancer cell signaling. *Int. J. Cancer*, **134** (7), 1517–1528.
57. Hirst, A.M., Frame, F.M., Maitland, N.J., and O'Connell, D. (2014) Low temperature plasma causes double-strand break DNA damage in primary epithelial cells cultured from a human prostate tumor. *IEEE Trans. Plasma Sci.*, **42** (10), 2740–2741.
58. Landsberg, K., Scharf, C., Darm, K., Wende, K., Daeschlein, G., Kindel, E., Weltmann, K.-D., and von Woedtke, T. (2011) Use of proteomics to investigate plasma–cell interactions. *Plasma Med.*, **1** (1), 55–63.
59. Barton, A., Wende, K., Bundscherer, L., Hasse, S., Schmidt, A., Bekeschus, S., Weltmann, K.-D., Lindequist, U., and Masur, K. (2013) Nonthermal plasma increases expression of wound healing related genes in a keratinocyte cell line. *Plasma Med.*, **3** (1–2), 125–136.
60. Eisuke, T., Tsuyoshi, K., Junpei, K., Satoshi, I., Shunsuke, Y., Kentaro, S., Hideya, K., Ryuichi, A., and Katsuhisa, K. (2014) Chemical modification of amino acids by atmospheric-pressure cold plasma in aqueous solution. *J. Phys. D: Appl. Phys.*, **47** (28), 285403.
61. Kosuke, T., Ken, C., Yuichi, S., Masaharu, S., Makoto, S., and Masaru, H. (2013) Investigations on plasma–biomolecules interactions as fundamental process for plasma medicine. *J. Phys. Conf. Ser.*, **441** (1), 012001.
62. Setsuhara, Y., Cho, K., Shiratani, M., Sekine, M., and Hori, M. (2013) Plasma interactions with aminoacid (l-alanine) as a basis of fundamental processes in plasma medicine. *Curr. Appl. Phys.*, **13** (Suppl. 1), S59–S63.
63. Russo, L., Zanini, S., Giannoni, P., Landi, E., Villa, A., Sandri, M., Riccardi, C., Quarto, R., Doglia, S., Nicotra, F., and Cipolla, L. (2012) The influence of plasma technology coupled to chemical grafting on the cell growth compliance of 3D hydroxyapatite scaffolds. *J. Mater. Sci. - Mater. Med.*, **23** (11), 2727–2738.
64. Çökeliler, D., Gökta, H., Tosun, P.D., and Mutlu, S. (2010) Infection free titanium alloys by stabile thiol based nanocoating. *J. Nanosci. Nanotechnol.*, **10** (4), 2583–2589.
65. Bazaka, K., Jacob, M., Truong, V.K., Crawford, R.J., and Ivanova, E.P. (2011) The effect of polyterpenol thin film surfaces on bacterial viability and adhesion. *Polymers*, **3** (4), 388–404.
66. Bazaka, K., Jacob, M.V., and Ostrikov, K. (2016) Sustainable life cycles of natural-precursor-derived nanocarbons. *Chem. Rev.*, **116** (1), 163–214.
67. Seo, D.H., Rider, A.E., Han, Z.J., Kumar, S., and Ostrikov, K. (2013) Plasma break-down and re-build: same functional vertical graphenes from diverse natural precursors. *Adv. Mater.*, **25** (39), 5638–5642.
68. Bazaka, K., Jacob, M.V., Truong, V.K., Wang, F., Pushpamali, W.A.A., Wang, J.Y., Ellis, A.V., Berndt, C.C., Crawford, R.J., and Ivanova, E.P. (2010) Plasma-enhanced synthesis of bioactive polymeric coatings from monoterpene alcohols: a combined experimental and theoretical study. *Biomacromolecules*, **11** (8), 2016–2026.
69. Bazaka, K., Jacob, M.V., and Ivanova, E.P. (2010) A study of a retention of

antimicrobial activity by plasma polymerized terpinen-4-ol thin films. *Mater. Sci. Forum*, **654–656**, 2261–2264.
70. Bazaka, K., Jacob, M.V., Taguchi, D., Manaka, T., and Iwamoto, M. (2011) Investigation of interfacial charging and discharging in double-layer pentacene-based metal-insulator-metal device with polyterpenol blocking layer using electric field induced second harmonic generation. *Chem. Phys. Lett.*, **503** (1–3), 105–111.
71. Bazaka, K., Jacob, M.V., and Bowden, B.F. (2011) Optical and chemical properties of polyterpenol thin films deposited via plasma-enhanced chemical vapor deposition. *J. Mater. Res.*, **26** (08), 1018–1025.
72. Ahmad, J., Bazaka, K., and Jacob, M.V. (2014) Optical and surface characterization of radio frequency plasma polymerized 1-isopropyl-4-methyl-1, 4-cyclohexadiene thin films. *Electronics*, **3** (2), 266–281.
73. Jacob, M.V., Olsen, N.S., Anderson, L., Bazaka, K., and Shanks, R.A. (2013) Plasma polymerised thin films for flexible electronic applications. *Thin Solid Films*, **546**, 167–170.
74. Shi, F.F. (1996) Recent advances in polymer thin films prepared by plasma polymerization synthesis, structural characterization, properties and applications. *Surf. Coat. Technol.*, **82** (1-2), 1–15.
75. Whittle, J.D., Short, R.D., Steele, D.A., Bradley, J.W., Bryant, P.M., Jan, F., Biederman, H., Serov, A.A., Choukurov, A., Hook, A.L., Ciridon, W.A., Ceccone, G., Hegemann, D., Körner, E., and Michelmore, A. (2013) Variability in plasma polymerization processes – an international round-robin study. *Plasma Processes Polym.*, **10** (9), 767–778.
76. Chan, C.-M. and Ko, T.-M. (1996) Polymer surface modification by plasmas and photons. *Surf. Sci. Rep.*, **24** (1-2), 1–54.
77. Alf, M.E., Asatekin, A., Barr, M.C., Baxamusa, S.H., Chelawat, H., Ozaydin-Ince, G., Petruczok, C.D., Sreenivasan, R., Tenhaeff, W.E., Trujillo, N.J., Vaddiraju, S., Xu, J., and Gleason, K.K. (2010) Chemical vapor deposition of conformal, functional, and responsive polymer films. *Adv. Mater.*, **22** (18), 1993–2027.
78. Chen, H.-Y. and Lahann, J. (2011) Designable biointerfaces using vapor-based reactive polymers. *Langmuir*, **27** (1), 34–48.
79. Ohl, A. and Schröder, K. (1999) Plasma-induced chemical micropatterning for cell culturing applications: a brief review. *Surf. Coat. Technol.*, **116–119**, 820–830.
80. Vargo, T.G., Bekos, E.J., Kim, Y.S., Ranieri, J.P., Bellamkonda, R., Aebisher, P., Margevich, D.E., Thompson, P.M., Bright, F.V., and Gardella, J.A. Jr., (1995) Synthesis and characterization of fluoropolymeric substrata with immobilized minimal peptide sequences for cell adhesion studies. *J. Biomed. Mater. Res.*, **29** (6), 767–778.
81. Lee, J.H., Lee, J.W., Khang, G., and Lee, H.B. (1997) Interaction of cells on chargeable funtional group gradient surfaces. *Biomaterials*, **18** (4), 351–358.
82. Parry, K.L., Shard, A.G., Short, R.D., White, R.G., Whittle, J.D., and Wright, A. (2006) ARXPS characterisation of plasma polymerised surface chemical gradients. *Surf. Interface Anal.*, **38** (11), 1497–1504.
83. Alexander, M.R., Whittle, J.D., Barton, D., and Short, R.D. (2004) Plasma polymer chemical gradients for evaluation of surface reactivity: epoxide reaction with carboxylic acid surface groups. *J. Mater. Chem.*, **14** (3), 408–412.
84. Leclair, A.M., Ferguson, S.S.G., and Lagugné-Labarthet, F. (2011) Surface patterning using plasma-deposited fluorocarbon thin films for single-cell positioning and neural circuit arrangment. *Biomaterials*, **32** (5), 1351–1360.
85. Mierczynska, A., Michelmore, A., Tripathi, A., Goreham, R.V., Sedev, R., and Vasilev, K. (2012) pH-tunable gradients of wettability and surface potential. *Soft Matter*, **8** (32), 8399–8404. doi: 10.1039/c2sm25221j
86. Goreham, R.V., Mierczynska, A., Pierce, M., Short, R.D., Taheri, S., Bachhuka, A., Cavallaro, A., Smith, L.E., and

Vasilev, K. (2013) A substrate independent approach for generation of surface gradients. *Thin Solid Films*, **528**, 106–110.
87. Leong, K., Boardman, A.K., Ma, H., and Jen, A.K.-Y. (2009) Single-cell patterning and adhesion on chemically engineered poly(dimethylsiloxane) surface. *Langmuir*, **25** (8), 4615–4620.
88. Rettig, J.R. and Folch, A. (2005) Large-scale single-cell trapping and imaging using microwell arrays. *Anal. Chem.*, **77** (17), 5628–5634.
89. Veiseh, M., Veiseh, O., Martin, M.C., Asphahani, F., and Zhang, M. (2007) Short peptides enhance single cell adhesion and viability on microarrays. *Langmuir*, **23** (8), 4472–4479.
90. Jiang, X., Bruzewicz, D.A., Wong, A.P., Piel, M., and Whitesides, G.M. (2005) Directing cell migration with asymmetric micropatterns. *Proc. Natl. Acad. Sci. U.S.A.*, **102** (4), 975–978.
91. Nakanishi, J., Kikunchi, Y., Inoue, S., Yamaguchi, K., Takarada, T., and Maeda, M. (2007) Spatiotemporal control of cell migration of single cells on a photoactivatable cell microarray. *J. Am. Chem. Soc.*, **129** (21), 6694–6695.
92. Tang, J., Peng, R., and Ding, J. (2010) The regulation of stem cell differentiation by cell–cell contact on micropatterned material surfaces. *Biomaterials*, **31** (9), 2470–2476.
93. Nelson, C.M. and Chen, C.S. (2002) Cell–cell signaling by direct contact increases cell proliferation via a PI3K-dependent signal. *FEBS Lett.*, **514** (2-3), 238–242.
94. Aronsson, B.-O., Lausmaa, J., and Kasemo, B. (1997) Glow discharge plasma treatment for surface cleaning and modification of metallic biomaterials. *J. Biomed. Mater. Res.*, **35** (1), 49–73.
95. Hermanson, G.T. (2008) *Bioconjugate Techniques*, Academic Press, New York.
96. Pirrung, M.C. and Huang, C.-Y. (1996) A general method for the spatially defined immobilization of biomolecules on glass surfaces using "caged" biotin. *Bioconjugate Chem.*, **7** (3), 317–321.
97. Strother, T., Knickerbocker, T., Russell, J.N. Jr., Butler, J.E., Smith, L.M., and Hamers, R.J. (2002) Photochemical functionalization of diamond films. *Langmuir*, **18** (4), 968–971.
98. Ulman, A. (1996) Formation and structure of self-assembled monolayers. *Chem. Rev.*, **96** (4), 1533–1554.
99. Inan, U.S. and Golkowski, M. (2011) *Principles of Plasma Physics for Engineers and Scientists*, Cambridge University Press, New York.
100. Lane, J.M. and Hourston, D.J. (1993) Surface treatments of polyolefins. *Prog. Org. Coat.*, **21** (4), 269–284.
101. Grace, J.M. and Gerenser, L.J. (2003) Plasma treatment of polymers. *J. Dispersion Sci. Technol.*, **24** (3–4), 305–341.
102. Oyane, A., Uchida, M., Yokomaya, Y., Choong, C., Triffitt, J., and Ito, A. (2005) Simple surface modification of poly(epsilon-capro-lactone) to induce its apatite-forming ability. *J. Biomed. Mater. Res. Part A*, **75A** (1), 138–145.
103. Kim, Y.J., Kang, I.K., Huh, M.W., and Yoon, S.C. (2000) Surface characterization and in vitro blood compatibility of poly(ethylene terephthalate) immobilized with insulin and/or heparin using plasma glow discharge. *Biomaterials*, **21** (2), 121–130.
104. Kong, J.S., Lee, D.J., and Kim, H.D. (2001) Surface modification of low-density polyethylene (LDPE) film and improvement of adhesion between evaporated copper metal film and LDPE. *J. Appl. Polym. Sci.*, **82** (7), 1677–1690.
105. Hu, Y.H., Winn, S.R., Krajbich, I., and Hollinger, J.O. (2003) Porous polymer scaffolds surface-modified with arginine-glycine-aspartic acid enhance bone cell attachment and differentiation in vitro. *J. Biomed. Mater. Res. Part A*, **64A** (3), 583–590.
106. Wang, M.J., Chang, Y.I., and Poncin-Epaillard, F. (2005) Acid and basic functionalities of nitrogen and carbon dioxide plasma-treated polystyrene. *Surf. Interface Anal.*, **37** (3), 348–355.
107. Aouinti, M., Bertrand, P., and Poncin-Epaillard, F. (2003) Characterization of polypropylene surface

treated in CO_2 plasma. *Plasma Polym.*, **8** (4), 225–236.
108. Švorčík, V., Kasálková, N., Slepička, P., Záruba, K., Král, V., Bačáková, L., Pařízek, M., Lisá, V., Ruml, T., Gbelcová, H., Rimpelová, S., and Macková, A. (2009) Cytocompatibility of Ar+ plasma treated and Au nanoparticle-grafted PE. *Nucl. Instrum. Methods Phys. Res., Sect. B*, **267** (11), 1904–1910.
109. Kuhn, G., Weidner, S., Decker, R., Ghode, A., and Friedrich, J. (1999) Selective surface functionalization of polyolefins by plasma treatment followed by chemical reduction. *Surf. Coat. Technol.*, **116–119**, 796–801.
110. Michelmore, A., Steele, D.A., Robinson, D.E., Whittle, J.D., and Short, R.D. (2013) The link between mechanisms of deposition and the physico-chemical properties of plasma polymer films. *Soft Matter*, **9** (26), 6167–6175.
111. Michelmore, A., Steele, D.A., Whittle, J.D., Bradley, J.W., and Short, R.D. (2013) Nanoscale deposition of chemically functionalised films via plasma polymerisation. *RSC Adv.*, **3** (33), 13540–13557.
112. Kuhn, G., Retzko, I., Lippitz, A., Unger, W., and Friedrich, J. (2001) Homofunctionalized polymer surfaces formed by selective plasma processes. *Surf. Coat. Technol.*, **142–144**, 494–500.
113. Michelmore, A., Gross-Kosche, P., Al-Bataineh, S.A., Whittle, J.D., and Short, R.D. (2013) On the effect of monomer chemistry on growth mechanisms of nonfouling PEG-like plasma polymers. *Langmuir*, **29** (8), 2595–2601.
114. Yasuda, H. (1985) *Plasma Polymerization*, Academic Press Inc., Orlanda, FL.
115. Nakajima, K., Bell, A.T., Shen, M., and Milllard, M.M. (1979) Plasma polymerization of tetrafluoroethylene. *J. Appl. Polym. Sci.*, **23** (9), 2627–2637.
116. Friedrich, J. (2011) Mechanisms of plasma polymerization – reviewed from a chemical point of view. *Plasma Processes Polym.*, **8** (9), 783–802.
117. Thompson, L.F. and Mayhan, K.G. (1972) The plasma polymerization of vinyl monomers. II. A detailed study of the plasma polymerization of styrene. *J. Appl. Polym. Sci.*, **16** (9), 2317–2341.
118. Clark, D.T., Dilks, A., and Shuttleworth, D. (1978) *Polymer Surfaces*, John Wiley & Sons, Inc., New York.
119. Oehr, C., Muller, M., Elkin, B., Hegemann, D., and Vohrer, U. (1999) Plasma grafting – a method to obtain monofunctional surfaces. *Surf. Coat. Technol.*, **116–119**, 25–35.
120. Yang, H.S., Park, K., Ahn, K.D., Kim, B.S., and Han, D.K. (2006) Optimal hydrophilization and chondrocyte adhesion of PLLA films and scaffolds by plasma treatment and acrylic acid grafting. *Polym. Korea*, **30** (2), 168–174.
121. Gupta, B., Hillborn, J.G., Bisson, I., and Frey, P. (2001) Plasma-induced graft polymerization of acrylic acid onto poly(ethylene terephthalate) films. *J. Appl. Polym. Sci.*, **81** (12), 2993–3001.
122. Vreuls, C., Zocchi, G., Thierry, B., Garitte, G., Griesser, S.S., Archambeau, C., Van de Weerdt, C., Martial, J., and Griesser, H. (2010) Prevention of bacterial biofilms by covalent immobilization of peptides onto plasma polymer functionalized substrates. *J. Mater. Chem.*, **20** (37), 8092–8098.
123. Coad, B.R., Jasieniak, M., Griesser, S.S., and Griesser, H.J. (2013) Controlled covalent surface immobilisation of proteins and peptides using plasma methods. *Surf. Coat. Technol.*, **233**, 169–177.
124. Cole, M.A., Voelcker, N.H., Thissen, H., and Griesser, H.J. (2009) Stimuli-responsive interfaces and systems for the control of protein-surface and cell–surface interactions. *Biomaterials*, **30** (9), 1827–1850.
125. Xia, Y., Boey, F., and Venkatraman, S.S. (2010) Surface modification of poly(L-lactic acid) with biomolecules to promote endothelialization. *Biointerfaces*, **5** (3), FA32–FA40.
126. Williams, S.K. (1995) Endothelial cell transplantation. *Cell Transplant.*, **4** (4), 401–410.
127. McGuigan, A.P. and Sefton, M.V. (2007) The influence of biomaterials

on endothelial cell thrombogenicity. *Biomaterials*, **28** (16), 2547–2571.

128. Peter, S., Graupner, K., Grambole, D., and Richter, F. (2007) Comparative experimental analysis of the a-C:H deposition processes using CH4 and C2H2 as precursors. *J. Appl. Phys.*, **102** (5), 053304.

129. Butter, R., Allen, M., Chandra, L., Lettington, A.H., and Rushton, N. (1995) In vitro studies of DLC coatings with silicon intermediate layer. *Diamond Relat. Mater.*, **4** (5–6), 857–861.

130. Hauert, R., Müller, U., Francz, G., Birchler, F., Schroeder, A., Mayer, J., and Wintermantel, E. (1997) Surface analysis and bioreactions of F and Si containing a-C:H. *Thin Solid Films*, **308–309**, 191–194.

131. Linder, S., Pinkowski, W., and Aepfelbacher, M. (2002) Adhesion, cytoskeletal architecture and activation status of primary human macrophages on a diamond-like carbon coated surface. *Biomaterials*, **23** (3), 767–773.

132. Maguire, P.D., McLaughlin, J.A., Okpalugo, T.I.T., Lemoine, P., Papakonstantinou, P., McAdams, E.T., Needham, M., Ogwu, A.A., Ball, M., and Abbas, G.A. (2005) Mechanical stability, corrosion performance and bioresponse of amorphous diamond-like carbon for medical stents and guidewires. *Diamond Relat. Mater.*, **14** (8), 1277–1288.

133. Krishnan, L.K., Varghese, N., Muraleedharan, C.V., Bhuvaneshwar, G.S., Derangère, F., Sampeur, Y., and Suryanarayanan, R. (2002) Quantitation of platelet adhesion to Ti and DLC-coated Ti in vitro using 125I-labeled platelets. *Biomol. Eng.*, **19** (2–6), 251–253.

134. Hasebe, T., Matsuoka, Y., Kodama, H., Saito, T., Yohena, S., Kamijo, A., Shiraga, N., Higuchi, M., Kuribayashi, S., Takahashi, K., and Suzuki, T. (2006) Lubrication performance of diamond-like carbon and fluorinated diamond-like carbon coatings for intravascular guidewires. *Diamond Relat. Mater.*, **15** (1), 129–132.

135. Okpalugo, T.I.T., Ogwu, A.A., Maguire, P.D., and McLaughlin, J.A.D. (2004) Platelet adhesion on silicon modified hydrogenated amorphous carbon films. *Biomaterials*, **25** (2), 239–245.

136. Saito, T., Hasebe, T., Yohena, S., Matsuoka, Y., Kamijo, A., Takahashi, K., and Suzuki, T. (2005) Antithrombogenicity of fluorinated diamond-like carbon films. *Diamond Relat. Mater.*, **14** (3–7), 1116–1119.

137. Logothetidis, S., Gioti, M., Lousinian, S., and Fotiadou, S. (2005) Haemocompatibility studies on carbon-based thin films by ellipsometry. *Thin Solid Films*, **482** (1–2), 126–132.

138. Lopez-Santos, C., Colaux, J.L., Laloy, J., Fransolet, M., Mullier, F., Michiels, C., Dogné, J.M., and Lucas, S. (2013) Bioactivity and hemocompatibility study of amorphous hydrogenated carbon coatings produced by pulsed magnetron discharge. *J. Biomed. Mater. Res. Part A*, **101A** (6), 1800–1812.

139. Hasebe, T., Ishimaru, T., Kamijo, A., Yoshimoto, Y., Yoshimura, T., Yohena, S., Kodama, H., Hotta, A., Takahashi, K., and Suzuki, T. (2007) Effects of surface roughness on anti-thrombogenicity of diamond-like carbon films. *Diamond Relat. Mater.*, **16** (4–7), 1343–1348.

140. Kwok, S.C.H., Wang, J., and Chu, P.K. (2005) Surface energy, wettability, and blood compatibility phosphorus doped diamond-like carbon films. *Diamond Relat. Mater.*, **14** (1), 78–85.

141. Roy, R.K. and Lee, K.-R. (2007) Biomedical applications of diamond-like carbon coatings: a review. *J. Biomed. Mater. Res. Part B*, **83B** (1), 72–84.

142. Hauert, R., Thorwarth, K., and Thorwarth, G. (2013) An overview on diamond-like carbon coatings in medical applications. *Surf. Coat. Technol.*, **233**, 119–130.

143. Orlanda, F.L., Yi, J.W., Moon, M.-W., Ahmed, S.F., Kim, H., Cha, T.-G., Kim, H.-Y., Kim, S.-S., and Lee, K.-R. (2010) Long-lasting hydrophilicity on nanostructured Si-incorporated diamond-like carbon films. *Langmuir*, **26** (22), 17203–17209.

144. Ahmed, M.H., Byrne, J.A., McLaughlin, J.A.D., Elhissi, A., and Ahmed, W. (2013) Comparison between FTIR and XPS characterization of amino acid

glycine adsorption onto diamond-like carbon (DLC) and silicon doped DLC. *Appl. Surf. Sci.*, **273**, 507–514.

145. Chou, C.-C., Wu, Y.-Y., Lee, J.-W., Yeh, C.-H., and Huang, J.-C. (2013) Characterization and haemocompatibility of fluorinated DLC and Si interlayer on Ti6Al4V. *Surf. Coat. Technol.*, **231**, 418–422.
146. Hauert, R. (2003) A review of modified DLC coatings for biological applications. *Diamond Relat. Mater.*, **12** (3–7), 583–589.
147. Ahmed, M.H., Byrne, J.A., McLaughlin, J., and Ahmed, W. (2013) Study of human serum albumin adsorption and conformational change on DLC and silicon doped DLC using XPS and FTIR spectroscopy. *J. Biomater. Nanobiotechnol.*, **4** (02), 194–203.
148. Ahmed, M.H., Byrne, J.A., and McLaughlin, J. (2012) Evaluation of glycine adsorption on diamond like carbon (DLC) and fluorinated DLC deposited by plasma-enhanced chemical vapour deposition (PECVD). *Surf. Coat. Technol.*, **209**, 8–14.
149. Ohgoe, Y., Hiratsuka, M., Sumikura, H., Fukunaga, K., Homma, A., Hirakuri, K.K., Funakubo, A., and Fukui, Y. (2013) Improved hemolytic performance of blood pump with fluorine-doped hydrogenated amorphous carbon coating. *Adv. Chem. Eng. Sci.*, **3** (03), 10–16.
150. Shiba, K., Ohgoe, Y., Hirakuri, K., Mizuno, J., Shoji, S., Ozeki, K., Sato, K., Fukata, N., and Alanazi, A. (2014) Hemocompatibility of DLC coating for blood analysis devices. 2014 International Conference on Electronics Packaging (ICEP), April 23–25, 2014, pp. 748–751.
151. Roy, R.K., Choi, H.W., Yi, J.W., Moon, M.W., Lee, K.R., Han, D.K., Shin, J.H., Kamijo, A., and Hasebe, T. (2009) Hemocompatibility of surface-modified, silicon-incorporated, diamond-like carbon films. *Acta Biomater.*, **5** (1), 249–256.
152. Yi, J.W., Moon, M.-W., Ahmed, S.F., Kim, H., Cha, T.-G., Kim, H.-Y., Kim, S.-S., and Lee, K.-R. (2010) Long-lasting hydrophilicity on nanostructured Si-incorporated diamond-like carbon films. *Langmuir*, **26** (22), 17203–17209.
153. Marciano, F.R., Bonetti, L.F., Mangolin, J.F., Da-Silva, N.S., Corat, E.J., and Trava-Airoldi, V.J. (2011) Investigation into the antibacterial property and bacterial adhesion of diamond-like carbon films. *Vacuum*, **85** (6), 662–666.
154. Lee, F.-P., Wang, D.-J., Chen, L.-K., Kung, C.-M., Wu, Y.-C., Ou, K.-L., and Yu, C.-H. (2013) Antibacterial nanostructured composite films for biomedical applications: microstructural characteristics, biocompatibility, and antibacterial mechanisms. *Biofouling*, **29** (3), 295–305.
155. Ren, D.W., Zhao, Q., and Bendavid, A. (2013) Anti-bacterial property of Si and F doped diamond-like carbon coatings. *Surf. Coat. Technol.*, **226**, 1–6.
156. Del-Prado, G., Pascual, F.-J., Terriza, A., Molina-Manso, D., Yubero, F., Puertolas, J.-A., Gomez-Barren, E., and Esteban, J. (2014) Staphylococcal biofilm formation on diamond-like carbon-coated UHMWPEs: a first approach. *Bone Joint J. Orthop. Proc. Suppl.*, **96** (Suppl. 11), 84.
157. Lan, W.-C., Ou, S.-F., Lin, M.-H., Ou, K.-L., and Tsai, M.-Y. (2013) Development of silver-containing diamond-like carbon for biomedical applications. Part I: microstructure characteristics, mechanical properties and antibacterial mechanisms. *Ceram. Int.*, **39** (4), 4099–4104.
158. Dearnaley, G. and Arps, J.H. (2005) Biomedical applications of diamond-like carbon (DLC) coatings: a review. *Surf. Coat. Technol.*, **200** (7), 2518–2524.
159. Grill, A. (2003) Diamond-like carbon coatings as biocompatible materials—an overview. *Diamond Relat. Mater.*, **12** (2), 166–170.
160. Wang, M., Zhao, Y., Xu, R., Zhang, M., Fu, R.K.Y., and Chu, P.K. (2013) Direct formation of amine functionality on DLC films and surface cyto-compatibility. *Diamond Relat. Mater.*, **38**, 28–31.
161. Ali, E. and Christophe, D. (2006) Tribology of diamond-like carbon films: recent progress and future

prospects. *J. Phys. D: Appl. Phys.*, **39** (18), R311–R327.

162. Liu, J., Wang, X., Wu, B.J., Zhang, T.F., Leng, Y.X., and Huang, N. (2013) Tribocorrosion behavior of DLC-coated CoCrMo alloy in simulated biological environment. *Vacuum*, **92**, 39–43.

163. Escudeiro, A., Polcar, T., and Cavaleiro, A. (2014) Adsorption of bovine serum albumin on Zr co-sputtered a-C(:H) films: implication on wear behaviour. *J. Mech. Behav. Biomed. Mater.*, **39**, 316–327.

164. Wang, L., Su, J.F., and Nie, X. (2010) Corrosion and tribological properties and impact fatigue behaviors of TiN- and DLC-coated stainless steels in a simulated body fluid environment. *Surf. Coat. Technol.*, **205** (5), 1599–1605.

165. Thorwarth, K., Thorwarth, G., Figi, R., Weisse, B., Stiefel, M., and Hauert, R. (2014) On interlayer stability and high-cycle simulator performance of diamond-like carbon layers for articulating joint replacements. *Int. J. Mol. Sci.*, **15** (6), 10527–10540.

166. Franta, L., Fojt, J., Joska, L., Kronek, J., Cvrcek, L., Vyskocil, J., and Cejka, Z. (2013) Hinge-type knee prosthesis wear tests with a mechanical load and corrosion properties monitoring. *Tribol. Int.*, **63**, 61–65.

167. Xu, Z.Y., Zheng, Y.J., Sun, H., Yong-xiang, L., and Huang, N. (2012) Numerical and experimental study of residual stress of multilayer diamond-like carbon films prepared by filtered cathodic vacuum arc deposition. *IEEE Trans. Plasma Sci.*, **40** (9), 2261–2266.

168. Sahoo, S., Pradhan, S.K., Jeevitha, M., Bagchi, S., and Barhai, P.K. (2014) A study of diamond like carbon/chromium films deposited by microwave plasma activated chemical vapor deposition. *J. Non-Cryst. Solids*, **386**, 14–18.

169. Taeger, G., Podleska, L.E., Schmidt, B., Ziegler, M., and Nast-Kolb, D. (2003) Comparison of diamond-like-carbon and alumina-oxide articulating with polyethylene in total hip arthroplasty. *Materialwiss. Werkstofftech.*, **34** (12), 1094–1100.

170. Joyce, T.J. (2007) Examination of failed ex vivo metal-on-metal metatarsophalangeal prosthesis and comparison with theoretically determined lubrication regimes. *Wear*, **263** (7–12), 1050–1054.

171. Hauert, R., Thorwarth, G., Müller, U., Stiefel, M., Falub, C.V., Thorwarth, K., and Joyce, T.J. (2012) Analysis of the in-vivo failure of the adhesive interlayer for a DLC coated articulating metatarsophalangeal joint. *Diamond Relat. Mater.*, **25**, 34–39.

172. Mikhalovska, L., Chorna, N., Lazarenko, O., Haworth, P., Sudre, A., and Mikhalovsky, S. (2011) Inorganic coatings for cardiovascular stents: in vitro and in vivo studies. *J. Biomed. Mater. Res. Part B*, **96B** (2), 333–341.

173. Seo, D.H., Rider, A.E., Kumar, S., Randeniya, L.K., and Ostrikov, K. (2013) Vertical graphene gas- and bio-sensors via catalyst-free, reactive plasma reforming of natural honey. *Carbon*, **60**, 221–228.

174. Seo, D.H., Han, Z.J., Kumar, S., and Ostrikov, K. (2013) Structure-controlled, vertical graphene-based, binder-free electrodes from plasma-reformed butter enhance supercapacitor performance. *Adv. Energy Mater.*, **3** (10), 1316–1323.

175. Jacob, M.V., Rawat, R.S., Ouyang, B., Bazaka, K., Kumar, D.S., Taguchi, D., Iwamoto, M., Neupane, R., and Varghese, O.K. (2015) Catalyst-free plasma enhanced growth of graphene from sustainable sources. *Nano Lett.*, **15** (9), 5702–5708.

176. Hu, W., Peng, C., Luo, W., Lv, M., Li, X., Li, D., Huang, Q., and Fan, C. (2010) Graphene-based antibacterial paper. *ACS Nano*, **4** (7), 4317–4323.

177. Liu, S., Zeng, T.H., Hofmann, M., Burcombe, E., Wei, J., Jiang, R., Kong, J., and Chen, Y. (2011) Antibacterial activity of graphite, graphite oxide, graphene oxide, and reduced graphene oxide: membrane and oxidative stress. *ACS Nano*, **5** (9), 6971–6980.

178. Gurunathan, S., Han, J., Dayem, A., Eppakayala, V., and Kim, J. (2012) Oxidative stress-mediated antibacterial activity of graphene oxide and reduced

graphene oxide in Pseudomonas aeruginosa. *Int. J. Nanomed.*, **2012** (7), 5901–5914.

179. Kumar, S., Mehdipour, H., and Ostrikov, K. (2013) Plasma-enabled graded nanotube biosensing arrays on a Si nanodevice platform: catalyst-free integration and in situ detection of nucleation events. *Adv. Mater.*, **25** (1), 69–74.

180. Ryoo, S.-R., Kim, Y.-K., Kim, M.-H., and Min, D.-H. (2010) Behaviors of NIH-3T3 fibroblasts on graphene/carbon nanotubes: proliferation, focal adhesion, and gene transfection studies. *ACS Nano*, **4** (11), 6587–6598.

181. Nayak, T.R., Andersen, H., Makam, V.S., Khaw, C., Bae, S., Xu, X., Ee, P.-L.R., Ahn, J.-H., Hong, B.H., Pastorin, G., and Özyilmaz, B. (2011) Graphene for controlled and accelerated osteogenic differentiation of human mesenchymal stem cells. *ACS Nano*, **5** (6), 4670–4678.

182. Li, N., Zhang, X., Song, Q., Su, R., Zhang, Q., Kong, T., Liu, L., Jin, G., Tang, M., and Cheng, G. (2011) The promotion of neurite sprouting and outgrowth of mouse hippocampal cells in culture by graphene substrates. *Biomaterials*, **32** (35), 9374–9382.

183. Patole, A.S., Patole, S.P., Jung, S.-Y., Yoo, J.-B., An, J.-H., and Kim, T.-H. (2012) Self assembled graphene/carbon nanotube/polystyrene hybrid nanocomposite by in situ microemulsion polymerization. *Eur. Polym. J.*, **48** (2), 252–259.

184. Fan, H., Wang, L., Zhao, K., Li, N., Shi, Z., Ge, Z., and Jin, Z. (2010) Fabrication, mechanical properties, and biocompatibility of graphene-reinforced chitosan composites. *Biomacromolecules*, **11** (9), 2345–2351.

185. Wang, J., Wang, C.-F., and Chen, S. (2012) Amphiphilic egg-derived carbon dots: rapid plasma fabrication, pyrolysis process, and multicolor printing patterns. *Angew. Chem. Int. Ed.*, **51** (37), 9297–9301.

186. Zhou, J., Booker, C., Li, R., Zhou, X., Sham, T.-K., Sun, X., and Ding, Z. (2007) An electrochemical avenue to blue luminescent nanocrystals from multiwalled carbon nanotubes (MWCNTs). *J. Am. Chem. Soc.*, **129** (4), 744–745.

5
Smart Electroactive Polymers and Composite Materials

T.P.D. Rajan and J. Mary Gladis

5.1
Introduction

Electroactive polymers (EAPs) are polymeric materials whose shapes are modified when a voltage is applied to them. They can be used as actuators or sensors. As actuators, they are characterized by the fact that they can undergo a large amount of deformation while sustaining large forces. Due to the similarities with biological tissues in terms of achievable stress and force, they are often called *artificial muscles*, and have the potential for application in the field of robotics, where large linear movement is often needed. When certain types of EAPs are physically flexed, they produce a voltage output. This effect allows EAPs to be used as potential sensors in various types of equipment. With the inherent flexible and durable nature of EAPs, long sensor life is expected. EAPs such as ionic polymer metal composites (IPMCs) are active materials that exhibit interesting bidirectional electromechanical coupling phenomena; for example, by bending an IPMC strip, a voltage output is obtained, while a voltage input is able to cause the strip to bend. Thus, they are also large motion sensors. The output voltage can be calibrated for a standard-size sensor and correlated to the applied loads or stresses. EAPs can be manufactured and cut into any size and shape. For example, for a structural health monitoring of a huge motor bridge against all vibrational, aerodynamics, or natural disturbances, a completely integrated and distributed computer controlled package of quickly installed, user-friendly IPMC sensor elements numbering 100 000 are required.

EAPs are a relatively new class of materials that can be used both as sensors and actuators. Conductive polymers (CP) and ionic metal polymer composites (IPMC) are categorized as electroactive polymeric materials that exhibit interesting sensing and actuating behaviors. They are among the best candidates for use in solar cells, sensors, and actuators (Otero and Teresa, 2001; Wallace *et al.*, 2003 [1, 2]), due to their (i) large strains of up to 39%, (ii) biocompatibility, (iii) micro- and nanoscale manufacturing feasibility and, (iv) relatively low actuation voltages; Jager *et al.*, 2000; Shahinpoor *et al.*, 2007; Hara *et al.*, 2005; Carpi and Smela, 2009 [3–8]. The possibility of tailoring the properties and the microstructure of EAPs,

Biomedical Applications of Polymeric Materials and Composites, First Edition.
Edited by Raju Francis and Sakthi Kumar.

allows new and challenging applications in the biomedical area both in device applications and in inducing targeted cell responses. EAPs are candidate materials for state-of-the-art applications in an array of devices ranging from biomedical appliances through artificial organs to micro-electromechanical systems (MEMS).

5.2
Types of Electroactive Polymers

EAPs can be classified into two major categories, namely, the ionic EAPs which are activated by an electrically induced transport of ions or molecules and the electronic EAPs which are activated by an external electric field and by coulombian forces. The ionic EAPs are polymer gels, conducting polymers, and ion polymer metal composites (IPMC). These materials can be activated by very low voltages (1 – 5 V) and can be operated only within a surrounding electrolyte medium. The electronic EAP are piezoelectric polymers, electrostrictive polymers, and dielectric elastomers (DEs).

5.3
Polymer Gels

Stimuli-responsive polymers and gels that swell or shrink in response to environmental changes have been developed and find application in biomimetic actuators or artificial muscles. They are expected to act as soft actuators because not only are they light, soft, and flexible materials, but they can also generate biomimetic motion without using mechanical parts such as motors and drive shafts, gears, and so on. Following the observation of volume phase transition of polymer gels by Tanaka [9], they have been used for application in various fields such as drug delivery systems, robotic hands, and transporting devices. The phase transition of polymer gel is induced by hydrogen bonds, coulomb, hydrophobic, and van der Waals interactions (Shingo *et al.*, 2010 [10]). Thus, by changing the external physicochemical conditions, these applications can be controlled. A major example is poly(*N*-isopropylacrylamide) (PNIPAAm), which is thermo-sensitive and undergoes a discontinuous volume change. In application, a microfluidic device using MEMS technology and PNIPAAm, could adsorb proteins from solution and release them due to the adsorption change of PNIPAAm by controlling resistive heating [11].

Gels exhibit a unique capability of undergoing spontaneous volume changes in response to oscillatory chemical reactions. For example, gels can undergo rhythmic swelling and shrinking in response to variations in the pH of the surrounding solution caused by an oscillating reaction. The pH oscillations were generated by the Landolt reaction [12] or by an enzymatic reaction [13]. Periodical volume changes were also observed in a pH-responsive gel, which exhibited bistability with diffusion of a reactive substrate into the gel [14]. In all these studies, the cause of the complex behaviors was outside of the gels.

The self-motion of the gel is produced by the dissipating chemical energy of the oscillatory Belousov–Zhabotinsky (BZ) reaction [15]. The BZ reaction is the most commonly known oscillating reactions. The overall process is the oxidation of an organic substrate such as citric or malonic acid by an oxidizing agent (bromate) in the presence of a metal catalyst under acidic condition. Metal ions or metal complexes with high redox potentials, such as cerium ion, ferroin, or ruthenium tris(2,2′-bipyridine) are widely used as catalysts. During the course of the reaction, the catalyst ion periodically changes its charge number to oscillate between the oxidized and reduced states for several hours as long as the substrate exists.

In an oscillating gel system, the polymer network itself takes part in the BZ reaction, because the metal catalyst is covalently bounded to the polymer chain. As a result, the reaction medium can change in time and space. In other words, the BZ reaction induces the structural changes. When the redox state of the metal catalyst moiety in the gel changed, the solubility of the polymer chain changed as well. As a result, the change in the osmotic pressure inside the gel causes the swelling or shrinking of the polymer gel. The displacement of the self-oscillating gel is several dozen micrometers [15] as shown in Figure 5.1. However, the mechanical displacement of the gel was too small to design the gel actuator. Therefore, in order to construct gel actuators, the displacement of the gel has to be improved greatly.

For realizing the large deformation of the gel, a gradient structure is introduced into the gel by Maeda *et al.* [16]. In order to make the gradient structure in the gel, the hydrophobic interaction between the $Ru(bpy)_3{}^{2+}$ moiety and the casting mold during the polymerization is used. As a result, the large deformation of the self-oscillating gel was achieved. During polymerization, the monomer solution faces two different surfaces of plates: a hydrophilic glass surface and a hydrophobic, Teflon surface. Since $Ru(bpy)_3{}^{2+}$ monomer is hydrophobic, it migrates easily to the Teflon surface side. As a result, a uniform distribution in the direction of the thickness is formed for the component, and the resulting gel has a gradient distribution for the content of each component in the polymer network. Thus, the hydrophilic 2-acrylamido-2-methylpropanesulfonic acid (AMPS) component at the glass side was higher than that at the Teflon side. In contrast, the hydrophobic $Ru(bpy)_3{}^{2+}$ moiety at the Teflon side was higher than that at the glass side. Therefore, as for the gel at the AMPS-rich side, the swelling ratio was higher than that at the opposite side (at the $Ru(bpy)_3{}^{2+}$ rich side). Consequently, the gel in the

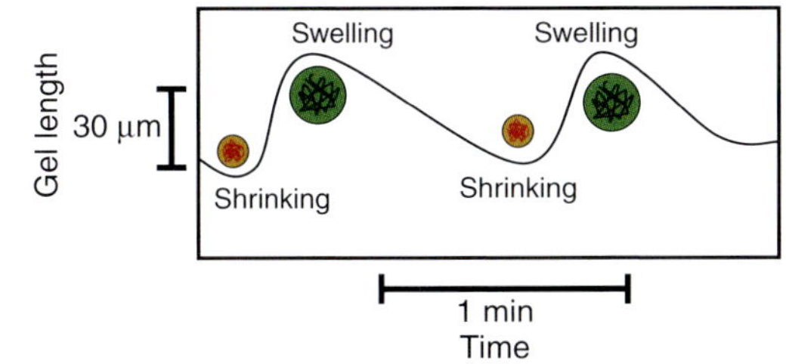

Figure 5.1 Conventional self-oscillating gel.

water bends to the direction of the surface which was made to face the Teflon plate during polymerization.

The development of stimuli-responsive gels was largely focused on their potential use as muscle-like actuators driven by chemicals, electric fields, or by electrochemical reactions. More recent work has addressed the development of drug delivery systems, micro fluidic components and circuits, sensors, biosensors, optical components, active membranes for separation, smart surfaces, and scaffolds for tissue engineering.

Hydrogels are hydrophilic macromolecular networks that swell in water or biological fluids. Hydrogels have been used in numerous biomedical disciplines, in ophthalmology as contact lenses and in surgery as absorbable sutures, as well as in many other areas of clinical practice to cure such illnesses as diabetes mellitus, osteoporosis, asthma, heart diseases and neoplasms. Poly-2-hydroxyethyl methacrylate is the first hydrogel synthesized by Lim and Wichterle, which is commonly used in contact lens production [17]. The main advantage of hydrogel is its stability under varying pH, temperature, and tonicity conditions. Hydrogel is considered to be a material that is produced when a water-insoluble polymer absorbs a large amount of water, or else it is simply a water-swollen polymer network. Chemical hydrogels are prepared either by cross-linking water-soluble polymers or by converting hydrophobic polymers into hydrophilic polymers that are then cross-linked to form a network. Cross-linking may be either physical (e.g., hydrogen bonding) or chemical (covalent, atomic, ionic).

The swelling of hydrogels is quite a complicated process and consists of a number of steps. In the first step, water molecules entering the hydrogel matrix hydrate the most polar, hydrophilic groups. This results in the appearance of primary bound water. In the second step, hydrophobic groups are exposed, and they interact with water molecules giving the so-called hydrophobically bound water or secondary bound water. Primary and secondary bound water together form the total bound water. In the third step, because the covalent or physical cross-links resist the osmotic driving force of the network toward infinite dilution, an additional amount of water is absorbed. The water absorbed up to the equilibrium swelling level is called bulk water or free water; it fills the space between the network chains and the centers of larger pores, macropores, or voids. The total amount of water absorbed by a hydrogel depends on the temperature and the specific interaction between the water molecules and polymer chains. Poly(hydroxyethyl methacrylate) (polyHEMA, PHEMA) (Figure 5.2) is one of the most important and most widely applied hydrogel biomaterials.

Poly(ethylene glycol) (PEG), is one of the most widely used hydrogels in medicine. PEG-based hydrogels are characterized by their high biocompatibility, lack of toxic influence on the surrounding tissue, and solubility in water, which makes them good candidates for drug delivery system applications. PEG hydrogel drug release systems are stimuli-sensitive and react in the presence of a physical or chemical agent [18]. Physical stimuli include temperature, solvent, light, radiation, pressure, and a magnetic, acoustic, or electrical field, while the chemical and biological stimuli include pH, specific ions, and molecular

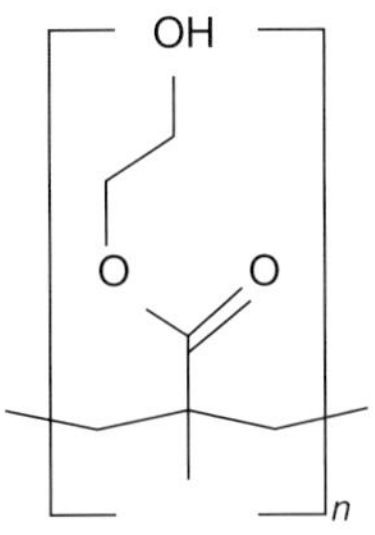

Figure 5.2 Poly(hydroxyethyl methacrylate).

recognition events. Polyvinyl alcohol (PVA)-based hydrogels are distinguished by their good mechanical properties and their ability to retain water in the structure, which ensures a prolonged moist environment. Other common hydrogels are polyvinylpyrrolidone, polyimide, polyacrylate, and polyurethane.

5.4 Conducting Polymers

Conducting polymers are conjugated polymers, namely organic compounds that have an extended p-orbital system, through which electrons can move from one end of the polymer to the other. Conducting polymers contain (π-electron backbone responsible for their unusual electronic properties such as electrical conductivity, low energy optical transitions, low ionization potential, and high electron affinity. This extended (π-conjugated system of the conducting polymers have single and double bonds alternating along the polymer chain. Electrochemical synthesis is rapidly becoming the preferred general method for preparing electrically conducting polymers because of its simplicity and reproducibility. The advantage of electrochemical polymerization is that the reactions can be carried out at room temperature. By varying either the potential or current with time the thickness of the film can be controlled. The great advantage of conductive polymers is that their chemical, electrical, and physical properties can be tailored to the specific needs of their application by incorporating antibodies, enzymes, and other biological moieties. Structures of common conducting polymers are given in Figure 5.3 and the conductivities in Table 5.1.

Electrochemical polymerization of conducting polymers is generally employed by: (i) constant current or galvanostatic; (ii) constant potential or potentiostatic; (iii) potential scanning/cycling or sweeping methods. Standard electrochemical technique that employs a divided cell containing a working electrode, a counter electrode, and a reference electrode generally produces the best films. The commonly used anodes are chromium, gold, nickel, palladium, titanium, platinum, and indium-tin oxide coated glass plates.

The most studied conductive polymer, as evidenced by the amount of literature published on its properties and applications, is the conjugated polymer polypyrrole (PPy). It has good *in vitro* and *in vivo* biocompatibility [21], good chemical

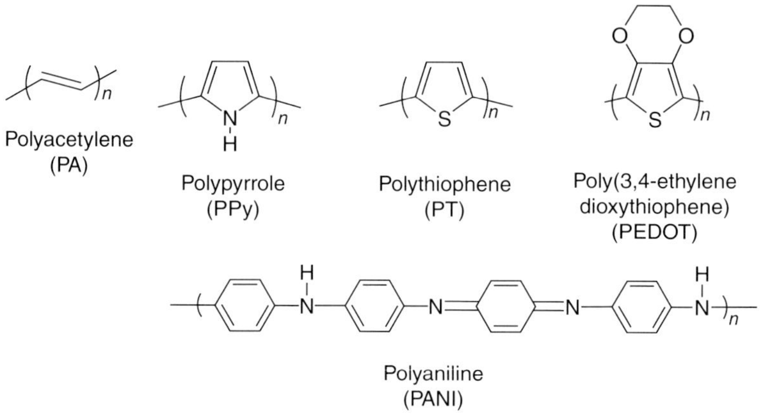

Figure 5.3 Structures of common conducting polymers.

Table 5.1 Conductivity of common CPs.[a)]

Conducting polymer	Maximum conductivity ($S\ cm^{-1}$)[b)]	Type of doping
Polyacetylene (PA)	200–1000	n,p
Polyparaphenylene (PPP)	500	n,p
Polyparaphenylene sulfide (PPS)	3–300	p
Polyparavinylene (PPv)	1–1000	p
Polypyrrole (PPy)	40–200	p
Polythiophene (PT)	10–100	p
Polyisothionaphthene (PITN)	1–50	p
Polyaniline (PANI)	5	n,p

a) Reproduced from [19, 20].
b) S = Siemens.

stability in, for example, air and water, and reasonably high conductivity under physiological conditions. PPy can be easily and flexibly synthesized in large quantities at room temperature in a wide range of solvents, including water. PPy is also stimulus-responsive, allowing the dynamic control of its properties by the application of an electrical potential.

Optimizing the material properties (e.g., roughness, porosity, hydrophobicity, conductivity, degradability) of conductive polymers and the binding of biological molecules (that makes conductive polymers so promising for biomedical applications) can be done by four major chemical ways, namely, through adsorption, by entrapping the molecule inside the polymer, by covalently bonding the molecule to the monomer of the polymer, and by exploiting the very doping process that renders conductive polymers conductive.

A wide range of biologically important molecules have been used to improve the bioactivity of PPy: for example, dermatan sulphate was used to increase keratinocyte viability, heparin was incorporated to promote endothelial cell proliferation, doping with laminin-derived peptides aided in neuron and astrocyte adhesion, NGF and poly-L-glutamic acid enhanced neuronal growth, while HA and CS were used for skeletal myoblast growth and differentiation [22].

5.5 Ionic Polymer–Metal Composites (IPMC)

An IPMC generally consists of a thin backbone polyelectrolyte membrane with noble metal electrodes chemically plated on both of its faces, and neutralized using the necessary amount of cations to balance the negative charges of the anions that are covalently fixed to the backbone ionomer. When the IPMC is hydrated, the positive ions in the Nafion polymer, such as sodium and calcium ions, bring water molecules, and migrate to the cathode side under an electric field, whereas the negative ions are permanently fixed to the carbon chain [23]. The ion transportation and water migration introduce swelling in the cathode side and shrinking in the anode side, which eventually cause the bending motion of the IPMC [24]. Figure 5.4 shows the typical mechanism of ionic polymer–metal composites.

When a strip of IPMC sample in the hydrated state is stimulated by a small (1–2 V) alternating current (AC), it shows a large bending vibration at the applied frequency. When the same IPMC membrane is suddenly bent, a small voltage of the order of millivolts is generated across its surface. Thus, IPMCs can serve as soft actuators and sensors [25]. IPMCs may have certain advantages over some of the traditional electroactive materials. They require only a modest operating voltage (1–2 V), show relatively fast responses (tenths of Hz), generate large bending tip displacements (up to 10% of the gauge length), have intrinsic sensor–actuator capabilities, and are light in weight, compact in design, and can operate in liquid or open air. Using these features, various prototype designs have been investigated

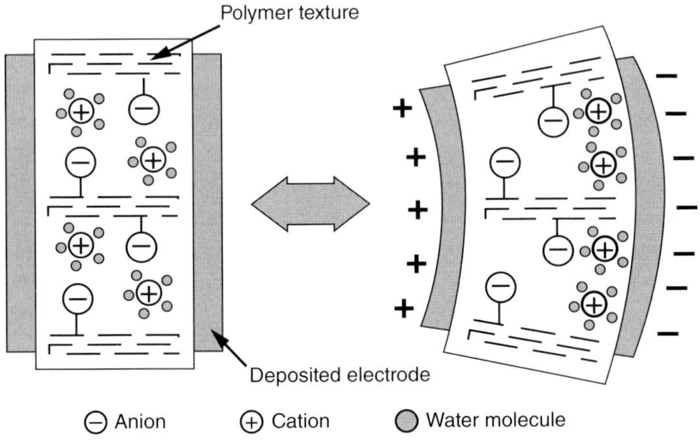

Figure 5.4 Mechanism of ionic polymer–metal composites.

for potential applications in the fields of micro-robotics [26], artificial muscles [3], biomedical devices [5], and control systems. Examples include robotic fingers and grippers for planetary missions, catheter tips for intravascular neurosurgery, a dust wiper developed for the Nanorover's camera window [27], and a robotic fish that can swim in water (EAMEX Corporation).

The ion-exchange reaction can be tailored in order to obtain IPMCs in a desired combined-cation form. For IPMCs in various Na–TBA cation compositions, the actuation behaviors as well as other physical properties show remarkable variations from those of the pure Na+-form to those of the pure TBA+-form. The duration of the initial bending toward the anode, and the subsequent relaxation toward the cathode of Nafion-based IPMCs can be controlled by properly adjusting the corresponding cation content. For Nafion-based IPMCs in the Na–TBA combined-cation forms, the actuation activities can be greatly improved. The actuation deformation of Flemion-based IPMCs is linearly related to the amount of charge accumulation at the cathode boundary. The time variation of the electromechanical response of an IPMC can be controlled by the application of electric fields with suitable time variation. Various DC and AC electric functions have been used to actuate IPMCs. By applying a slowly increasing potential field, the Nafion-based IPMCs' initial displacement toward the anode can be controlled and actually eliminated.

5.6
Conjugated Polymer

Conjugated polymers are electroactive polymers and have found applications as artificial muscles. Conventional polymers, plastics, have been used traditionally because of their attractive chemical, mechanical, and electrically insulating properties, and not for their electronic properties. Although the idea of using polymers for their electrically conducting properties dates back at least to the 1960s, the use of organic n-conjugated a polymers as electronic materials in molecular-based electronics is relatively new. While behaving as insulators or semiconductors in the pristine form, conjugated polymers can reach metallic-like electrical conductivity when doped (in chemical terminology, when oxidized or reduced).

The charge transport of conjugated polymers has been studied for nearly two decades. Early work focused on developing conjugated polymers as plastic conductors and tried to increase the conductivity to that of inorganic metals. This was accomplished by highly doping the polymer and stretch orienting the films. Polyacetylene, polyaniline, and polythiophene were the predominant polymers studied for conductor applications. More recently, conjugated polymers are finding use in perhaps the area of highest activity to date for these materials, that of electronic applications. In particular, conjugated polymers as well as n-conjugated oligomers play a central role in organic-based transistors and integrated circuits, photovoltaic devices, especially in organic-based light emitting devices. Even solid-state lasers are under development.

In conjugated polymers, there exists a continuous network, often a simple chain, of adjacent unsaturated carbon atoms, that is, carbon atoms in the sp^2 (or sp) hybridized state. Each of these sp^2 C-atoms has three p-bonds, and a remaining pz atomic orbital that exhibits n-overlap with the pz-orbitals of the nearest neighbor, the sp^2 hybridized C-atoms. This chain of atoms with n-overlap of the atomic pz-orbitals leads to the formation of n-states delocalized along the polymer chain. In a system with one-dimensional periodicity, these n-states form the frontier electronic bands, with an n-band gap, E' (n)(E' (p), accounting for optical absorption at lower photon energies. The essential properties of the delocalized n-electron system, which differentiate a typical conjugated polymer from a conventional polymer with p-bands, are as follows: (i) the electronic band gap, E', is relatively small (1 – 4 eV), leading to low-energy electronic excitations and semiconductor behavior; (ii) the polymer chains can be rather easily oxidized or reduced, usually through charge transfer with molecular dopant species; (iii) carrier mobilities are large enough that high electrical conductivities are realized in the doped (chemically oxidized or reduced) state; and (iv) charge carrying species are not free electrons or holes, but quasi-particles, which may move relatively freely through the material, or at least along uninterrupted polymer chains. Although both positively and negatively charged species can exist, mostly negatively charged species formed by the addition of electrons are discussed, because these species are directly accessible through photoelectron spectroscopy (while hole states are not easily studied by photoelectron spectroscopy). Finally, since few polymers are crystalline, macroscopic electrical conductivity in finite samples requires hopping between chains.

Blood vessel connecters, which are used during surgery to connect the blood vessel quickly, are developed using the conjugated polymer of PPy/Au bilayer. The blood vessel connecter is made by rolling up a micro-fabricated PPy bilayer into a cylinder by applying the reduced potential. The tube is inserted into two severed ends. PPy spontaneously returns to its oxidation state when the potential is removed, so that the tube expands *in situ*. The spring-like force on the walls of the blood vessel holds the two ends together when they heal [5].

5.7 Piezoelectric and Electrostrictive Polymers

The piezoelectric effect is the phenomena where some materials generate an electric potential in response to an applied mechanical stress. Figure 5.5 shows the schematic of the piezoelectric effect. "Piezo" is derived from the Greek word piezein, which means to squeeze or press. Piezoelectricity was discovered by Pierre and Jacques Curie in 1880. Based on crystal symmetry and Neumann's principle, it is known that the piezoelectric effect only exists in crystals that do not have a center of symmetry. Piezoelectric materials play an important role in MEMS and nano-electromechanical systems (NEMS). Polyvinylidene difluoride (PVDF) has been widely used in engineering applications due to its favorable

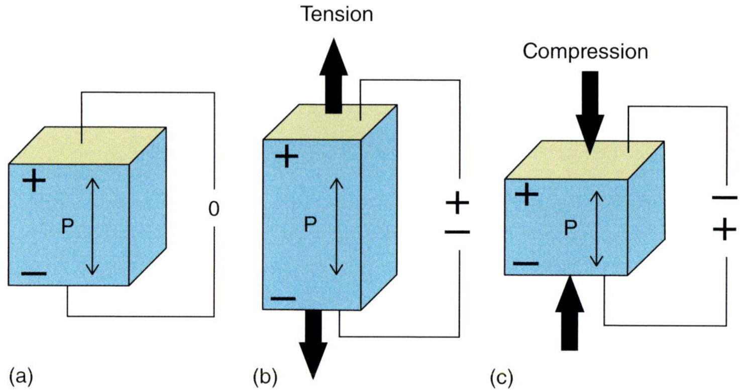

Figure 5.5 Schematic of direct piezoelectric effect; (a) piezoelectric material, (b) energy generation under tension, (c) energy generation under compression.

chemical and mechanical properties. Properties such as high piezoelectric coefficient, good flexibility, biocompatibility, low acoustic, and mechanical impedance, and light weight, are especially unique for MEMS applications. The polymer PVDF is one of the most widely used piezoelectric materials in the fluoropolymer family. Its piezoelectricity was discovered in 1969. However, the mechanism of piezoelectricity has not been clearly explained. This uncertainty has hindered the development of MEMS or NEMS.

Polymers are researched extensively as piezoelectrics because of their unique properties and advantages over other piezoelectrics. The piezoelectric response of polymers is less pronounced than those of single crystal inorganics, but polymers do have their advantages. Poly(vinylidene fluoride), in particular, has high chemical resistance, and high efficiency in converting mechanical energy to electrical energy. Polymers are easier to manufacture, often at lower temperatures, and can be customized more easily into shapes for use in complex operations. In addition, polymers are inherently flexible, have relatively low modulus and low mechanical impedance, with high sensitivity to mechanical loads. These properties make them more versatile than other piezoelectric materials for sensing and actuation. There are a few other semicrystalline organic materials that show piezoelectric properties, but none have shown the same magnitude of response as poly(vinylidene fluoride) and its copolymers.

Poly(vinylidene fluoride) (PVDF) has received an increasing amount of attention because it exhibits the strongest piezoelectric response of any commercially available polymer. These piezoelectric properties have proved useful as actuators and sensors. Current manufacturing processes limit PVDF to thin films and restricting their uses largely to sensors. Further applications using the diversity in mechanical properties of piezoelectric polymers. Evaluating to what extent the mechanical properties will change with applied electric field and finding new ways to manufacture PVDF will lead to new applications of piezoelectric polymers.

There are different polymer categories that can be considered piezoelectric. The first category of piezoelectric polymers is the bulk polymer. These are solid polymer films that have the piezoelectric mechanism because of their molecular structure and its arrangement. The second category is the piezoelectric composite polymer. These are polymer structures with integrated piezoelectric ceramics from which the piezoelectric effect is generated. These composites make use of the mechanical flexibility of polymers and the high electromechanical coupling of the piezoelectric ceramics. The third type is the voided charged polymer, a radically different type of piezoelectric polymer than the first two categories. This is a polymer film in which gas voids are introduced and surfaces are charged so as to form internal dipoles [28].

The use of polymer materials in different MEMS and microfluidics applications has had increasing interest due to the advantages the polymer materials have. These advantages include the mechanical flexibility that is necessary in certain applications as compared to silicon. In addition, polymer-based devices are commonly less expensive in terms of material cost and processing technology, which includes soft lithographic techniques that do not commonly require advanced microfabrication facilities. The commonly used polymers in many microfabricated devices are generally electrically insulating and mechanically flexible compared to inorganic materials. Piezoelectric tactile sensors, a device that can measure a physical phenomenon through contact and touch, find application in robotics and medicine. Piezoelectric polymers are relevant for such applications in measuring force or pressure. $BaTiO_3$ NP/MW-CNT/PDMS composite is used for power generation from human motion [29].

5.8 Dielectric Elastomers

Dielectric elastomers (DEs) are smart electroactive polymers that can generate large strains. Dielectric elastomers consist of a sheet of stretched rubber, or elastomer, coated on both sides with compliant electrode materials; application of a voltage generates an electrostatic pressure that deforms the elastomer. When a voltage is applied across the compliant electrodes, the elastomer film shrinks in thickness and expands in area, that is, in the film plane directions as shown in Figure 5.6. The elastomer comes back to its original position when the voltage is removed. The electrodes must be compliant to allow the film to strain in area as well as in thickness. They are essentially soft parallel plate capacitors. They can function as soft generators, sensors, or actuators. Dielectric elastomers, also known as *artificial muscles* find a large number of potential applications, ranging from entertainment to medicine and space exploration. Intensive research is conducted worldwide to develop these materials due to large strain (up to 380%) and very high energy density ($3.4\,J\,g^{-1}$), which is unmatched by any other smart materials such as ferroelectrics and piezoelectrics [30]. They also posses large stresses (3.2 MPa), high speed of response (10^{-3} s) and high peak strain rate ($34\,000\%\,s^{-1}$).

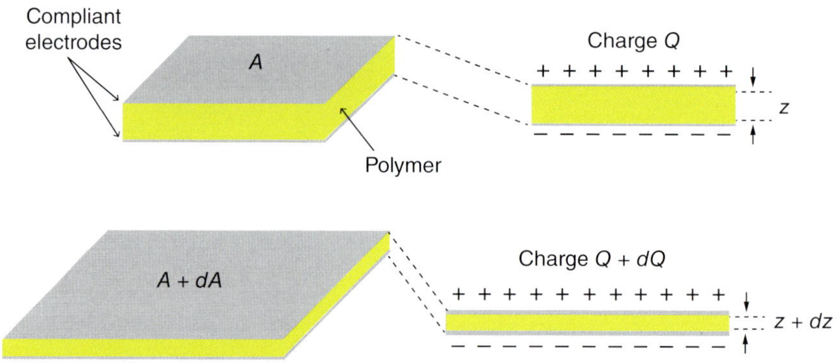

Figure 5.6 Principle of dielectric elastomer actuators.

They transform electrical energy directly into mechanical work and produce large strains.

Dielectric polymers having a low elastic modulus and subjected to a high electric field exhibit large deformations, mainly due to a Coulombian effect, that is by means of the electrostatic interactions among the free charges on the electrodes [31]. Acrylic and silicone rubbers are the most representative materials of the dielectric elastomer class for actuation purposes. Such kinds of polymers are very compliant and show the highest actuating deformations among all EAP materials [32]. The performance of elastomer actuators can be tailored by choosing different types of elastomers, changing the cross-linking chemistry of polymer chains, adding functional entities, and improving fabrication techniques with ease and versatility in most cases. Elastomers are lightly cross-linked polymers. Without cross-linking, the polymer chains have no chemical bonds between chains and, therefore, the polymer may flow upon heating over the glass transition temperature. If the polymer is densely cross-linked, the chains cannot flow upon heating, and a large deformation cannot be expected upon stretching. The mechanical behavior of an elastomer depends strongly on its cross-link density. When an uncross-linked elastomer is stressed, chains may readily slide past one another and disentangle. As cross-linking is increased further, the gel point is eventually reached, where a complete three-dimensional network is formed. The elastomer properties, especially the modulus, are significantly changed by the cross-link density in most elastomer systems, and thus the actuator performance can be adjusted by controlling the degree of elastomer vulcanization (degree of cross-link density). The cross-link density can be adjusted by the kinetic variables of vulcanization reactions such as sulfur (or peroxide) content, reaction time, reaction temperature, and catalyst.

DEs function as electromechanical transducers, operating through several regimes. As energy harvesters, dielectric elastomer generators (DEGs) convert mechanical work into electrical energy. In this mode, energy can be generated either through a constant charge or a constant voltage process. The performance of elastomer actuators can be tailored by choosing different types of elastomers, changing the cross-linking chemistry of polymer chains, adding functional entities, and improving fabrication techniques with ease and versatility in most cases.

The important biomedical applications of dielectric elastomers are active microfluidic devices [33–35], cell bioreactors [36], anti-biofouling surfaces [37], diaphragm blood pumps [38], refreshable haptic displays [39], surgical robotics training [40], rehabilitation orthotics [41], artificial limbs [42, 43], and soft robots that can walk, crawl, hop, and fly [44, 45].

The dielectric elastomer is a highly versatile biomimetic smart material with an impressively wide area of engineering applications due to its high strain, variable stiffness, and noiseless operation devoid of moving parts. Because it shares many of the same intrinsic mechanical properties of living muscle, it finds quite a natural niche in biomedical engineering technologies. Smart DE surfaces can help the blind to read, improve your touch screen sensory experience, or even cast barnacles off boats. Dielectric elastomer sensors can gently sense how tight neural prostheses clamp nerves; or help physical therapists, prosthetists, and researchers analyze gait and posture. DE generators can even harvest the bioenergy of the pedestrian masses. DEAs can also manipulate surgical equipment and provide a surgeon remote tactile feedback, find use in compliant rehabilitation robotics and orthotics, and potentially give rise to the next generation of prosthetic limbs and artificial organs. DEA-driven hyper-redundant binary robotic manipulator prototype has been developed by Wingert and colleagues at MIT [46].

5.9 Summary

Biomedical applications of EAPs are one of the most promising fields that take advantage of the inherent characteristics of these smart polymers. Various electroactive smart polymers such as polymer gels, conductive polymers, ionic metal polymer composites, conjugated polymer, dielectric elastomers, piezoelectric, and electrostrictive polymers have been developed and they are used for varieties of biomedical applications. Significant advances have taken place in understanding the gel responses to electrical fields and in the design of polymer gels with superior properties. Conducting polymers have attracted much interest in the development of biosensors. Piezocomposites are more advantageous when it comes to choosing a piezoelectric polymer material for an energy harvesting application due to their highest coupling coefficients.

References

1. Otero, T.F., and Teresa Cortes, M. (2001) Characterization of triple layers Smart Structures and Materials: Electroactive Polymer Actuators and Devices. *Proc. SPIE 4329, Smart Structures and Materials: Electroactive Polymer Actuators and Devices*, Newport Beach, CA, USA.

2. Gordon, G.W., Geoffrey, M.S., Leon, A.P.K., and Peter, R.T. (2003) Conductive Electroactive Polymers - Intelligent Materials Systems, CRC PRESS.
3. Madden, J.D.W., Vandesteeg, N.A., Anquetil, P.A., Madden, P.G.A., Takshi, A., Pytel, R.Z., Lafontaine, S.R., Wieringa, P.A., and Hunter, I.W. (2004) Artificial muscle technology: physical principles and naval prospects. *IEEE J. Oceanic Eng.*, **29** (3), 706–728.
4. Jager, E., Smela, E., and Inganas, I. (2000) Microfabricating conjugated polymer actuators, *Science*, **290**, 1540–1545.
5. Smela, E. (2003) Conjugated polymer actuators for biomedical applications. *Adv. Mater.*, **15** (6), 481–494.
6. Shahinpoor, M., Kim, J.K., and Mojarrad, M. (2007) *Artificial muscles: applications of Advanced Polymeric Nanocomposites*, CRC Press LLC, Boca Raton, FL, USA.
7. Hara, S., Zama, T., Takashima, W., and Kaneto, K. (2005) Free-standing gel-like polypyrrole actuators doped with bis (perfluoroalkylsulfonyl) imide exhibiting extremely large strain, *Smart Mater. Struct.* **14** (6), 481–494.
8. Carpi, F. and Smela, E. (2009) *Biomedical Applications of Electroactive Polymer Actuators*, John Wiley & Sons Ltd., London, UK.
9. Tanaka, T. (1981) *Gels. Sci. Am.*, **244**, 110–116.
10. Shingo, M., Yusuke, H., Ryo, Y., and Shuji, H. (2010) Active Polymer Gel Actuators. *Int. J. Mol. Sci.*, **11**, 52–66.
11. Huber, D.L., Manginell, R.P., Samara, M.A., Kim, B., and Bunker, B.C. (2003) Programmed adsorption and released of proteins in a microfluidic device. *Science*, **301** (5631), 352–354.
12. Crook, C.J., Smith, A., Jones, A.L., and Ryan, A.J. (2002) Chemically induced oscillations in a pH-responsive hydrogel. *Phys. Chem. Chem. Phys.*, **4** (8), 1367–1369.
13. Lerox, J.C. and Siegel, R.A. (1999) Autonomous gel/enzyme oscillator fueled by glucose: preliminary evidence for oscillations. *Chaos*, **9** (2), 267–275.
14. Labrot, V., De Kepper, P., Boissonade, J., Szalai, I., and Gauffre, F. (2005) Wave patterns driven by chemomechanical instabilities in responsive gels. *J. Phys. Chem. B*, **109** (46), 21476–21480.
15. Zaikin, A.N. and Zhabotinsky, A.M. (1970) Concentration wave propagation in two-dimensional liquidphase self-oscillating system. *Nature*, **225**, 535–537.
16. Maeda, S., Hara, Y., Yoshida, R., and Hashimoto, S. (2008) Control of the dynamic motion of a gel actuator driven by the Belousov-Zhabotinsky reaction. *Macromol. Rapid Commun.*, **29** (5), 401–405.
17. Wichterle, O. and Lim, D. (1960) Hydrophilic gels for biological use. *Nature*, **185**, 117–118.
18. Wona, G. and Helena, J. (2010) Review: synthetic polymer hydrogels for biomedical applications. *Chem. Chem. Technol.*, **4** (4), 297.
19. Collier, J.H., Camp, J.P., Hudson, T.W., and Schmidt, C.E. (2000) Synthesis and characterization of polypyrrole–hyaluronic acid composite biomaterials for tissue engineering applications. *J. Biomed. Mater. Res.*, **50** (4), 574–584.
20. Guimard, N.K., Gomez, N., and Schmidt, C.E. (2007) Conducting polymers in biomedical engineering. *Prog. Polym. Sci.*, **32** (8-9), 876–921.
21. Kim, D.H., Richardson-Burns, S.M., Hendricks, J.L., Sequera, C., and Martin, D.C. (2007) Effect of immobilized nerve growth factor on conductive polymers: electrical properties and cellular response. *Adv. Funct. Mater.*, **17** (1), 79–86.
22. Balint, R., Cassidy, N.J., and Cartmell, S.H. (2014) Conductive polymers: towards a smart biomaterial for tissue engineering. *Acta Biomater.*, **10**, 2341–2353.
23. Nemat-Nasser, S. and Li, J. (2000) Electromechanical response of ionic polymer–metal composites. *J. Appl. Phys.*, **87** (7), 3321–3331, ISSN: 0021–8979..
24. Shahinpoor, M. and Kim, K.J. (2001) Ionic polymer–metal composites: I. Fundamentals. *Smart Mater. Struct.*, **10** (4), 819–833.
25. Nemat-Nasser, S. and Wu, Y. (2006) Tailoring the actuation of ionic

polymer–metal composites. *Smart Mater. Struct.*, **15** (4), 909–923.
26. Paquette, J.W. and Kim, K.J. (2004) Ionomeric electroactive polymer artificial muscle for naval applications. *IEEE J. Oceanic Eng.*, **29** (3), 729–737.
27. Bar-Cohen, Y., Leary, S.P., Yavrouian, A., Oguro, K., Tadokoro, S., Harrison, J.S., Smith, J.G., and Su, J. (2000) Challenges to the application of IPMC as actuators of planetary mechanisms. Proceedings of SPIE, vol. 3987, p. 140.
28. Ramadan, K.S., Sameoto, D., and Evoy, S. (2014) A review of piezoelectric polymers as functional materials for electromechanical transducers. *Smart Mater. Struct.*, **23** (3), 033001.
29. Park, K. *et al.* (2012) Flexible nanocomposite generator made of $BaTiO_3$ nanoparticles and graphitic carbons. *Adv. Mater.*, **24** (22), 2999–3004.
30. Liu, Y., Liu, L., Zhang, Z., and Leng, J. (2009) Dielectric elastomer film actuators: characterization, experiment and analysis. *Smart Mater. Struct.*, **18** (9), 095024.
31. De Rossi, D., Carpi, F., and Mazzoldi, A. (2004) Electrically responsive polymers as materials for "artificial muscles", in *Soft Actuators – Aiming at Realizations of Artificial Muscles* (ed. Y. Osada), NTS Inc..
32. Pelrine, R., Kornbluh, R., Pei, Q., and Joseph, J. (2000) High-speed electrically actuated elastomers with strain greater than 100%. *Science*, **287** (5454), 836–839.
33. Maffli, L., Rosset, S., and Shea, H. (2013) Zipping dielectric elastomer actuators: characterization, design and modeling. *Smart Mater. Struct.*, **22** (10), 104013.
34. Murray, C., McCoul, D., Sollier, E., Ruggiero, T., Niu, X., Pei, Q., and Di Carlo, D. (2013) Electro-adaptive microfluidics for active tuning of channel geometry using polymer actuators. *Microfluid. Nanofluid.*, **14** (1–2), 345–358.
35. Price, A.K. and Culbertson, C.T. (2009) Generation of nonbiased hydrodynamic injections on microfluidic devices using integrated dielectric elastomer actuators. *Anal. Chem.*, **81** (21), 8942–8948.
36. Akbari, S. and Shea, H. (2012) Microfabrication and characterization of an array of dielectric elastomer actuators generating uniaxial strain to stretch individual cells. *J. Micromech. Microeng.*, **22** (4), 045020.
37. Shivapooja, P., Qang, Q., Orihuela, B., Rittschof, D., López, G.P., and Zhao, X. (2013) Bioinspired surfaces with dynamic topography for active control of biofouling. *Adv. Mater.*, **25** (10), 1430–1434.
38. Goulbourne, N., Frecker, M.I., Mockensturm, E.M., and Snyder, A.J. (2003) Modeling of a dielectric elastomer diaphragm for a prosthetic blood pump. Proceedings of SPIE, Smart Structures and Materials 2003: Electroactive Polymer Actuators and Devices (EAPAD), July 28, 2003, vol. 5051, p. 319, doi: 10.1117/12.484388.
39. Niu, X., Brochu, P., Salazar, B., and Pei, Q. (2011) Refreshable tactile displays based on bistable electroactive polymer. SPIE Smart Structures and Materials Nondestructive Evaluation and Health Monitoring, International Society for Optics and Photonics.
40. Carpi, F., Frediani, G., and De Rossi, D. (2009) Electroactive elastomeric haptic displays of organ motility and tissue compliance for medical training and surgical force feedback. *IEEE Trans. Biomed. Eng.*, **56** (9), 2327–2330.
41. Herr, H.M. and Kornbluh, R.D. (2004) New horizons for orthotic and prosthetic technology: artificial muscle for ambulation *Proc.*, SPIE 5385 1–9.
42. Biddiss, E. and Chau, T. (2008) Dielectric elastomers as actuators for upper limb prosthetics: challenges and opportunities. *Med. Eng. Phys.*, **30** (4), 403–418.
43. Kovacs, G., Lochmatter, P., and Wissler, M. (2007) An arm wrestling robot driven by dielectric elastomer actuators. *Smart Mater. Struct.*, **16** (2), S306–S317.
44. Jung, K., Koo, J.C., Lee, Y.K., and Choi, H.R. (2007) Artificial annelid robot driven by soft actuators. *Bioinspiration Biomimetics*, **2** (2), S42–S49.
45. Pei, Q., Pelrine, R., Rosenthal, M.A., Stanford, S., Prahlad, H., and Kornbluh,

R.D. (2004) Recent progress on electroelastomer artificial muscles and their application for biomimetic robots. Proceedings of SPIE – The International Society for Optical Engineering, vol. 5385, pp. 41–50.

46. Wingert, A., Lichter, M.D., Dubowsky, S., and Hafez, M. (2002) Hyper-redundant robot manipulators actuated by optimized binary-dielectric polymers. SPIE's 9th Annual International Symposium on Smart Structures and Materials, International Society for Optics and Photonics.

6
Synthetic Polymer Hydrogels

Anitha C. Kumar and Harikrishna Erothu

6.1
Introduction

Polymer hydrogels are a rapidly developing group of materials, gaining wide application in different fields, such as pharmaceuticals, medicine, and agriculture. Since the 1950s, many reports have been published in scientific literature about new chemical and physical structures, properties, and applications of polymer hydrogels [1]. This chapter provides information and a clear classification of synthetic polymer hydrogels in accordance with their chemical structure, properties, and applications.

6.2
Polymer Hydrogels

The term gel, originating from *gelatin* refers to a jelly-like material that can have properties ranging from soft and weak to hard and tough [2]. A polymeric hydrogel is a three-dimensionally cross-linked network of flexible polymer chains that contain water. They are water-insoluble due to chemical or physical cross-linking and are often found as colloids in the dispersion of aqueous medium. Water plays an important role in determining the physico-chemical properties of the hydrogels. Due to high hydrophilicity, the hydrogels can imbibe large quantities of water or aqueous solutions. The three-dimensional network is able to retain the liquids forming a swollen gel phase and the liquid prevents the polymer network from collapsing into a compact mass. A gel forms when the homogeneous dispersion present in the initial sol rigidifies. This process of gelation prevents the development of inhomogeneities within the material. A sol, or a solution, can be transformed into a polymeric (or colloidal) gel at the gel-point. Practically, it is at this point that the sol abruptly changes from a viscous liquid state to a solid phase called the gel.

Biomedical Applications of Polymeric Materials and Composites, First Edition.
Edited by Raju Francis and Sakthi Kumar.

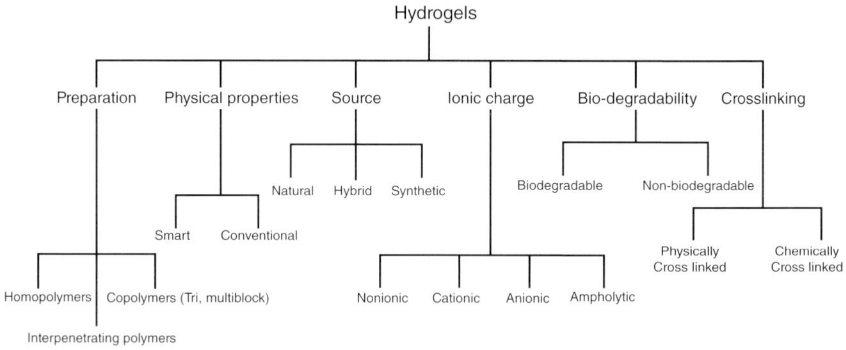

Figure 6.1 Classification of hydrogels.

Gels can be differentiated by the nature of cross-linking into:

a) Physical gels
b) Chemical gels

A number of polymers and polyampholytes can form gels without chemical cross-linking. These are called *physical gels*; almost all biopolymeric gels are physical gels [3]. Physical gels are formed and stabilized in the solvent through secondary forces such as hydrogen bonding, van der Waal's forces, hydrophobic interactions, and so on. These are fragile compared to *chemical gels* that are formed as a result of covalent bonding [4]. In chemical gels, the implantation of cross-links in a system of chains tends to induce segregation between the chains and the solvent. Each cross-link forces the two chains to come into proximity.

Hydrogels may display reversible sol–gel transitions, which is induced by changes in the environmental conditions such as temperature, pH, ionic strength, phase separation, wavelength of light, crystallinity, and so on; these are known as *stimuli responsive, smart,* or *intelligent hydrogels* [5]. These reversible gels are physical gels.

Depending on the preparation methods, ionic charges, sources, nature of swelling with changes in the environment, rate of biodegradation, and the nature of cross-linking, hydrogels can be classified in several ways. Figure 6.1 shows the chart for hydrogel classification [6].

6.3 Synthetic Polymer Hydrogels

Synthetic polymer hydrogels differ in their characteristics due to various chemical structures, synthesis technique, and water content or cross-linking. It is still possible to design new hydrogels that can fulfill specific functions for specific needs. A change in chemical composition, or even a change in one of the synthesis factors (cross-linking method, cross-linking agent, synthesis method, conditions of the synthesis) may lead to new intelligent biomaterials.

Thus, any technique that can be used to create a cross-linked polymer can be used to produce a hydrogel. Copolymerization/cross-linking free-radical polymerizations are commonly used to produce hydrogels by reacting hydrophilic monomers with multifunctional cross-linkers. Water-soluble linear polymers of both natural and synthetic origin are cross-linked to form hydrogels in a number of ways.

6.3.1 Methods to Synthesis Hydrogels

Cross-linked networks of synthetic polymers or natural biopolymers have been reported. The general methods to produce physical and chemical gels are described in the following text.

6.3.1.1 Physical Cross-Linking

Due to relative ease of production, there has been increased interest in physical or reversible gels and the advantage of not using cross-linking agents. These agents affect the integrity of substances to be entrapped as well as the need for their removal before application. Careful selection of hydrocolloid type, concentration, and pH can lead to the formation of a broad range of gel textures and is currently an area receiving considerable attention, particularly in the food industry [7]. The various methods reported in literature to obtain physically cross-linked hydrogels are have been dealt with in the following sections.

Heating/Cooling a Polymer Solution Physically cross-linked gels are formed when cooling hot solutions of gelatin or carrageenan. The gel formation is due to helix formation, association of the helices, and forming junction zones [8]. Carrageenan in hot solution above the melting transition temperature is present as random coil conformation. Upon cooling, it transforms to rigid helical rods. In the presence of salt (K^+, Na^+, etc.), due to screening of repulsion of sulfonic group (SO^{-3}), double helices further aggregate to form stable gels.

Hydrogel can also be obtained by simply warming the polymer solutions, which causes the coil to globule transition (e.g., poly(*N*-isopropylacrylamide) (PNIPAM)) [9] or block copolymerization (e.g., polyethylene oxide-polypropylene oxide [10], polyethylene glycol–polylactic acid hydrogel [11]).

Ionic Interaction Ionic polymers can be cross-linked by the addition of di- or tri-valent counterions. This method underlies the principle of gelling a polyelectrolyte solution (e.g., Na^+ alginate$^-$) with a multivalent ion of opposite charges (e.g., $Ca^{2+} + 2Cl^-$). Some other examples are chitosan-polylysine [12], chitosan-glycerol phosphate salt [13], chitosan-dextran hydrogels [11].

Complex Coacervation Complex coacervate gels can be prepared by mixing a polyanion with a polycation. This method is based on the principle that polymers with opposite charges stick together and form soluble and insoluble complexes depending on the concentration and pH of the respective solutions. Coacervating polyanionic xanthan with polycationic chitosan [14] is one such example. Below its isoelectric point, proteins are positively charged and are likely to associate with anionic hydrocolloids to form polyion complex hydrogels (complex coacervate) [15].

Hydrogen Bonding Hydrogen bonding is a strong intermolecular force that forms a special type of dipole–dipole attraction. Hydrogen bonds are stronger than normal dipole–dipole interactions and dispersion forces but they remain weaker than covalent and ionic bonds. In hydrogels, the structure and stability of water molecules are highly affected by the bonds. The polar groups in the polymer strongly bind water molecules and form hydrogen bonds that also cause hydrophobic effects to occur [16]. The hydrophobic effects combined with the hydrophilic effects within the hydrogel structure can be balanced through dangling side chains that mediate the hydrogen bonding that occurs between two separate hydrogel pieces or across a ruptured hydrogel. H-bonded hydrogel can be obtained by lowering the pH of aqueous solution of polymers carrying carboxyl groups. Poly acrylic acid (PAA) and poly methacrylic acid (PMA) form complexes with poly ethylene glycol (PEG) from the hydrogen bonds between the oxygen of the PEG and the carboxylic group of PMA [11]. This interaction allows for the complex to absorb liquids and swell at low pH, which transforms the system into a gel. Another example is carboxymethyl cellulose (CMC) [17].

Freeze–Thawing Cycle Physical cross-linking of a polymer to form its hydrogel can also be achieved by using freeze–thaw cycles. The mechanism involves the formation of microcrystals in the structure due to freeze–thawing. Examples of this type of gelation are freeze–thawed gels of polyvinylalcohol (PVA) and xanthan [10, 18]. The preparation of pure PVA hydrogels by freezing–thawing technique was first reported by Peppas in 1975 [19].

6.3.1.2 Chemical Cross-Linking

The cross-linking of polymers can be achieved through the reaction of their functional groups (such as OH, COOH, and NH_2) with cross-linkers such as aldehyde (e.g., glutaraldehyde, adipic acid dihydrazide). A number of methods to obtain chemically cross-linked permanent hydrogels are reported in the literature [11].

6.3.1.3 Radiation Cross-Linking

Radiation cross-linking is a widely used technique since it does not involve the use of chemical additives, thereby retaining the biocompatibility of the biopolymer. In addition, modification and sterilization can be achieved in a single step and, therefore, modification of biopolymers for their end use, specifically in biomedical applications, is a cost-effective process [20]. The technique mainly relies on producing free radicals in the polymer following exposure to the high-energy source such as gamma ray, X-ray, or electron beam. The action of radiation (direct or indirect) will depend on the polymer environment (i.e., dilute solution, concentrated solution, solid state).

6.3.2 Examples of Synthetic Polymer Hydrogels

Depending on the method of synthesis, hydrogels can be classified into:

a) *Homopolymer hydrogels* – cross-linked networks of one type of hydrophilic monomer unit. For example: PAA, PVA, PNIPAM.
b) *Copolymer hydrogels* – produced by cross-linking of two co-monomer units, at least one of which must be hydrophilic, to render them swellable. For example: Poly(ethylene glycol methacrylate) (PEG-PEGMA) by free-radical photopolymerization using tetra (ethylene glycol) dimethacrylate as cross-linker.
c) *Multipolymer hydrogels* – produced from three or more co-monomers reacting together
For example: poly(ethylene glycol)–poly(ε-caprolactone)–poly(ethylene glycol).
d) *Interpenetrating polymeric hydrogels* – produced by preparing a first network that is then swollen in a monomer. The latter reacts to form a second intermeshing network structure. For example: cross-linked chitosan/PNIPAM, poly(ethyleneglycol diacrylate) (PEGDA) hydrogels modified with
β-chitosan .

Poly(acrylic acid) and its derivatives, poly(ethylene oxide) and its copolymers, poly(vinyl alcohol), poly(vinyl pyrrolidone) and polypeptides are the main class of synthetic polymer hydrogels and are discussed in detail.

6.3.2.1 Poly(acrylic acid) and its Derivatives

Poly(acrylamide) (PAAm) Hydrogels PAAm hydrogel can be synthesized by using acrylamide monomer (AAm) and *N,N′*-methylenebisacrylamide (MBAAm) cross-linker mixed in deionized water. The monomer–cross-linker solution gently swirls with a magnetic bar on a stirring plate until all reactants are completely dissolved. The monomer solution deoxygenates for 15 min to prevent the reaction between oxygen and the initiators. Following this, ammonium persulfate (APS) solution and *N,N,N′,N′*-tetramethylethylenediamine (TEMED) initiator are added and the solution is spun gently five or six times by hand to mix all the reactants and is poured into a polypropylene petri dish under nitrogen atmosphere. The solution polymerizes at room temperature for 2 h. The synthesized gel is immersed in deionized water for 5 days, with water changed three times a day to remove any unreacted monomers [21].

Poly(*N*-isopropylacrylamide) (PNIPAM) Hydrogels PNIPAM is a chemical isomer of poly-leucine, having a polar peptide group in the side chain rather than in the back bone as shown in Figure 6.2.

Aqueous solutions of PNIPAM show a reversible temperature-induced phase separation. When an aqueous solution of PNIPAM is heated to 32 °C (the cloud point (CP) or LCST), the polymer precipitates from the solution leading to a two-phase system. The macroscopic phase separation reflects the collapse of individually solvated coils into dehydrated globules that aggregate to form a polymer-rich phase, which is insoluble in water. The temperature-induced phase transition of PNIPAM is an ideal tool to investigate the physical properties of the formed thermoreversible hydrogels in the presence of H_2O and in aqueous solvent mixtures [22].

Figure 6.3 shows the photograph of PNIPAM solution before and after sol–gel transition. Below the sol–gel transition temperature, it is a clear solution. This solubility is due to the formation of a hydrogen bond between the amide group of PNIPAM and water. Above the LCST, due to the coil-to-globule transition, a phase separation occurs and, due to the hydrophobic interaction, all the globules aggregate and form a macrogel.

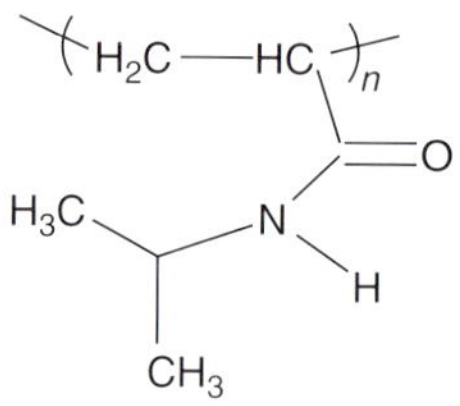

Figure 6.2 Structure of PNIPAM.

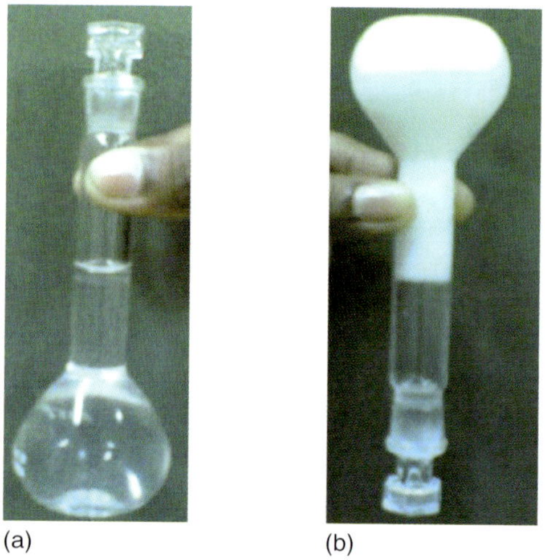

Figure 6.3 PNIPAM solution (a) below and (b) above sol–gel transition temperature [23].

Poly(acrylic acid) (PAA) Hydrogels Polyacrylic acid (PAA) is another homopolymeric hydrogel [24]. Commercial version of its hydrogel contains 2.5 % of PAA and 97.5 % of water. It is stable and has optimal elasticity property. When used as an endoprosthesis, it was designed to be nontoxic, noninflammatory and to imitate the surrounding soft tissue (Figure 6.4).

Duran *et al.* [25] synthesized the acrylic acid-acrylamide hydrogels from different compositions of AAm/AAcmole ratios (AAm/AAc mole ratios, 15/85, 20/30, 30/70). These solutions were placed in poly (vinylchloride) (PVC) straws of 3 mm diameter and irradiated in air at ambient temperature in a Gammacell 220 type γ irradiator. Doses of 2.6, 3, 4, 8, 12, 16, 20 kGy were applied at a fixed dose rate of 0.16 kGy h^{-1}. Hydrogels obtained in long cylindrical shapes were cut, washed with distilled water to remove unreacted monomers and dried in air and in vacuum and stored for later evaluations. The percent conversion was determined gravimetrically.

Poly(2-hydroxyethyl methacrylate) (HEMA) Poly(2-hydroxyethyl methacrylate) (HEMA) is one of the most studied synthetic hydrogels. The permeability and hydrophilicity of this gel is dependent on the cross-linking agents [26]. Macroporous poly(HEMA) gels can be prepared by freeze/thaw, or particulate leaching techniques for cartilage replacement [27]. Many different types of molecules and cells have also been encapsulated into poly(HEMA)gels, and this approach has been reported to be successful for delivery of insulin or other proteins into the body [28]. Poly(HEMA) gels are not degradable in physiological conditions (Figure 6.5), while dextran-modified poly(HEMA) gels have been synthesized, and reported to be degradable by enzymes [29].

Poly(HEMA) gels can also be prepared by using 2-hydroxyethylmethacrylate (HEMA) [30] as a monomer, polyethylene glycoldimethacrylate as the cross-linking agent, and benzoinisobutyl ether (BIE) as the UV-sensitive initiator. Deionized water appropriate for the desired concentration should then be added to the system prepared from the listed components. The final products are obtained in the form of films or membranes by treating them with UV radiation

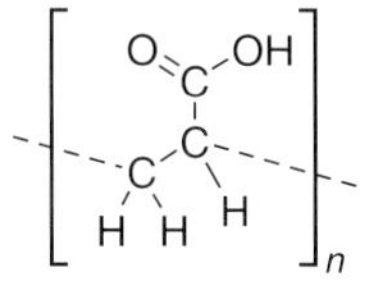

Figure 6.4 Structure of poly acrylic acid.

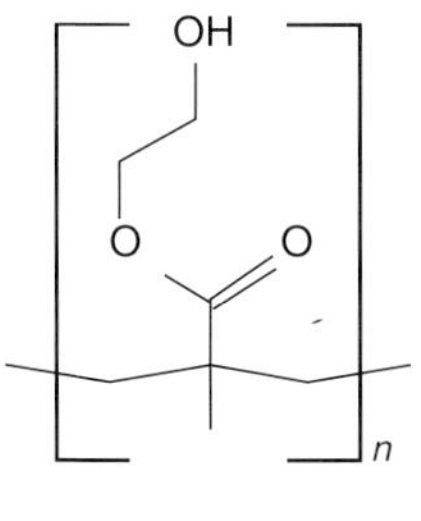

Figure 6.5 Structure of poly(HEMA).

(4 lamps, 20 W, $\lambda = 253.7$ nm, 11 mm distance from the source, 20 min). Another cross-linking agent used in poly(HEMA)manufacturing is a low molecular weight 1,1,1-trimethylolpropane trimethacrylate. The hydrogel obtained with this agent is soft and contains 30–40% of water and is distinguished by its high oxygen permeability [31].

6.3.2.2 Poly(ethylene oxide) (PEO) and its Copolymers

Poly(ethylene oxide) (PEO) otherwise known as *poly(ethylene glycol) (PEG)* is one of the major classes of synthetic polymer hydrogels. It has been approved by the Food and Drug Administration (FDA) for several medical applications due to its biocompatibility and low toxicity [32]. PEO itself is very hydrophilic and can be synthesized by anionic or cationic polymerization of ethylene oxide (Figure 6.6). PEO gels can be prepared by UV photopolymerization of the precursor and consist of PEO with acrylate termini at each end in the presence of R-hydroxy acid [33].

Poly(ethyleneglycolmethacrylate) (PEGMA) and Poly(ethyleneglycol dimethacrylate) (PEGDMA) Foulger *et al.* [34] prepared the hydrogel from PEGMA and PEGDMA by using PEG-MA, $M_n = 360$ as monomer and PEG-DMA, $M_n = 550$ as cross-linker. 2,2-Diethoxyacetophenone(DEAP) is used as a photoinitiator. This mixture was injected between two quartz plates separated by a para film spacer and then polymerized by exposure to a UV source for 4 min (Figure 6.7).

Poly(ethylene oxide) and Poly(propylene oxide) Triblock Copolymer (PEO-*b*-PPO-*b*-PEO) This is known by the trade name pluronics or poloxamers, and is commercially available in various lengths and compositions. These polymers form thermally reversible gels without any permanent cross-links. In addition, it was reported that PEO–PPO–PEO triblock copolymers could be designed to form gels at body temperature by forming a liquid crystalline phase [35]. They form hydrogels in aqueous solutions in response to temperature changes.

Poly(ethylene glycole)–Poly(ethylene glycol methacrylate) (PEG–PEGMA) Kim and Peppas [36] prepared copolymers of methacrylic acid (MAA) with a mixture of

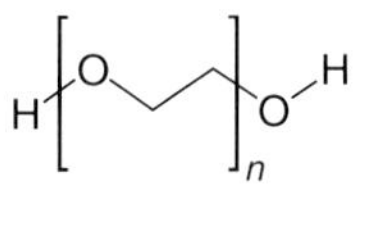

Figure 6.6 Structure of PEG.

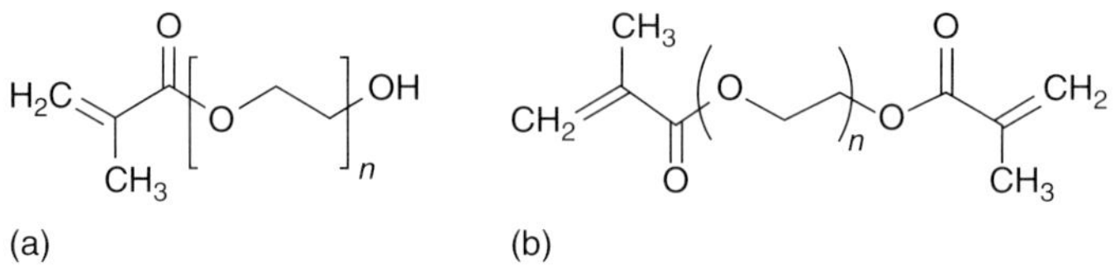

Figure 6.7 Structure of (a) poly(ethylene glycol methacrylate) (PEGMA) and (b) poly(ethylene glycol dimethacrylate) (PEGDMA).

PEG-PEGMA in a free-radical photo polymerization using tetra(ethylene glycol)dimethacrylate as a cross-linker. The cross-linking occurred in the presence of an initiator1-hydroxycyclohexyl phenyl ketone under a nitrogen atmosphere during a 30-min exposure to UV light. The authors claim that the swelling behavior and consequently the rate of release strongly depend on the molecular weight of PEG (Figure 6.8). These hydrogels were successfully used in insulin release systems [37].

Poly(ethylene glycol)–Poly(ε-caprolactone)–Poly(ethylene glycol) (PEG–PCL–PEG) (PECE) Gong *et al.* [38] synthesized the biodegradable triblock PEG–PCL–PEG (PECE), hydrogel copolymers for developing drug delivery systems by the ring-opening copolymerization of ε-caprolactone. mPEG was used as the initiator, stannousoctoate as catalyst and hexamethylene diisocyanate (HMDI) as coupling agent during triblock formation for the synthesis. Thermosensitive PECE hydrogels formed *in situ* can be easily applied in controlled drug delivery, cell encapsulation, and tissue repair. In a number of experiments, they demonstrated its specific biodegradability ratio and biocompatibility. Both hydrophilic and hydrophobic drugs, as well as protein drugs are released slowly from a PECE hydrogel over a sustained time period. It is an alternative to the commercially available Pluronic F-127 hydrogel.

Poly(oligoethylene glycol methacrylate) (POEGMA) POEGMA is synthesized via free radical copolymerization [39, 40]. The hydrazide-functionalized POEGMA precursors (PO100Hy) were synthesized by copolymerizing OEGMA475 (EO repeat units, $n = 8-9$) with acrylic acid (AA) and subsequent post-polymerization modification using 1-ethyl-3-(3-dimethylaminopropyl)carbodiimide (EDC) chemistry with a large excess of adipic acid dihydrazide. The aldehyde-functionalized

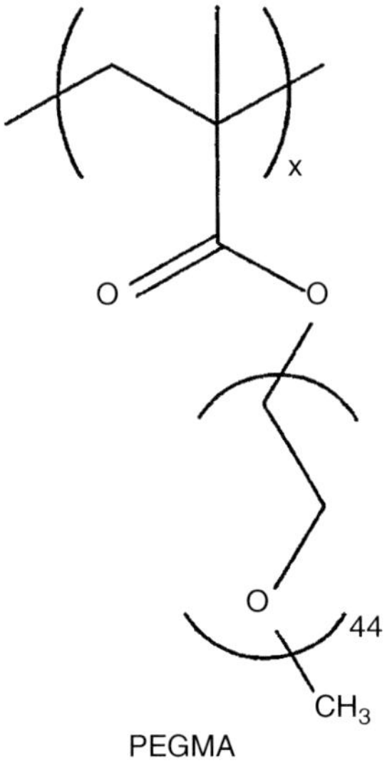

Figure 6.8 Structure of PEGMA.

POEGMA precursors (PO100Ay) were synthesized by copolymerizing OEGMA475 with afunctional acetal monomer (*N*-(2,2-dimethoxyethyl) methacrylamide, DMEMAm) and subsequently converting the acetal to the corresponding aldehyde by acid-catalyzed hydrolysis. The PEG-analog hydrogels are based on hydrazide and aldehyde functionalized POEGMA precursors that rapidly form a hydrogel network via reversible hydrazone bond formation upon coextrusion [41, 42]. POEGMA hydrogels were prepared by coextruding PO100Hy andPO100Ay solutions in 10 mM PBS using a double-barrel syringe. Gelation occurs over time frames ranging from several hours (~8 h) to a few minutes (<10 min) depending on the functional group content and polymer concentration. The hydrogels swell in PBS following preparation, indicating high water affinity. For POEGMA hydrogels prepared with precursors containing 25, 30, or 40 mol% functional groups (both hydrazide and aldehyde), the equilibrium mass-based swelling ratio (Qm) is reached within 30 hand decreases with both the degree of chain functionalization and the concentration of precursor polymers systematically used to prepare the hydrogel. The injectable, *in situ* gelling nature of this system is useful to circumvent many of the issues concerning surgical implantation of bulk hydrogel-based materials [43].

PEG–Polyester Copolymer Hydrogels Aliphatic polyesters including poly(glycolic acid) (PGA), poly(lactic acid) (PLA), and copolymers (PLGA) of these materials are the most widely used synthetic polymers [44, 45] (Figure 6.9).

PLA or poly(lactide-co-glycolide)(PLGA)–PEG copolymer forms amphiphilic micelles in aqueous solution, which transform into a hydrogel due to physical cross-linking influenced by swelling, hydration, and self-assembly of polymers responding to temperature [46]. In 2001, Fujiwara and Kimura introduced the stereo complex mechanism to prepare specifically the "thermosensitive hydrogels" from triblock copolymers, PLA–PEG–PLA [47]. Aqueous micelle solutions from enantiomeric triblock copolymers with a particular molecular weight, PLLA–PEG–PLLA (1300–4600–1300) and PDLA–PEG–PDLA (1100–4600–1100), exhibited sol-to-gel transition between 25 and 37 °C, which was considered to be a promising injectable hydrogel.

6.3.2.3 Poly(vinyl pyrrolidone) (PVP)

PVP results from the polymerization of vinylpyrrolidone. Different chain lengths yield in different viscosities. Traditionally, the degree of polymerization is characterized by the *K*-value, which is essentially a function of the viscosity in aqueous solution (PVP K-25, K-30, and PVP K-90). PVP is a very widely used excipient for the preparation of solid dosage forms. The main application is related to its

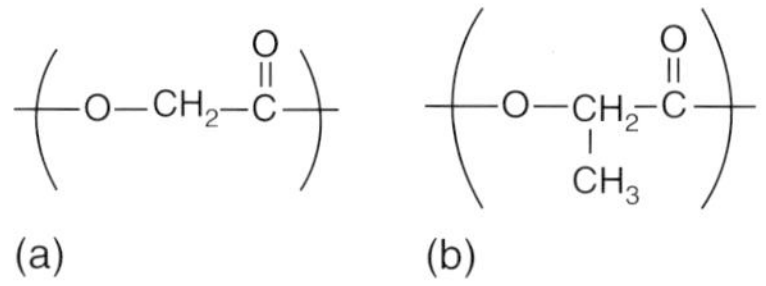

Figure 6.9 Chemical structure of (a) poly(glycolic acid), (b) poly(lactic acid).

function as a binder in wet granulation. It is also useful for the preparation of effervescent tablets or in direct compression applications. Many other uses, including nonparenteral applications, have been described in the very long history of this polymer [48]. Benamer *et al.* irradiated PVP solutions using a ^{60}Co source at a dose rate of 3.2 Gy min^{-1} to produce hydrogels [49]. Lugao *et al.* [50] obtained PVP hydrogels using different irradiation doses (5–15 KGy) and different additives: PEG (MW 600, 6000), PEO (400 000), and glycerol. Glycol and PEO used as additives reduce the cross-linking density of the PVP network, whereas PEG is nontoxic and increases the elasticity of the gels as a result of the plasticizing effect. Moreover, PVP/PEG hydrogels are sterile and noncytotoxic, which makes PEG an ideal addition to biomedical hydrogels designed as dressings. The additives such as agar enhance the mechanical properties of PVP hydrogel [51] (Figure 6.10).

6.3.2.4 Poly(vinyl alcohol) (PVA) Hydrogel

PVA is chemically inert in many organic solvents and optically transparent in the UV-Vis region. The alcohol units are proton donors and can interact by hydrogen bonding with the amide carbonyl groups of the tertiary polyamide. The possibility of hydrogen bond formation between hydroxyls and neighboring carbonyls in the copolymer imply a short-scale competition of specific interactions.

PVA is not prepared by the polymerization of the corresponding monomer, because of the unstable nature of vinyl alcohol becoming acetaldehyde and because it does not exist in the free form. PVA is synthesized by various methods but the most widely used method is from vinyl acetate [52].

PVA films can be prepared by pouring 4% (w/v) PVA solution into flat-bottomed dishes in such a manner that a uniform thin layer of liquid covers the surface. These dishes were kept in a vacuum desiccator and films were allowed to dry. The dry polymer film could be easily detached from the dish [53].

PVA hydrogels can be obtained by alternating cycles of freezing and thawing. This method first reported by Peppas in 1975 [19]. This was preparedby freezing the aqueous solution of PVA between 2.5% and 15% w/v at −20 °C and thawing it back to room temperature to its crystalline stage. The crystallinity can be characterized by measuring the turbidity change in the PVA sample. The crystallinity related to the concentration of PVA solution, freezing time and thawing time. The PVA material prepared by this method has greater mechanical strength than that obtained by UV radiation or by crosslinking agent. Functional groups of PVA are more accessible which broadens its range of application.

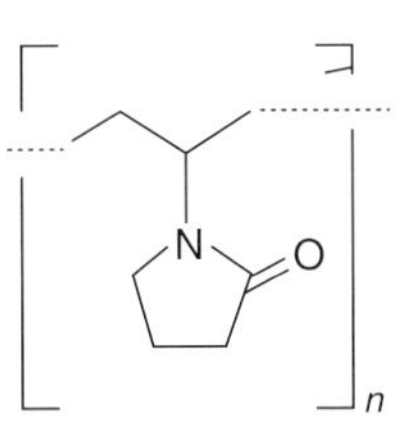

Figure 6.10 Structure of Polyvinyl pyrrolidone.

Zhang *et al.* [54] prepared the series of PVA-PNIPAM semi-interpenetrating polymeric network (semi-IPN) hydrogels by incorporating PVA into cross-linked PNIPAM. These semi-IPN hydrogels showed faster responsive rates compared to conventional PNIPAM hydrogels and undergo full deswelling in 1 min. They lose about 95% water within 1 min, when the temperature is raised above their LCST. These semi-IPN hydrogels have larger equilibrium swelling ratios at room temperature because of the incorporation of PVA, which forms water-releasing channels and results in increased hydrophilicity into the PNIPAM hydrogel networks.

PVA hydrogels can be prepared by simply mixing with borax hydrated sodium tetraborate, ($Na_2B_4O_7 \cdot 10H_2O$)) solution in a 10 : 1 ratio.

Borax is a known nontoxic food additive. Han *et al.* [55] incorporated cellulose nanoparticle (CNP) into PVA-borax (PB) hydrogels.

6.3.2.5 Polypeptide Hydrogels

Peptides are naturally occurring biological molecules. They are short chains of amino acid monomers linked by peptide (amide) bonds. Polymer-peptide conjugate (PPC) hydrogels are physically bonded networks capable of imbibing large quantities of water. As with proteins, the physical bonding can lead to secondary structure formation, for example, α-helices and β-sheets, which can lead to tertiary structure formation. The advantage of using PPC hydrogels for biomaterials is that the best properties of peptides and those of synthetic polymers can be combined [55]. The peptide component provides increased functional control, well-defined homogeneous hierarchical structures, consistent mechanical properties, and supportive folding/unfolding transitions [56, 57]. Stupp's group [58, 59] have made pioneering steps in this field using peptide amphiphiles. A peptide amphiphile is a hydrophilic peptide attached to a hydrophobic polymer chain. These materials will supra-molecularly self-assemble (i.e., they reversibly bind together so that they can be formed or destroyed depending on external conditions) to form nanoscale fibers, which entangle to form a 3-D supramolecular hydrogel [60–63].

Common methods of self-assembly to give PPC hydrogels include solvent exchange, direct rehydration, temperature-switch, and salt-triggered processes. Various structures can be obtained depending upon the conditions of assembly, for example, temperature, solvent, or molar ratio of polymer to peptide.

Cui *et al.* [64] synthesized the biodegradable hydrogels from water-soluble ABA triblock ionic polypeptides, by mixing poly(L-glutamic acid)-*block*-poly(ethylene glycol)-*block*-poly(L-glutamic acid)(PGA–PEG–PGA) with poly (L-lysine)–*block*-poly(ethylene glycol)–*block*-poly(L-lysine) (PLL–PEG–PLL). PGA–PEG–PGA and PLL–PEG–PLL were synthesized through ring-opening polymerization (ROP) of BLG-NCA and ZLL-NCA in DMF using NH2–PEG–NH2 as initiator and followed by deprotection reaction, respectively.

Dave Adams and group synthesized low molecular weight dipeptide hydrogels by using 2-thiophene diphenylalanine. They made a solution of 2-thiophene diphenylalanine in deionized water at pH 11 using sodium hydroxide that resulted in a transparent solution. Glucono-δ-lactone (GdL) was then used to lower the pH slowly and trigger gelation. After 1 h, the initially transparent solution became turbid. After 6 h, an opaque self-supporting gel formed. This gel turned to a completely transparent gel after 3 days [65].

6.3.3
Properties of Synthetic Polymer Hydrogels

The structural properties of gels make them useful for various kinds of applications. Hydrogel structure and, thus, the hydrogel properties are closely related to the conditions under which the hydrogels are formed, that is, the cross-linker concentration, the initial degree of dilution of the monomers, and the chemistry of the units building the network structure.

6.3.3.1 Smart Polymer Hydrogels

Certain hydrogels can undergo a volume change in response to a change in the surrounding conditions, such as pH [66, 67], temperature [5a,b], and ionic strength [68] and these are known as smart hydrogels or stimuli-responsive hydrogels or intelligent hydrogels.

Thermoreversible Gels Among the various types of stimuli-responsive gels, those sensitive to small temperature changes, known as *thermoreversible gels*, have attracted much attention. Thermosensitive hydrogels can be divided generally into two categories: those, which exhibit an increase in swelling with temperature (upper critical solution temperature – UCST) and those, which show a decrease in swelling capacity with temperature (lower critical solution temperature – LCST). The solution is homogeneous at low temperature and a macroscopic phase separation appears when the temperature exceeds a critical value called the *cloud point* (*CP*) of the mixture. The LCST can be thus considered as the lowest CP of the system as it corresponds to the minimum in the phase diagram [22]. LCST is principally an entropic process in contrast to the conjugated phenomenon of UCST, which is principally enthalpic.

Prominent examples for water soluble polymers displaying inverse solubility upon heating (LCST) are PNIPAM [9], methylhydroxypropyl cellulose (MHPC) [68], poly(vinylcaprolactam) (PVCa) [69], poly(vinyl methyl ether) (PVME) [70] and poly(propelene glycol) [71]. Among this, PNIPAM is the widely studied polymer having an LCST of ~32 °C [22].

pH Sensitive Gels When a hydrogel is composed of both weakly acidic and weakly basic polymers, it may be highly swollen at high and low pH, while its lowest swellability will be observed in the pH 4–5 region. For example, since pK_a of acrylic acid is between 4.5 and 5.0, PAA hydrogels swell significantly above pH 5, which is the pH of the small intestine. However, they do not swell significantly below pH 4, which is the pH of the stomach. Therefore, one of the major applications of acrylic acid gels is in sustained gastro-intestinal drug delivery systems [72, 73].

Ion Responsive Hydrogels Cross-linked PNIPAM-co-benzo-18-crown-6-acrylamide (PNIPAM-co-BCAm) smart hydrogels exhibiting both ion-recognition and thermoresponsive characteristics were prepared via thermally initiated free-radical cross-linking copolymerization by Ju *et al.* [74] Crown ethers have remarkable properties of selectively recognizing specific ions and forming stable "host-guest" complexes. If the crown ether groups are introduced into the thermosensitive PNIPAM hydrogel, it is able to prepare an ion-recognition hydrogel that responds to both temperature and specific ion stimuli.

Glucose-Responsive Hydrogels Glucose-sensitive holographic sensor was synthesized by Lee *et al.* [75]. This sensor consisted of copolymers of 3-acrylamido-phenyl boronic acid (3APB) and of acrylamide, cross-linked by *N,N′*-methylenebisacrylamide. The equilibrium complexation of glucose or of other cis-diols with the boronic group of 3-APB depends on their concentration in the investigated solution. It is quantitatevely reflected by the degree of swelling of the hydrogel. Lapeyre *et al.* [76] investigated the microgels with the PNIPAM core and the PNIPAM-co-p3APB shell, which were used for the determination of glucose concentration at 25 °C. Swelling of the shell was coupled with the swelling of the core. Maximal overall swelling, at pH 8.5 and at constant glucose concentration, was observed when the molar concentration of the boron containing polymer (p3APB) in the copolymer was in the vicinity of 5 mol. Kang and Bae [77] prepared a glucose-responsive hydrogel by attaching glucose oxidase and catalase to a pH-sensitive hydrogel based on the *N,N*-diacrylsulfonamide, which undergoes transition in the pH range 7.5–6.55. This transition is very sharp when the pH of the solution decreases from 7.4 to 7.2 because of the enzymatically catalyzed oxidation of glucose to gluconic acid. This gel exhibits reversible glucose concentration-dependent swelling at this pH range, with no hysteresis.

6.3.3.2 Swelling Property

Water plays an important role in determining the physico-chemical properties of the hydrogels. Due to high hydrophilicity, the hydrogels can imbibe large quantities of water or aqueous solutions. The swelling behavior of polymer hydrogels has significant effect on their applications in different fields [4].

The total amount of water absorbed by a hydrogel depends on the temperature and the specific interaction between water molecules and polymer chains; it can be described by the Flory-Huggins solution theory. The free energy of the mixing (ΔGm) of polymer chains and water molecules is expressed by equation.

$$\Delta Gm = kT\ [n_w \ln \phi_w + \ln(1 - \phi_w) + \chi n_w(1 - \phi_w)]$$

where χ is the apparent interaction (water molecules–polymer) parameter dependent on chemical structure, which can be calculated from experimental data of the equilibrium water uptake of the network in the presence of a vapor phase containing water; n_w is the number of molecules; and ϕ_w is the water volume [78, 79].

Depending on the degree of association between water and polymer, the behavior of water can change. Three different states of water have been identified in swollen hydrogels, that is, nonfreezable bound-water, freezable bound-water, and free water. From the DSC study of partially swollen PVA hydrogels, Li *et al.* [80], differentiated the relative content of these water states. Nagura *et al.* [81] suggested the existence of three different ice forms in a frozen PVA hydrogel by DSC measurements. The total weight of water present in a swollen hydrogel is the sum of two main parts, the weight of freezable water and that of nonfreezable water. It was suggested that the nonfreezable bound water molecule has two hydrogen bonds directly fixed to a polymer network chain and could not freeze to ice upon cooling. When more water is introduced to the gel, these two end fixed hydrated water gradually change to one end fixed hydrated water and merged with the freezable hydrated water. The free hydrogen atom of the one end fixed hydrated water may join with another free water molecule; the mobility of the molecule is partially retained and could freeze upon cooling.

6.4 Applications of Synthetic Polymer Hydrogels

The structural properties of gels make them useful for various kinds of applications such as sensors, contact lenses, artificial organs, and drug delivery systems [4]. It was found that, poly(methylmethacrylate) (PMMA) based gel electrolytes are the most preferred potential candidates as electrolytes in electrochromic windows due to their high transparency as well as good gelatinizing and solvent-retention ability [82]. Electrophoresis through agarose or poly(acrylamide) gels is the standard method that is used to separate, identify, and purify DNA or RNA fragments [83–85].

The first hydrogel with potential biomedical application was poly HEMA, used – soon after its discovery – in contact lens production by Professors Lim and Wichterle of Prague, Czech Republic in 1955 [10, 86]. They are also used in many drug delivery applications [87].

The LCST of PNIPAM in water is approximately 32 °C and can be matched to body temperature by copolymerization [22]. Therefore, the use of PNIPAM and its copolymers in tissue engineering would be very beneficial as one can easily prepare a mixed solution of cells and the polymer at room temperature or even at a lower temperature and inject it into the desired site.

PEG is nontoxic, and is thus ideal for biological applications, and can be injected into the body without adverse effects. It is also an FDA approved material for use in humans. PEG and its "stealth" properties, that is once it is attached to certain formulations, it allows slow release of the formulation, thus enabling controlled release, as well as reduced uptake of harmful immunoglobulins. This allows longer dosage and reduces immunogenicity of substances such as adenosine deaminase (ADA) and asparaginase [88]. Table 6.1 shows the applications of different synthetic polymer hydrogels.

Table 6.1 Applications of synthetic polymer hydrogels.

Synthetic polymer hydrogel	Applications
Poly(acrylic acid) and its derivatives	Disposible diapers, ion exchange resins and adhesives, drug delivery Thickening, dispersing, suspending, and emulsifying agents in pharmaceuticals, cosmetics, and paints [89] Artificial organs
Poly HEMA films	Contact lens, artificial skin manufacturing, burn dressings, drug delivery systems, marrow and spinal cord cell regeneration scaffolds for promoting cell adhesion, and in artificial cartilage production [90–97]
Polyethylene oxide and derivatives	Cell culture, biosensor materials, as drug carriers in the efficient and controlled release systems of drugs, scaffolds for protein recombination, and functional tissue production [36, 38, 98, 99]
Poly(vinylpyrrolidone)	Preparation of synthetic plasma and as a carrier for drug delivery [49, 100] binder in wet granulation [48]
Poly(vinyl alcohol)	Tissue engineering, drug delivery, optical films [101]
Polypeptide	Injectable polymeric systems, spinal cord treatment, cell culture [58, 62]

6.5 Conclusion

This chapter discusses the synthesis, properties, and applications of synthetic polymer hydrogels. It is still possible to use Synthetic polymer hydrogels to design new hydrogels to fulfill the particular needs of specific functions. They differ in their characteristics due to various chemical structures, synthesis technique, and water content or cross-linking. A change in chemical composition, or even a change in one of the synthesis factors (cross-linking method, cross-linking agent, synthesis method, and conditions of the synthesis) may lead to new intelligent biomaterials.

Abbreviations

3APB	3-acrylamido-phenylboronic acid
AAm	acrylamide
ADA	adenosine deaminase
APS	ammonium persulfate
BIE	benzoin isobutyl ether
CMC	carboxymethyl cellulose
CNP	cellulose nanoparticle
CP	cloud point
DEAP	2,2-diethoxyacetophenone
DMEMAm	*N*-(2,2-dimethoxyethyl)methacrylamide

EDC	1-ethyl-3-(3-dimethylaminopropyl)carbodiimide
FDA	Food and Drug Administration
HEMA	(2-hydroxyethyl methacrylate)
HMDI	hexamethylenediisocyanate
LCST	lower critical solution temperature
MBAAm	*N*,*N′*-methylenebisacrylamide
MHPC	methylhydroxypropyl cellulose
PAA	poly acrylic acid
PAAm	poly(acrylamide)
PEG	poly(ethylene glycol)
PEGDA	poly(ethylene glycol diacrylate)
PEGDMA	poly(ethylene glycol dimethacrylate)
PEGMA	poly(ethylene glycol methacrylate)
PEO	poly(ethylene oxide)
PGA	poly(glycolic acid)
PGA–PEG–PGA	poly(L-glutamicacid)–*block*-poly(ethyleneglycol)–*block*-poly(L-glutamic acid)
PLA	poly(lactic acid)
PLGA	poly(lactide-co-glycolide)
PLL–PEG–PLL	poly(L-lysine)–*block*-poly(ethylene glycol)–*block*-poly(L-lysine)
PMA	poly(methacrylic acid)
PNIPAM	poly(*N*-isopropylacrylamide)
PPC	polymer-peptide conjugate
PPG	poly(propelene glycol)
PVA	poly(vinyl alcohol)
PVC	poly(vinyl chloride)
PVCa	poly(vinylcaprolactam)
PMMA	poly(methyl methacrylate)
PVME	poly(vinyl methyl ether)
PVP	poly(vinyl pyrrolidone)
ROP	ring-opening polymerization
TEMED	*N*,*N*,*N′*,*N′*-tetramethylethylenediamine
UCST	upper critical solution temperature

References

1. Guenet, J.-M. (1992) *Thermoreverible Gelation of Polymers and Biopolmers*, Academic Press, London.
2. Harper, D. (2013) Online Etymology Dictionary. Retrieved 09 December 2013.
3. Nijenhuis, K. (1997) Thermoreversible networks-viscoelastic properties and structure of gels. *Adv. Polym. Sci.*, **130**, 267.
4. Bohidar, H.B. (2001) Dynamics in thermoreversible polymer gels. *Curr. Sci.*, **80** (8), 1008–1017.
5. (a) Senel, S., I-sik-Yuruksoy, B., Ciaek, H., and Tuncel, A. (1997) Thermoresponsive N-isopropylacrylamide-vinylpyrrolidone copolymer by radiation polymerization. *J. Appl. Polym. Sci.*, **64**, 1775–1784; (b) Akkas, P., Sari, M., Sen, M., and Guven, O.

(1999) The effect of external stimuli on the bovine serum albumin adsorption capacity of poly(acrylamide/maleic acid) hydrogels prepared by gamma rays. *Radiat. Phys. Chem.*, **55**, 717–721.
6. Patel, A. and Mequanint, K. (2011) in *Biomedical Engineering – Frontiers and Challenges* (ed. R. Fazel-Rezai), InTech, p. 386, Chapters published August 01, 2011 under CC BY-NC-SA 3.0license, doi: 10.5772/1019, ISBN: 978-953-307-309-5..
7. Gulrez, S.K.H., Al-Assaf, S., and Phillips, G.O. (2011) Hydrogels: methods of preparation, characterisation and applications, in *Progress in Molecular and Environmental Bioengineering – From Analysis and Modeling to Technology Applications* (ed. A. Carpi), InTech. ISBN: 978-953-307-268-5
8. Funami, T., Hiroe, M., Noda, S., Asai, I., Ikeda, S., and Nishimari, K. (2007) Influence of molecularstructure imaged with atomic force microscopy on the rheological behavior of carrageenan aqueous systems in the presence or absence of cations. *Food Hydrocolloids*, **21**, 617–629.
9. Schild, H.G. (1992) Poly(*N*-isopropylacrylamide): experiment, theory and application. *Prog. Polym. Sci.*, **17**, 163–249.
10. Hoffman, A.S. (2002) Hydrogels for biomedical applications. *Adv. Drug Delivery Rev.*, **43**, 3–12.
11. Hennink, W.E. and Nostrum, C.F. (2002) Novel crosslinking methods to design hydrogels. *Adv. Drug Delivery Rev.*, **54**, 13–36.
12. Bajpai, A.K., Shukla, S.K., Bhanu, S., and Kankane, S. (2008) Responsive polymers in controlled drug delivery. *Prog. Polym. Sci.*, **33**, 1088–1118.
13. Zhao, Q.S., Ji, Q.X., Xing, K., Li, X.Y., Liu, C.S., and Chen, X.G. (2009) Preparation and characteristics of novel porous hydrogel films based on chitosan and glycerophosphate. *Carbohydr. Polym.*, **76**, 410–416.
14. Esteban, C. and Severian, D. (2000) Polyionic hydrogels based on xanthan and chitosan forstabilising and controlled release of vitamins. Patent WO0004086 (A1) (ed. U. United States Patent), Kemestrielnc [CA], USA.
15. Magnin, D., Lefebvre, J., Chornet, E., and Dumitriu, S. (2004) Physicochemical and structural characterization of a polyionic matrix of interest in biotechnology, in the pharmaceutical and biomedical fields. *Carbohydr. Polym.*, **55**, 437–453.
16. Tanaka, H., Tamai, Y., and Nakanishi, K. (1996) Molecular dynamics study of polymer–water interaction in hydrogels. 2. Hydrogen-bond dynamics. *Macromolecules*, **29** (21), 6761–6769.
17. Takigami, M., Amada, H., Nagasawa, N., Yagi, T., Kasahara, T., Takigami, S., and Tamada, M. (2007) Preparation and properties of CMC gel. *Trans. Mater. Res. Soc. Jpn.*, **32** (332), 713–716.
18. Giannouli, P. and Morris, E.R. (2003) Cryogelation of xanthan. *Food Hydrocolloids*, **17**, 495–501.
19. Peppas, N.A. (1975) Turbidimetric studies of aqueous PVA solutions. *Macromol. Chem.*, **176**, 3433.
20. Lugao, A.B. and Malmonge, S.M. (2001) Use of radiation in the production of hydrogels. *Nucl. Instrum. Methods Phys. Res., Sect. B*, **185**, 37–42.
21. Kim, S., Iyer, G., Nadarajah, A., Frantz, J.M., and Spongberg, A.L. (2010) Polyacrylamide hydrogel properties for horticultural applications. *Int. J. Polym. Anal. Charact.*, **15**, 307–318.
22. Heskins, M. and Guillet, J.E. (1968) Solution properties of poly(N- isopropylacrylamide). *J. Macromol. Sci. Chem.*, **A2**, 1441–1455.
23. Kumar, A.C. and Mishra, A.K. (2006) Fluorescence studies on poly(*N*-isopropylacrylamide) (PNIPAM) thermoreversible gel. Proceedings of International Conference on Molecules to Materials, Longowal, Chandigarh, March 3–4, 2006, pp. 382–386.
24. Christensen, L., Breiting, V., Vuust, J., and Hogdall, E. (2006) Adverse reactions following injection with a permanent facial filler polyacrylamide hydrogel (Aquamid): causes and treatment. *Eur. J. Plast. Surg.*, **28**, 464–471.

25. Duran, S., Solpan, D., and Guven, O. (1999) Synthesis and characterization of acrylamide-acrylic acidhydrogels and adsorption of some textile dyes. *Nucl. Instrum. Methods Phys. Res., Sect. B*, **151**, 196–199.
26. Kost, J. and Langer, R. (1987) in *Hydrogels in Medicine and Pharmacy*, vol. 3 (ed. N. Peppas), CRC Press, Boca Raton, FL, p. 95.
27. Oxley, H.R., Corkhill, P.H., Fitton, J.H., and Tighe, B.J. (1993) Macroporous hydrogels for biomedical applications: methodology and morphology. *Biomaterials*, **14**, 1064.
28. Sefton, M.V., May, M.H., Lahooti, S., and Babensee, J.E.J. (2000) Making microencapsulation work: conformal coating, immobilization gels and in vivo performance. *J. Controlled Release*, **65**, 173–186.
29. Meyvis, T.K.L., De Smedt, S.C., Demeester, J., and Hennink, W.E. (2000) Influence of the degradation mechanism of hydrogels on their elastic and swelling properties during degradation. *Macromolecules*, **33**, 4717.
30. Young, C., Wu, J.-R., and Tsou, T.-L. (1998) Fabrication and characteristics of polyHEMA artificial skin with improved tensile properties. *J. Membr. Sci.*, **146**, 83.
31. Cretu, A., Gattin, R., Brachais, L., and Barbier-Baudry, D. (2004) Synthesis and degradation of poly (2-hydroxyethyl methacrylate)-graft-poly (ε-caprolactone) copolymers. *Polym. Degrad. Stab.*, **83**, 399.
32. Zalipsky, S. (1995) Functionalized poly(ethylene glycols) for preparation of biologically relevant conjugates. *Bioconjugate Chem.*, **6**, 150.
33. West, J.L. and Hubbell, J.A. (1995) Photopolymerized hydrogel materials for drug delivery applications. *React. Polym.*, **25**, 139.
34. Foulger, S.H., Jiang, P., Lattam, A.C., Smith, D.W. Jr., and Ballato, J. (2001) Mechanochromic response of poly(ethylene glycol) methacrylate hydrogel encapsulated crystalline colloidal arrays. *Langmuir*, **17**, 6023–6026.
35. Alexandridis, P., Zhou, D., and Khan, A. (1996) Lyotropic liquid crystallinity in amphiphilic block copolymers: temperature effects on phase behavior and structure of poly(ethylene oxide)-b-poly(propylene oxide)-b-poly(ethylene oxide) copolymers of different compositions. *Langmuir*, **12**, 2690.
36. Kim, B. and Peppas, N. (2003) PEG-containing hydrogel micrparticles for oral protein delivery applications. *Biomed. Microdevices*, **5**, 333–341.
37. Gibas, I. and Janik, H. (2010) Review: synthetic polymer hydrogels for biomedical applications. *Chem. Chem. Technol.*, **4** (4), 297–304.
38. Gong, C., Shi, S., Dong, P.-W. *et al.* (2009) Synthesis and characterization of PEG-PCL-PEG thermosensitive hydrogel. *Int. J. Pharm.*, **365** (99), 89.
39. Luzon, M., Boyer, C., Peinado, C., Corrales, T., Whittaker, M., Tao, L.E.I., and Davis, T.P. (2010) Water-soluble, thermoresponsive, hyperbranched copolymers based on PEG-methacrylates: synthesis, characterization, and LCST behaviour. *J. Polym. Sci., Part A: Polym. Chem.*, **48**, 2783–2792.
40. Soeriyadi, A.H., Li, G.-Z., Slavin, S., Jones, M.W., Amos, C.M., Becer, C.R., Whittaker, M.R., Haddleton, D.M., Boyerand, C., and Davis, T.P. (2011) Synthesis and modification of thermoresponsive poly(oligo(ethylene glycol) methacrylate) via catalytic chain transfer polymerization and thiol–ene Michael addition. *Polym. Chem.*, **2**, 815–822.
41. Patenaude, M. and Hoare, T. (2012) Injectable, degradable thermoresponsive poly(N-isopropylacrylamide) hydrogels. *ACS Macro Lett.*, **1**, 409–413.
42. Ito, T., Yeo, Y., Highley, C.B., Bellas, E., and Kohane, D.S. (2007) Dextran-based in situ cross-linked injectable hydrogels to prevent peritoneal adhesions. *Biomaterials*, **28**, 3418–3426.
43. Smeets, N.M.B., Bakaic, E., Patenaude, M., and Hoare, T. (2014) Injectable and tunable poly(ethylene glycol) analogue hydrogels based on poly(oligoethylene glycol methacrylate). *Chem. Commun.*, **50**, 3306–3309.
44. Harris, L.D., Kim, B.-S., and Mooney, D.J. (1998) Open pore biodegradable

matrices formed with gas foaming. *J. Biomed. Mater. Res.*, **42**, 396–402.
45. Thomson, R.C., Mikos, A.G., Beahm, E., Lemon, J.C., Satterfield, W.C., Aufdemorte, T.B., and Miller, M.J. (1999) Guided tissue fabrication from periosteum using preformed biodegradable polymer scaffolds. *Biomaterials*, **20**, 2007.
46. Abebe, D.G. and Fujiwara, T. (2012) Controlled thermoresponsive hydrogels by stereo complexed PLA-PEG-PLA prepared via hybrid micelles of premixed copolymers with different PEG lengths. *Biomacromolecules*, **13**, 1828–1836.
47. Fujiwara, T., Mukose, T., Yamaoka, T., Yamane, H., Sakurai, S., and Kimura, Y. (2001) Novel thermoresponsive formation of a hydrogel by stereo-complexation between PLLA-PEG-PLLA and PDLA-PEG-PDLA block copolymers. *Macromol. Biosci.*, **1**, 204–208.
48. Harke Pharma http://www.harke.com/index.php?id=0&L=1&bc=131;198;164;408;411&tx_hkcatalog_pi1%5btest42%5d=1&tx_hkcatalog_pi1%5bproductid%5d=646&tx_hkcatalog_pi1%5bcountry%5d=156&tx_hkcatalog_pi1%5blegal%5d=294&tx_hkcatalog_pi1%5bmn%5d=44;id11&tx_hkcatalog_pi1%5bnewsid%5d=-1&PHPSESSID=uu6kpcag37bivvddhd5o064garbvt3hvm0281bosm631ia6b2h60 (accessed 22 June 2016).
49. Benamer, S., Mahlous, M., Boukrif, A., Mansouri, B., and Larbi Youcef, S. (2006) Synthesis and characterisation of hydrogels based on poly(vinyl pyrrolidone). *Nucl. Instrum. Methods Phys. Res., Sect. B*, **248**, 284–290.
50. Lugao, A., Rogero, S., and Malmonge, S. (2002) Rheological behaviour of irradiated wound dressing poly(vinyl pyrrolidone) hydrogels. *Radiat. Phys. Chem.*, **63**, 543–546.
51. Ajji, Z., Othoman, I., and Rosiak, J. (2005) Production of hydrogel wound dressings using gamma radiation. *Nucl. Instrum. Methods Phys. Res., Sect. B*, **229**, 375–380.
52. http://what-when-how.com/forensic-sciences/types/ (accessed 18 April 2016).
53. Kumar, A.C. and Mishra, A.K. (2007) 1-Naphthol as an excited state proton transfer fluorescent probe for sensing bound – water hydration of polyvinyl alcohol. *Talanta*, **71**, 2003–2006.
54. Zhang, J.T., Cheng, S.X., and Zhuo, R.X. (2003) Poly(vinyl alcohol)/poly(N-isopropylacrylamide) semi-interpenetrating polymer network hydrogels with rapid response to temperature changes. *Colloid. Polym. Sci.*, **281** (6), 580–583.
55. Han, J., Lei, T., and Wu, Q. (2013) Facile preparation of mouldable polyvinyl alcohol-borax hydrogels reinforced by well-dispersed cellulose nanoparticles: physical, viscoelastic and mechanical properties. *Cellulose*, **20**, 2947–2958.
56. Klok, H.-A. (2009) Peptide/protein–synthetic polymer conjugates: quo vadis. *Macromolecules*, **42** (21), 7990–8000.
57. Van Hest, J.C.M. (2007) Biosynthetic-synthetic polymer conjugates. *J. Macromol. Sci. Part C Polym. Rev.*, **47** (1), 63–92.
58. Stupp, S.I. (2010) Self-assembly and biomaterials. *Nano Lett.*, **10**, 4783–4786.
59. Angeloni, N.L., Bond, C.W., Tang, Y., Harrington, D.A., Zhang, S., Stupp, S.I., McKenna, K.E., and Podlasek, C.A. (2011) Regeneration of the cavernous nerve by sonic hedgehog using aligned peptide amphiphile nanofibers. *Biomaterials*, **32**, 1091–1101.
60. Langer, R. and Vacanti, J. (1993) Tissue engineering. *Science*, **260**, 920–926.
61. Wang, Y., Ameer, G.A., Sheppard, B.J., and Langer, R. (2002) A tough biodegradable elastomer. *Nat. Biotechnol.*, **20**, 602–606.
62. Almany, L. and Seliktar, D. (2005) Biosynthetic hydrogel scaffolds made from fibrinogen and polyethylene glycol for 3D cell cultures. *Biomaterials*, **26**, 2467–2477.
63. Tessmar, J.K. and Gopferich, A.M. (2007) Matrices and scaffolds for protein delivery in tissue engineering. *Adv. Drug Delivery Rev.*, **59**, 274–291.
64. Cui, H., Zhuang, X., He, C., Wei, Y., and Chen, X. (2015) High performance

and reversible ionic polypeptide hydrogel based on charge-driven assembly for biomedical applications. *Acta Biomater.*, **11**, 183–190.
65. Draper, E.R., McDonald, T.O., and Adams, D.J. (2015) A low molecular weight hydrogel with unusualgel aging. *Chem. Commun.*, **51**, 6595–6597.
66. Sen, M., Yakar, A., and Gven, O. (1999) Determination of average molecular weight between cross-links from swelling behaviours of diprotic acid-containing hydrogels. *Polymer*, **40**, 2969–2974.
67. Lee, W. and Shieh, C. (1999) pH-thermoreversible hydrogels. I. Synthesis and swelling behaviors of the (*N*-isopropylacrylamide-*co*-acrylamide-*co*-2-hydroxyethyl methacrylate) copolymeric hydrogels. *J. Appl. Polym. Sci.*, **71**, 221–231.
68. Klug, E.D. (1971) Some properties of water-soluble hydroxyalkyl celluloses and their derivatives. *J. Polym. Sci., Part C: Polym. Symp.*, **36**, 491–508.
69. Eisele, M. and Burchard, W. (1990) Hydrophobic water-soluble polymers 1. Dilute solution properties of poly(1-vinyl-2-piperidone) and poly(*N*-vinylcaprolactam). *Makromol. Chem.*, **191**, 169–184.
70. Yoshioka, H., Mikami, M., Mori, Y., and Tsuchida, E. (1994) A synthetic hydrogel with thermoreversible gelation. II: effect of added salts. *J. Macromol. Sci.*, **A31** (1), 121–125.
71. Malcolm, G. and Rowlinson, J. (1957) Thermodynamic properties of aqueous solutions of polyethylene glycole, poly propylene glycole and dioxane. *Trans. Faraday Soc.*, **53**, 921–931.
72. Gurny, R. and Junginger, H.E. (eds) (1990) *Bioadhesion: Possibilities and Future Trends*, WissenSchaftlicheVerlagsgesellschaft, Stuttgart, p. 14.
73. Lenaert, V. and Gurny, R. (eds) (1990) *Bioadhesive Drug Delivery Systems*, CRC Press, Boca Raton, FL, pp. 1–2419.
74. Ju, X.-J., Chu, L.-Y., Liu, L., Mi, P., and Lee, Y.M. (2008) A novel thermoresponsive hydrogel with ion-recognition property through supramolecular host–guest complexation. *J. Phys. Chem. B*, **112** (4), 1112–1118.
75. Lee, M.-C., Marshall, A.J., Kabilan, S., Blyth, J., and Lowe, C.R. (2004) Glucosesensitive holographic sensors for monitoring bacterial growth. *Anal. Chem.*, **76** (19), 5748–5755.
76. Lapeyre, V., Ancla, C., Catargi, B., and Ravaine, V. (2008) Glucose-responsive microgels with a core shell structure. *J. Colloid Interface Sci.*, **327**, 316–323.
77. Kang, S.I. and Bae, Y.H. (2003) A sulfonamide-based glucose-responsive hydrogel with covalently immobilized glucose oxidase and catalase. *J. Controlled Release*, **86**, 115–121.
78. Pradas, M., Gomez Ribelles, J., Serrano Aroca, A. *et al.* (2001) Interaction between water and polymer chains in poly(hydroxyethyl acrylate) hydrogels. *Colloid. Polym. Sci.*, **279**, 323–330.
79. Ferrer, G., Pradas, M., Gomez Ribelles, J., and Sanchez, M. (2004) Thermodynamical analysis of the hydrogel state in poly(2-hydroxyethyl acrylate). *Polymer*, **45**, 6207–6217.
80. Li, W., Xue, F., and Cheng, R. (2005) States of water in partially swollen poly(vinyl alcohol) hydrogels. *Polymer*, **46**, 12026–12031.
81. Nagura, M., Takagi, N., Katakami, H., Gotoh, Y., Ohkoshi, Y., Koyano, T., and Minoura, N. (1997) States of water in poly(viny1 alcohol) hydrogels. *Polym. Gels Networks*, **5**, 455–468.
82. Deepa, M., Agnihotry, S.A., Gupta, D., and Chandra, R. (2004) Ion-pairing effects and ion-solvent-polymer interactions in LiN(CF3SO2)2-PC-PMMA electrolytes: a FTIR study. *Electrochim. Acta*, **49**, 373–383.
83. Sambrook, J. and Russell, D.W. (2001) *Molecular Cloning: A Laboratory Manual*, 3rd edn, Cold Spring Harbor Laboratory Press, Cold Spring Harbor, NY.
84. Helling, R.B., Goodman, H.M., and Boyer, H.W. (1974) Analysis of endonucleaseR- SEco RI fragments of DNA from lambdoidbacteriophagesand other viruses by agarose-gel electrophoresis. *J. Virol.*, **14**, 1235–1244.

85. Ausubel, F.M., Brent, R., Kingstone, R.E., Moore, D.D., Seidman, J.G., Smith, J.A., and Struhl, K. (eds) (1987) *Current Protocols in Molecular Biology*, vol. **1**, John Wiley & Sons, Inc., New York.
86. Wichterle, O. and Lim, D. (1960) Hydrophilic gels for biological use. *Nature*, **185**, 117–118.
87. Lu, S.X. and Anseth, K.S.J. (1999) Photopolymerization of multilaminatedpoly(HEMA) hydrogels for controlled release. *J. Controlled Release*, **57**, 291–300.
88. Russell, R.J. *et al.* (2001) Mass transfer in rapidly photopolymerizedpoly(ethylene glycol) hydrogels used for chemical sensing. *Polymer*, **42** (11), 4893–4901.
89. http://pslc.ws/macrog/acrylate.htm (accessed 18 April 2016).
90. Syková, E., Jendelová, P., Urdzíková, L., Lesný, P., and Hejčl, A. (2006) Bone marrow stem cells and polymer hydrogels-two strategies for spinal cord injury repair. *Cell. Mol. Neurobiol.*, **26** (7), 1111–1127.
91. Kuo, S., Liou, C., Chang, S., and Wang, Y.-J. (2001) Synthesis and characterizations of hydrogel based on PVA-AE and HEMA. *J. Polym. Res.*, **83**, 169–174.
92. Pavlyuchenko, V., Ushakov, N., Novikov, S. *et al.* (2006) Polymer hydrogels based on 2-hydroxyethyl methacrylate: modification, sorption, and desorption of aminoglycosides. *Russ. J. Appl. Chem.*, **79**, 584–589.
93. Saika, S., Miyamoto, T., and Ohnishi, Y.J. (2003) Histology of anterior capsule opacification with a poly-HEMA/HOHEXMA hydrophilic hydrogel intraocular lens compared to poly(methyl methacrylate), silicone, and acrylic lenses. *J. Cataract. Refract. Surg.*, **29**, 1198–1203.
94. Kubinova, S., Horak, D., Kozubenko, N. *et al.* (2010) The use of superporous Ac-CGGASIKVAVS-OH-modified PHEMA scaffolds to Promote cell adhesion and the differentiation of human fetal neural precursors. *Biomaterials*, **31**, 5966–5975.
95. Kubinova, S., Horak, D., and Sykova, E. (2009) Cholesterol-modified superporouspoly(2-hydroxyethyl methacrylate) scaffolds for tissue engineering. *Biomaterials*, **30**, 4601–4609.
96. Kumar, N., Ganapathy, H., Kim, J. *et al.* (2008) Preparation of poly 2-hydroxyethyl methacrylate functionalized carbon nanotubes as novel biomaterial nanocomposites. *Eur. Polym. J.*, **44**, 579–586.
97. Bavaresco, V., Zavaglia, C., Reis, M., and Gomes, J. (2008) Study on the tribological properties of pHEMA hydrogels for use in artificial articular cartilage. *Wear*, **265**, 269–277.
98. Rizzi, S., Halstenberg, S., and Hubbell, J. (2001) Synthetic, enzymatically degradable extracellular matrices formed from engineered recombinant protein-(poly)ethyleneglycol. *Eur. Cells Mater.*, **2**, 82–83.
99. Lin, C. and Anseth, K. (2009) PEG hydrogels for the controlled release of biomolecules in regenerative medicine. *Pharm. Res.*, **26**, 631–643.
100. Kaplan, H. and Guner, A. (2000) Characterization and determination of swelling and diffusion characteristics of poly(N-vinyl-2-pyrrolidone) hydrogels in water. *J. Appl. Polym. Sci.*, **78**, 994–999.
101. Lee, J. (1990) Competitive ionic hydration involving outer-shell solvent: temperature dependence. *J. Phys. Chem.*, **94**, 258–262.

7 Hydrophilic Polymers

Harikrishna Erothu and Anitha C. Kumar

7.1 Introduction

A polymer is a large molecule (macromolecules) composed of repeating structural units. These subunits are typically connected by covalent chemical bonds. A hydrophilic (water loving) polymer has a tendency to interact with or be dissolved by water and other polar substances [1]. Hydrophilic polymers contain polar or charged functional groups, rendering them soluble in water. These polymers with various architectures are of great interest in the field of polymer science due to their wide range of possible applications. In this chapter, the hydrophilic polymers have been divided into three categories (i) Natural (i.e., isolated from plant, microbial, or animal sources), (ii) semisynthetic, and (iii) synthetic.

Global consumption of synthetic hydrophilic polymer began in the year 2010, and China is the world's largest consumer of synthetic hydrophilic polymers, accounting for 31% of the world market. Western Europe is the second-largest market with 24% of consumption, followed by the United States with 18% [2].

7.2 Classification

Polymers can be classified based on any of the following categories: (i) source (natural, semi synthetic, synthetic); (ii) structure of the polymer (linear, branched chain, cross-linked, or network polymers); (iii) type of polymerization (addition, condensation polymers); (iv) molecular forces (elastomers, fibers, thermoplastic, thermosetting); (v) chain growth polymerization (free radical governed); (vi) degradability (biodegradable, non-biodegradable), and so on However, this chapter focuses mostly on the classification based on source [3] (Figure 7.1).

Biomedical Applications of Polymeric Materials and Composites, First Edition.
Edited by Raju Francis and Sakthi Kumar.

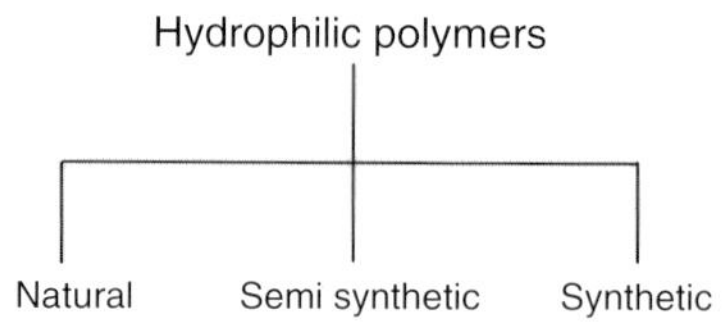

Figure 7.1 Classification of hydrophilic polymers based on source.

7.2.1
Natural Hydrophilic Polymers

Natural hydrophilic polymers are again classified into (i) plant origin and (ii) animal origin.

7.2.1.1 Natural Hydrophilic Polymers from Plant Origin

Guar gum [4–7], xanthan gum [8–12], starch [13], pectin [14–18], dextran [19–27], carrageenan (CRG) [28–33], algin [34], agarose, inulin are the natural hydrophilic polymers from plant origin. Most of these polymers are explained in the chapter *natural biopolymers*.

Agarose is extracted from seaweed and it is a linear polysaccharide made up of the repeating unit of a disaccharide, agarobiose (Figure 7.2). Agarose is one of the two principal components of agar, and is purified from agar by removing agar's other component, agaropectin [35].

Agarose forms thermoreversible gels in water at a concentration as low as 0.1% and at temperatures considerably below the temperature of gel melting (Tgelation ~40 °C and Tmelting ~90 °C) depending on the presence of substituents [36].

Agarose is frequently used in molecular biology for the separation of large molecules, especially DNA, by electrophoresis. Slabs of agarose gels (usually 0.7–2%) for electrophoresis are readily prepared by pouring the warm, liquid solution into a mold. A wide range of different agaroses, of varying molecular weights and properties are commercially available for this purpose.

Inulin is a polysaccharide linked by β (2 → 1) linkages of D-fructose with the end of glucose residue [37] and was discovered by German scientist Valentin Rose in 1804 [38]. Because of this special β-linkage configuration between fructose monomers, inulin-type fructans cannot be degraded by the human digestive system and, therefore, blood sugar levels are not affected [39, 40]. Inulin has a unique range of molecular weight with the degree of polymerization (DP) varying from 2 to 100. The length, composition, and polydispersity of inulin depend on plant species, harvesting time, and extraction and post-extraction processes [41].

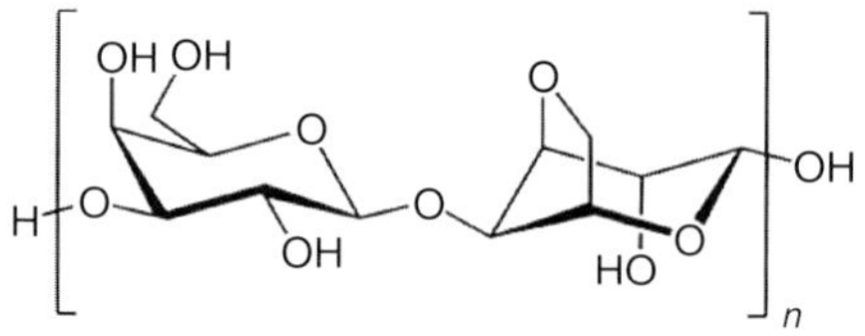

Figure 7.2 Structure of Agarose.

Industrially, it is most commonly extracted from the plant chicory [42]. Inulin is a natural storage carbohydrate present in more than 36 000 species of plants, including wheat, onion, bananas, garlic, asparagus, sunchoke, and chicory [43, 44] (Figure 7.3).

7.2.1.2 Natural Hydrophilic Polymers from Animal Origin

Chitosan (CS) CS is a linear polysaccharide composed of randomly distributed β-(1−4)-linked D-glucosamine and *N*-acetyl-D-glucosamine. It is prepared by treating shrimp and other crustacean shells with the alkali sodium hydroxide [45] (Figure 7.4).

While chitin is insoluble in neutral water, CS is readily soluble in dilute acidic solutions below pH 6.0. This is because CS can be considered a strong base as it possesses primary amino groups with a pK_a value of 6.3. The presence of the amino groups indicates that pH substantially alters the charged state and properties of CS [46]. At low pH, these amines get protonated and become positively charged and that renders CS a water-soluble cationic polyelectrolyte. On the other hand, as the pH increases above 6, CS's amines become deprotonated and the polymer loses its charge and becomes insoluble. The soluble–insoluble transition occurs at its pK_a value around pH between 6 and 6.5 [47] (Figure 7.5).

The dissolution constant K_a of the amine group is obtained from the equilibrium:

$$-NH_2 + H_2O \leftrightarrow -NH_3^{\,+} + OH^-$$

$$K_a = [-NH_2][H_3O\_]/[NH_3^{\,+}] \text{ and } pK_a = -\log K_a \text{ [48].}$$

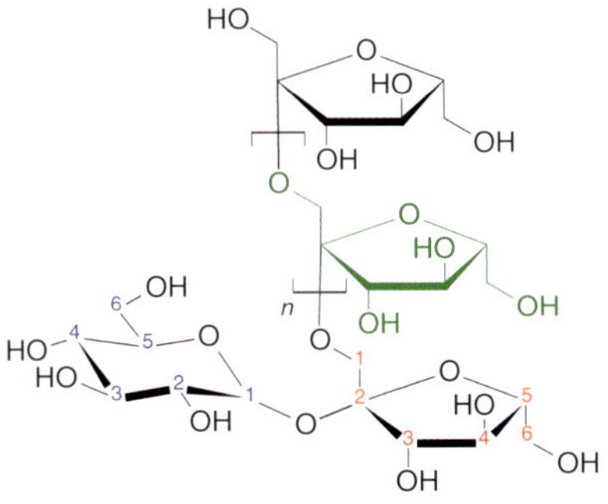

Figure 7.3 Structure of inulin.

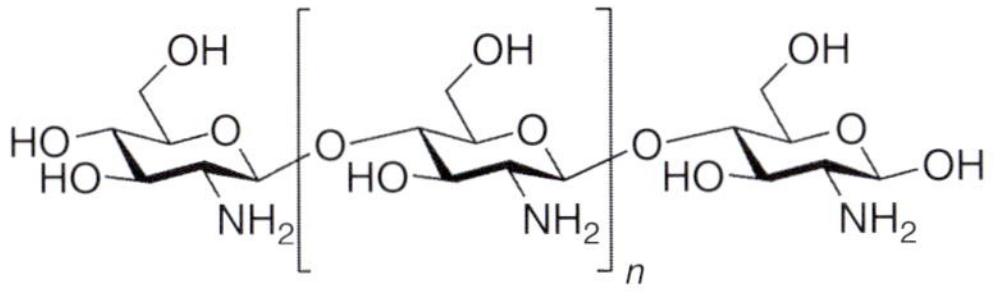

Figure 7.4 Structure of chitosan.

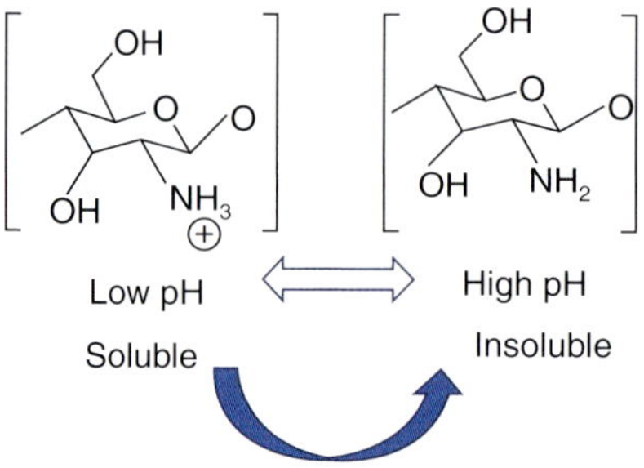

Figure 7.5 Schematic illustration of chitosan's versatility. At low pH (less than about 6), chitosan's amine groups are protonated conferring polycationic behavior to chitosan. At higher pH (above about 6.5), chitosan's amines are deprotonated and reactive.

Chitosan has a number of potential commercial and biomedical uses. It can be used in agriculture as a seed treatment and biopesticide, helping plants to fight off fungal infections. In wine making it can be used as a fining agent, and also helps to prevent spoilage. In industry, it can be used in a self-healing polyurethane paint coating. In medicine, it is used in bandages to reduce bleeding and as an antibacterial agent; it can also be used to help deliver drugs through the skin [48].

Albumin The *albumin* family consists of globular proteins that are water-soluble, the most common of which are serum albumins. Substances containing albumins, such as egg white, are called *albuminoids* [49].

Serum albumins are the most abundant transport proteins in blood plasma. They are the major constituents of the circulatory system. They perform multiple physiological functions that include transportation and disposition of endogenous and exogenous compounds [50, 51]. They are capable of regulating ligand sequestration and transportation, which influence many biological functions, such as membrane penetration, metabolism, half-life, as well as influence several other pharmacokinetic properties. Bovine serum albumin (BSA) and human serum albumin (HSA) are the two most abundant multifunctional serum proteins, accounting for about 52–60% of the plasma [52].

7.2.2 Semisynthetic Hydrophilic Polymers

Semisynthetic water-soluble polymers are derived by either chemical modification of natural polymers or from microbial sources. Most natural hydrophilic polymers are polysaccharides, which vary substantially in their basic sugar units, linkages, and substituents. Derivatives are obtained by substitution, oxidation, cross-linking or partial hydrolysis. The products from animal sources are proteinaceous analogs of the more commonly used polysaccharide-based vegetable polymers.

7.2.2.1 Modified Cellulose

Cellulose is a natural polysaccharide found in all plants. It is composed of repeating D-glucopyranose units bound by β-1,4-glycosidic linkages [53]. Due to strong intramolecular hydrogen bonding, pure cellulose is insoluble in water. If cellulose is converted to cellulose esters or cellulose ethers, they become hydrophilic and are soluble in water. These water-soluble cellulose derivatives are used in a wide range of applications (Figure 7.6).

Hydroxypropylmethyl Cellulose (HPMC) HPMC is a solid, and is a slightly off-white to light brown powder in appearance and may be formed into granules. The addition of methyl and hydroxypropyl substituents to HPMC disrupts the crystalline structure of native cellulose, making cellulose water-soluble [54]. For the synthesis of HPMC, cellulose from wood pulp is extracted using an alkaline base at high temperatures [55] followed by the addition of alkyl halides or oxiranes to supply the methyl and hydroxypropyl substituents. Methyl oxide, methyl chloride, and propylene oxide are generally used and the final proportions of substituents can be altered by changing the molar ratio of these sources [56]. HPMC is used routinely as a coating for pharmaceutical tablets because of its ability to coat using an aqueous system that improves environmental safety [57]. HPMC is approved by the Food and Drug Administration (FDA) as both a direct and an indirect food additive, and is approved for use as a food additive by the EU (Figure 7.7).

Hydroxyethyl Cellulose (HEC) HEC is commercially produced by reaction of alkali cellulose with ethylene oxide (EO) in a heterogeneous process. It is one of the most important types of cellulose because of its wonderful properties and chemical composition. It has a large amount of easily accessible hydroxyl units that can be bonded with a number of functional groups [58, 59]. Depending on the etherification degrees, HEC shows different solubility and is generally classified as water-soluble or alkali-soluble. Water-soluble HEC has been extensively used as a stabilizer in food and cosmetic products, binder in tablets, thickener in latex paints, water-binder in welding rods or glazes of ceramics, and in building materials applications in industry [60, 61] (Figure 7.8).

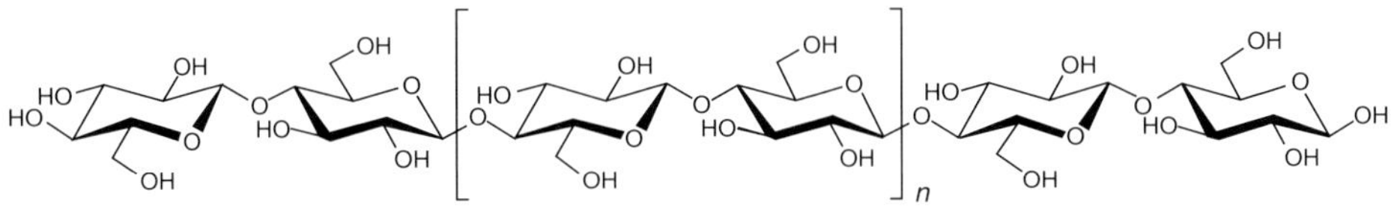

Figure 7.6 Structure of cellulose.

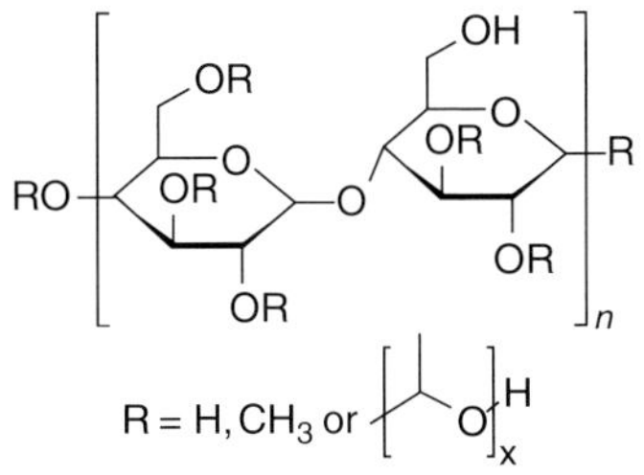

Figure 7.7 Structure of HPMC.

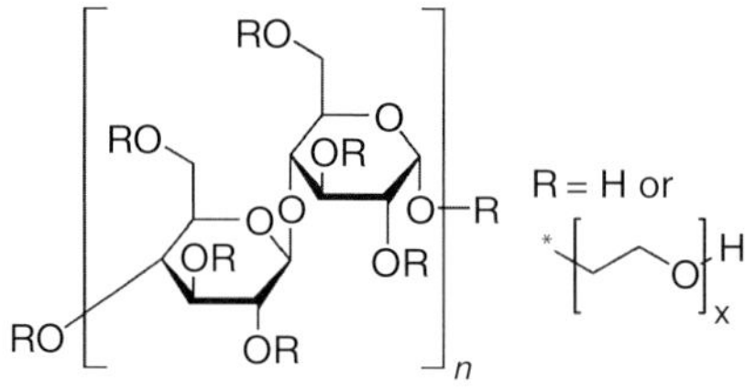

Figure 7.8 Structure of HEC.

Sodium Carboxy Methyl Cellulose (Na-CMC) *Na-CMC* can be prepared from cellulose by treatment with alkali and monochloro-acetic acid or its sodium salt under rigidly controlled conditions. It was commercially introduced in 1946 by Hercules in the United States [62] Structure of Na-CMC is illustrated in Figure 7.9.

It easily absorbs moisture and dissolves in cold or hot water to form a colloidal solution. Their solution characteristics depend on the average chain length or DP as well as the degree of substitution. As the molecular weight increases, the viscosity of Na-CMC solutions increases rapidly. The degree of neutralization of carboxymethyl groups also impacts viscosity. In solution, the degree of neutralization is controlled by the pH [62].

7.2.2.2 Modified Chitosan

Chitosan is insoluble in water at neutral pH and dissolves only in acidic solutions. Therefore, water-soluble derivatives of chitosan have been synthesized by various researchers by chemical modification [63–66]. Chitosan become water soluble through a chemical modification.

Chitosan-PEG hybrid Masatoshi *et al.* [63] synthesized the water-soluble chitosan–PEG hybrid by the following method. Chitosan was dissolved in a mixture of aqueous 2% acetic acid solution and methanol. An aqueous solution of PEG-aldehyde was added to the above chitosan solution and stirred for 30 min at room temperature. Then the pH of chitosan/PEG-aldehyde solution was adjusted to 6.5 with aqueous 1 M NaOH solution and stirred for 60 min at room temperature. At this time, the solution was still pale yellow and did not precipitate. Sodium cyanoborohydride (NaCNBH) in water was added to the reaction mixture dropwise for 20 min and the solution was stirred for 18 h at room temperature. The reaction mixture was dialyzed with dialysis membrane against aqueous 0.05 M NaOH solution and water alternately. When the pH of

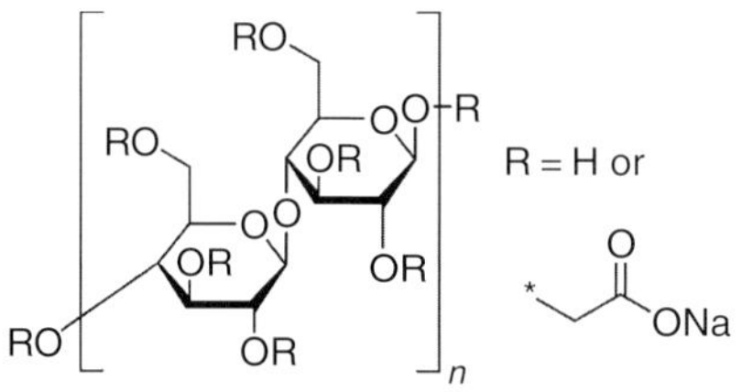

Figure 7.9 Structure of Na-CMC [62].

the outer solution reached 7.5, the inner solution was centrifuged for 20 min. The supernatant was freeze-dried and washed twice with 100 ml acetone. Unreacted PEG was removed by washing with acetone. After drying in vacua, a white powder was obtained as water-soluble chitosan-PEG hybrid.

N-[(2-hydroxy-3-trimethylammonium)propyl]chitosan Chloride (HTCC) Lim *et al.* [64] reported the synthesis of water-soluble chitosan derivative HTCC. It is synthesized by reacting chitosan with glycidyltrimethylammonium chloride (GTMAC) in a neutral aq. condition, in which the hydroxyl groups of chitosan are not sufficiently nucleophilic to induce ring opening of GTMAC, whereas the amino group of chitosan is nucleophilic enough to do that. The HTCC was further modified by reacting with *N*-methylolacrylamide (NMA) to prepare a fiber-reactive chitosan derivative, *O*-acrylamidomethyl-HTCC (NMA–HTCC). The optimal reaction conditions for introducing higher amounts of the fiber-reactive (acrylamidomethyl) groups on chitosan backbone are also reported by this group. HTCC shows water solubility as well as excellent antimicrobial activity [67, 68].

Half N-Acetylated Chitosan Kubota *et al.* [65] synthesized the water-soluble half N-acetylated chitosan by degradation followed by N-acetylation of chitosan. Chitosan is degraded by treatment with sodium perborate ($NaBO_3$), N-acetylated with acetic anhydride in aqueous acetic acid. They investigated the relationship between the molecular weight and water solubility of the obtained N-acetylated chitosan as well as the solubility of the half N-acetylated chitosan in some organic solvents. They concluded that the half N-acetylated chitosan thus obtained had a random distribution of the *N*-acetyl groups, and that the lower the molecular weight, the higher the water solubility. Furthermore, the solubility of the half N-acetylated chitosan in aqueous organic solvents also increased with decreasing molecular weight.

Hydroxypropyl Chitosan (HPCTS) Water-soluble chitosan derivative *HPCTS* was synthesized from chitosan and propylene epoxide under alkali conditions by Xie *et al.* [66]. Purified chitosan was added to 50 wt% NaOH solution and placed at −18 °C for alkalization. Alkali chitosan and isopropyl alcohol were mixed and stirred for 1 h at 40 °C. Then propylene epoxide was added, and refluxed for 2 h at 60 °C with continuous stirring. The reaction mixture was adjusted to pH 7.0 by adding 1:1 (v/v) HCl, filtrated, and the obtained product was repeatedly washed by acetone and 95% (v/v) alcohol and then dried under vacuum at 60 °C for 48 h (Figure 7.10).

Chitosan with Phenolic Hydroxyl Groups (Chit-Ph) Sakai *et al.* conjugated chitosan with 3-(*p*-hydroxyphenyl)propionic acid using aqueous-phase carbodiimide activation chemistry to produce Chit-Ph[69]. Chi-Ph is soluble in water at neutral pH and gelated via an enzymatic reaction by consuming H_2O_2 within seconds. The time necessary for gelation decreased with increasing content of Ph groups,

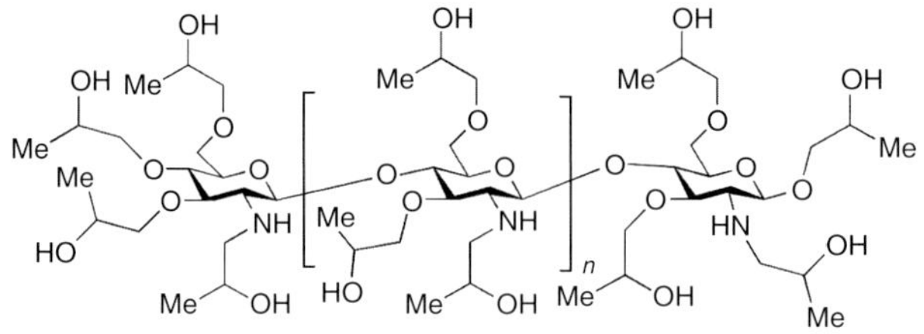

Figure 7.10 Structure of HPCTS.

temperature, peroxidase concentration, and decreasing H_2O_2 concentration. Chit-Ph has the potency for use as injectable hydrogels in applications such as tissue engineering and drug delivery.

Carboxymethyl Chitosan Carboxymethylation is another method to improve the water solubility of chitosan [70]. Chitosan has reactive amino, primary hydroxyl, and secondary hydroxyl groups, which can be used for chemical modifications under mild reaction conditions to alter its properties. carboxymethylchitosan are of three types: (i) *N-carboxymethyl chitosan* (*NCMC*) [71], (ii) *O-carboxymethyl chitosan* (*OCMC*), and (iii) *N,O-carboxymethyl chitosan* (*NOCMC*) [72–74].

One way to synthesize the *N-carboxymethyl chitosan* is to treat chitosan with glyoxylic acid, and then hydrogenate by reacting it with NaBH4 or NaCNBH3(reductive alkylation).In this method partially di-substituted *N*-carboxymethyl chitosan (*N,N-diCMC*) [75] is unavoidably produced, even under mild conditions; therefore, the term *N*-carboxymethyl chitosan should imply that a substantial fraction is di-substituted. Muzzarelli *et al.* [71], who first reported this method, found an alternative for this. They dissolved chitosan in 1% acetic acid to get approximately 1–1.5 w/v solution, then treated with solution of glyoxylic acid in molar ratio 1 : 1–1 : 3 of amine:acid followed by reduction with portions of sodium borohydride to obtain pH of 4–5 without precipitation in the reaction mixture. The viscous solution was then dialyzed against water and lyophilized to get *N*-carboxymethyl chitosan.

An *et al.* [76] reacted chitosan 1% w/v swollen in water with monochloroacetic acid in a 1 : 4 ratio of amine:acid (by weight) at pH 8–8.5 at a temperature of 90 °C to get *N,N-dicarboxymethylchitosan.*

For synthesis of *OCMC* and *NOCMC*, the chitosan is soaked in alkaline solution at freezing or room temperature for 2–24 h. For this purpose, the concentration of chitosan commonly reported is 4–20% w/v in 40–50% w/v solution of NaOH. The activated chitosan is then reacted with monochloroacetic acid in solid or solution form. The concentration of monochloroacetic acid used is 1 : 1–1 : 6 by weight in isopropanol/ethanol and the reaction is carried out at 0–60 °C for 2–24 h [72–74]. The product is precipitated by solvent as acetone, ethanol, and desalted by pH adjustment or dialysis.

Carboxybutyl Chitosan Another chitosan derivative, *N*-carboxybutyl chitosan, is an amphoteric polymer that is soluble under acidic, neutral, and basic conditions [77] (Figure 7.11).

It is synthesized by the reaction of levulinic acid on chitosan [78]. Depending on the chemical conditions, the reaction tends to form *N*-carboxybutyl chitosan or 5-methylpyrrolidinone chitosan [79, 80], a cyclic product.5-methylpyrrolidinone chitosan dissolves only in acidic condition similarly to pure chitosan. *N*-carboxybutyl chitosan is used for wound healing, cosmetic production, and so on.

7.2.3 Synthetic Hydrophilic Polymers

Natural hydrophilic polymers were not always suitable because their properties were not always reproducible for many applications. Therefore, a lot of interest has been devoted to the design of polymeric materials for many applications. Synthetic hydrophilic polymers have different applications in pharmacology, biotechnology, and chemistry. In this chapter, some examples of synthetic hydrophilic polymers have been provided.

7.2.3.1 Poly(acrylamide) (PAAM)

The acrylamide monomer used for the synthesis of polyacrylamide was first reported in 1894 by Moureu [81]. It is mostly prepared by radical polymerization using peroxide or persulfate as initiators [82]. PAAM is chemically inert, stable in the pH range 3–11 and is used in a wide range of applications such as microanalysis to macro-fractionation for proteins, nucleic acid, and other biomolecules, and is nowadays the medium of choice in all electrophoretic techniques, cosmetic products (moisturizers, lotions, creams, self-tanning products, etc.) drug delivery, and so on [83–87]. PAAM with less than 0.2% acrylamide monomer is approved by the FDA (Figure 7.12).

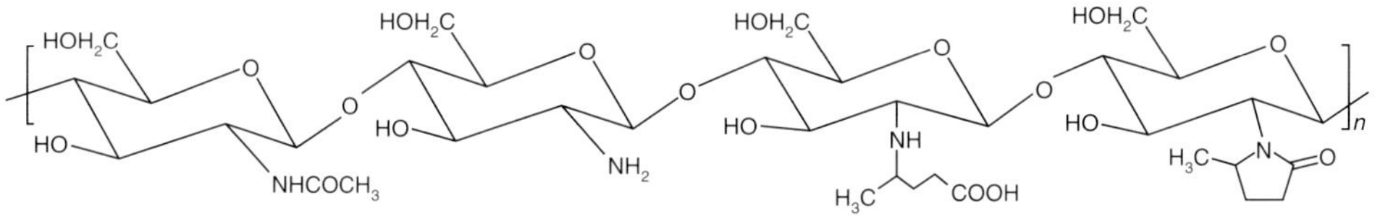

Figure 7.11 *N*-Carboxybutyl chitosan and 5-methylpyrrolidinone chitosan.

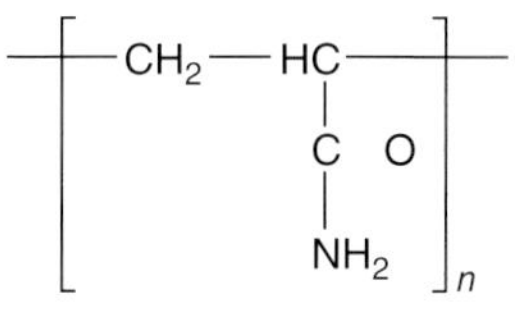

Figure 7.12 Structure of PAAM.

7.2.3.2 Poly(acrylic acid) (PAA)

PAA is the homopolymer of acrylic acid, cross-linked with an allyl ether pentaerythritol, allyl ether of sucrose or allyl ether of propylene. It has the ability to absorb and retain water and swell to many times its original volume and, therefore, it is used in disposable diapers [88]. For many applications, PAAs are used in the form of alkali metal or ammonium salts, for example, sodium polyacrylate (Figure 7.13).

7.2.3.3 Poly(ethylene Oxide) (PEO) or Poly(ethylene Glycol) (PEG)

PEO is produced by the interaction of ethylene oxide with water, ethylene glycol, or ethylene glycol oligomers [3, 89]. It has been approved by the FDA for several medical applications due to its biocompatibility and low toxicity [90].

$$HOCH_2CH_2OH + n(CH_2CH_2O) \rightarrow HO(CH_2CH_2O)n + 1H$$

Polymerization can be cationic or anionic depending on the catalyst type. The process of both covalent and non-covalent attachment or amalgamation of PEG polymer chains to molecules and macrostructures, such as a drug, therapeutic protein, or vesicle is known as *PEGylation* (also often styled *pegylation*) and was first introduced in the late 1970s [91–94]. PEG prolongs the circulation half-life of therapeutic proteins, liposomes, or nanoparticles and reduces their immunogenicity by providing a steric barrier against interactions with plasma proteins, opsonins, and cells of the mononuclear phagocyte system (stealth property) [95–97] (Figure 7.14).

7.2.3.4 Poly[(organo)phosphazenes]

Poly[(organo)phosphazenes] are inorganic/organic hybrid polymers. The polymer backbone consists of alternating phosphorus and nitrogen atoms and organic substituents are linked to the phosphorus atoms as side groups [98] (Figure 7.15).

The major precursor, polydichlorophosphazene, is extremely hydrolytically unstable but can be readily substituted with nucleophilic substituents to give a wide range of stable poly[(organo)phosphazenes] [99]. Some of the most important water-soluble polyphosphazenes are poly[di(carboxylatophenoxy) phosphazene] (PCPP), poly[di(methoxyethoxyethoxy) phosphazene] (MEEP)

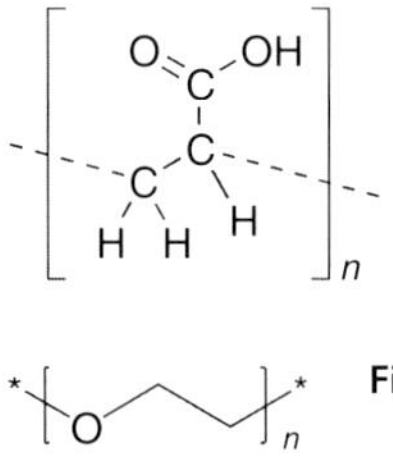

Figure 7.13 Structure of PAA.

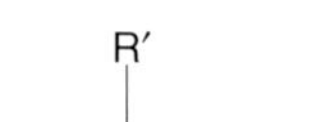

Figure 7.14 Structure of PEO.

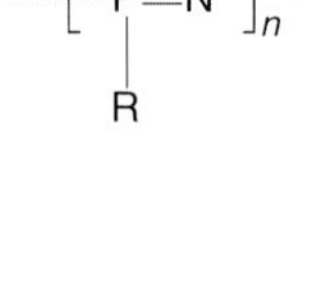

Figure 7.15 Generic structure of poly[(organo)phosphazenes].

have been studied by Allcock and his coworkers [100, 101]. Poly[(organo) phosphazenes] are used for tissue engineering and drug delivery, as hydrogels, shape memory polymers, and as stimuli-responsive materials [98].

7.2.3.5 Poly[*N*-(2-hydroxypropyl) methacrylamide] (PHPMA)

This is a highly hydrophilic, nonimmunogenic and nontoxic polymer and resides well in blood circulation. PHPMA can be synthesized by a variety of polymerization techniques including conventional radical polymerization [102], atom transfer radical polymerization (ATRP) [103], and reversible addition-fragmentation chain transfer (RAFT) polymerization of *N*-(2-hydroxypropyl) methacrylamide (HPMA) [104] (Figure 7.16).

The first HPMA copolymer–drug [*N*-(4-aminobenzensulfonyl)-*N*′-butylurea] conjugate was presented at the Prague Microsymposium on Polymers in Medicine in 1977 by Obereigner *et al.* [105, 106]. This is an alternative hydrophilic polymer that incorporates functionality via a secondary hydroxyl group, which has been shown to be a viable alternative to PEG in many applications in the field of nanomedicine [107].

7.2.3.6 Divinyl Ether-Maleic Anhydride (DIVEMA)

The copolymer DIVEMA, which is also known as pyran copolymer, is used in drug delivery systems. It acts as an antitumor, antiviral, antifungal, and antibacterial agent. Its biological activity depends on the molecular weight. At a molecular weight of 10 000, DIVEMA exhibits antitumor activity, and a higher molecular weight activitates antibacterial activity. The preparation of 1 : 2 divinyl ether-maleic anhydride copolymer was first reported by Butler. It is synthesized by the radical polymerization of monomers and the low molecular

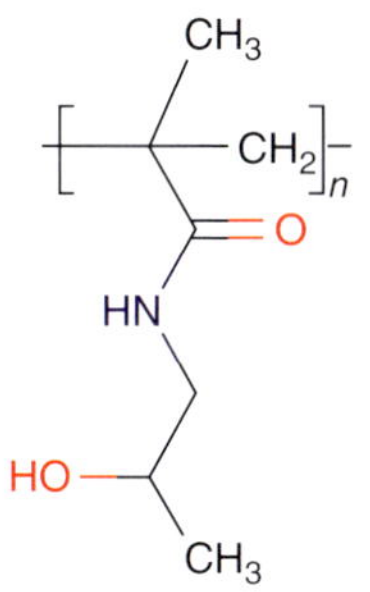

Figure 7.16 Structure of PHPMA.

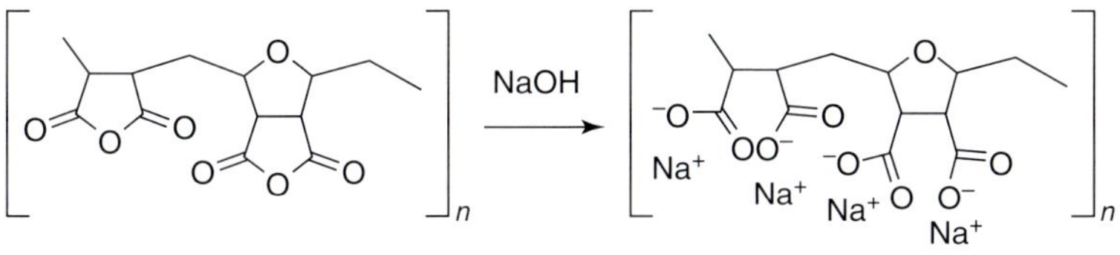

Figure 7.17 Structure of DIVEMA and sodium salt of DIVEMA.

weight impurities is removed by the extraction of ether [108]. It is readily soluble in water by alkaline hydrolysis [109] (Figure 7.17).

7.2.3.7 Poly(oxazoline) (POZ)

Polyoxazoline polymers are nonionic, stable, and highly soluble in water and organic solvents. They are prepared by the living cationic polymerization method. Different methods have been reported in the literature. One is the stoichiometric addition of an electrophile initiator like alkyl tosylate or alkytriflate to the oxazo line monomer that is dissolved in a dry organic solvent and in an inert atmosphere [110, 111]. The propagation phase is conducted at 80 °C for approximately 1 to 3 days. Another one is the polymerization that is carried out with microwave energy to reduce the propagation time from days to hours [112, 113]. In both cases, the living cation is terminated by the introduction of a nucleophile such as OH, NH, COO, or S. Termination is conducted with aqueous sodium carbonate to give a hydroxyl terminal group or by reacting with a secondary amine such as morpholine or piperidine to give a terminal tertiary amine.

It was first developed as a food additive in the early 1980s [114]. POZ has the same "stealth" properties as PEG and, therefore, can be used in multiple pharmaceutical and medical applications1 [115, 116]. The generic chemical structures of polymethy-loxazoline (PMOZ), polyethyloxazoline (PEOZ), and polypropy-loxazoline (PPOZ) are shown in Figure 7.18.

7.2.3.8 Poly(vinyl pyrrolidone) (PVP)

PVP is synthesized by the polymerization of vinylpyrrolydone in water or isopropanol and has a molecular weight ranging from 40 000 to 360 000. PVP is FDA approved and the main use of PVP is as a binder in tablet formation and it is available in different grades based on molecular weight. It was found that acetaminophen (paracetamol) tablets formulated with 4% PVP 90 000 as a binder released the drug more quickly than did tablets with gelatin or hydroxypropyl cellulose [118–120] (Figure 7.19).

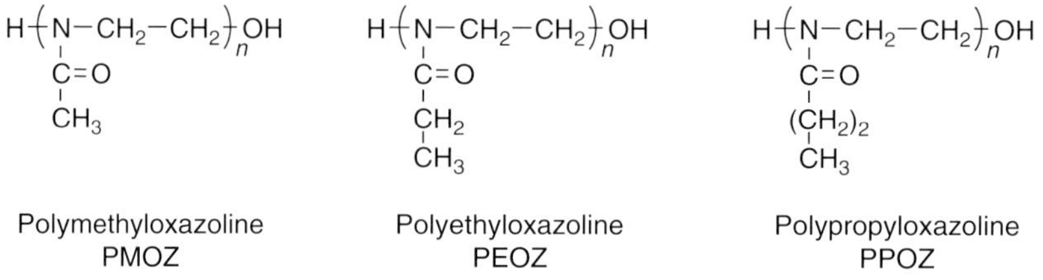

Figure 7.18 Chemical structures of three types of POZ [117].

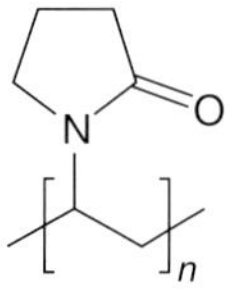

Figure 7.19 Structure of PVP.

7.2.3.9 Poly(*N*-isopropylacrylamide) (PNIPAM)

PNIPAM is a chemical isomer of poly-leucine, having a polar peptide group in the side chain rather than in the back bone as shown in Figure 7.20. It is a temperature-responsive polymer that shows lower critical solution temperature (LCST) and was first synthesized in the 1950s [121] from *N*-isopropylacrylamide by free-radical polymerization and is readily functionalized making it useful in a variety of applications. PNIPAM is used in biochemical or biomedical applications [122] (Figure 7.20).

7.2.3.10 Poly(vinyl alcohol) (PVA)

PVA is synthesized by the polymerization of vinyl acetate to polyvinyl acetate (PVAc), which is then hydrolyzed to get PVA. Water is the most important solvent for PVA. It is also soluble in highly polar and hydrophilic solvents, such as dimethyl sulfoxide (DMSO), ethylene glycol (EG), and *N*-methyl pyrrolidone (NMP).They form tough, clean films that have high tensile strength and abrasion resistance. PVA is widely used in industry in the manufacture of pharmaceuticals, optical films, and so on [123]. A number of investigators developed PVA hydrogels for biomedical applications, in particular, transdermal drug delivery systems [124]. It is a particularly interesting polymer system for such applications because of its low toxicity, high biocompatibility, and high degree of swelling in water. PVA is chemically inert in many organic solvents and optically transparent in the UV-Visible region. The alcohol units are proton donors and can interact by hydrogen bonding with the amide carbonyl groups of the tertiary polyamide. The possibility of hydrogen bond formation between hydroxyls and neighboring carbonyls in the copolymer imply a short-scale competition of specific interactions (Figure 7.21).

7.3 Applications of Hydrophilic Polymers

The interest evinced on hydrophilic polymers is because of its vast area of applications such as food, pharmaceuticals, paint, textiles, paper, constructions, adhesives, coatings, water treatment, dispersing and suspending agents,

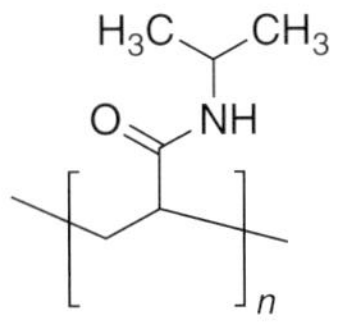

Figure 7.20 Structure of PNIPAM.

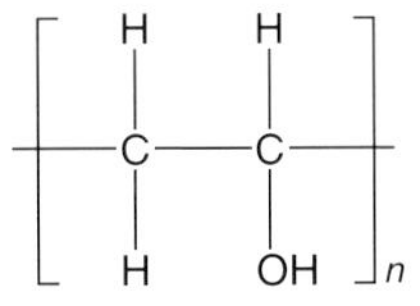

Figure 7.21 Structure of PVA.

stabilizers, thickeners, gellants, flocculants and coagulants, film-formers, humectants, binders and lubricants, personal care, building products, detergents, oil field products, and mineral processing [3].

Many cellulose and chitosan derivatives are used in food materials as gelling agents, thickening agents, and so on (Table 7.1).

Hydrophilic polymers are promising biomaterials intended to replace conventional products. Soluble grades of PVP and polyvinyl pyrrolidone-vinyl acetate (PVP-VA) copolymer have been used to improve the bioavailability of many poor water-soluble drugs such as indomethacin, tolbutamide, and nifedipine [126, 127]. The "stealth" properties of PEO and POZ make them very useful in biomedical applications like drug carriers [128]. Studies show that radiolabeled POZ suggests that the polymer is rapidly excreted by the kidney with no significant accumulation in tissues [129, 130]. The super absorbent polymers, polyacrylates and sodium polyacrylates, are used in disposable diapers [88]. The use of hydrophilic polymers-starch-based soil additives for container-grown plants helps reduce water consumption and irrigation frequency [131].

Hydrophilic polymers have many different roles in the field of tissue engineering. They are applied as delivery vehicles for bioactive molecules and as space filling agents. As space filling scaffolds, hydrogels maintain the desired volume and structural integrity for the required time [132]. Space filling agents are the simplest group of scaffolds and are used in bulking, adhesion prevention, as a biological "glue," promotion of angiogenesis, and encapsulation of secretory cells. Hydrogel scaffolds can engineer every tissue in the body, including cartilage, bone, and smooth muscle. Scaffolds composed of alginate, chitosan, and collagen show potential for use as general bulking agents. Synthetic hydrogels are often appropriate materials for use as anti-adhesives because, if designed appropriately, proteins cannot be readily absorbed by them. PEG has been used to prevent post-operative adhesions and to protect arteries from intimal thickening after damage [133–135].

Different types of chitosan-based scaffolds are available such as chitosan-based hydrogel scaffolds, chitosan-based nanofiber scaffolds, polymer-based composite chitosan scaffolds for *in vivo* evaluation, chitosan–calcium phosphate composite scaffolds, and chitosan-based scaffolds with enhanced functionality for bone tissue engineering applications [136]. Chitosan is especially attractive as a bone

Table 7.1 Use of cellulose and chitosan derivatives [125].

Material	Function of material
Cellulose derivatives	
CMC	Thickener
HPC	Thickener and emulsifier
HOMC	Thickener
MC	Thickener, emulsifier, and gelling agent
Chitosan	Gelling agent
	Antimicrobials

scaffold material as it supports the attachment and proliferation of bone-forming osteoblast cells *in vitro* [137]. In addition, modified chitosan scaffolds are bioactive and biodegradable, and exhibit osteo conductivity *in vivo* in surgically created bone defects [138, 139].

Alginate hydrogels in pharmaceutics serve as thickening, gel forming, and stabilizing agents, as alginate can play a significant role in wound healing [140], drug delivery [141], protein delivery [142], and tissue engineering applications to date, as these gels exhibit structural similarity to the extracellular matrices in tissues and can be manipulated to play several critical roles [143]. Oral dosage forms are currently the most frequent use of alginate in pharmaceutical applications, but the use of alginate hydrogels as depots for tissue-localized drug delivery is growing. Kong *et al.* reported that alginate gels release condensed plasmid DNA (size ~100 nm) at the degradation time. Cells must migrate out of alginate hydrogels, and/or be released as the gel degrades [144]. Alginate gels are also being actively investigated for their ability to mediate the regeneration and engineering of a variety of other tissues and organs, including skeletal muscle, pancreas, and liver and those in the central and peripheral nerve systems. Current strategies for skeletal muscle regeneration using alginate gels include cell transplantation, growth factor delivery, or a combination of both approaches [145, 146]. A combined delivery of VEGF and insulin-like growth factor-1 (IGF-1) from alginate gels was used to modulate both angiogenesis and myogenesis [147].

7.4 Conclusions

Polymeric Sciences has a history spanning many years in hydrophilic materials. Water-soluble polymers have a distinguished record of clinical relevance. Hydrophilic polymers are important because of their use in a variety of applications. Scientists are still trying to synthesize new polymers and improve its properties. This chapter discusses the synthesis, properties, and applications of different hydrophilic polymers. The nature of thr polymer depends on its molecular weight, crystallinity, chemical composition, and macromolecular topology or architecture. By varying these parameters, hydrophilic polymers can be useful for many more applications.

Abbreviations

Chit-Ph	chitosan with phenolic hydroxyl groups
CRG	carrageenan
CS	chitosan
DIVEMA	divinyl ether-maleic anhydride
DMSO	dimethyl sulfoxide
DP	degree of polymerization

EG	ethylene glycol
EO	ethylene oxide
FDA	Food and Drug Administration
GTMAC	glycidyltrimethylammonium chloride
HEC	hydroxyethyl cellulose
HPCTS	hydroxypropyl chitosan
HPMA	*N*-(2-hydroxypropyl) methacrylamide
HPMC	hydroxypropylmethyl cellulose
HTCC	*N*-[(2-hydroxy-3-trimethylammonium) propyl]chitosan chloride
LCST	lower critical solution temperature
MEEP	poly[di(methoxyethoxyethoxy) phosphazene]
$NaBO_3$	sodium perborate
Na-CMC	sodium carboxy methyl cellulose
NaCNBH	sodium cyanoborohydride
NCMC	*N*-carboxymethyl chitosan
NMA	*N*-methylolacrylamide
NMA–HTCC	*O*-acrylamidomethyl-HTCC
NMP	*N*-methyl pyrrolidone
NOCMC	*N*,*O*-carboxymethyl chitosan
OCMC	*O*-carboxymethyl chitosan
PAA	poly(acrylic acid)
PAAM	poly(acrylamide)
PCPP	poly[di(carboxylatophenoxy) phosphazene]
PEG	poly(ethylene glycol)
PEO	poly(ethylene oxide)
PHPMA	poly[*N*-(2-hydroxypropyl) methacrylamide]
PNIPAM	poly(*N*-isopropylacrylamide)
POZ	poly(oxazoline)
PVA	poly(vinyl alcohol)
PVAc	poly(vinyl acetate)
PVP	poly(vinyl pyrrolidone)
PVP-VA	poly(vinyl pyrrolidone)-vinyl acetate
RAFT	reversible addition-fragmentation chain transfer

References

1. (a) IUPAC (1997) *Compendium of Chemical Terminology*, 2nd edn (the "Gold Book"). Compiled by A.D. McNaught and A. Wilkinson, Blackwell Scientific Publications, Oxford; (b)XML on-line corrected version: http://goldbook.iupac.org (2006) created by M. Nic, J. Jirat, and B. Kosata; updates compiled by A. D. Jenkins.
2. Will, R., Loechner, U., and Yokose, K. (2011) Synthetic Water Soluble Polymers, http://www.sriconsulting.com/CEH/Public/Reports/582.0000/ (accessed 28 June 2011).
3. Kadajji, V.G. and Betageri, G.V. (2011) Water soluble polymers for pharmaceutical applications. *Polymers*, **3**, 1972–2009.

4. Guar Gum http://www.fao.org/ag/agn/jecfa-additives/specs/monograph3/additive-218.pdf (accessed 18 April 2011).
5. Goldstein, A.M., Alter, E.N., and Seaman, J.K. (1973) in *Industrial Gums, Polysaccharides and their Derivatives* (ed. R.L. Whistler), Academic Press, New York, pp. 303–321.
6. Berner-Strzelczyk, A., Koodziejska, J., and Zgoda, M. (2006) Application of guar gum biopolymer in the prescription of tablets with sodium ibuprofen–quality tests and pharmaceutical availability in vitro. *Polim. Med.*, **36**, 3–11.
7. Diytrade http://www.diytrade.com/china/pd/5131458/Fast_Hydrating_Guar_Gum.html (accessed 18 April 2016).
8. Barrére, G.C., Barber, C.E., and Daniels, M.J. (1986) Molecular cloning of genes involved in the production of the extracellular polysaccharide xanthan by *Xanthomonas campestris* pv. *campestris*. *Int. J. Biol. Macromol.*, **8** (6), 372–374.
9. Fooducate http://blog.fooducate.com/2010/09/23/10-facts-about-xantham-gum-a-very-popular-food-additive/ (accessed 18 April 2016).
10. Garcia-Ochoa, F., Santos, V.E., Casas, J.A., and Gomez, E. (2000) Xanthan gum: production, recovery and properties. *Biotechnol. Adv.*, **18**, 549–579.
11. All Allergy Substance Info (and synonyms): Xanthan gum. http://www.allallergy.net/fapaidfind.cfm?cdeoc=2322 (accessed 19 May 2010).
12. Sharma, B.R., Naresh, L., Dhuldhoya, N.C., Merchant, S.U., and Merchant, U.C. (2006) Xanthan gum-a boon to food industry. *Food Promot. Chron.*, **1**, 27–30.
13. Pareta, R. and Edirisinghe, M.J. (2006) A novel method for the preparation of starch films and coatings. *Carbohydr. Polym.*, **63**, 425–431.
14. Braconnot, H. (1825) Investigations into a new acid spread throughout all plants. *Ann. Chim. Phys.*, **2** (28), 173–178.
15. Keppler, F., Hamilton, J.T., Brass, M., and Röckmann, T. (2006) Methane emissions from terrestrial plants under aerobic conditions. *Nature*, **439**, 187–191.
16. Stephen, A.M. and Phillips, G.O. (2006) *Food Polysaccharides and their Applications*, Taylor & Francis, Boca Raton, FL.
17. Sriamornsak, P. (2003) Chemistry of pectin and its pharmaceutical uses: a review. *Silpakorn Univ. Int. J.*, **3** (1–2), 206–228.
18. Silvateam http://en.silvateam.com/Products-Services/Food-Ingredients/Pectin/Main-applications (accessed 18 April 2016).
19. Pasteur, L. (1861) On the viscous fermentation and the butyrous fermentation. *Bull. Soc. Chim. Paris*, **11**, 30–31 (in French) ISSN: 0037–8968..
20. Nácher-Vázquez, M., Ballesteros, N., Canales, Á., Saint-Jean, S.R., Pérez-Prieto, S.I., Prieto, A., Aznar, R., and López, P. (2015) Dextrans produced by lactic acid bacteria exhibit antiviral and immunomodulatory activity against salmonid viruses. *Carbohydr. Polym.*, **124**, 292–301.
21. http://www.ncbi.nlm.nih.gov/pmc/articles/PMC422963/ (accessed 18 April 2016).
22. Lewis, S.L. (2010) *Medical Surgical Nursing*, 8th edn, Elsevier, ISBN: 978–0323079150.
23. Hosseinkhani, H., Aoyama, T., Ogawa, O., and Tabata, Y. (2003) RETRACTED: tumor targeting of gene expression through metal-coordinated conjugation with dextran. *J. Controlled Release*, **88** (2), 297–312.
24. Anitha, A., Deepagan, V.G., Rani, V.V.D., Menon, D., Nair, S.V., and Jayakumar, R. (2011) Preparation, characterization, *in vitro* drug release and biological studies of curcumin loaded dextran sulphate–chitosan nanoparticles. *Carbohydr. Polym.*, **84**, 1158–1164.
25. Ritcharoen, W., Thaiying, Y., Saejeng, Y., Jangchud, I., Rangkupan, R., Meechaisue, C., and Supaphol, P. (2008) Electrospun dextran fibrous membranes. *Cellulose*, **15**, 435–444.
26. Cutiongco, M.F.A., Tan, M.H., Ng, M.Y.K., Le Visage, C., and Yim, E.K.F. (2014) Composite pullulan–dextran

polysaccharide scaffold with interfacial polyelectrolyte complexation fibers: a platform with enhanced cell interaction and spatial distribution. *Acta Biomater.*, **10**, 4410–4418.

27. Sun, G.M., Zhang, X.J., Shen, Y.I., Sebastian, R., Dickinson, L.E., Fox-Talbot, K., Reinblatt, M., Steenbergen, C., Harmon, J.W., and Gerecht, S. (2011) Dextran hydrogel scaffolds enhance angiogenic responses and promote complete skin regeneration during burn wound healing. *Proc. Natl. Acad. Sci. U.S.A.*, **108**, 20976–20981.
28. Bixler, H.J. (1994) The carrageenan connection IV. *Br. Food J.*, **96** (3), 12–17.
29. Necas, J. and Bartosikova, L. (2013) Carrageenan: a review. *Vet. Med.*, **58** (4), 187–205.
30. van de Velde, F., Knutsen, S.H., Usov, A.I., Rollema, H.S., and Cerezo, A.S. (2002) ^{1}H and^{13}C high resolution NMR spectroscopy of carrageenans: application inresearch and industry. *Trends Food Sci. Technol.*, **13** (3), 73–92.
31. Pavli, M., Baumgartner, S., Kos, P., and Kogej, K. (2011) Doxazosin-carrageenan interac-tions: a novel approach for studying drug-polymer interactions and relation to controlled drug release. *Int. J. Pharm.*, **421** (1), 110–119.
32. Campo, V.L., Kawano, D.F., da Silva, D.B., and Carvalho, I. (2009) Carrageenans: bio-logical properties, chemical modifications and structural analysis-a review. *Carbohydr. Polym.*, **77** (2), 167–180.
33. Liu, J., Zhan, X., Wan, J., Wang, Y., and Wang, C. (2015) Review for carrageenan-based pharmaceutical biomaterials: favourable physical features versus adverse biological effects. *Carbohydr. Polym.*, **121**, 27–36.
34. Rowe, R.C., Sheskey, P.J., and Quinn, M.E. (2009) *Handbook of Pharmaceutical Excipients*, 6th edn, Pharmaceutical Pr, pp. 11–12. ISBN: 0-85369-792-2
35. Fisheries and Aquaculture Department (2003) Agar, Food and Agricultural Organization of the United Nations, Rome, http://www.fao.org/docrep/006/y4765e/y4765e06.htm (accessed 23 June 2016).
36. Garcia, R.B., Vidal, R.R.L., and Rinaudo, M. (2000) Preparation and structural characterization of O-acetyl agarose with low degree of substitution. *Polímeros*, **10** (3), 155–161.
37. Causey, J.L., Feirtag, J.M., Gallaher, D.D., Tuqland, B.C., and Slavin, J.L. (2000) Effects of dietary inulin on serum lipids, blood glucose and the gastrointestinal environment in hypercholesterolemic men. *Nutr. Res.*, **20**, 191–201.
38. Boeckner, L.S., Schnepf, M.I., and Tungland, B.C. (2001) Inulin: a review of nutritional and health implications. *Adv. Food Nutr. Res.*, **43**, 1–63.
39. Bach, V., Jensen, S., Clausen, M.R., Bertram, H.C., and Edelenbos, M. (2013) Enzymatic browning and after-cooking darkening of *Jerusalem artichoke* tubers (*Helianthus tuberosus* L). *Food Chem.*, **14**, 1445–1450.
40. Li, L.L., Li, L., Wang, Y.P., Du, Y.G., and Qin, S. (2013) Biorefinery products from the inulin-containing crop *Jerusalem artichoke. Biotechnol. Lett.*, **35** (4), 471–477.
41. Ronkart, S.N., Blecker, C.S., Fourmanoir, H., Fougnies, C., Deroanne, C., Herck, J.V. *et al.* (2007) Isolation and identification of inulooligosaccharides resulting from inulin hydrolysis. *Anal. Chim. Acta*, **604** (1), 81–87.
42. Roberfroid, M.B. (2007) Inulin-type fructans: functional food ingredients. *J. Nutr.*, **137** (11), 2493S–2502S.
43. Niness, K.R. (1999) Inulin and oligofructose: what are they? *J. Nutr.*, **129** (7), 1402S–1406S.
44. Kalyani Nair, K., Kharb, S., and Thompkinson, D.K. (2010) Inulin dietary fiber with functional and health attributes-a review. *Food Rev. Int.*, **26** (2), 189–203.
45. http://en.wikipedia.org/wiki/Chitosan (accessed 18 April 2016).
46. Yi, H., Wu, L.-Q., Bentley, W.E., Ghodssi, R., Rubloff, G.W., Culver, J.N. *et al.* (2005) Biofabrication with chitosan. *Biomacromolecules*, **6**, 2881–2894.

47. Cho, Y.-W., Jang, J., Park, C.R., and Ko, S.-W. (2000) Preparation and solubility in acid and water of partially deacetylated chitins. *Biomacromolecules*, **1**, 609–614.
48. Pillai, C.K.S., Paul, W., and Sharma, C.P. (2009) Chitin and chitosan polymers: chemistry, solubility and fiber formation. *Prog. Polym. Sci.*, **34** (7), 641–678.
49. http://en.wikipedia.org/wiki/Albumin (accessed 18 April 2016).
50. Ghuman, J., Zunszain, P.A., Petitpas, I., Bhattacharya, A.A., Otagiri, M., and Curry, S. (2005) Structural basis of the drug-binding specificity of human serum albumin. *J. Mol. Biol.*, **353**, 38–52.
51. Kratochwil, N.A., Huber, W., Muller, F., Kansy, M., and Gerber, P.R. (2002) Predicting plasma protein binding of drugs: a new approach. *Biochem. Pharmacol.*, **64**, 1355–1374.
52. Carter, D.C., He, X., Munson, S.H., Twigg, P.D., Gernert, K.M., Broom, M.B. *et al.* (1989) Three-dimensional structure of human serum albumin. *Science*, **244**, 1195–1198.
53. Updegraff, D.M. (1969) Semimicro determination of cellulose in biological materials. *Anal. Biochem.*, **32** (3), 420–424.
54. Thielking, H. and Schmidt, M. (2000) Cellulose ethers, in *Ullmann's Encyclopedia of Industrial Chemistry*, Wiley-VCH Verlag GmbH & Co. KGaA.
55. Adden, R., Müller, R., and Mischnick, P. (2006) Analysis of the substituent distribution in the glucosyl units and along the polymer chain of hydroxypropylmethyl celluloses and statistical evaluation. *Cellulose*, **13** (4), 459–476.
56. Viridén, A., Wittgren, B., Andersson, T., Abrahmsen-Alami, S., and Larsson, A. (2009) Influence of substitution pattern on solution behavior of hydroxypropyl methylcellulose. *Biomacromolecules*, **10** (3), 522–529.
57. Aulton, M.E., Abdul-Razzak, M.H., and Hogan, J.E. (1981) The mechanical properties of hydroxypropylmethylcellulose films derived from aqueous systems part 1: the influence of plasticizers. *Drug Dev. Ind. Pharm.*, **7**, 649–668.
58. Erkselius, S. and Karlsson, O.J. (2005) Free radical degradation of hydroxyethyl cellulose. *Carbohydr. Polym.*, **62** (4), 344–356.
59. Liedermann, K. and Lapčıćk, L. Jr., (2000) Dielectric relaxation in hydroxyethyl cellulose. *Carbohydr. Polym.*, **42** (4), 369–374.
60. Adden, R., Müller, R., Brinkmalm, G., Ehrler, R., and Mischnick, P. (2006) Comprehensive analysis of the substituent distribution in hydroxyethyl celluloses by quantitative MALDI-ToF-MS. *Macromol. Biosci.*, **6** (6), 435–444.
61. Guo, J., Skinner, G., Harcum, W., and Barnum, P. (1998) Pharmaceutical applications of naturally occurring water-soluble polymers. *Pharm. Sci. Technol. Today*, **1** (6), 254–261.
62. AQUALON® CMC An Anionic Water-Soluble Polymer, www.aqualon.com
63. Masatoshi, S., Minoru, M., Hitoshi, S., Hiroyuki, S., and Yoshihiro, S. (1998) Preparation and characterization of water-soluble chitin and chitosan derivatives. *Carbohydr. Polym.*, **36**, 49–59.
64. Lim, S.-H. and Hudson, S.M. (2004) Synthesis and antimicrobial activity of a water-soluble chitosan derivative with a fiber-reactive group. *Carbohydr. Res.*, **339** (2), 313–319.
65. Kubota, N., Tatsumotoa, N., Sanoa, T., and Toyab, K. (2000) A simple preparation of half N-acetylated chitosan highly soluble in water and aqueous organic solvents. *Carbohydr. Res.*, **324** (4), 268–274.
66. Xie, W., Xu, P., Wang, W., and Liu, Q. (2002) Preparation and antibacterial activity of a water-soluble chitosan derivative. *Carbohydr. Polym.*, **50** (1), 35–40.
67. Daly, W.H. and Guerrini, M.M. (1998) Antimicrobial properties of quaternary ammonium cellulose and chitosan derivatives. *Polym. Mater. Sci. Eng.*, **79**, 220–221.
68. Kim, Y.H., Choi, H.-M., and Yoon, J.H. (1998) Synthesis of a quaternary

ammonium derivative of chitosan and its application to a cotton antimicrobial finish. *Text. Res. J.*, **68**, 428–434.
69. Sakai, S., Yamada, Y., Zenke, T., and Kawakami, K. (2009) Novel chitosan derivative soluble at neutral pH and in-situ gellable via peroxidase-catalyzed enzymatic reaction. *J. Mater. Chem.*, **19**, 230–235.
70. Mourya, V.K., Inamdar, N.N., and Tiwari, A. (2010) Carboxymethyl chitosan and its applications. *Adv. Mater. Lett.*, **1** (1), 11–33.
71. Muzzarelli, R.A.A., Tanfani, F., Emanuelli, M., and Mariotti, S. (1982) N-(carboxymethylidene) chitosans and N-(carboxymethyl) chitosans: novel chelating polyampholytes obtained from chitosansglyoxylate. *Carbohydr. Res.*, **107**, 199–219.
72. Zhu, A., Liu, J., and Ye, W. (2006) Effective loading and controlled release of camptothecin by O-carboxymethylchitosan aggregates. *Carbohydr. Polym.*, **63**, 89.
73. Chen, L., Tian, Z., and Du, Y. (2004) Synthesis and pH sensitivity of carboxymethyl chitosan-based polyampholyte hydrogels for protein carrier matrices. *Biomaterials*, **25**, 3725.
74. Chen, X.G. and Park, H.J. (2003) Chemical characteristics of O-carboxymethyl chitosan related to its preparation conditions. *Carbohydr. Polym.*, **53**, 355.
75. Rinaudo, M., Dung, P.L., and Milas, M. (1992) Substituent distribution on O, N-carboxymethylchitosans by ^{1}H and ^{13}C NMR. *Int. J. Biol. Macromol.*, **14**, 122.
76. An, N.T., Dung, P.L., Thien, D.T., Dong, N.T., and Nhi, T.T.Y. (2008) An improved method for synthesizing N,N-dicarboxymethyl chitosan. *Carbohydr. Polym.*, **73**, 261–264.
77. Rinaudo, M., Desbrieres, J.L., Dung, P., Thuy, B.P., and Dong, N.T. (2001) NMR investigation of chitosan derivatives formed by the reaction of chitosan with levulinic acid. *Carbohydr. Polym.*, **46**, 339.
78. Muzzarelli, R.A.A., Ramos, V., Stanic, V., Dubini, B., Mattioli-Belmonte, M., Tosi, G., and Giardino, R. (1998) Osteogenesis promoted by calcium phosphate dicarboxyboxymethyl chitosan. *Carbohydr. Polym.*, **36**, 267–276.
79. Inouye, K., Yamaguchi, T., Iwasaki, M., Ohto, K., and Yoshizuka, K. (1995) Adsorption of some platinum group metals on some complexane types of chemically modified chitosan. *Sep. Sci. Technol.*, **30**, 2477–2489.
80. Muzzarelli, R.A.A., Ilari, P., and Tomasetti, M. (1993) Preparation and characteristic properties of 5-methylpyrrolidinone chitosan. *Carbohydr. Polym.*, **20**, 99–105.
81. Moureu, C. (1894) The first reported synthesis of polyacrylamide by acrylamide monomer. *Anj. Chim. Phys.*, **2**, 175.
82. Bartoň, J. and Juraničová, V. (2000) Polymerization of acrylamide in styrenecontaining inverse microemulsions: polymerization kinetics and polymer productcomposition studies. *Polym. Int.*, **49**, 1483–1491.
83. Raymond, S. (1964) Protein purification by elution convection electrophoresis. *Science*, **146**, 406–407.
84. Chrambach, A. and Rodbard, D. (1971) Polyacrylamide gel electrophoresis. *Science*, **172**, 440–451.
85. Davis, B.K. (1972) Control of diabetes with polyacrylamide implants containing insulin. *Experientia*, **28**, 348.
86. Hussain, M.D., Rogers, J.A., Mehvar, R., and Vudathala, G.K. (1999) Preparation and release of ibuprofenfrom polyacrylamide gels. *Drug Dev. Ind. Pharm.*, **25**, 265–271.
87. Sairam, M., Babu, V.R., Vijaya, B., Naidu, K., and Aminabhavi, T.M. (2006) Encapsulation efficiency and controlled release characteristics of crosslinked polyacrylamide particles. *Int. J. Pharm.*, **320**, 131–136.
88. http://pslc.ws/macrog/acrylate.htm (accessed 18 April 2016).
89. http://chemindustry.ru/Polyethylene_Glycol.php (accessed 18 April 2016).
90. Zalipsky, S. (1995) Functionalized poly(ethylene glycols) for preparation of biologically relevant conjugates. *Bioconjugate Chem.*, **6**, 150.

91. Bhadra, D., Bhadra, S., Jain, P., and Jain, N.K. (2002) Pegnology: a review of PEG-ylated systems. *Pharmazie*, **57**, 5–29.
92. Delgado, C., Francis, G.E., and Fisher, D. (1992) The uses and properties of PEG-linked proteins. *Crit. Rev. Ther. Drug Carrier Syst.*, **9**, 249–304.
93. Hamidi, M., Azadi, A., and Rafiei, P. (2006) Pharmacokinetic consequences of pegylation. *Drug Delivery*, **13**, 399–409.
94. Harris, J.M. and Chess, R.B. (2003) Effect of pegylation on pharmaceuticals. *Nat. Rev. Drug Discovery*, **2**, 214.
95. Storm, G., Belliot, S.O., Daemen, T., and Lasic, D.D. (1995) Surface modification of nanoparticles to oppose uptake by the mononuclear phagocyte system. *Adv. Drug Delivery Rev.*, **17**, 31–48.
96. Wattendorf, U. and Merkle, H.P. (2008) PEGylation as a tool for the biomedical engineering of surface modified microparticles. *J. Pharm. Sci.*, **97**, 4655–4669.
97. Knop, K., Hoogenboom, R., Fischer, D., and Schubert, U. (2010) Poly(ethylene glycol) in drug delivery: pros and cons as well as potential alternatives. *Angew. Chem. Int. Ed.*, **49**, 6288–6308.
98. Teasdale, I. and Brüggemann, O. (2013) Polyphosphazenes: multifunctional, biodegradable vehicles for drug and gene delivery. *Polymers*, **5**, 161–187.
99. Allcock, H.R. (2003) *Chemistry and Applications of Polyphosphazenes*, John Wiley & Sons, Inc., Hoboken, NJ.
100. Allcock, H.R. and Kwon, S. (1989) An ionically crosslinkable polyphosphazene: poly[bis(carboxylatophenoxy) phosphazene] and its hydrogels and membranes. *Macromolecules*, **22**, 75–79.
101. Allcock, H.R., Austin, P.E., Neenan, T.X., Sisko, J.T., Blonsky, P.M., and Shriver, D.F. (1986) Polyphosphazenes with etheric side groups: prospective biomedical and solid electrolyte polymers. *Macromolecules*, **19**, 1508–1512.
102. Kopeček, J. and Bailová, H. (1973) Poly[N-(2-hydroxypropyl) methacrylamide]-I. Radical polymerization and copolymerization. *Eur. Polym. J.*, **9** (1), 7–14.
103. Teodorescu, M. and Matyjaszewski, K. (1999) Atom transfer radical polymerization of (Meth)acrylamides. *Macromolecules*, **32**, 4826–4831.
104. Scales, C.W., Vasilieva, Y.A., Convertine, A.J., Lowe, A.B., and McCormick, C.L. (2005) Direct, controlled synthesis of the nonimmunogenic, hydrophilic polymer, poly (N-(2-hydroxypropyl) methacrylamide) via RAFT in aqueous media. *Biomacromolecules*, **6**, 1846–1850.
105. Obereigner, B., Burešová, M., Vrána, A., and Kopeček, J. (1977) Preparation of polymerizable derivatives of N-(4-aminobenzenesulfonyl)-N′-butylurea. 17th Prague Microsymposium on Macromolecules, July 1977, Institute of Macromolecular Chemistry Prague.
106. Obereigner, B., Burešová, M., Vrána, A., and Kopeček, J. (1979) Preparation of polymerizable derivatives of N-(4-aminobenzenesulfonyl)-N′-butylurea. *J. Polym. Sci. Polym. Symp.*, **66**, 41–52.
107. Kopecek, J. and Kopecková, P. (2010) HPMA copolymers: origins, early developments, present, and future. *Adv. Drug Delivery Rev.*, **62**, 122–149.
108. Volkova, I.F., Gorshkova, M.Y., Ivanov, P.E., and Stotskaya, L.L. (2002) New scope for synthesis of divinyl ether and maleic anhydride copolymer with narrow molecular mass distribution. *Polym. Adv. Technol.*, **13**, 1067–1070.
109. Izumrudov, V.A., Gorshkova, M.Y., and Volkova, I.F. (2005) Controlled phase separations in solutions of soluble polyelectrolyte complex of DIVEMA (copolymer of divinyl ether and maleic anhydride). *Eur. Polym. J.*, **41** (6), 1251–1259.
110. Kobayashi, S., Mureo, K., Sawada, S., and Saegusa, T. (1985) Synthesis of poly(2-methyl-2-oxazoline) macromers. *Polym. Bull.*, **13**, 447–451.
111. Liu, Q., Konas, M., and Riffle, J.S. (1993) Investigations of 2-ethyl-2-oxazoline polymerizations in chlorobenzene. *Macromolecules*, **26**, 5572–5576.

112. Hoogenboom, R., Leenen, M.A.M., Wiesbrock, F., and Schubert, U.S. (2005) Microwave accelerated polymerization of 2-phenyl-2-oxazoline: microwave or temperature effects? *Macromol. Rapid Commun.*, **26**, 1773–1778.
113. Wiesbrock, F., Hoogenboom, R., Leenen, M.A.M., Meier, M.A.R., and Schubert, U.S. (2005) Investigation of the living cationic ring-opening polymerization of 2-methyl, 2-ethyl, 2-nonyl, and 2-phenyl- 2-oxazoline in a single-mode microwave reactor. *Macromolecules*, **38**, 5025–5034.
114. The Dow Chemical Company (1985) Food Additive Petition for Polyethyloxazoline, May 8, 1985.
115. Adams, N. and Schubert, U.S. (2007) Poly(2-oxazolines) in biological and biomedical application contexts. *Adv. Drug Delivery Rev.*, **59**, 1504–1520.
116. Hoogenboom, R. (2009) Poly(2-oxazoline)s: a polymer class with numerous potential applications. *Angew. Chem. Int. Ed.*, **48**, 7978–7994.
117. Viegas, T.X., Bentley, M.D., Harris, J.M., Fang, Z., Yoon, K., Dizman, B., Weimer, R., Mero, A., Pasut, G., and Veronese, F.M. (2011) Polyoxazoline: chemistry, properties, and applications in drug delivery. *Bioconjugate Chem.*, **22**, 976–986.
118. Chowhan, Z.T. (1980) Role of binders in moisture-induced hardness increase in compressed tablets and its effect on in vitro disintegration and dissolution. *J. Pharm. Sci.*, **69**, 1–4.
119. Chowhan, Z.T., Amaro, A.A., and Ong, J.T.H. (1992) Punch geometry and formulation considerations in reducing tablet friability and their effect on in vitro dissolution. *J. Pharm. Sci.*, **81**, 290–294.
120. Jun, Y.B., Min, B.H., Kim, S.I., and Kim, Y.I.J. (1989) Preparation and evaluation of acetaminophen tablets. *Korean Pharm. Sci.*, **19**, 123–128.
121. Schild, H.G. (1992) Poly(N-isopropylacrylamide): experiment, theory and application. *Prog. Polym. Sci.*, **17** (2), 163–249.
122. De Rossi, D., Kajiwara, K., Osada, Y., and Yamauchi, A. (1991) *Polymer Gels: Fundamentals and Biomedical Applications*, Plenum Press, New York.
123. Lee, J. (1990) Competitive ionic hydration involving outer-shell solvent: temperature dependence. *J. Phys. Chem.*, **94**, 258–262.
124. Urushizaki, F., Yamguchi, H., Nakamura, K., Numajiri, S., Sugibayashi, K., and Morimoto, Y. (1990) Swelling and mechanical properties of poly(vinyl alcohol) hydrogels. *Int. J. Pharm.*, **58**, 135–142.
125. http://cdn.intechopen.com/pdfs-wm/29151.pdf (accessed 18 April 2016).
126. Forster, A., Hempenstall, J., and Rades, T. (2001) Characterization of glass solutions of poorly water-soluble drugs produced by melt extrusion with hydrophilic amorphous polymers. *J. Pharm. Pharmacol.*, **53**, 303–315.
127. Jijun, F., Lishuang, X., Xiaoli, W., Shu, Z., Xiaoguang, T., Xingna, Z., Haibing, H., and Xing, T. (2011) Nimodipine (NM) tablets with high dissolution containing NM solid dispersions prepared by hot-melt extrusion. *Drug Dev. Ind. Pharm.*, **37**, 934–944.
128. Mero, A., Pasut, G., Dalla Via, L., Fijten, M.W., Schubert, U.S., Hoogenboom, R., and Veronese, F.M. (2008) Synthesis and characterization of poly(2-ethyl 2-oxazoline)-conjugates with proteins and drugs: suitable alternatives to PEG-conjugates? *J. Controlled Release*, **2**, 87–95.
129. Goddard, P., Hutchinson, L.E., Brown, J., and Brookman, L.J. (1989) Soluble polymeric carriers for drug delivery. Part 2. Preparation and in vivo behaviour of N-acylethylenimine copolymers. *J. Controlled Release*, **10**, 5–16.
130. Gaertner, F.C., Luxenhofer, R., Blechert, B., Jordan, R., and Essler, M. (2007) Synthesis, biodistribution and excretion of radiolabeled poly(2-oxazoline)s. *J. Controlled Release*, **119**, 291–300.
131. Furuta, T. and Autio, R.E. (1988) Hydrophilic polymers in potting soil mix. *Calif. Agric.*, **42** (3), 19.
132. Drury, J.L. and Mooney, D.J. (2003) Hydrogels for tissue engineering: scaffold design variables and applications. *Biomaterials*, **24**, 4337–4351.

133. West, J.L., Chowdhury, S.M., Sawhney, A.S., Pathak, C.P., Dunn, R.C., and Hubbell, J.A. (1996) Efficacy of adhesion barriers: resorbable hydrogel, oxidized regenerated cellulose and hyaluronic acid. *J. Reprod. Med.*, **41**, 149–154.
134. Elbert, D.L. and Hubbell, J.A. (1998) Reduction of fibrous adhesion formation by a copolymer formation possessing an affinity for anionic surfaces. *J. Biomed. Mater. Res.*, **42**, 55–65.
135. West, J.L. and Hubbell, J.A. (1996) Separation of the arterial wall from blood contact using hydrogel barriers reduces intimal thickening after balloon injury in the rat: the roles of medial and luminal factors in arterial healing. *Proc. Natl. Acad. Sci. U.S.A.*, **93**, 13188–13193.
136. Levengood, S.K.L. and Zhang, M. (2014) Chitosan-based scaffolds for bone tissue engineering. *J. Mater. Chem. B*, **2**, 3161–3184.
137. Seol, Y.J., Lee, J.Y., Park, Y.J., Lee, Y.M., Young, K., Rhyu, I.C., Lee, S.J., Han, S.B., and Chung, C.P. (2004) Chitosan sponges as tissue engineering scaffolds for bone formation. *Biotechnol. Lett.*, **26**, 1037–1041.
138. Muzzarelli, R.A., Mattioli-Belmonte, M., Tietz, C., Biagini, R., Ferioli, G., Brunelli, M.A., Fini, M., Giardino, R., Ilari, P., and Biagini, G. (1994) Stimulatory effect on bone formation exerted by a modified chitosan. *Biomaterials*, **15**, 1075–1081.
139. Venkatesan, J. and Kim, S.K. (2010) Chitosan composites for bone tissue engineering—an overview. *Mar. Drugs*, **8**, 2252–2266.
140. Rabbany, S.Y., Pastore, J., Yamamoto, M., Miller, T., Rafii, S., Aras, R., and Penn, M. (2010) Continuous delivery of stromal cell-derived factor-1 from alginate scaffolds accelerates wound healing. *Cell Transplant.*, **19**, 399–408.
141. Chan, A.W. and Neufeld, R.J. (2010) Tuneable semi-synthetic network alginate for absorptive encapsulation and controlled release of protein therapeutics. *Biomaterials*, **31**, 9040–9047.
142. Lee, K.Y. and Mooney, D.J. (2012) Alginate: properties and biomedical applications. *Prog. Polym. Sci.*, **37**, 106–126.
143. Zhang, X.L., Hui, Z.Y., Wan, D.X., Huang, H.T., Huang, J., Yuan, H., and Yu, J.H. (2010) Alginate microsphere filled with carbon nanotube as drug carrier. *Int. J. Biol. Macromol.*, **47**, 389–395.
144. Kong, H.J., Kim, E.S., Huang, Y.C., and Mooney, D.J. (2009) Design of biodegradable hydrogel for the local and sustained delivery of angiogenic plasmid DNA. *Pharm. Res.*, **25**, 1230–1238.
145. Saxena, A.K., Marler, J., Benvenuto, M., Willital, G.H., and Vacanti, J.P. (1999) Skeletal muscle tissue engineering using isolated myoblasts on synthetic biodegradable polymers: preliminary studies. *Tissue Eng.*, **5**, 525–532.
146. Levenberg, S., Rouwkema, J., Macdonald, M., Garfein, E.S., Kohane, D.S., Darland, D.C., Marini, R., van Blitterswijk, C.A., Mulligan, R.C., D'Amore, P.A., and Langer, R. (2005) Engineering vascularized skeletal muscle tissue. *Nat. Biotechnol.*, **23**, 879–884.
147. Cristina, B., Hannah, S., Frank, B., Dmitry, S., Christine, C., Jeff, W.L., Herman, H.V., and David, J.M. (2009) Functional muscle regeneration with combined delivery of angiogenesis and myogenesis factors. *Proc. Natl. Acad. Sci. U.S.A.*, **107**, 3287–3292.

8
Properties of Stimuli-Responsive Polymers

Raju Francis, Geethy P. Gopalan, Anjaly Sivadas, and Nidhin Joy

8.1
Introduction

The most energizing and rising class of materials that can react to an external stimulus is referred to as stimuli-responsive polymers. A lot of work has been devoted to developing ecologically delicate macromolecules that can be created into novel smart materials. They can be classified according to the stimuli they respond to such as temperature, pH, ionic strength, light, electric, and magnetic field. Some polymers respond to a combination of two or more stimuli. Another basis of classifying these polymers is their physical form, that is, free chains in solutions, chains grafted on a surface, covalently cross-linked gels, and reversible or physical gels. Stimuli responsive changes in shape, surface qualities, dissolvability, and arrangement of a perplexing molecular self-assembly and a sol – gel transition have empowered a few novel applications in the conveyance of therapeutics, cell culture, tissue engineering, sensor or actuator frameworks, bioseparations, immobilized biocatalysts, drug conveyance, bioseparations, thermoresponsive surfaces, biomimetic actuators, and bioconjugates [1, 2].

Stimuli are commonly classified into three categories – physical, chemical, and biological [3, 4] – as shown in Figure 8.1 [5]. Physical stimuli, such as temperature, ultrasound, magnetic, light, mechanical, electrical, and so on, generally transform chain dynamics, but chemical stimuli, such as solvent, electrochemical, pH, ionic strength, and so on, modulate the molecular interactions, whether between polymer and dissolvable particles or between polymer chains. Biological stimuli such as enzymes and receptors impact the actual functioning of molecules, that is, enzymatic reactions and receptor recognition of molecules. Moreover, there are dual-responsive polymers that concurrently respond to more than one stimulus.

Biomedical Applications of Polymeric Materials and Composites, First Edition.
Edited by Raju Francis and Sakthi Kumar.

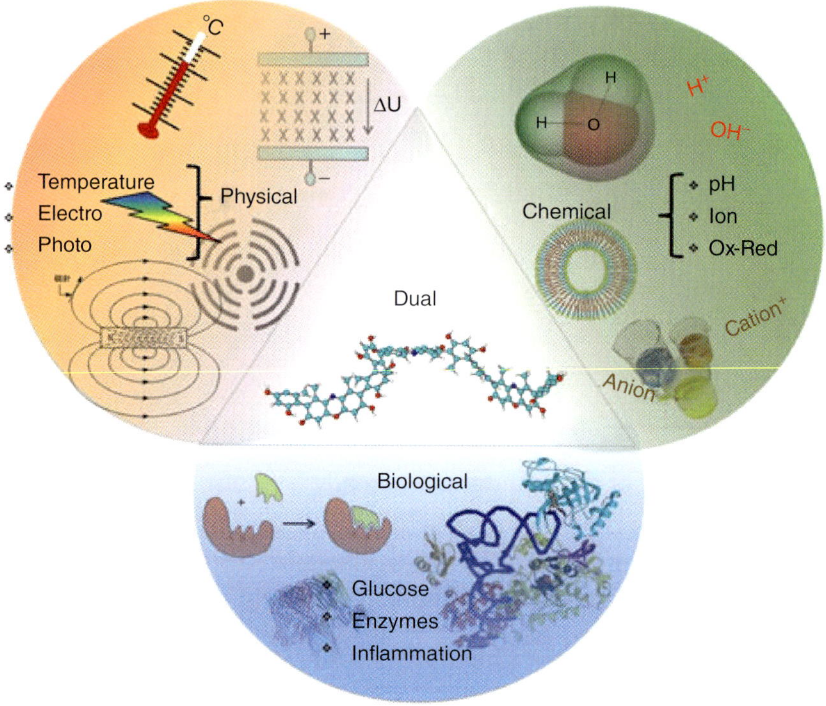

Figure 8.1 Classification of stimuli-responsive polymers. (Cabane 2012 [5]. Reproduced with permission from American Institute of Physics.)

8.2 Physically Dependent Stimuli

Physically dependent stimuli mainly include temperature, electric field, light, magnetic field, and mechanical deformation.

8.2.1 Temperature

Temperature-responsive polymers have gained very much attention in the fields of bioengineering and biotechnology applications since certain diseases are apparent due to temperature changes [6]. In general these copolymers are characterized by a critical solution temperature around which the hydrophilic and hydrophobic interactions between the aqueous media and the polymeric chains rapidly change within a little temperature change. This affects interruption of intra- and intermolecular electrostatic and hydrophobic interactions and results in a volume phase transition. Normally, the polymer solutions acquire an upper critical solution temperature. On the other hand, polymer solutions that appear as monophasic below a specific temperature and biphasic above it generally possess this so-called lower critical solution temperature (LCST). A variety of temperature-responsive polymers have been reported on the basis of the chemistry of the groups and their mechanism: poly(*N*-alkyl-substituted acrylamides), such as poly(*N*-isopropylacrylamide) (PNIPAM) [7]; poly(*N*-vinylalkylamides), such as poly(*N*-vinylcaprolactam) (PNVC) [8]; and copolymers, for example, poly(L-lactic acid)–poly(ethylene glycol)–poly(L-lactic acid) (PLLA–PEG–PLLA) triblock copolymers [9] and poly(ethylene oxide)–poly(propylene oxide)–poly(ethylene oxide)(PEO–PPO–PEO) copolymers [10].

8.2.1.1 Poly(*N*-isopropylacrylamide)(PNIPAM)

PNIPAM is the most widely recognized and thermally responsive smart polymer system that has been studied [11]. It is the most strongly examined polymer with reference to biomedical applications because of its LCST being near to body temperature and its quick on-off exchange. PNIPAM shows turbidity at about 32 °C in pure water. On heating the solution above 32 °C, it becomes phase separated which occurs at a temperature slightly lower than that of physiologic saline. Above the LCST, a cross-linked PNIPAM hydrogel will suddenly contract and excrete its aqueous swelling solution, and a very wettable PNIPAM-coated surface will abruptly be hydrophobic. When the stimulus is reversed, so are the above phenomena, even though reversal rates can vary depending on the composition and the geometry of the system. The kinetics of the phase transitions also depends on the structure in the case of hydrogels. Yoshida *et al.* [12] demonstrated that macromonomers of NIPAM could be utilized to shape a water-swollen, cross-linked "comb-type" hydrogel. At the point when that gel was heated above the LCST of PNIPAM, it shrank considerably more quickly than conventional cross-connected hydrogels of PNIPAM, which are broken down gradually. Since it naturally appears when the temperature is increased above the LCST, the free energy drop must be driven by an entropy expansion. Additionally, if the solution of polyacrylamide can be heated, no phase separation will happen. In this manner, the temperature-induced phase partition of PNIPAM is because of an increase in entropy with respect to the isopropyl groups of PNIPAM. As isopropyl groups aggregate jointly at the LCST, it is best understood as being driven by the release of the hydrophobically bound water molecules around the isopropyl groups. Frequently, the rate of reversion back to the hydrated state might be slower than the collapse, since in the reverse procedure the hydrophobic groups of the polymer must be rehydrated one by one, and that procedure is thermodynamically contradicted by the resultant decrease in the entropy of the water molecules. The general reswelling process above the LCST is favored by the increase in entropy as the polymer chain grows in addition to the (small but positive) exothermic hydration of the hydrophobic groups. The rate of dehydration or rehydration of such smart polymer systems can also depend on the dimensions of the system. For smaller systems, the phase separation will be faster, that is, microscopic systems were slower than nanosystems, which are in turn quicker than macroscopic systems. In terms of "smart cell culture surfaces," Okano, Yamato and associates are the pioneers [13, 14]. Utilizing an electron accelerator, they radiation-grafted

PNIPAM to polystyrene (PS) cell culture surfaces and cultured cells to confluent sheets on the surfaces at 37 °C, which is above the LCST of the polymer. Above LCST, the grafted PNIPAM chains collapsed due to its hydrophobic behaviour. This lead to physical adsorption of cell adhesion proteins from the culture medium. This improves the cell culture process at the polymer surface as the cells grew to confluent cell sheets. Then, when the temperature was lowered below LCST, the PNIPAM chains became rehydrated, and the confluent cell sheets were released from the surface along with the cell adhesion proteins that remained bound to the cell surfaces. They lately found that if the fixed NIPAM chains were framed as brushes and ended with COOH groups, the cells developed to juncture all the more quickly at 37 °C, and they likewise discharged all the more quickly and all the more neatly from the surface at room temperature. These stimulating [15] new applications of smart surface cell sheets are being connected for corneal and myocardial tissue recreation by Okano and associates [3, 4]. Nanoparticle-based diagnostic frameworks utilize PNIPAM coatings on microfluidic channels, on gold nanoparticles, and on magnetic nanoparticles [16–24]. For clinical immunoassay applications, these smart nanoscale systems were produced. At the point when a smart polymer is crosslinked to form a gel, the gel will collapse and reswell in water as a function of heat stimulus. If the drug is stacked into the gel, the breakdown can discharge the medication in a burst. The potential of PNIPAM hydrogels as biomaterials was initially recognized by Hoffman and coworkers who found that smart gels could be used for entrapping drugs and delivering them. Using smart gels can entrap the enzymes and cells, and by inducing cyclic swelling and collapse of the gel, the enzymes or the enzymes within the cells could be switched "on" and "off" [25–28]. In the late 1980s and 1990s, studies about smart hydrogels were actively done by Kim, Okano, Bae, and coworkers. Smart gels containing entrapped cells which are applicable for artificial organs were successfully explored [29]. By controlling the polymer composition and topology, the coil-to-globule transition could be kinetically and thermodynamically controlled. Copolymerization of NIPAM with hydrophobic butyl methacrylate decreases the LCST of aqueous copolymer solution and copolymerization with hydrophilic comonomers, such as acrylic acid or hydroxyethyl methacrylate (HEMA), and results in an increase in LCST [30]. Depending on the content of hydrophilic moieties of poly(NIPAM–co–acrylic acid) and poly(NIPAM)-*b*-poly(ethylene glycol) (PNIPAM-*b*-PEG) at 37 °C, polymers exhibit sol–gel transition rather than precipitation [31, 32]. Aoyagi *et al.* described an interesting example of molecular design of LCST polymers [33]. When 5 mol% of 2-carboxyisopropyl acrylamide (CIPAAm) was copolymerized with NIPAM, the copolymer showed little or no change in LCST, whereas 5 mol% of acrylic acid resulted in LCST increases of ~10 °C, as measured in Phosphate-Buffered Saline (PBS) at pH 7.4. By increasing the ratio of the hydrophobic PPGMA to hydrophilic POEGMA, the thermal transition temperature was decreased to below 37 °C in a phosphate buffer solution at pH 7.4. Both carboxylic acid groups and thermosensitivity are needed for this molecular design concept, and it is very useful. Polymer systems with more than one transition can be obtained by controlling polymer architecture. For example, hydrogels containing different LCST oligomer grafts showed dual swelling transitions with increasing temperature. The first transition resulted from oligo-NIPAM at 32 °C, and the second transition occurred at 36 °C owing to the presence of oligo(*N*-vinylcaprolactam) [34]. Control of deswelling kinetics was also achieved by using graft copolymer structure. The comb-type grafted hydrogels of cross-linked P(NIPAM) grafted with oligo-NIPAM [12] and poly(NIPAM-*g*-PEG) [35] exhibited fast response to temperature. Changes of NIPAM copolymers focused on biological applications such as separations, enzyme immobilization, gene delivery, and cell culture [36–41]. Hoffman *et al.* reviewed the progress in smart bioconjugates that use stimuli-responsive properties of PNIPAM [2]. In a related application, the PNIPAM polymers were investigated for on–off control of avidin–biotin binding. Below the transition temperature of 32 °C, NIPAM copolymers are in a fully extended conformation in water because of favorable polymer–water interactions. The PNIPAM with fully extended conformation interferes with the biotin-binding site on the avidin, whereas above the transition temperature, the polymers collapsed and cannot interfere with the binding sites. In a related research aimed at the design of new bioseparation methods, PNIPAMs were conjugated to trypsin and chymotrypsin [36, 37], which demonstrated specific enzyme activity–temperature profiles. Cell manipulation techniques using temperature-responsive culture surfaces grafted with PNIPAM were also investigated [39]. A decrease in culture temperature below the LCST resulted in the release of cardiac myocyte sheets from the cell culture dishes without enzymatic treatment. In another cell culture-related application, PNIPAM–acrylic acid copolymers were used as a three-dimensional cell culture matrix for preservation of the phenotype of articular chondrocytes. The chondrocytes cultured in a monolayer lost their phenotype, whereas those cultured in the PNIPAM–acrylic acid gel kept the phenotype and rounded shape of the cells. PNIPAM–acrylic acid copolymers were also used for entrapping islets of Langerhans for a refillable biohybrid artificial pancreas [40]. Poly(*N*-isopropylacrylamide)-grafted hyaluronan (PNIPAM-HA) and PNIPAM-grafted gelatin (PNIPAM-gelatin) shown in Figure 8.2, which exhibited sol–gel transformation at physiological temperature, were applied as control of tissue adhesions: tissue adhesion prevention material and hemostatic aid, respectively.

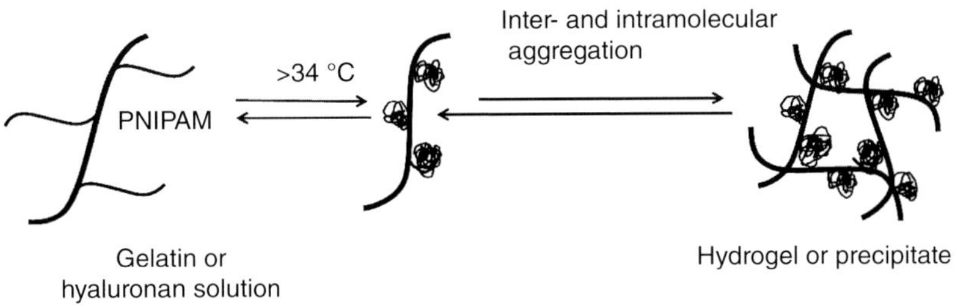

Figure 8.2 Thermoresponsive gelation mechanisms of PNIPAM-HA and PNIPAM-gelatin [7].

Okuyama *et al.* wrote an initial paper on the swelling energy of NIPAM with butyl methacrylate (BMA), P(NIPAM-co-BMA), remarking on the requirement for zero-order drug discharge profiles and found that after a burst arrival of drug from the external part of the hydrogel, a maintained discharge can be acquired [42]. Coughlan and Corrigan demonstrated the significance of comprehending the nature of a stacked drug in a polymer system with the cross-linker fixation and drug interaction with the polymer having a huge effect on the rate of arrival of medications from PNIPAM gels [43, 44]. Jones *et al.* and coworkers synthesized various types of PNIPAM conetworks, which are applicable for the delivery of microbial agents in combination with medicinal gadgets. PNIPAM and HEMA conetworks showed LCST at 34 °C suitable for *in vivo* applications [42] such as drug release and mechanical strength. A comparative study by Jones *et al.* observed the incorporation of zinc tetraphenylporphyrin (Zn-TPP) into PNIPAM-co-PHEMA. They demonstrated that above the LCST the Zn-TPP discharge rate drastically diminished. Once discharged, the Zn-TPP was free for photoinduced antimicrobial activity. After a careful observation, Jones demonstrated that an on–off drug release can be accomplished for different applications by controlling the concentration of polymer and therefore the LCST [45]. Xiao *et al.* synthesized a biodegradable hydrogel, which includes thermoresponsive PNIPAM with cleavable lactic acid and dextran units [46]. Zhao *et al.* and others also done a similar work with grafting PNIPAM and PNVC-HEMA onto a dextran chain producing injectable and biodegradable hydrogels. This gel was equipped for delivering drugs more than a few days with insignificant cytotoxicity [47]. Ma *et al.* synthesized conetworks of PNIPAM, lactic acid, and PHEMA, and its LCSTs of 10–20 °C with PNIPAM contents of 80% or more were found [48]. The gels exhibited good mechanical properties and degraded slowly with no cytotoxic by-products when used in tissue engineering. Investigation by Ratner *et al.* utilized templating strategies to create cross-linked PNIPAM hydrogels with a characterized pore size [49]. Exchanging pore size with temperature took into consideration the embodiment of cells inside the gel for consequent uses as a part of tissue designing. A thermoresponsive star block copolymer based on L-lactide and NIPAM was successfully synthesized by Wei *et al.* In water, these star polymers self-assemble into large micelle structures, which demonstrated a quick on–off drug switching with respect to temperature [50].

8.2.1.2 **Polyethylene Glycol (PEG)**

Polyethylene oxide (PEO), or more commonly known as poly(ethylene glycol) (PEG), has an LCST of around 85 °C. Kim *et al.* develop a group of thermally gelling, hydrolytically degradable triblock copolymers that were physically blended with medications and infused subcutaneously or intramuscularly to produce stage-isolated, degradable, Q14 drug depot masses at body conditions [29, 51–53]. These triblock copolymers were made out of exchanging ABA or BAB blocks, for example, PLGA–PEG–PLGA or PEG–PLGA–PEG blocks. The thermally produced gelation of these block copolymer-drug mixtures is most probably motivated by the mechanism which is comparable to that of PNIPAM. This is due to the large entropy gain caused by the discharge of bound water molecules from the hydrophobic PLGA blocks at 37 °C. The PLGA blocks aggregate together and the phase-separated region then slowly releases the drug by dissolution and diffusion of the drug. This was accompanied and enhanced by the hydrolytic degradation of the PLGA–PEG–PLGA triblock copolymer into PEG, lactic acid, and glycolic acid. Kan *et al.* developed a zero-order drug release which was prepared by integrating a smart polymer, such as PEG-*b*-PLGA-*b*-PEG, into an oil–water emulsion. Above the LCST of the polymer, the water phase produced a hydrogel over a 20–30 °C range, which entraps the oil droplets. Drug release using these droplets demonstrated a controlled rate with no burst discharge [54]. A sequence of degradable PEG–alt–thiol hydrogels with differing LCSTs which are applicable for tissue engineering was developed by Wang and his collaborators. For the degradation of the hydrogels *in vivo*, thiol groups gave suitable sites [55]. Conjugation of Pluronics® to peptide moieties enhances cell interaction, adhesion and growth within the tissue scaffold [56]. PoligoGel® is like Pluronics® which utilizes PEG and poly(propylene glycol) (PPG) blocks and appears to be nontoxic to cells with an LCST close to body temperature [57]. Cohn *et al.* used the formation of micelles above the LCST of PEG-*b*-PPG-*b*-PEG triblock copolymers, where PPG was the hydrophobic PPG block, also called poly(propylene oxide) (PPO), to form functional nanoshells. As shown in the succeeding figure, a methacrylate group is integrated onto every end of the block copolymers and cross-linking them, while a collapsible and expandable shell structure was molded with large void spaces capable of encapsulating various moieties in the case of micellar configuration [58]. Cohn *et al.* reported that the thermoresponsive polymers with significant PEG content are particularly interesting from a biomedical perspective, given their low toxicity/immunogenicity and high biocompatibility. Once the temperature is reduced below critical micellization temperature (CMT), the individual chains tend to revert to their unimeric state, but since the triblocks are covalently cross-linked, this process is prevented from nearing completion, generating remarkably expanded nanostructures. Conversely, when heated up above the transition temperature, they shrink dramatically, as the supramolecular constructs revert to their micellar array, driven by the forces common to all micellization processes. This reversible phenomenon is schematically shown in Figure 8.3.

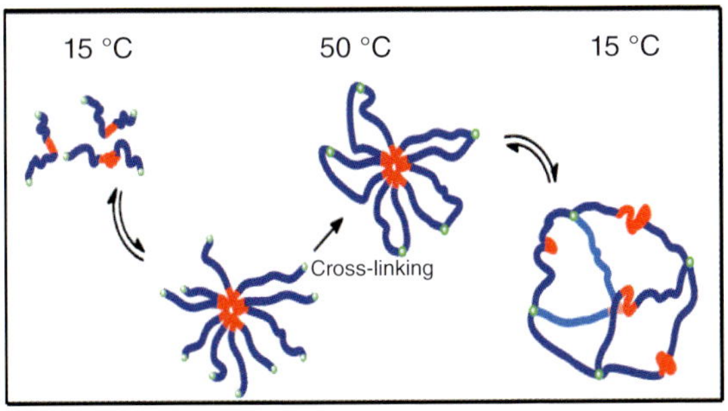

Figure 8.3 Formation of nanocages from polymers of PEG (blue), PPG (red), and methacrylate groups (green). (Cohn 2009 [58]. Reproduced with permission from Elsevier.)

8.2.1.3 Elastin

Elastin-like peptides (ELPs) have been studied extensively for biomaterial/biomedical applications. This is because they phase-separate when heated, similarly to PNIPAM. But since they are based on a natural protein, they may be more "biocompatible" than a synthetic polymer, especially PNIPAM. These polymers depend on the temperature-affected phase separation conduct of a repeating peptide chain inside a hydrophobic domain of elastin. The most widely recognized sequence in elastin is valine-proline-glycine-X-glycine, or (VPGXG)m, where X can be any amino acid other than proline and m is the number of units. There are numerous variations of ELPs that seem to show elastin-like properties, yet the pentapeptide motif of VPGXG has generally been examined. Side groups fit for adding usefulness to the ELP, for instance, cysteine, can be added to take into consideration conjugation of bioactive atoms, while lysine residues have been added to take into consideration cross-linking. Chilkoti and colleagues have widely studied these brilliant polypeptides [59–62]. These smart polypeptides later on may find rewarding applications as biomaterials. Elastin-like polymers with polypeptide repeat units were developed by Bessa *et al.* [63] and Rincon *et al.* [64]. It is a thermoresponsive polypeptide that has a special thermoresponsive capacity. Above its LCST of 30 °C, chains itself fold to form a nanoparticle, but below its LCST, it is solvated and extended in solution. Specifically, it forms nanoparticles that entrap particles inside their structure, permitting them to be utilized as a drug delivery vector. Bessa demonstrated that bone morphogenetic proteins could be encapsulated along these lines and conveyed sustainedly for 14 days to advance bone arrangement. Another intriguing point is that these elastin particles are not identified by the immune system giving a nontoxic vector without further alteration. Thermoresponsive elastin-like polypeptide–doxorubicin (DOX) conjugate has also been employed for temperature-mediated tumor suppression [65].

8.2.1.4 Poly(*N*-vinylisobutyramide)

Poly(*N*-vinylisobutyramide) (poly(NVIBA)), a thermoresponsive water-soluble polymer, showed an LCST at 39 °C. This thermoresponsive synthetic polymer exhibits both hydrogen-bonding and hydrophobic properties, which causes changes in their molecular level states (coil to collapse) in an aqueous solution [66]. Poly(NVIBA) has been considered to represent a simple but relevant protein model.

8.2.1.5 Poly(diethyl vinylphosphonate) (PDEVP)

Poly(diethyl vinylphosphonate) (PDEVP) homopolymer was prepared by group transfer polymerization using rare earth metal complexes. It is amphiphilic, and its aqueous solutions exhibit a cloud point of 40–46 °C, depending on the molar mass and concentration [67]. Biocompatibility makes PDEVP an interesting alternative compared to established thermoresponsive polymers. Therefore, thermoresponsive PDEVPs are promising candidates in biomedical applications, for example, for controlled cell growth and cell release.

8.2.1.6 Poly(*N*-vinylcaprolactam)

PNVC [68–70] has an LCST between 25 and 35 °C. PNVC contains a seven-membered lactam ring and has a repeat unit consisting of a hydrophilic heterocyclic amide ring. Of potential interest for biomedical applications, PNVC offers benefits of low toxicity, water and organic solubility, high complexing ability, and good film-forming properties [71–74].

8.2.1.7 Poly(*N*,*N*-diethylacrylamide) (PDEAAm)

Poly(*N*,*N*-diethylacrylamide) (PDEAAm) is a well-known thermoresponsive polymer which shows an LCST over the range of 25–32 °C. A number of other thermoresponsive monomers have been utilized for preparing hydrogel including poly(dimethyl acrylamide) (PDMAAm), PEG [75–77]. Martellini *et al.* developed a PDMAAm-co-poly(methoxyethyl acrylate) and demonstrated that at body temperature this hydrogel releases drug after a Fickian diffusion process with a linear relationship in respect to the square root of time. In another study, Bradley *et al.* demonstrated the application of PDEAM in nanomechanical cantilever sensors [78]. Lowe and coworkers have reported numerous examples of PDEAM-thermoresponsive systems. Lowe and Ishihara *et al.* reported a doubly responsive block copolymer of PDEAM and poly(2-(methacryloyloxy)ethyl phosphorylcholine) (PMPC), a biocompatible and zwitterionic polymer containing anionic phosphate and quaternary amine functional groups in the same monomer unit [79].

8.2.1.8 Poly(*N*-alkyl methacrylamides)

Tunable thermoresponsive polymers based on acid-labile poly(*N*-alkyl methacrylamides were reported by Li *et al.* using a similar approach to those based on pendant cyclic orthoester groups [80]. Poly(*N*-(2-methoxy-1,3-dioxan-5-yl) methacrylamide) (PNMM) (L10) and poly(*N*-(2-ethoxy-1,3-dioxan-5-yl) methacrylamide) (PNEM) (L11) were determined to have transition temperatures of 22 and 52 °C, respectively. Varying the composition of statistical (co)polymers based on these two repeat units allowed the thermal transition to be tuned between these two values. Moreover, the presence of labile orthoester groups in the side chain allowed further tuning of the thermoresponsive nature by controlled hydrolysis under mildly acidic conditions. Hydrolysis of the polymers above the cloud point resulted in the hydrophobic polymer becoming more hydrophilic and eventually water soluble, suggesting the potential for being employed as site-specific drug delivery systems that target mildly acidic sites. The same research group reported additional examples of acid-labile thermoresponsive (meth)acrylamide polymers that contained pendant six-membered cyclic acetal moieties [81]. Bioerodible thermoresponsive copolymers were prepared by copolymerization of *N*-isopropylmethacrylamide and a methacrylamide monomer containing hydrophobic *n*-alkyl groups attached via a hydrolytically labile hydrazone bond (L14) [82]. The cloud point of these copolymers could be adjusted to between 13 and 44 °C by varying the copolymer composition. However, upon hydrolytic cleavage of the hydrazone bonds, even the most hydrophobic of the copolymers exhibited transition temperatures greater than 44 °C, leading to complete solubility at body temperature. These thermoresponsive polymers were targeted to serve as carriers in radiotherapeutic applications.

8.2.1.9 Oligo(ethylene Glycol)-Based Polymers

Oligo(ethylene glycol)-based polymers with intermediate side chain lengths generally exhibit cloud points in aqueous solution that are lower than high molecular weight PEG due to the increase in hydrophobicity of the hydrocarbon polymer backbone. For instance, poly(2-(2-methoxyethoxy)ethylmethacrylate) (PMEO2MA) (2 ethylene oxide units) (L27) and PMEO3MA (3 ethylene oxide units) (L28) have transition temperatures around 26 and 52 °C, respectively [83]. Poly(oligo(ethylene glycol) methacrylate)s (POEGMA) (L29) with longer side chains (4–9 ethylene oxide units) exhibit transitions in the range 60–90 °C [83, 84]. A variety of thermoresponsive OEGMA-based polymers and their use in diverse biologically relevant applications have recently been highlighted by Lutz as shown in Figure 8.4 [85]. These copolymers combine the advantages of PEG (i.e., biocompatibility) and thermoresponsive polymers (i.e., LCST behavior in water) in a single macromolecular structure. Moreover, these polymers have inherent advantages such as (i) an excellent biorepellency below LCST (i.e., antifouling behavior), (ii) reversible phase transitions (i.e., no marked hysteresis), and (iii) bioinert properties (i.e., no specific interactions with biological materials).

A thermoresponsive biocompatible copolymer was prepared from POEGMA and poly(propylene glycol) methacrylate (PPGMA) via atom transfer radical polymerization (ATRP) and conventional free-radical polymerization. The cloud point of the copolymers was varied by changing the ratios of comonomers. By increasing the ratio of the hydrophobic PPGMA to hydrophilic POEGMA, the thermal transition temperature was decreased to below 37 °C in a phosphate buffer solution (PBS) at pH 7.4. These P(OEGMA-co-PGMA) copolymers were further entrapped into poly(lactic acid-co-glycolic acid) (PLGA) particles to form thermoresponsive biodegradable microparticles [86] that could be useful for specific cell delivery and tissue engineering applications.

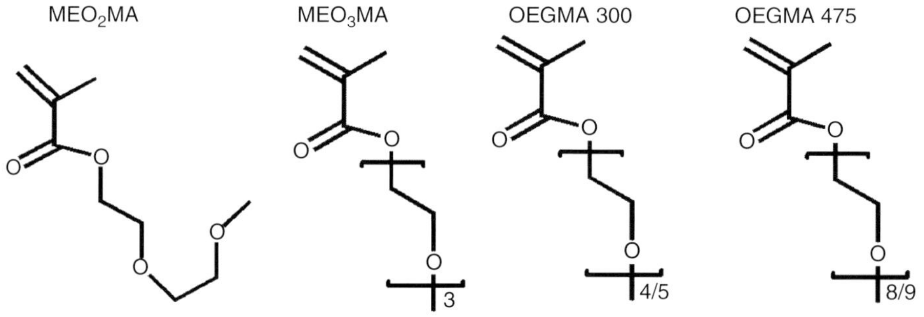

Figure 8.4 Molecular structures of oligo(ethylene glycol) methacrylates frequently used for synthesizing thermoresponsive biocompatible polymers [85].

8.2.1.10 Poly(*N*-substituted α/β-asparagine)

Poly(*N*-substituted α/β-asparagine) exhibits a sol–gel–sol phase transition, and by incorporating *N*,*N*-dimethylaminopropyl side chains, the transition temperatures could be tuned between room temperature and approximately the boiling point of water. In addition, not only a physical gelation in a concentrated aqueous solution but also a phase separation in a dilute aqueous solution was observed in the polymers with the tertiary amine in the terminal moieties of the hydrophilic side chains. These polymer aqueous solutions formed a hydrogel without any additives, and these materials are expected to be applicable for controlled release of drugs and tissue engineering [87]. L-Asparaginase inhibition of glycoprotein synthesis in leukemic cells *in vitro* has been described [88]. The structures of both L-asparagines and aspartic acid are shown in Figure 8.5 [89]. The mechanism of action of L-asparaginase is based on the fact that lymphocytic leukemic cells are deficient in L-asparagine synthesis and hence are dependent on an exogenous supply of L-asparagine. On treatment with L-asparaginase, which catalyzes the conversion of L-asparagine to L-aspartate and ammonia, the growth of these cells is critically affected with the rapid depletion of L-asparagine from the blood supply and the surrounding tissue. Cells require a steady supply of the amino acid L-asparagine to build proteins. Most cells use the enzyme asparagine synthetase to make their own asparagine. The enzyme takes L-aspartate and adds an amine, forming the characteristic amide group of asparagine. Thus, most cells can make their own supplies of asparagine and do not need to obtain it in their diet. L-Asparaginase performs the opposite reaction; it takes L-asparagine and pulls off its amine, releasing L-aspartate and ammonia [90]. As a result of the hydrolysis of L-asparagine, accumulation of large amount of L-aspartic acid and ammonia has been reported.

8.2.2 Pressure

The concept that hydrogels may undergo pressure-induced volume phase transition came from thermodynamic calculations based on uncharged hydrogel theory. According to the theory, hydrogels that are collapsed at low pressure would expand at higher pressure.

Pressure-modulated adhesion between flat, stiff objects and an elastomeric surface with sharp pyramidal features was presented [91]. Rogers and coworkers fabricated elastomeric micropyramidal structures on a square surface, specifically

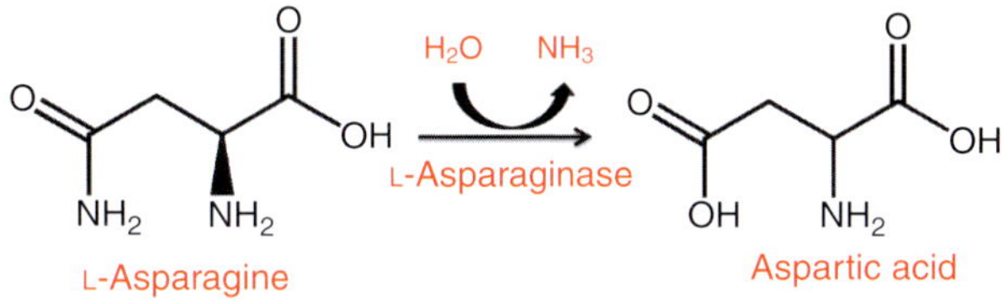

Figure 8.5 L-Asparagines and aspartic acid [89].

designed for transfer printing applications. To pick up some object, the pressure was applied to deform and collapse the region between the pyramids and make a big contact area with the object. After pickup the sample relaxes, and the picked-up object exhibits a contact just with the pyramids. Therefore, the contact area is quite small, which makes it possible to detach the object easily by gently pressing it on a receiver surface. In such a way, the adhesion strength could be switched by more than three orders of magnitude in a reversible fashion.

8.2.2.1 Poly(*N*-isopropylacrylamide) (PNIPAM)

Experiments with poly(*N*-isopropylacrylamide) hydrogels confirmed this prediction [92]. The degree of swelling of poly(*N*-isopropylacrylamide) hydrogels increased under hydrostatic pressure when the temperature is close to its LCST. Other hydrogels, such as poly(*N*-*n*-propylacrylamide), poly(*N*,*N*-diethylacrylamide), and poly(*N*-isopropylacrylamide), all showed the pressure sensitivity near their LCSTs. The pressure sensitivity appeared to be a common characteristic feature of temperature-sensitive gels. It was concluded that the pressure sensitivity of the temperature-sensitive gels was due to an increase in their LCST value with pressure [93].

8.2.3 Magnetic Field

Magnetic field-responsive polymers have been investigated as a form of hydrogels to have swelling, shrinking, or bending behavior in response to an external field. These properties of such polymers have been applied for biological applications such as drug delivery systems, artificial muscle, or biomimetic actuators [94].

8.2.3.1 Poly(*N*-isopropylacrylamide) (PNIPAM)

Magnetic field-sensitive gels were obtained by incorporating colloidal magnetic particles into cross-linked PNIPAM-co-poly(vinyl alcohol) hydrogels [95]. The gel beads formed straight chain-like structures in uniform magnetic fields, while they aggregated in nonhomogeneous fields. The rapid and controllable shape changes of these gels are expected to mimic muscular contraction.

Micrometer- and submicrometer-sized thermoresponsive polymer magnetic microspheres based on a copolymer of styrene and *N*-isopropylacrylamide have been synthesized previously. The preparation of magnetic thermoresponsive microspheres using a two-step method, in which iron oxide nanoparticles were absorbed onto previously synthesized PNIPAM-co-styrene microspheres and then the obtained microspheres were encapsulated by PNIPAM through a soap-free polymerization process, was reported by Sauzedde and coworkers. The process of preparation is not easily controllable, as this two-step method could lead to thermoresponsive polymer magnetic composite microspheres. Ding and his coworkers prepared thermoresponsive polymer magnetic microspheres based on the dispersion copolymerization of styrene and PNIPAM in the presence of iron oxide nanoparticles [96].

8.2.3.2 Poly(ethylene glycol) methacylate (PEGMA)

Meenach and his colleagues developed the hydrogels of PEGMA-containing iron oxide particles for the possible drug delivery applications. Upon increasing the temperature these hydrogels showed thermoresponsive property with a deswelling of the gels. Moreover, these gels exhibited magneto responsive property. The application of an external alternating magnetic field lead to rapid heating and deswelling of the gel [97]. Papaphilippou and collaborators combined PEGMA hydrogels by the consolidation of magnetic nanoparticles with superparamagnetic properties during polymerization. These hydrogels demonstrated a deswelling on elevating temperature and a tunable superparamagnetic character reliant on the amount of magnetite fused [98].

8.2.4 Light

Light-responsive polymers have had considerable attention, compared to other physical stimuli such as temperature. Light has specific physical characteristics whereby it can be localized in time and space [99]. Light-responsive polymers undergo a phase transition in response to exposure to light. The major advantages of light-sensitive polymers are that they are water soluble, biocompatible, and biodegradable. Another advantage is their capacity for instantaneous delivery of the sol–gel stimulus, making light-responsive polymers important for various engineering and biomedical applications. Light-responsive polymers are very attractive for triggering drug release because of their ability to control the spatial and temporal triggering of the release. This means that the encapsulated drug can be released or activated after irradiation with a light source from outside the body. Limitations of light-sensitive polymers include inconsistent response due to the leaching of noncovalently bound chromophores during swelling or contraction of the system and the slow response of hydrogel toward the stimulus. One of the drawbacks of light-responsive polymer is dark toxicity. On the basis of the wavelength of light, these polymers are classified into UV sensitive and visible light sensitive, and that triggers their phase transition. Visible light-sensitive polymers are comparatively preferred over UV-sensitive polymers because of their availability, safety, and ease of use [100].

8.2.4.1 Poly(*N*-isopropylacrylamide) (PNIPAM)

Recently, the Winnik and Ikeda group showed that the reversible photo-controlled phase separation of an azobenzene end-group-functionalized PNIPAM polymer could be dramatically intensified through the addition of dioxane to water, which enabled the reversible conversion from a turbid suspension into a clear solution upon photo-irradiation [101].

Visible light-sensitive hydrogels were prepared by introducing a light-sensitive chromophore (e.g., trisodium salt of copper chlorophyllin) to poly(*N*-isopropylacrylamide) hydrogels [102]. When light (e.g., 488 nm) is applied to the hydrogel, the chromophore absorbs light that is then dissipated locally as heat by radiationless transitions, increasing the "local" temperature of the hydrogel. The temperature increase alters the swelling behavior of poly(*N*-isopropylacrylamide) hydrogels, which are thermosensitive hydrogels. The temperature increase is proportional to the light intensity and the chromophore concentration. If an additional functional group, such as an ionizable group of PAA, is added, the light-sensitive hydrogels become responsive to pH changes as well [103]. This type of hydrogel can be activated (i.e., induced to shrink) by visible light and can be deactivated (i.e., induced to swell) by increasing pH.

8.2.5 Solvent

The successful control of wettability of self-adapted polymer systems by exposing them to different solvents was examined by Minko *et al.* [104]. The heterogeneous binary polymer brushes were sensitive to toluene, ethanol, and water. The adaptive behavior of the polymer chains was amplified by the microscale roughness of the material. As a result, the wettability of the mixed brushes could be switched from complete superhydrophilic to superhydrophobic states. Biocompatible and biodegradable polymer brushes of PEG and polydimethylsiloxane (PDMS) were recently fabricated by the group of Minko as shown in Figures 8.6 and 8.7 [105]. These brushes are widely used in medicine and the food and cosmetic industry. At room temperature, these polymers have very mobile chains because of low glass transition temperature (*T*g), and they are able to immediately adapt their properties to changes in environmental conditions. It was demonstrated that PDMS–PEG brushes exhibit low adhesion in both wet and dry states.

Müller *et al.* synthesized core–shell cylindrical polymer brushes with poly (*t*-butyl acrylate)-*b*-poly(*n*-butyl acrylate), which were hydrolyzed later [106]. Due to the responsive nature of the PAA blocks toward different kinds of solvent,

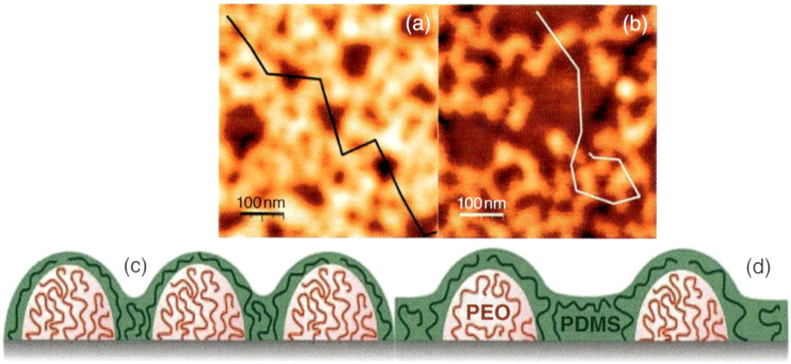

Figure 8.6 (a, b) AFM topographical images and (c, d) schematics of PDMS–PEO brushes ((a, c) 33% PDMS, (b, d) 56% PDMS) in air *z* scale – 10 nm. (Sheparovych 2008 [105]. Reproduced with permission from American Chemical Society.)

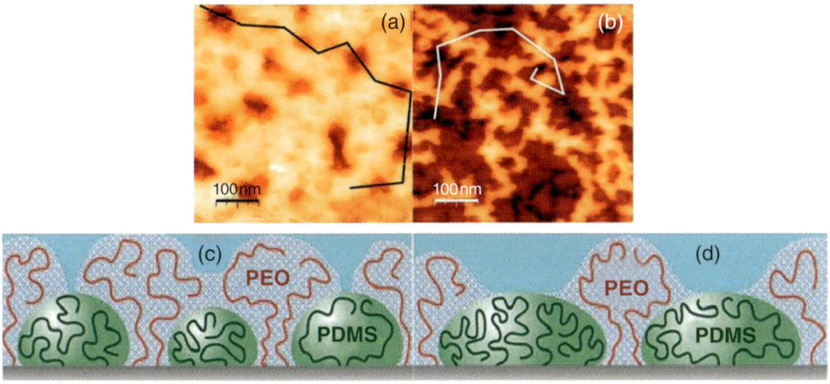

Figure 8.7 (a, b) AFM topographical images and (c, d) schematics of PDMS–PEO brushes ((a, c) PDMS 33%, (b, d) PDMS 56%) in water z scale – 25 nm. (Sheparovych 2008 [105]. Reproduced with permission from American Chemical Society.)

conformational transitions were observed as a function of solvent quality. Fischer and Schmidt made cylindrical brushes with PS side chains and studied solvent-induced length variation of the molecular brushes [107]. They found that the lengths of the backbone and side chains become shorter in a poor solvent as compared to a good solvent. It is argued that the repulsion of the side chains represents the extension force, which acts against the entropic contraction force of the main chain. The adhesive properties of binary heterogeneous polymer brushes made from end-functionalized PS and poly(2-vinylpyridine) (P2VP) chains have been investigated by Creton *et al.* [108, 109]. The adhesion and wetting properties can be reversibly switched by exposure of the system to selective solvents for PS (toluene) and for P2VP (acidic water).

8.2.6 Mechanical Stress

Suh and coworkers have used a wrinkled PDMS sheet with a thickness of 1 mm with built-in micropillars as shown in Figure 8.8. The wrinkles were generated through oxygen plasma treatment of the extended PDMS sheet and subsequent strain release. Active, dynamic control of normal and shear adhesion was achieved: relatively strong normal and shear forces were obtained for a fully extended (strained) PDMS sheet, whereas the forces could be rapidly reduced to nearly zero once the strain was released. Durability tests showed the ability of such systems to be switched in more than 100 attachment and detachment cycles. Nadermann *et al.* showed structures with a fibrillar PDMS surface terminated by a continuous film that can be switched between two metastable states. In the first one, the film is stretched and held up by fibrils and demonstrates strong adhesion compared to an unstructured flat PDMS. In the second state, the film collapses and adheres to the substrate between fibrils. To switch the system, the terminal

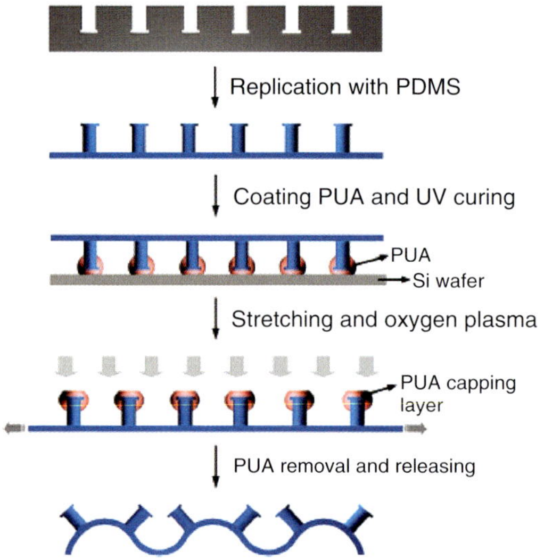

Figure 8.8 Schematic illustration for fabricating a stretchable dry adhesive with micropillars. (Jeong 2010 [112]. Reproduced with permission from American Chemical Society.)

film was then sucked in using air pressure or mechanical pressure. As a result, the surface gets rough due to periodic arrays of bumps. The contact area as well as the adhesion force will decrease. The surface can be switched again by removal of the pressure or through blowing up the film, and the properties will be recovered [110]. Micropatterned PDMS surfaces in the work of Paretkar *et al.* [111] were fabricated using photolithography and molding. The adhesion properties of the surface of 30 μm length and 10 μm diameter fibrils can be switched reversibly with a compressive preload as an external stimulus. Adhesion forces were measured with a flat probe as a function of preload. At low or moderate compression, there is good contact between the surfaces; the adhesion force is big, whereas at high compressive preloads, adhesion dropped to very low values. It can be explained by bending and buckling of the fibrils under high pressure and a subsequent loss of contact with the probe surface. The elasticity of PDMS contributes to the pillar recovery to regain the upright position upon removal of preload enabling repeatability of the switch. The switch can be controlled by fibril aspect ratio, tip shape, and alignment to the test surface. The folding of end flaps at the tip of the fibrils facilitates larger difference in adhesion strength between the adhesive and nonadhesive states. Jeong reported that regularly ordered surface wrinkles were generated by a strain mismatch due to oxygen plasma treatment on a prestrained (or extended) PDMS sheet and subsequent strain release. Although surface wrinkling has been proposed as a tool for adhesion control using a nonpatterned flat surface, a versatile use for the gecko-like hairy structures in active adhesion control has not been demonstrated. By employing well-defined micro-pillars and surface wrinkling, one can use real-time control of normal and shear adhesion with strong attachment and rapid, easy detachment [112].

8.3 Chemically Dependent Stimuli

Chemically dependent stimuli comprise pH, specific ions, redox, and so on.

8.3.1 pH

Polymers containing ionizable functional groups that respond to change in pH are called *pH-sensitive polymers*. By generating the charge along the polymer backbone, the electrostatic repulsion results in an increase in the hydrodynamic volume of the polymer. Polyacrylic acid, polymethacrylic acid (PMAA), poly(ethylene imine), poly(L-lysine), and poly(*N*,*N*-dimethyl aminoethyl methacrylamide) are typical examples of pH-sensitive polymers. When we consider the pH variation in our body, the gastrointestinal tract (GI tract) is an important site for the application of pH-sensitive polymers. The gastric pH is ~2, whereas intestinal pH is ~7.4 or 7.8. pH-sensitive polymers have been regaining attention for applications in gene delivery and gene therapy research. In physiological conditions, as a result of negative charges and the huge size of DNA molecules, the movement of the exposed DNA into a cell is difficult. Therefore, positively charged polymers are used to balance out the charge and condense the DNA to nanoparticles of ~100 nm in size (Table 8.1) [113–118].

8.3.1.1 Methacrylic Acid (MAAc)

Enteric coatings on medication tablets have been accessible over the counter for over 60 years. There are two main types of smart enteric polymer coatings used

Table 8.1 Various applications of pH-sensitive polymers for drug delivery systems.

Polymer	Application	References
Poly(ethylene glycol)-*block*-poly(propylene glycol)-poly(ethylene glycol)	Prolongation of survival time in comparison with single drug therapy	[113]
Poly(*n*-isopropylacrylamide-co-propylacrylic acid-co-butyl acrylate)	To improve angiogenesis in infracted myocardium	[114]
Poly(acrylamide)-*g*-carrageenan and sodium alginate	For colon-targeted delivery	[115]
Poly(methoxyl ethylene glycol-caprolactone-co-methacrylic acid-co-poly(ethylene glycol) methylethylenemethacrylate)	For oral drug delivery	[116]
Alginate and chemically modified carboxymethyl chitosan	For oral delivery	[117]

today. One type depends on copolymers of pH-sensitive methacrylic monomers such as methacrylic acid (MAAc) and hydrophobic methacrylate monomers such as methyl methacrylate (MMA). Another sort of enteric polymer depends on a cellulosic polymer backbone, where a few $-CH_2OH$ groups are esterified with phthalic anhydride. Both sorts of polymers are hydrophobic at stomach or gastric pHs, since carboxyl groups are protonated and nonionized and become hydrophilic at intestinal or enteric pHs where carboxyl groups are ionized. In this way, the drug is not delivered in the stomach, where it could irritate or inflame the stomach lining, yet is quickly released once it reaches the intestines where the pH elevates to physiologic pH levels. The coatings are likewise valuable for shielding "delicate" drugs from stomach acid and gastric compounds. A graft PMAA-g-PEG copolymer was assessed for calcitonin delivery to the intestines.

8.3.1.2 Polyacrylic Acid

Poly(acrylic acid) polymers have been formulated into drug-loaded particles for oral drug delivery where they retain their therapeutic cargo in the acidic environment of the stomach but release the encapsulated drug in the alkaline environment of the small intestine due to ionization of the carboxylic acid groups and swelling of the polymer matrix [119]. Poly(acrylic acid) copolymers incorporating hydrophobic MMA or butyl methacrylate (BMA) monomers were synthesized where the chemical structure and percentage of the hydrophobic monomer influenced the polymer's pK_a value. For example, Barba *et al.* [120] synthesized a range of poly(MMA-co-AA) copolymers with an increasing volumetric ratio of MMA monomer (0%, 25%, 30%, 40%, 50%, 60%, 70%, 75%, 100%) and examined their dissolution at different pH values. The results showed that the increase in MMA content in a given polymer increased the pH necessary to dissolve this polymer (pH 4.0–6.8; copolymers with 75% and higher MMA content were not soluble), which indirectly indicates the increase in the polymer's pK_a with the increase in MMA content. Carbopol® is the most widely recognized mucoadhesive polymer, which is an enrolled trademark of the Lubrizol Corporation for a group of polymers that are utilized as thickeners, suspending agents, and stabilizers. They have been utilized in different vaginal drug delivery formulations, especially to improve residence time of the medication in the vagina. Most Carbopol® polymers are high molecular weight polyacrylic acid chains that are lightly cross-linked and are accessible as powders or fluids [121]. Another study by Licea-Claverie *et al.* showed that the insertion of a variable number of methylene groups in a poly(MMA) polymer increases the polymer's pK_a (1–10 CH_2 spacers; MW range: 43–90 KDa; pK_a range: 3.8–7.3) due to the formation of hydrophobic microdomains that act as a cross-linker that minimizes the polymer's dissolution and swelling [122]. One example that clearly indicates the effect of solution pH on poly(acrylic acid) polymers is reported by Guan *et al.* who used poly(acrylic acid-9-aminoacridine-co-acrylamide) as a pH sensor in biological applications. This application depends on the polymer's (MW 3.5 KDa) ability to change its fluorescence intensity as it transitions from double to single protonation to amino and finally to imino forms as a function of environment pH (pH 0–13.71) [123]. Ethyl acrylic acid (EAAc) and propyl acrylic acid (PAAc) form pH-sensitive polymers and copolymers. They showed phase transition when pH is lowered through their pKa, which is within the pH range of early endosomes. When these polymers act as drug carriers and endocytosed into target cells, they can disrupt the lipid bilayer of the endosome as pH drops within the endosome, facilitating the "escape" of the polymer-drug carrier into the cytosol [124–130]. This intracellular drug delivery technology is still under trial. It can be postulated that, if such smart materials and methods could show significantly enhanced delivery of drugs such as siRNA, they might be used in clinical testing. Bae and coworkers have also developed interesting temperature and pH-sensitive polymers useful for stimulating endosomal release of drug formulations [131, 132]. PPA and poly(ethacrylic acid) (PEA) are also examples of pH-sensitive polymers applied in gene delivery. Both polymers demonstrate an abrupt conformational change at pH of ~5–6 [124]. Using red blood cells, membrane fusion efficacy was confirmed for both polymers at endosomal pH. Hemolytic activity of PEA and PPA increases rapidly as pH decreases from 6 to 5, whereas there is no hemolytic activity at pH 7.4 [125].

8.3.1.3 Poly(L-lysine)

Poly(L-lysine)-*g*-poly(histidine) is a membrane fusion polymer designed and investigated for DNA delivery [133]. The poly(L-lysine) parts are positively charged at physiological pH and used for DNA condensing, whereas poly(histidine) parts are supposed to act as endosomal fusion polymers. The pK_a of poly(histidine) is 6.0, and therefore it undergoes conformational changes at endosomal pH. Poly(L-lysine)-*g*-poly(histidine) graft copolymer demonstrated enhanced transfection efficiency in comparison with poly(L-lysine) for 293 T cells, supporting the concept of poly(histidine) function in this system.

8.3.1.4 Polysulfonic Acid

The second group of pH-sensitive polymers with acidic functional groups includes poly(sulfonic acid) polymers and their derivatives. These polymers have pendant sulfonate groups ($-SO_3H$) with pK_a values of 2–3 that become ionized over a wide pH range [134]. Polysulfonates are often used as cross-linking agents of other polymers such as styrene and vinyl-based polymers to tune the pK_a of the formulated particles for a specific application. For example, McCormick *et al.* synthesized hydrogel-based particles using 3-[*N*-(2-methacroyloyethyl)-*N*,*N*-dimethylammonio]propanesulfonate (MW 49 KDa; polydispersity index (PDI) = 1.04) via controlled polymerization techniques. These particles were synthesized using an aqueous salt solvent system, which is an unconventional method for synthesis of acrylic-based polymers that typically require an organic solvent. These particles are attractive for drug delivery applications due to their biocompatibility, ease of production in aqueous salt solvent systems, and narrow distribution of molecular weight [135].

8.3.2
Ionic Strength

The characteristic property of polymers containing ionized groups is their responsiveness to ionic strength. These polymer frameworks show strange rheological behavior due to the attractive Coulombic interactions between oppositely charged species, which may render the polymer insoluble in deionized water yet soluble in critical concentration of added electrolytes where the attractive charge/charge interactions are protected [136–138]. Therefore, changes in ionic strength cause changes in the length of the polymer chains, the polymer solubility, and the fluorescence quenching kinetics of chromophores bound to electrolytes [139, 140].

8.3.2.1 Poly(*N*-isopropylacrylamide) (PNIPAM)

Ionic strength-responsive polymers undergo their phase transitions, resulting from the different concentration of salts (e.g., ionic strength). Cu(II) metal ion was immobilized on poly(NIPAM-co-vinylimidazole) for protein separation using the affinity binding of specific proteins to Cu(II) [141]. When the ionic strength was increased, the polymer chains binding the proteins becomes precipitated while not interfering with protein–metal ion interactions and reducing the nonspecific binding of foreign proteins to polymer chains. The proposed mechanism was that the high salt concentration reduced the repulsive electrostatic strength of the copolymer, resulting in an increase of hydrophobic interactions, leading to the precipitation.

8.3.3
Redox-Responsive Polymers

Redox-responsive biodegradable or bioerodible systems are prepared using polymer with labile groups. Redox-responsive stimuli were induced by the acid labile moieties inside anhydrides [142, 143], PLGA [144], and poly(*b*-amino esters) (PbAEs)[145]. Disulfide groups have additionally been utilized to actuate redox responsiveness, since they are unsteady in a reducing atmosphere, being cleaved for thiol groups [146, 147]. Reductive amino acid-based molecules are the polymers with disulfide cross-links which were degraded when exposed to cysteine or glutathione [148]. Another average redox-responsive polymer is poly(NIPAM-co-Ru(bpy)3), which can create a chemical wave by the intermittent redox change of Ru(bpy)3 into an oxidized state of lighter color [149]. This redox response modifies the hydrophobic and hydrophilic properties of the polymer chains and results in deswelling and swelling of the polymer.

8.4
Biologically Dependent Stimuli

Biologically responsive polymer systems are increasingly important in various biomedical applications. The major advantage of bioresponsive polymers is that they can respond to the stimuli that are inherently present in the natural system. Bioresponsive polymeric systems mainly arise from common functional groups that are known to interact with biologically relevant species, and in other instances the synthetic polymer is conjugated to a biological component. Analytes and biomacromolecules such as glucose, enzymes, and overproduced metabolites in inflammation are major examples of biologically dependent stimuli.

8.4.1
Enzyme-Responsive Polymers

Enzyme-responsive polymers form the basis for hydrogels that are responsive only to specific enzymes. These enzymes are used as signals for monitoring several physiological changes and have very successfully been used as signals for site-specific delivery of various drugs to specific organs. Enzymes play a central role in cell regulation and, therefore, are important targets for drug development and in therapeutics. When the enzymatic activity is associated to a particular tissue or the enzyme is found at higher concentrations at the target site, the nanomaterial can be programmed to deliver drugs via enzymatic conversion of the carrier [150]. Moreover, the detection of enzyme activity can be an extremely useful tool in diagnostics, since dysregulation of enzyme expression is a characteristic feature of numerous diseases [151].

8.4.1.1 Polyethylene Glycol (PEG)
Amir and Hawker *et al.* [152] reported enzyme-triggered self-assembly from an initially water-soluble diblock copolymer consisting of PEG and a phosphorylated poly(4-vinylphenol) (PVPh) block, which was synthesized by nitroxide-mediated polymerization (NMP) using a PEG-based mediating agent. The precursor diblock copolymer is molecularly dissolved in aqueous media due to the presence of hydrophilic phosphate residues on the enzyme-reactive block. In the presence of acid phosphatase (AP), enzyme-catalyzed cleavage of phosphate moieties at pH 5 leads to the formation of an amphiphilic diblock copolymer due to which the PVPh block is insoluble under mildly acidic pH.

A similar strategy was also employed to achieve enzyme-triggered sol–gel transition from enzyme-responsive diblock copolymers, as reported by Zhao and coworkers [153]. In that case, they synthesized an ABA triblock copolymer, P(DEGEA-co-OPBA)-*b*-PEG-*b*-P(DEGEA-co-OPBA), consisting of a PEG middle block and two outer blocks of randomly copolymerized ethoxydi(ethylene glycol) acrylate (DEGEA) and ((dihydroxyphosphoryl)oxy)butyl acrylate (OPBA), via ATRP by using a PEG-based difunctional macroinitiator. AP-assisted dephosphorylation reaction at 37 °C in the thermoresponsive P(DEGEA-co-OPBA) block led to the decrease of the LCST or CMT for the ABA triblock copolymer. At relatively high polymer concentration (7.9 wt% in aqueous media), enzyme-triggered cleavage of phosphate residues led to sol–gel transition at 37 °C. Note that both before and after enzymatic reactions, the transition between gel and sol states can be tuned by temperatures, although differing in critical gelation temperatures.

8.4.2 Glucose-Responsive Polymers

A glucose-responsive polymer system for insulin-controlled release has been intensively investigated due to its huge potential in the biomedical market. When the concentration of glucose in the blood becomes high due to improper control of metabolism by the hormone insulin, a patient suffering from diabetes mellitus usually needs a supply of insulin that has to be administrated via periodic injection. However, blood glucose levels cannot be maintained in the normal range by this treatment. The glucose-responsive hydrogel system can provide self-regulating insulin release in response to the concentration of glucose in the blood, which can control the concentration of insulin within a normal range.

8.4.2.1 *N,N*-Dimethylaminoethyl Methacrylate (DMAEMA)

N,N-Dimethylaminoethyl methacrylate (DMAEMA), a weak cationic moiety, was introduced into copolymer hydrogels [154]. The hydrogels were obtained by copolymerization of 2-hydroxyethyl methacrylate and DMAEMA and immobilization of glucose oxidase and catalase. When excessive glucose diffuses into the hydrogels, glucose oxidase catalyzes the glucose conversion to gluconic acid. The gluconic acid lowers the pH within the hydrogel network and protonates the tertiary amine groups of DMAEMA, resulting in the swelling of the hydrogels due to increased electrostatic repulsion force. The swollen hydrogels result in an increased network mesh size and consequent increased release of insulin from the matrix. The incorporated catalase reconverts hydrogen peroxide to oxygen, which is required for glucose oxidization, and reduces the hydrogen peroxide inhibition of glucose oxidase. The effect of cross-links on the swelling and release was investigated. *In vivo* experiments on rats confirmed that this glucose-responsive insulin release system was effective in reducing blood glucose levels.

Horbett *et al.* [155–157] entrapped glucose oxidase within HEMA-DMAEMA copolymer hydrogel membranes to construct a glucose-sensitive delivery system. To obtain high insulin permeability, the hydrogel membranes were made porous under conditions that induced a phase separation during polymerization. The addition of glucose resulted in swelling of the membranes and an enhanced permeation of insulin from a reservoir via diffusion through the swollen hydrogel membranes.

8.4.2.2 **Polyethylene Glycol (PEG)**

Poly(ethylene oxide)-*block*-poly(2-glucosyl-oxyethyl acrylate) (PEO-*b*-PGEA) was designed for a glucose-responsive micellar structure to disrupt the micellar structure and release entrapped insulin when the glucose concentration in the blood is high [158]. This diblock copolymer was synthesized by ATRP with a methoxy-end-capped PEO macroinitiator. This diblock copolymer and its mechanism of glucose-responsive micellization. This water-soluble diblock copolymer showed reversible micellar association/dissociation at dilute concentration in response to glucose concentration. However, this study requires to further determine conditions such as optimal concentration of concanavalin A (ConA) and glucose for proper timing of insulin release after it is loaded.

8.5
Dual Stimuli

Smart polymers are characterized by their stimuli-responsive behavior, which is essentially dictated by the functional groups present on or within a polymer chain. In fact, a broad library of such functionalities have been studied and are covered appropriately in the literature. Different functionalities respond to different stimuli, and the most commonly used stimuli are temperature, pH, light, ionic strength, electron transfer (redox), and host–guest interactions. In this context, the combination of several functional moieties within one polymer that can respond to different stimuli is a relatively new occurrence. As a result, dual- or multistimuli-responsive polymers are obtained, which is the starting point to more sophisticated applications, due to the variability that is introduced to the responsiveness [159].

The dual- and multistimuli-responsive polymeric nanoparticles are particles that react to the combination of two or more signals, for example, pH/redox, pH/magnetic field, temperature/reduction, pH/temperature, double pH, pH and diols, temperature/enzyme, and temperature/magnetic field. Temperature/pH/magnetic, temperature/pH/redox, pH/redox/magnetic, temperature/redox/guest molecules, and temperature/pH/guest molecules are multistimuli which are recently created. Strikingly, these consolidated reactions occur either at the same time at the pathological site or in an orderly way from nanoparticle preparation such as nanoparticle transporting pathways to cell compartments. These dual- and multistimuli-responsive polymeric nanoparticles have demonstrated extraordinary control over drug delivery and release, resulting in a predominant *in vitro* and/or *in vivo* anticancer efficacy. With programmed site-specific drug delivery features, dual- and multistimuli-responsive nanoparticulate drug formulations have huge potential for focused tumor treatment [160].

8.5.1 Thermo- and pH-Responsive Polymers

The changes in pH have been established as an additional trigger within thermo responsive polymers [161]. These materials attracted great attention in the field of drug delivery because both variables are subject to changes within cancer tissue, which can be used to trigger an autonomous response. In such dual-responsive systems, functional groups that can either dissociate into ionic groups or form ionic groups upon protonation are incorporated into the backbone of an LCST polymer.

pH- and temperature-responsive nanoparticles are among the most studied dual-sensitive nanosystems. Many pH- and temperature-responsive polymers are designed and prepared by incorporating pH-sensitive components such as weak acids into thermosensitive PNIPAM, which afford copolymers with pH-dependent LCST. This fine-tuning of phase transition by subtle pH change has enabled the development of tumor pH-sensitive drug release systems.

Yang *et al.* reported that pH- and temperature-sensitive core shell nanoparticles self-assembled from poly(-NIPAM-co-*N*,*N*-dimethylacrylamide-co-10-undecenoic acid) (P(NIPAM-co-DMAAm-co-UA)) terpolymer were stable in a normal physiological condition (pH 7.4, 37 °C) while they deformed and precipitated in an acidic environment [162]. The *in vitro* release studies showed that DOX was released much faster at mildly acidic pH of 6.6 (simulating tumor microenvironment) than at pH 7.4. The conjugation of cholesterol to the hydrophobic segment of P(NIPAM-co-DMAAm-co-UA) and folic acid to the free amine group yielded stable and tumor-targeting nanoparticles that efficiently delivered and released DOX into folate-receptor-overexpressing cancer cells including 4T1 and KB cells, resulting in further improved antitumor activity [163].

Jiang *et al.* constructed thermo and pH dual-responsive nanoparticles based on poly(-NIPAM-co-acrylic acid)-*b*-PCL (P(NIPAM-co-AA)-*b*-PCL) diblock copolymer [164]. Interestingly, these nanoparticles could encapsulate up to 30 wt% of paclitaxel (PTX) and aggregated at pH 6.9 and 37 °C. Faster drug release was observed at higher temperature and lower pH. Hsiue *et al.* reported that temperature and pH dual-responsive micelles based on a mixture of methoxy-PEG-*b*-P(*N*-(2-hydroxypropyl) methacrylamide dilactate)-co-(*N*-(2-hydroxy propyl) methacrylamide-co-histidine) (mPEG-*b*-P(HPMA-Lac-co-His)), mPEG-*b*-PLA, and cy5.5–PEG–PLA copolymers displayed a specific targeting efficiency and an improved *in vivo* antitumor activity as compared to free DOX in Balb/c nude mice bearing human cervical tumors [165].

Hsiue *et al.* reported that pH- and thermoresponsive nanoparticles based on biodegradable poly(D,L-lactide)-*g*-poly(NIPAM-co-methacrylic acid) (PLA-*g*-P(NIPAM-co-MAA)) graft copolymers had an LCST above 37 °C and a high loading of 5-fluorouracil (5-FU) [166]. The release of 5-FU was significantly enhanced at pH 5.0 than at pH 7.4 as a result of pH-triggered collapse of

P(NIPAM-co-MAA) shells. Lu *et al.* developed pH and thermal dual-responsive ionically assembled nanoparticles based on poly(ionic liquid-co-NIPAM) and deoxycholic acid [167]. The *in vitro* release results showed that 80% of DOX was released in 48 h at pH 5.2 and 43 °C due to structural collapse of nanoparticles. In contrast, only 30% of DOX was released in 48 h at pH 7.4 and 37 °C. pH and temperature dual stimuli-responsive hollow nanogels were prepared from self-assembling of poly(AA-co-2-methacryloylethyl acrylate) (P(AA-co-MEA)) grafted with PNIPAM and mPEG at pH 3.0 and 25 °C followed by cross-linking via radical polymerization [168].

8.5.2 pH- and Redox-Responsive Polymers

pH and redox are the two most appealing stimuli, as they both exist naturally in certain pathological sites as well as in all cancer cells [169, 170]. A redox stimulus is defined as an electrochemical addressing of the redox-sensitive group, which causes a change in its oxidation state. Indeed, this kind of stimulus is more common in inorganic chemistry, especially with respect to transition metals. pH and redox dual-sensitive nanoparticles have been designed and developed to facilitate nanoparticle formation in aqueous environments through change of pH, to increase *in vivo* stability of nanoparticles via disulfide cross-linking, to trigger drug release or enhance tumor cell uptake via reversal of surface charges at tumor pH, to release the drug in the endo/lysosomal compartments, and/or to achieve fast drug release in the cytoplasm and nucleus. For example, pH and reduction dual-bioresponsive nanosized polymersomes were readily prepared from PEG-SS-poly(2-(diethylamino)ethyl methacrylate) (PEG-SS-PDEAEMA) double hydrophilic diblock copolymers by simply increasing their solution pH to 7.4 [171].

Wang *et al.* prepared pH and redox dual-responsive nanogels from MAA and *N,N*-bis(acryloyl)cystamine cross-linker via distillation–precipitation polymerization [172]. These nanogels could efficiently load DOX (up to 42.3 wt%) at physiological pH due to the presence of strong electrostatic interactions between nanogels and drug. The *in vitro* release studies showed that over 80% of DOX was released in 24 h at pH 5.0 and/or in the presence of 10 mM GSH, whereas drug release was less than 15% at pH 7.4 under otherwise the same conditions. CCK-8 assays indicated that DOX-loaded dual-sensitive nanogels had comparable antitumor activity to free DOX in U251MG cells.

Zhang *et al.* prepared redox and pH dual-sensitive cross-linked polyelectrolyte nanocapsules from cysteamine-conjugated chitosan (CS-SH) and dextran sulfate (DS) through layer-by-layer (LbL) assembly on b-cyclodextrin (b-CD)-functionalized silica spheres followed by oxidative cross-linking and core removal [173]. The *in vitro* release studies showed that protein release from gradient cross-linked nanocapsules while insignificant at pH 1.4 (simulating the pH in the stomach) and pH 6.8 (simulating the extracellular pH) was fast under pH 6.8 and

10 mM GSH conditions. The cell uptake results displayed that these nanocapsules could effectively deliver and release FITC-labeled BSA into the cytosol of Caco-2 cells.

The pH- and redox-responsive cross-linked micelles were developed based on poly(2-(2-pyridyldisulfide)ethylmethacrylate)-*b*-PHPMA (PDSM-*b*-PHPMA) block copolymer by conjugating maleimide-hydrazone-DOX derivative and simultaneous core cross-linking using tris(2-carboxyethyl)phosphine as a catalyst [174].

8.5.3 Thermo- and Redox-Responsive Polymers

Dual-responsive (thermo and redox) materials based on PNIPAM have been presented by Phillips and Gibson [175]. These systems consist of PNIPAM macromonomers, which were linked via disulfide units. Disulfide linkages were introduced into poly(*N*-isopropylacrylamide) by the polycondensation of a RAFT-derived, telechelic macromonomer to give degradable but vinyl-based polymers. These polymers displayed a redox-sensitive LCST with the shorter, degraded product displaying a higher LCST than its nondegraded counterpart.

Morimoto *et al.* prepared dual-responsive nanogels from pullulan lightly grafted with thiol-terminated PNIPAM by increasing its solution temperature from 25 to 50 °C followed by oxidative cross-linking of thiol ends [176]. The resulting nanogels could be destructed either upon cooling to room temperature or upon treatment with a reducing agent. In a similar way, temperature and redox dual-responsive nanogels have been prepared from dextran grafted with thiol-terminated PNIPAM [177] and thiolated hydroxypropyl cellulose (HPC-SH) [178].

8.5.4 pH- and Magnetic-Responsive Polymers

Magnetic nanoparticles have received enormous interests due to their several potential biomedical applications including targeted drug delivery, magnetic thermotherapy (hyperthermia), magnetic resonance imaging (MRI), and separation of proteins and cells [179–181].

Yan *et al.* prepared pH-responsive Fe_3O_4-cored nanoparticles using PEG-*b*-PMAA-*b*-poly(glycerol monomethacrylate) (PEG-*b*-PMAA-*b*-PGMA) triblock copolymers as coatings [174]. These nanoparticles efficiently loaded DOX at pH 7.4 likely due to the presence of ionic and hydrophobic interactions with PMAA. Under acidic conditions (<pH 5.5), however, DOX was rapidly released due to diminishing ionic interactions between DOX and PMAA ($pK_a = 5.6$). The following studies showed that folate-decorated DOX-loaded pH-responsive magnetic nanoparticles were efficiently taken up by HeLa cells via receptor-mediated endocytosis process, resulting in markedly enhanced antitumor activity [182].

8.5.5 Thermo- and Light-Responsive Polymers

The majority of examples describing a serial impact of multiple stimuli deal with the combination of thermoresponsive polymers with light-responsive molecules, which are attached onto the polymer chain to photo-control the LCST [183]. A prime example was reported by Kungwatchakun and Irie in 1988 [184]. They synthesized thermoresponsive copolymers by polymerization of *N*-isopropylacrylamide (NIPAM) with an *N*-(4-phenylazophenyl) acrylamide monomer. The intention of this work was to photo-control the phase separation temperature of aqueous solutions of PNIPAM by introducing photochromic azobenzene moieties. Consequently, a shift in the phase separation temperature from initial 21 to 27 °C after UV-light irradiation was observed, and this reversible LCST change was explained by the change of the dipole moment from 0 to 3 debye due to the trans-to-cis isomerization of the chromophoric azobenzene moieties. The initial phase transition temperature of 21 °C was reobtained after exposure to visible light, demonstrating the reversibility of the system [101, 185, 186].

8.6 Multistimuli-Responsive Materials

Multiresponsive materials are not only important in life sciences but also equally essential for new developments in information technology. These types of materials, bearing more than two responsive groups, combined in one polymer; the combinatorial impact of two or more stimuli-responsive groups can be parallel, serial, or causal. Over the years, examples for all cases have been presented. Using these terms, parallel means that the response of one group does not affect the response of the other and vice versa.

The selected examples of polymers responsive to two stimuli demonstrate impressively the strength of combining several stimuli within one polymer. In addition to dual-responsive nanoparticles, several multiresponsive nanoparticles have recently been developed. However, recent research activities aimed at adding one more stimulus, that is, triple-stimuli-responsive polymers, have gained momentum. The addition of one more stimulus is particularly advantageous because it can improve the degree of precision, enlarge the switching window, or even change the switching conditions due to the higher level of complexity of the polymer.

8.6.1 Light-, pH-, and Temperature-Responsive Polymers

As already mentioned previously, one way to obtain triple-stimuli-responsive polymers with a serial interplay is the combination of building blocks that are both

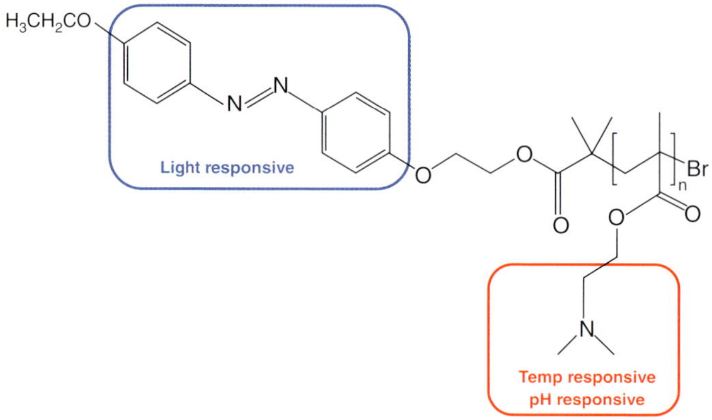

Figure 8.9 PDMAEMA polymer end functionalized with azobenzene, which can be stimulated by light, temperature, and change of the pH value [187].

pH and thermo sensitive, for example, PDMAEMA, with another responsive moiety (Figure 8.9) [187].

As designed, the polymer exhibited responsiveness toward pH, temperature, and light and was considered to be triple stimuli responsive. Indeed, changing the pH value could alter the LCST characteristic. At pH = 4 the dimethylamino functionality was fully protonated, resulting in an increased polarity, and thus no LCST was observed. By decreasing the proton concentration, that is, increasing the pH, the LCST was lowered to 68 °C at pH = 7 and to 30 °C at pH = 11, which was attributed to the consecutive deprotonation of the dimethylamino group. The additional effect of the azobenzene end group due to its photoisomerization at different pH values led to a slightly higher LCST after irradiation with UV light in comparison with the LCST before irradiation at the corresponding pH value. The process was fully reversible. The less pronounced impact of the light-responsive moiety is not the consequence of the azobenzene group *per se*, but is rather attributed to the small fraction of azobenzene per polymer.

Zhang *et al.* demonstrated a very interesting approach recently. They used a thermo-, pH-, and light-responsive hyperbranched polymer on the basis of hyperbranched polyethylenimine (HPEI) [188]. Termination of HPEI with isobutyramide groups, followed by supramolecular complexation of 4-(phenylazo)benzoic acid (PABA), led to a structure that was serial responsive to all three stimuli, similar to the linear copolymer.

It is significant that, as a single functional group, PDMAEMA is responsive to two stimuli, namely, pH and temperature. This might be advantageous, because the density of responsive groups within one polymer can be increased. However, it has to be mentioned that the two stimuli cannot be applied independently, which might be unfavorable in some applications. It is therefore possible that the subsequently applied second stimulus is suppressed by the state that was generated by the impact of the first applied stimulus. In the case of the poly

(NIPAM-co-NHMA-co-DNQ) polymer, each responsive moiety can be stimulated independently, even after the application of one orthogonal stimulus. In other words, the LCST can still be shifted by increasing or decreasing the pH value, even after UV irradiation. Clearly, one drawback in this system is the irreversibility of the photo induced rearrangement, which led to an increase of the LCST, but this change has permanently no chance to recover the initial LCST values.

8.6.2 Light-, Redox-, and Temperature-Responsive Polymers

Depending on the redox-active moiety employed, different classes of triple light-, redox- and temperature-responsive polymers can be defined. At first, the redox-active group 2,2,6,6-tetramethylpiperidine-1-oxyl (TEMPO) is discussed. Theato *et al.* prepared PNIPAM copolymers, containing 4-amino-2,2,6,6-tetramethylpiperidine-1-oxyl (amino-TEMPO) and amino-functionalized azobenzene moieties linked via an amide bond of the polymer backbone, which can be considered as a system with serial interplay [189]. The TEMPO moiety is redox sensitive and can be reduced and reoxidized in a reversible fashion, either chemically using ascorbic acid as a mild reducing agent and red prussiate as an oxidizing agent or electrochemically. The reduction of the TEMPO moiety to the corresponding hydroxylamine resulted in a shift of the hydrophilic/hydrophobic balance to an increased hydrophilicity and thus led to an increase in LCST. It is noteworthy that the LCST could be fine-tuned simply by the degree of reduction of the TEMPO moieties. Additional irradiation with UV light in order to stimulate the azobenzene chromophore led to a further increase of LCST. The independent addressing of the two responsive groups was investigated by the sequence of the applied stimuli. Although there was no difference in terms of the final LCST, a huge difference in the "intermediate" LCST was observed depending on the stimulation sequence.

8.6.3 Environmental-, pH-, and Temperature-Responsive Polymers

The group of Uchiyama prepared a random copolymer composed of PNIPAM, poly(dimethylaminopropyl acrylamide) (PDMAPAM) and *N*-{2-[(7-*N*,*N*-dimethylaminosulfonyl)-2,1,3-benzoxadiazol-4-yl-](methyl)amino}ethyl-*N*-methylacrylamide (DBD-AA) (Figure 8.10) [190].

Besides the already well-known PNIPAM, the PDMAPAM moiety belongs to the class of pH-responsive groups, while the benzofurazan derivative is considered as a polarity-sensitive fluorophore. Keeping the temperature fixed at 50 °C (i.e., above LCST of PNIPAM), the copolymer existed in the hydrated open form under acidic conditions, due to the high hydrophilicity induced by the protonated dimethylamino group. As soon as the pH was increased, the copolymer chains collapsed. The improved hydrophobic interaction between PNIPAM and DMAPAM units led to an increase of the DBD-AA fluorescence, because the water

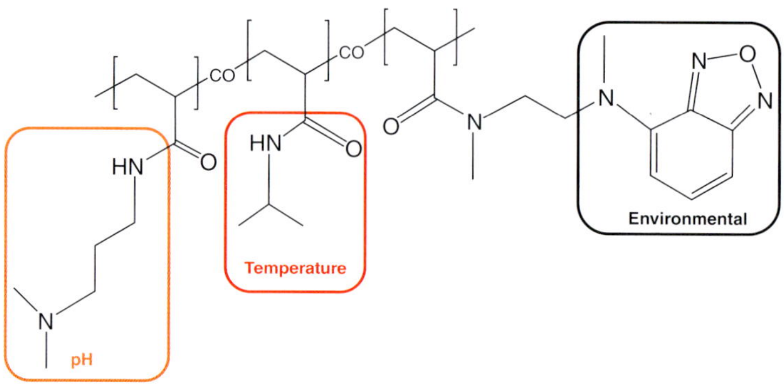

Figure 8.10 Stimuli-responsive polymer system with causal interaction [190].

molecules were repelled from the collapsed polymer chain. For the hydrophobic collapsed polymer chain, the fluorescence intensity was 6.6-fold stronger compared to the hydrophilic regime and exhibited a very sharp and distinct transition (within almost one unit), which suggests that these materials are advanced pH sensors. They found that the pH range can be fine-tuned by varying the ionic moiety: incorporation of a weaker proton receptor resulted in a transition under more acidic conditions, while a stronger proton receptor led to a shift of the fluorescence response at more basic pH values.

8.6.4
Redox-, pH-, and Temperature-Responsive Polymers

Thayumanavan *et al.* designed a triple-stimuli-sensitive nanoparticle based on a block copolymer comprising an acid-sensitive tetrahydropyran-protected 2-hydroxyethyl methacrylate (THP-protected HEMA) hydrophobic block, thermo sensitive PNIPAM hydrophilic block, and an intervening redox-sensitive disulfide linker [191].

These micellar nanoparticles were sensitive to redox, acid, and temperature: (i) increasing temperature to above its LCST led to precipitation of nanoparticles as the hydrophilic shell turned water insoluble, (ii) lowering pH resulted in dissolution of nanoparticles due to the transformation of the hydrophobic core into a hydrophilic core, and (iii) a reducing environment disrupted the assembly owing to scission of block copolymer into individual homopolymers.

Li *et al.* prepared temperature-, pH-, and redox-responsive nanogels by miniemulsion copolymerization of monomethyl oligo(ethylene glycol) acrylate (OEGA), 2-(5,5-dimethyl-1,3-dioxan-2-yloxy) ethyl acrylate (DMDEA) which contains an acid-labile orthoester bond, and bis(2-acryloyloxyethyl) disulfide (BADS) (Figure 8.5) [192]. These nanogels displayed a fast thermoresponsive property and were shrunk to 17–35 nm upon increasing the temperature to 37 °C. Notably, nanogels swelled quickly and significantly upon incubation in weakly acidic media (pH 4–6) due to acid-triggered hydrolysis of the orthoester groups or in response to 20 mM DTT at pH 7.4 owing to cleavage of disulfide cross-linkers. The *in vitro* release profiles of PTX, Nile red, and DOX pointed out that drug release was low at pH 7.4 but was greatly accelerated by decreasing media pH to 5.0 or 6.0. The drug release rate increased in response to 20 mM DTT, though to a less extent. MTT assays showed that PTX-loaded multiresponsive nanogels displayed a concentration-dependent cytotoxicity to MCF-7 cells.

8.6.5
Magnetic-, pH-, and Redox-Responsive Polymers

The magnetic-, pH-, and redox-sensitive particles using a sacrificial template-directed synthesis procedure followed by chemical deposition of magnetic nanocrystals via coprecipitation were obtained by Kordas *et al.* [193]. These multisensitive nanoparticles displayed a high encapsulation efficiency of approximately 98% for daunorubicin hydrochloride (DNR). The release of DNR was low (15% release in 24 h) at physiological pH but was enhanced at pH 5.0 (40% release in 24 h). The fastest drug release was observed in 20 mM GSH (94% release in 24 h) due to a complete rupture of the shell. These particles with good magnetic response could serve as multiresponsive drug carriers that also induce local heating in a controllable manner via magnetic hyperthermia.

8.6.6
Temperature-, pH-, and Magnetic-Responsive Polymers

Yang *et al.* prepared the thermo and pH dual-sensitive polymer poly (*N*-isopropylacrylamide-co-methacrylic acid), coated with magnetic MSN via precipitation polymerization [194]. The volume phase transition temperature were shown to be dependent on solution pH. The *in vitro* release studies showed that 37.1% and 80.2% of DOX were released at 37 °C in 24 h at pH 6.5 and pH 5.0, respectively, whereas only 7.2% of DOX was released at pH 7.4 under otherwise the same conditions, indicating facile control of drug release. MTT assays revealed that DOX-loaded multisensitive nanoparticles had a similar cytotoxicity to HeLa cells to free DOX. These multisensitive nanoparticles have the potential to overcome the lack of selectivity of anti cancer drugs and combining with EPR/magnetic targeting to increase the therapeutic efficacy.

8.7
Conclusion

In summary, thermoresponsive polymers have found applications in diverse biomedical uses: from tissue engineering to the delivery of therapeutic molecules, for example, drugs or genes. Cellular toxicity of the smart polymers, especially for applications involving intracellular delivery of biomolecular drugs such as peptide, protein, and nucleic acid drugs, mainly act within cells. The use of stimuli-responsive polymers in modified-release pharmaceutical dosage forms has many advantages, including the release and distribution of the drug in a specific target, thus reducing the side effects or adverse systemic reactions. The dual-stimuli responsiveness of new synthetic polymers such as elastin-like systems and acrylic homopolymers and copolymers are discussed in terms of characteristics and possible applications in the biomedical field.

Smart materials such as dual- or multiresponsive materials are not only important in life science but also equally important for new developments in many fields. These multifunctional materials are capable of addressing the challenging issues of current nanoparticulate drug formulations including aspects of preparation and drug loading, *in vivo* stability, tumor targetability, tumor cell uptake, and intracellular drug release. These features have offered unprecedented control over drug delivery and release profiles leading to superior *in vitro* and/or *in vivo* anticancer effects. Even though these materials are attractive for their potentials, they have to overcome several barriers – rapid response, mechanical strength, reproducibility, biocompatibility, biodegradability, nontoxicity, and so on – according to their applications. In recent years, many trials to achieve these requirements have been reported. Therefore, we expect that this chapter will assist to extend new stimuli-responsive polymers or polymeric systems that could be reliably developed in real-life applications.

Abbreviations

amino-TEMPO	4-amino-2,2,6,6-tetramethylpiperidine-1-oxyl
AP	acid phosphatase
BADS	bis(2-acryloyloxyethyl) disulfide
b-CD	b-cyclodextrin
BMA	butyl methacrylate
CIPAAm	2-carboxyisopropylacrylamide
CMT	critical micellization temperature
ConA	concanavalin A
CS-SH	cysteamine-conjugated chitosan
DEGEA	ethoxydi(ethylene glycol) acrylate
DMAEMA	*N*,*N*-dimethylaminoethyl methacrylate
DMDEA	2-(5,5-dimethyl-1,3-dioxan-2-yloxy) ethyl acrylate
DNR	daunorubicin hydrochloride
DOX	doxorubicin
DS	dextran sulfate
EAAc	ethyl acrylic acid
ELPs	elastin-like peptides
GI-tract	gastrointestinal tract
HEMA	hydroxyethyl methacrylate
HPEI	hyperbranched polyethylenimine
LbL	layer-by-layer

LCST	lower critical solution temperature
MAAc	methacrylic acid
MMA	methyl methacrylate
mNP	magnetic nanoparticles
MRI	magnetic resonance imaging
NMP	nitroxide-mediated polymerization
OEGMA	oligo(ethylene glycol) methacrylate
OPBA	((dihydroxyphosphoryl) oxy) butyl acrylate
P(AA-co-MEA)	poly(AA-co-2-methacryloylethyl acrylate)
P2VP	polystyrene (PS) and poly(2-vinylpyridine)
PAAc	propylacrylic acid
PABA	4-(phenylazo)benzoic acid
PbAEs	poly(*b*-amino esters)
PBS	phosphate-buffered saline
PDEAAm	poly(*N*,*N*-diethylacrylamide)
PDEVP	poly(diethyl vinylphosphonate)
PDMAPAM	poly(dimethylaminopropyl acrylamide)
PDMS	polydimethylsiloxane
PEG	poly(ethylene glycol)
PEGMA	poly(ethylene glycol) methacrylate
PEG-SS-PDEAEMA	PEG-SS-poly(2-(diethylamino)ethyl methacrylate)
PEO	poly(ethylene oxide)
PEO-*b*-PGEA	poly(ethylene oxide)-*block*-poly(2-glucosyl-oxyethyl) acrylate)
PEO–PPO–PEO	poly(ethylene oxide)–poly(propylene oxide)–poly(ethylene oxide)
PLGA	poly(lactic acid-co-glycolic acid)
PLLA-PEG-PLLA	(L-lactic acid)–poly(ethylene glycol)–poly(L-lactic acid)
PMAA	polyacrylic acid, polymethacrylic acid
PMEO2MA	poly(2-(2-methoxyethoxy)ethylmethacrylate)
PMPC	poly(2-(methacryloyloxy)ethyl phosphorylcholine)
PNEM	poly(*N*-(2-ethoxy-1,3-dioxan-5-yl) methacrylamide)
PNIPAM	poly(*N*-isopropylacrylamide)
PNIPAM-*b*-PEG	poly(NIPAM)-*b*-poly(ethylene glycol)
PNIPAM-HA	poly(*N*-isopropylacrylamide)-grafted hyaluronan
PNMM	poly(*N*-(2-methoxy-1,3-dioxan-5-yl) methacrylamide)
PNVC	poly(*N*-vinylcaprolactam)
POEGMA	poly(oligo(ethylene glycol) methacrylate)s
Poly(NVIBA)	poly(*N*-vinylisobutyramide)
PPG	poly(propylene glycol)
PPGMA	poly(propylene glycol) methacrylate
PPO	poly(propylene oxide)
PVPh	phosphorylated poly(4-vinylphenol)
TEMPO	2,2,6,6-tetramethylpiperidine-1-oxyl
Tg	glass transition temperature

UCST	upper critical solution temperature
VPGXG	valine-proline-glycine-X-glycine
Zn-TPP	zinc tetraphenylporphyrin

References

1. Galaev, I.Y. and Mattiasson, B. (1999) Smart polymers and what they could do in biotechnology and medicine. *Trends Biotechnol.*, **17**, 335–340.
2. Hoffman, A.S. *et al.* (2000) Really smart bioconjugates of smart polymers and receptor proteins. *J. Biomed. Mater. Res.*, **52**, 577–586.
3. Gil, E.S. and Hudson, S.M. (2004) Stimuli-responsive polymers and their bioconjugates. *Prog. Polym. Sci.*, **29**, 1173–1222.
4. Delcea, M., Möhwald, H., and Skirtach, A.G. (2011) Stimuli-responsive LbL capsules and nanoshells for drug delivery. *Adv. Drug Delivery Rev.*, **63**, 730–747.
5. Cabane, E., Zhang, X., Langowska, K., Palivan, C.G., and Meier, W. (2012) Stimuli-responsive polymers and their applications in nanomedicine. *Biointerphases*, **7**, 1–27.
6. Zhang, L., Xu, T., and Lin, Z. (2006) Controlled release of ionic drug through the positively charged temperature-responsive membranes. *J. Membr. Sci.*, **281**, 491–499.
7. Ohya, S., Sonoda, H., Nakayama, Y., and Matsuda, T. (2005) The potential of poly(N-isopropylacrylamide) (PNIPAM)-grafted hyaluronan and PNIPAM-grafted gelatin in the control of post-surgical tissue adhesions. *Biomaterials*, **26** (6), 655–659.
8. Suwa, K., Morishita, K., Kishida, A., and Akashi, M. (1997) Synthesis and functionalities of poly(*N*-vinylalkylamide). V. Control of a lower critical solution temperature of poly(*N*-vinylalkylamide). *J. Polym. Sci., Part A: Polym. Chem.*, **35**, 3087–3094.
9. Na, K., Lee, K.H., Lee, D.H., and Bae, Y.H. (2006) Biodegradable thermo-sensitive nanoparticles from poly(L-lactic acid)/poly(ethylene glycol) alternating multi block copolymer for potential anti cancer drug carrier. *Eur. J. Pharm. Sci.*, **27**, 115–122.
10. Sosnik, A. and Cohn, D. (2004) Ethoxysilane-capped PEO-PPO-PEO triblocks: a new family of reverse thermo-responsive polymers. *Biomaterials*, **25**, 2851–2858.
11. Heskins, H. and Guillet, J.E. (1968) Solution properties or poly(N-isopropyl acrylamide). *J. Macromol. Sci. Chem. A2*, **6**, 1209.
12. Yoshida, R., Uchida, K., Kaneko, Y., Sakai, K., Kikcuhi, A., and Okano, T. (1995) Comb-type grafted hydrogels with rapid deswelling response to temperature changes. *Nature*, **374**, 240–242.
13. Shimizu, T., Yamato, M., Kikuchi, A., and Okano, T. (2003) Cell sheet engineering for myocardial tissue reconstruction. *Biomaterials*, **24**, 2309–2316.
14. Yamato, M. and Okano, T. (2001) Cell sheet engineering for regenerative medicine. *Macromol. Chem. Symp.*, **14**, 21–29.
15. Takahashi, H., Matsuzaka, N., Nakayama, M., Kikuchi, A., Yamato, M., and Okano, T. (2012) Terminally functionalized thermo-responsive polymer brushes for simultaneously promoting cell adhesion and cell sheet harvest. *Biomacromolecules*, **13**, 253–260.
16. Golden, A.L., Battrell, C.F., Pennell, S., Hoffman, A.S., Lai, J.J., and Stayton, P.S. (2010) Simple fluidic system for purifying and concentrating diagnostic biomarkers using stimuli responsive antibody conjugates and membranes. *Bioconjugate Chem.*, **21**, 1820–1826.
17. Lai, J.J., Nelson, K.E., Nash, M.A., Hoffman, A.S., Yager, P., and Stayton,

P.S. (2009) Dynamic bio processing and micro fluidic transport control with smart magnetic nanoparticles in laminar-flow devices. *Lab Chip*, **9**, 1997–2002.
18. Lai, J.J., Hoffman, A.S., and Stayton, P.S. (2007) Dual magnetic-temperature responsive nanoparticles for micro fluidic separations and assays. *Langmuir*, **23**, 7385–7391.
19. Malmstadt, N., Yager, P., Hoffman, A.S., and Stayton, P.S. (2003) A smart micro fluidic affinity chromatography matrix composed of poly(N-isopropylacrylamide)-coated beads. *Anal. Chem.*, **75**, 2943–2949.
20. Malmstadt, N., Hyre, D., Ding, Z., Hoffman, A.S., and Stayton, P.S. (2003) Affinity thermo precipitation and recovery of biotinylated biomolecules via a mutant streptavidin smart polymer conjugate. *Bioconjugate Chem.*, **14**, 575–580.
21. Malmstadt, N., Hoffman, A.S., and Stayton, P.S. (2004) Smart mobile affinity matrix for micro fluidic immunoassays. *Lab Chip*, **4**, 412–415.
22. Nash, M.A., Yager, P., Hoffman, A.S., and Stayton, P.S. (2010) Mixed stimuli-responsive magnetic and gold nanoparticle system for rapid purification, enrichment, and detection of biomarkers. *Bioconjugate Chem.*, **21**, 2197–2204.
23. Nash, M.A., Lai, J.J., Hoffman, A.S., Yager, P., and Stayton, P.S. (2010) "Smart" diblock copolymers as templates for magnetic-core gold-shell nanoparticle synthesis. *Nano Lett.*, **10**, 85–91.
24. Nash, M.A., Hoffman, J.M., Stevens, D.Y., Hoffman, A.S., Stayton, P.S., and Yager, P. (2010) Laboratory-scale protein striping system for patterning biomolecules onto paper based immuno chromatographic test strips. *Lab Chip*, **10**, 2279–2282.
25. Dong, L.C. and Hoffman, A.S. (1986) Thermally reversible hydrogels: III. Immobilization of enzymes for feedback reaction control. *J. Controlled Release*, **4**, 223–227.
26. Dong, L.C. and Hoffman, A.S. (1991) A novel approach for preparation of pH-and temperature sensitive hydrogels for enteric drug delivery. *J. Controlled Release*, **15**, 141–152.
27. Park, T.G. and Hoffman, A.S. (1988) Effect of temperature cycling on the activity and productivity of immobilized β-galactosidase in a thermally reversible hydrogel bead reactor. *Appl. Biochem. Biotechnol.*, **19**, 1–9.
28. Park, T.G. and Hoffman, A.S. (1992) Synthesis and characterization of pH-and/or temperature sensitive hydrogels. *J. Appl. Polym. Sci.*, **46**, 659–671.
29. Vernon, B., Kim, S.W., and Bae, Y.H. (2000) Thermo reversible copolymer gels for extracellular matrix. *J. Biomed. Mater. Res.*, **51**, 69–79.
30. Kujawa, P. and Winnik, F.M. (2001) Volumetric studies of aqueous polymer solutions using pressure perturbation calorimetry: A new look at the temperature-induced phase transition of poly(*N*-isopropylacrylamide) in water and D_2O. *Macromolecules*, **43**, 4130–4135.
31. Ahn, Y.H. *et al.* (2001) Reversible gelling culture media for in-vitro cell culture in three dimensional matrices. US Patent US6103528.
32. Topp, M.D.C. *et al.* (1997) Thermo sensitive micelle forming block copolymers of poly(ethylene glycol) and poly(N-isopropylacrylamide). *Macromolecules*, **30**, 8518–8520.
33. Aoyagi, T. *et al.* (2000) Novel bifunctional polymer with reactivity and temperature sensitivity. *J. Biomater. Sci., Polym. Ed.*, **11**, 101–110.
34. Inoue, T. *et al.* (1997) Temperature sensitivity of a hydrogel network containing different LCST oligomers grafted to the hydrogel backbone. *Polym. Gels Networks*, **5**, 561–575.
35. Kaneko, Y. *et al.* (1998) Rapid deswelling response of poly(*N*-isopropylacrylamide) hydrogels by the formation of water release channels using poly(ethylene oxide) graft chains. *Macromolecules*, **31**, 6099–6105.
36. Bulmus, V. *et al.* (2000) Site-specific polymer–streptavidin bioconjugate for pH controlled binding and triggered release of biotin. *Bioconjugate Chem.*, **11**, 78–83.

37. Lee, H. and Park, T.G. (1998) Conjugation of trypsin by temperature-sensitive polymers containing a carbohydrate moiety: thermal modulation of enzyme activity. *Biotechnol. Progr.*, **14**, 508–516.
38. Kim, H.K. and Park, T.G. (1999) Synthesis and characterization of thermally reversible bioconjugates composed of α-chymotrypsin and poly(*N*-isopropylacrylamide-co-acrylamido-2-deoxy-D-glucose). *Enzyme Microb. Technol.*, **25**, 31–37.
39. Shimizu, T. *et al.* (2001) Two-dimensional manipulation of cardiac myocyte sheets utilizing temperature-responsive culture dishes augments the pulsatile amplitude. *Tissue Eng.*, **7**, 141–151.
40. Vernon, B. *et al.* (1999) Insulin release from islets of Langerhans entrapped in a poly(*N*-isopropylacrylamide-co-acrylic acid) polymer gel. *J. Biomater. Sci., Polym. Ed.*, **10**, 183–198.
41. Oya, T. *et al.* (1999) Reversible molecular adsorption based on multipoint interaction by shrinkable gels. *Science*, **286**, 1543–1545.
42. Okuyama, Y., Yoshida, R., Sakai, K., Okano, T., and Sakurai, Y. (1993) Swelling controlled zero-order and sigmoidal drug release from thermoresponsive poly(*N*-isopropylacrylamide-co-butyl methacrylate) hydrogel. *J. Biomater. Sci., Polym. Ed.*, **4**, 545–556.
43. Coughlan, D.C. and Corrigan, O.I. (2008) Release kinetics of benzoic acid and its sodium salt from a series of poly(*N*-isopropylacrylamide) matrices with various percentage crosslinking. *J. Pharm. Sci.*, **97**, 318–330.
44. Coughlan, D.C. and Corrigan, O.I. (2006) Drug-polymer interactions and their effect on thermoresponsive poly (*N*-isopropylacrylamide) drug delivery systems. *Int. J. Pharm.*, **313**, 163–174.
45. Jones, D.S., Lorimer, C.J., Andrews, G.P., McCoy, C.P., and Gorman, S.P. (2007) An examination of the thermo rheological and drug release properties of zinc tetraphenylporphyrin-containing thermoresponsive hydrogels, designed as light activated antimicrobial implants. *Chem. Eng. Sci.*, **62**, 990–999.
46. Xiao, H., Nayak, B.R., and Lowe, T.L. (2004) Synthesis and characterization of novel thermoresponsive-co-biodegradable hydrogels composed of *N*-isopropylacrylamide, poly(L-lactic acid), and dextran. *J. Polym. Sci., Part A: Polym. Chem.*, **42**, 5054–5066.
47. Wu, D.Q., Qiu, F., Wang, T., Jiang, X.J., Zhang, X.Z., and Zhuo, R.X. (2009) Toward the development of partially biodegradable and injectable thermoresponsive hydrogels for potential biomedical applications. *ACS Appl. Mater. Interfaces*, **1**, 319–327.
48. Ma, Z.W., Nelson, D.M., Hong, Y., and Wagner, W.R. (2010) Thermally responsive injectable hydrogel incorporating methacrylate-polylactide for hydrolytic lability. *Biomacromolecules*, **11**, 1873–1881.
49. Galperin, A., Long, T.J., and Ratner, B.D. (2010) Degradable, thermo-sensitive poly(N-isopropyl acrylamide)-based scaffolds with controlled porosity for tissue engineering applications. *Biomacromolecules*, **11**, 2583–2592.
50. Wei, H., Zhang, X.Z., Chen, W.Q., Cheng, S.X., and Zhuo, R.X. (2007) Self-assembled thermosensitive micelles based on poly(L-lactide-star block-N-isopropylacrylamide) for drug delivery. *J. Biomed. Mater. Res. Part A*, **83A**, 980–989.
51. Jeong, B., Kim, S.W., and Bae, Y.H. (2002) Thermosensitive sol–gel reversible hydrogels. *Adv. Drug Delivery Rev.*, **54**, 37–51.
52. Lee, D.S., Shim, M.S., Kim, S.W., Lee, H., Park, I., and Chang, T. (2001) Novel thermoreversible gelation of biodegradable PLGA-block-PEO-block-PLGA triblock copolymers in aqueous solution. *Macromol. Rapid Commun.*, **22**, 587–592.
53. Shim, W.S., Kim, J.H., Park, H., Kim, K., Kwon, I.C., and Lee, D.S. (2006) Biodegradability and biocompatibility of a pH- and thermo-sensitive hydrogel formed from a sulphonamide modified poly(ε-caprolactone-co-lactide)–poly(ethylene glycol)–poly(ε-caprolactone-co-lactide) block copolymer. *Biomaterials*, **27**, 5178–5185.

54. Kan, P., Lin, X.Z., Hsieh, M.F., and Chang, K.Y. (2005) Thermogelling emulsions for vascular embolization and sustained release of drugs. *J. Biomed. Mater. Res. Part B*, **75B**, 185–192.
55. Wang, N., Dong, A., Radosz, M., and Shen, Y.Q. (2008) Thermoresponsive degradable poly(ethylene glycol) analogues. *J. Biomed. Mater. Res. Part A*, **84A**, 148–157.
56. Garty, S., Kimelman-Bleich, N., Hayouka, Z., Cohn, D., Friedler, A., Pelled, G., and Gazit, D. (2010) Peptide-modified "smart" hydrogels and genetically engineered stem cells for skeletal tissue engineering. *Biomacromolecules*, **11**, 1516–1526.
57. Borden, B.A., Yockman, J., and Kim, S.W. (2010) Thermoresponsive hydrogel as a delivery scaffold for transfected rat mesenchymal stem cells. *Mol. Pharm.*, 7, 963–968.
58. Cohn, D., Sagiv, H., Benyamin, A., and Lando, G. (2009) Engineering thermoresponsive polymeric nanoshells. *Biomaterials*, **30**, 3289–3296.
59. Chow, D., Nunalee, M.L., Lim, D.W., Simnick, A.J., and Chilkoti, A. (2008) Peptide-based biopolymers in biomedicine and biotechnology. *Mater. Sci. Eng., R*, **62**, 125–155.
60. MacEwan, S.R. and Chilkoti, A. (2010) Elastin-like polypeptides: biomedical applications of tunable biopolymers. *Biopolymers*, **94**, 60–77.
61. Meyer, D.E. and Chilkoti, A. (1999) Purification of recombinant proteins by fusion with thermally-responsive polypeptides. *Nat. Biotechnol.*, **17**, 1112–1115.
62. Meyer, D.E., Kong, G.A., Dewhirst, M.W., Zalutsky, M.R., and Chilkoti, A. (2001) Targeting a genetically engineered elastin-like polypeptide to solid tumors by local hyperthermia. *Cancer Res.*, **61**, 1548–1554.
63. Bessa, P.C., Machado, R., Nurnberger, S., Dopler, D., Banerjee, A., Cunha, A.M., Rodriguez-Cabello, J.C., Redl, H., van Griensven, M., Reis, R.L. *et al.* (2010) Thermoresponsive self-assembled elastin-based nanoparticles for delivery of bmps. *J. Controlled Release*, **142**, 312–318.
64. Rincon, A.C., Molina-Martinez, I.T., de Las Heras, B., Alonso, M., Bailez, C., Rodriguez-Cabello, J.C., and Herrero-Vanrell, R. (2006) Biocompatibility of elastin-like polymer poly(VPAVG) microparticles: in vitro and in vivo studies. *J. Biomed. Mater. Res. Part A*, **78A**, 343–351.
65. Dreher, M.R., Raucher, D., Balu, N., Michael Colvin, O., Ludeman, S.M., and Chilkoti, A. (2003) Evaluation of an elastin-like polypeptide-doxorubicin conjugate for cancer therapy. *J. Controlled Release*, **91**, 31–43.
66. Kunugi, S., Tada, T., and Yamazak, Y. (2000) Thermodynamic studies on coil – globule transitions of poly(N vinylisobutyramide- co -vinylamine) in aqueous solutions. *Langmuir*, **16**, 2042–2044.
67. Zhang, N., Salzinger, S., and Rieger, B. (2012) Poly(vinylphosphonate)s with widely tunable LCST: a promising alternative to conventional thermoresponsive polymers. *Macromolecules*, **45**, 9751–9758.
68. Vihola, H., Laukkanen, A., Tenhu, H., and Hirvonen, J. (2008) Drug release characteristics of physically cross-linked thermosensitive poly(N-vinylcaprolactam) hydrogel particles. *J. Pharm. Sci.*, **97**, 4783–4793.
69. Vihola, H., Marttila, A.K., Pakkanen, J.S., Andersson, M., Laukkanen, A., Kaukonen, A.M., Tenhu, H., and Hirvonen, J. (2007) Cell-polymer interactions of fluorescent polystyrene latex particles coated with thermosensitive poly(N-isopropylacrylamide) and poly(N-vinylcaprolactam) or grafted with poly(ethylene oxide)-macromonomer. *Int. J. Pharm.*, **343**, 238–246.
70. Vihola, H., Laukkanen, A., Valtola, L., Tenhu, H., and Hirvonen, J. (2005) Cytotoxicity of thermosensitive polymers poly(N-isopropylacrylamide), poly(N-vinylcaprolactam) and amphiphilically modified poly(N-vinylcaprolactam). *Biomaterials*, **26**, 3055–3064.

71. Maeda, Y., Nakamura, T., and Ikeda, I. (2002) Hydration and phase behavior of poly(*N*-vinylcaprolactam) and poly(*N*-vinylpyrrolidone) in water. *Macromolecules*, **35**, 217–222.
72. Laukkanen, A., Valtola, L., Winnik, F.M., and Tenhu, H. (2004) Formation of colloidally stable phase separated poly (*N*-vinylcaprolactam) in water: a study by dynamic light scattering, microcalorimetry, and pressure perturbation calorimetry. *Macromolecules*, **37**, 2268–2274.
73. Makhaeva, E.E., Tenhu, H., and Khokhlov, A.R. (1998) Conformational changes of poly(vinylcaprolactam) macromolecules and their complexes with ionic surfactants in aqueous solution. *Macromolecules*, **31**, 6112–6118.
74. Alzari, V., Monticelli, O., Nuvoli, D., Kenny, J.M., and Mariani, A. (2009) Stimuli responsive hydrogels prepared by frontal polymerization. *Biomacromolecules*, **10**, 2672–2677.
75. Yoon, J.A., Gayathri, C., Gil, R.R., Kowalewski, T., and Matyjaszewski, K. (2010) Comparison of the thermoresponsive deswelling kinetics of poly(2-(2-methoxyethoxy)ethyl methacrylate) hydrogels prepared by atrp and frp. *Macromolecules*, **43**, 4791–4797.
76. Kiremitçi, A.S., Ciftçi, A., Ozalp, M., and Gümüeşderelioglu, M. (2007) Novel chlorhexidine releasing system developed from thermosensitive vinyl ether-based hydrogels. *J. Biomed. Mater. Res. Part B*, **83B**, 609–614.
77. Yang, H. and Kao, W.Y.J. (2006) Thermoresponsive gelatin/monomethoxy poly(ethylene glycol)-poly(D, 1lactide) hydrogels: formulation, characterization, and antibacterial drug delivery. *Pharm. Res.*, **23**, 205–214.
78. Martellini, F., Mei, L.H.I., Balino, J.L., and Carenza, M. (2003) Water and drug transport in radiation-crosslinked poly(2-methoxyethylacrylate-co-dimethyi acrylamide) and poly(2-methoxyethylacrylate-co-acrylamide) hydrogels. *Radiat. Phys. Chem.*, **66**, 155–159.
79. Yu, B., Lowe, A.B., and Ishihara, K. (2009) RAFT synthesis and stimulus-induced self-assembly in water of copolymers based on the biocompatible monomer 2-(methacryloyloxy)ethyl phosphorylcholine. *Biomacromolecules*, **10**, 950–958.
80. Huang, X., Du, F., Ju, R., and Li, Z. (2007) Novel acid-labile, thermoresponsive poly(methacrylamide)s with pendent ortho ester moieties. *Macromol. Rapid Commun.*, **28**, 597–603.
81. Huang, X.-N., Du, F.-S., Zhang, B., Zhao, J.-Y., and Li, Z.-C. (2008) Acid-labile, thermoresponsive (meth)acrylamide polymers with pendant cyclic acetal moieties. *J. Polym. Sci., Part A: Polym. Chem.*, **46**, 4332–4343.
82. Hruby, M., Kucka, J., Lebeda, O., Mackova, H., Babic, M., Konak, C., Studenovsky, M., Sikora, A., Kozempel, J., and Ulbrich, K. (2007) New bioerodable thermoresponsive polymers for possible radiotherapeutic applications. *J. Controlled Release*, **119**, 25–33.
83. Lutz, J.-F. (2008) Polymerization of oligo(ethylene glycol) (meth)acrylates: toward new generations of smart biocompatible materials. *J. Polym. Sci., Part A: Polym. Chem.*, **46**, 3459–3470.
84. Mertoglu, M., Garnier, S., Laschewsky, A., Skrabania, K., and Storsberg, J. (2005) Stimuli responsive amphiphilic block copolymers for aqueous media synthesised via reversible addition fragmentation chain transfer polymerisation (RAFT). *Polymer*, **46**, 7726–7740.
85. Lutz, J.-F. (2011) Thermo-switchable materials prepared using the OEGMA-platform. *Adv. Mater.*, **23**, 2237–2243.
86. Wang, W., Liang, H., Cheikh Al Ghanami, R., Hamilton, L., Fraylich, M., Shakesheff, K.M., Saunders, B., and Alexander, C. (2009) Biodegradable thermoresponsive microparticle dispersions for injectable cell delivery prepared using a single-step process. *Adv. Mater.*, **21**, 1809–1813.
87. Watanabe, E., Tomoshige, N., and Uyama, H. (2007) New biodegradable and thermoresponsive polymers based

on amphiphilic poly(asparagine) derivatives. *Macromol. Symp.*, **249–250**, 509–514.
88. Bosmann, H.B. and Kessel, D. (1970) Inhibition of glycoprotein synthesis in L5178Y mouse leukaemic cells by L-asparaginase in vitro. *Nature*, **226**, 850–851.
89. El-Naggar, N.E.-A., El-Ewasy, S.M., and El-Shweihy, N.M. (2014) Microbial L-asparaginase as a potential therapeutic agent for the treatment of acute lymphoblastic leukemia: the pros and cons. *Int. J. Pharmacol.*, **10** (4), 182–199.
90. Hosamani, R. (2012) Studies on the production of *L*-asparaginase an antitumor agent from filamentous fungus-Fusarium equiseti. PhD thesis. Karnatak University, Dharwad, India.
91. Kim, S., Wu, J., Carlson, A., Jin, S.H., Kovalsky, A., Glass, P., Liu, Z., Ahmed, N., Elgan, S.L., Chen, W., Ferreira, P.M., Sitti, M., Huang, Y., and Rogers, J.A. (2010) Microstructured elastomeric surfaces with reversible adhesion and examples of their use in deterministic assembly by transfer printing. *Proc. Natl. Acad. Sci. U.S.A.*, **107**, 17095–17100.
92. Lee, K.K., Cussler, E.L., Marchetti, M., and McHugh, M.A. (1990) Pressure-dependent phase transitions in hydrogels. *Chem. Eng. Sci.*, **45**, 766–767.
93. Zhong, X., Wang, Y.-X., and Wang, S.-C. (1996) Pressure dependence of the volume phase transition of temperature-sensitive gels. *Chem. Eng. Sci.*, **51**, 3235–3239.
94. Shiga, T. (1997) Deformation and viscoelastic behavior of polymer gels in electric fields. *Adv. Polym. Sci.*, **134**, 131–163.
95. Zrinyi, M. (2000) Intelligent polymer gels controlled by magnetic fields. *Colloid. Polym. Sci.*, **278**, 98–103.
96. Deng, Y.H., Yang, W.L., Wang, C.C., and Fu, S.K. (2003) A novel approach for preparation of thermoresponsive polymer magnetic microspheres with core shell structure. *Adv. Mater.*, **15** (20), 1729–1732.
97. Meenach, S.A., Anderson, K.W., and Hilt, J.Z. (2010) Synthesis and characterization of thermoresponsive poly(ethylene glycol)-based hydrogels and their magnetic nanocomposites. *J. Polym. Sci., Part A: Polym. Chem.*, **48**, 3229–3235.
98. Papaphilippou, P.C., Pourgouris, A., Marinica, O., Taculescu, A., Athanasopoulos, G.I., Vekas, L., and Krasia-Christoforou, T. (2011) Fabrication and characterization of superparamagnetic and thermoresponsive hydrogels based on oleic-acid-coated Fe_3O_4 nanoparticles, hexa(ethylene glycol) methyl ether methacrylate and 2-(acetoacetoxy)ethyl methacrylate. *J. Magn. Magn. Mater.*, **323**, 557–563.
99. Schumers, J.-M., Fustin, C.-A., and Gohy, J.-F. (2010) Light-responsive block copolymers. *Macromol. Rapid Commun.*, **31**, 1588–1607.
100. You, J., Shao, R., Wei, X., Gupta, S., and Li, C. (2010) Near-infrared light triggers release of paclitaxel from biodegradable microspheres: photothermal effect and enhanced antitumor activity. *Small*, **6**, 1022–1031.
101. Ishii, N., Mamiya, J.-I., Ikeda, T., and Winnik, F.M. (2011) Solvent induced amplification of the photoresponsive properties of α,ω-di-[4-cyanophenyl-4′-(6-hexyloxy)-azobenzene]-poly(*N*-isopropylacrylamide) in aqueous media. *Chem. Commun.*, **47**, 1267–1269.
102. Suzuki, A. and Tanaka, T. (1990) Phase transition in polymer gels induced by visible light. *Nature*, **346**, 345–347.
103. Suzuki, A., Ishii, T., and Maruyama, Y. (1996) Optical switching in polymer gels. *J. Appl. Phys.*, **80**, 131–136.
104. Minko, S., Muller, M., Motornov, M., Nitschke, M., Grundke, K., and Stamm, M. (2003) Two-level structured self-adaptive surfaces with reversibly tunable properties. *J. Am. Chem. Soc.*, **125** (13), 3896–3900.
105. Sheparovych, R., Motornov, M., and Minko, S. (2008) Adapting low-adhesive thin films from mixed polymer brushes. *Langmuir*, **24**, 13828–13832.
106. Zhang, M. and Müller, A. (2003) Amphiphilic cylindrical brushes with

poly(acrylic acid) core and poly(n-butyl acrylate) shell and narrow length distribution. *Polymer*, **44**, 1449–1458.
107. Fischer, H. (2001) The persistent radical effect: a principle for selective radical reactions and living radical polymerizations. *Chem. Rev.*, **101**, 3581–3610.
108. Retsos, H., Kiriy, A., Senkovskyy, V., Stamm, M., Feldstein, M.M., and Creton, C. (2006) Controlling tack with bicomponent polymer brushes. *Adv. Mater.*, **18**, 2624–2628.
109. Retsos, H., Gorodyska, G., Kiriy, A., Stamm, M., and Creton, C. (2005) Adhesion between chemically heterogeneous switchable polymeric brushes and an elastomeric adhesive. *Langmuir*, **21**, 7722–7725.
110. Nadermann, N., Ning, J., Jagota, A., and Hui, C.Y. (2010) Active switching of adhesion in a film-terminated fibrillar structure. *Langmuir*, **26**, 15464–15471.
111. Paretkar, D., Kamperman, M., Schneider, A.S., Martina, D., Creton, C., and Arzt, E. (2011) Bioinspired pressure actuated adhesive system. *Mater. Sci. Eng., C*, **31**, 1152–1159.
112. Jeong, H.E., Kwak, M.K., and Suh, K.Y. (2010) Stretchable, adhesion-tunable dry adhesive by surface wrinkling. *Langmuir*, **26** (4), 2223–2226.
113. Zhao, L., Zhu, L., Liu, F., Liu, C., Shan-Dan , Wang, Q. *et al.* (2011) pH triggered injectable amphiphilic hydrogel containing doxorubicin and paclitaxel. *Int. J. Pharm.*, **410**, 83–91.
114. Garbern, J.C., Minami, E., Stayton, P.S., and Murry, C. (2011) Delivery of basic fibroblast growth factor with a pH-responsive, injectable hydrogel to improve angiogenesis in infarcted myocardium. *Biomaterials*, **32**, 2407–2416.
115. Kulkarni, R.V., Boppana, R., Krishna, M.G., Mutalik, S., and Kalyane, N.V. (2012) pH-responsive inter penetrating network hydrogel beads of poly(acrylamide)-*g*-carrageenan and sodium alginate for intestinal targeted drug delivery: synthesis, in vitro and in vivo evaluation. *J. Colloid Interface Sci.*, **367**, 509–517.
116. Wang, K., Xu, X., Wang, Y., Yan, X., Guo, G., Huang, M. *et al.* (2010) Synthesis and characterization of poly(methoxyl ethyleneglycol-caprolactone-co-methacrylic acid-co-poly(ethyleneglycol) methylether methacrylate) pH sensitive hydrogel for delivery of dexamethasone. *Int. J. Pharm.*, **389**, 130–138.
117. El-Sherbiny, I.M. (2010) Enhanced pH-responsive carrier system based on alginate and chemically modified carboxymethyl chitosan for oral delivery of protein drugs: preparation and in-vitro assessment. *Carbohydr. Polym.*, **80**, 1125–1136.
118. Jeong, B. and Gutowska, A. (2002) Lessons from nature: stimuli-responsive polymers and their biomedical applications. *Trends Biotechnol.*, **20** (7), 305–311.
119. Duncan, R., Ferruti, P., Sgouras, D., Tuboku-Metzger, A. *et al.* (1994) A polymer-triton X-100 conjugate capable of pH-dependent red blood cell lysis: a model system illustrating the possibility of drug delivery within acidic intracellular compartments. *J. Drug Targeting*, **2**, 341–347.
120. Barba, A.A., Dalmoro, A., De Santis, F., and Lamberti, G. (2009) Synthesis and characterization of p(MMAAA) copolymers for targeted oral drug delivery. *Polym. Bull.*, **62** (5), 679–688.
121. Lubrizol [Admix Corp] http://www.admix.com/carbopol (accessed 21 April 2016).
122. Licea-Claverie, A., Rogel-Hernandez, E., Salgado-Rodriguez, R., Lopez-Sanchez, J.A. *et al.* (2004) The use of hydrophobic spacers in the development of new temperature- and pH-sensitive polymers. *Macromol. Symp.*, **207**, 193–215.
123. Guan, X., Liu, Z., and Su, Z. (2007) Synthesis and photophysical behaviors of temperature/pH-sensitive polymeric materials. *Eur. Polym. J.*, **43** (7), 3094–3105.
124. Lackey, C.A., Murthy, N., Press, O.W., Tirrell, D.A., Hoffman, A.S., and Stayton, P.S. (1999) Hemolytic activity of pH-responsive polymer–streptavidin

bioconjugates. *Bioconjugate Chem.*, **10**, 401–405.
125. Murthy, N., Stayton, P.S., Robichaud, J.R., Tirrell, D.A., and Hoffman, A.S. (1999) The design and synthesis of polymers for eukaryotic membrane disruption. *J. Controlled Release*, **61**, 137–143.
126. Murthy, N., Campbell, J., Fausto, N., Hoffman, A.S., and Stayton, P.S. (2003) Bioinspired polymeric carriers that enhance intracellular delivery of biomolecular therapeutics. *Bioconjugate Chem.*, **14**, 412–419.
127. Murthy, N., Campbell, J., Fausto, N., Hoffman, A.S., and Stayton, P.S. (2003) Design and synthesis of pH-responsive polymeric carriers that target uptake and enhance the intracellular delivery of oligonucleotides to hepatocytes. *J. Controlled Release*, **89**, 365–374.
128. Stayton, P.S. and Hoffman, A.S. (2008) Smart pH-responsive carriers for intracellular delivery of biomolecular drugs, in *Multifunctional Pharmaceutical Nanocarriers* (ed. V. Torchilin), Springer-Verlag.
129. Tirrell, D. (1987) Macromolecular switches for bilayer membranes. *J. Controlled Release*, **6**, 15–21.
130. Yin, X., Stayton, P.S., and Hoffman, A.S. (2006) Temperature- and pH-responsiveness of poly(Nisopropylacrylamide-co-propylacrylic acid) copolymers prepared by RAFT polymerization. *Biomacromolecules*, **7**, 1381–1385.
131. Kang, H.C. and Bae, Y.H. (2007) pH-tunable endosomolytic oligomers for enhanced nucleic acid delivery. *Adv. Funct. Mater.*, **17**, 1263–1272.
132. Na, K., Lee, D.H., Hwang, D.J., Lee, K.H., and Bae, Y.H. (2006) pH-sensitivity and pH-dependent structural change in polymeric nanoparticles of poly(vinyl sulfadimethoxine)- deoxycholic acid conjugate. *Eur. Polym. J.*, **42**, 2581–2588.
133. Benns, J.M. *et al.* (2000) pH-sensitive cationic polymer gene delivery vehicle: *N*-Ac-poly(Lhistidine)- graft-poly(L-lysine) comb shaped polymer. *Bioconjugate Chem.*, **11**, 637–645.
134. Neumann, M.G., Pastre, I.A., Chinelatto, A.M., and El Seoud, O.A. (1996) Effects of the structure of anionic polyelectrolytes on surface potentials of their aggregates in water. *Colloid. Polym. Sci.*, **274** (5), 475–481.
135. Donovan, M.S., Sumerlin, B.S., Lowe, A.B., and McCormick, C.L. (2002) Controlled/living polymerization of sulfobetaine monomers directly in aqueous media via raft. *Macromolecules*, **35**, 8663–8666.
136. Corpart, J.M. and Candau, F. (1993) Aqueous solution properties of ampholytic copolymers prepared in microemulsions. *Macromolecules*, **26**, 1333–1343.
137. Kathmann, E.E.L., White, L.A., and McCormick, C.L. (1997) Electrolyte and pH responsive zwitterionic copolymer of 4-[(2acrylamido-2-methylpropyl)-dimethylammonio] butanoate with 3-[(2acrylamido-2-methylpropyl dimethylammonio] propane sulfonate. *Macromolecules*, **30**, 5297–5304.
138. Salamone, J.C., Rodriguez, E.L., Lin, K.C., Quach, L., Watterson, A.C., and Ahmed, I. (1985) Aqueous salt absorption by ampholytic polysaccharides. *Polymer*, **26**, 1234–1238.
139. Morrison, M.E., Dorfman, R.C., Clendening, W.D., Kiserow, D.J., Rossky, P.J., and Webber, S.E. (1994) Quenching kinetics of anthracene covalently bound to a polyelectrolyte 1. Effect of ionic strength. *J. Phys. Chem.*, **98**, 5534–5540.
140. Szczubiałka, K., Jankowska, M., and Nowakowska, M. (2003) Smart polymeric nanospheres as new materials for possible biomedical applications. *J. Mater. Sci. - Mater. Med.*, **14**, 699–703.
141. Kumar, A., Galaev, I.Y., and Mattiasson, B. (1998) Affinity precipitation of a-amylase inhibitor from wheat meal by metal chelate affinity binding using cu(II)-loaded copolymers of L-vinylimidazole with *N*-isopropylacrylamide. *Biotechnol. Bioeng.*, **59**, 695–704.
142. Leong, K.W., Brott, B.C., and Langer, R. (1985) Bioerodible polyanhydrides as drug carrier matrices I: characterization, degradation, and release

characteristics. *J. Biomed. Mater. Res.*, **19**, 941–955.

143. Mathiowitz, E., Jacob, J.S., Jong, Y.S., Carino, G.P., Chickering, D.E., Chaturvedi, P., Santos, C.A., Vijayaraghavan, K., Montgomery, S., Bassett, M., and Morrell, C. (1997) Biologically erodable microspheres as potential oral drug delivery systems. *Nature*, **386**, 410–414.
144. Cohen, S., Yoshioka, T., Lucarelli, M., Hwang, L.H., and Langer, R. (1991) Controlled delivery systems for proteins based on poly(lactic/glycolic acid)microspheres. *Pharm. Res.*, **8**, 713–720.
145. Shenoy, D., Little, S., Langer, R., and Amiji, M. (2005) Polyethylene oxide modified poly beta-amino ester)nanoparticles as a pH sensitive system for tumor targeted delivery of hydrophobic drugs: part 2. In vivo distribution and tumor localization studies. *Pharm. Res.*, **22**, 2107–2114.
146. Cerritelli, S., Velluto, D., and Hubbell, J.A. (2007) PEG-SS-PPS: reduction sensitive disulfide block copolymer vesicles for intracellular drug delivery. *Biomacromolecules*, **8**, 1966–1972.
147. Oh, J.K., Siegwart, D.J., Lee, H.-I., Sherwood, G., Peteanu, L., Hollinger, J.O., Kataoka, K., and Matyjaszewski, K. (2007) Biodegradable nanogels prepared by atom transfer radical polymerization as potential drug carrier: synthesis biodegradation, in vitro release and bioconjugation. *J. Am. Chem. Soc.*, **129**, 5939–5945.
148. Matsumoto, S., Christie, R.J., Nishiyama, N., Miyata, K., Ishii, A., Oba, M., Koyama, H., Yamasaki, Y., and Kataoka, K. (2008) Environment-responsive block copolymer micelles with a disulfide cross-linked core for enhanced siRNA delivery. *Biomacromolecules*, **10**, 119–127.
149. Yoshida, R., Yamaguchi, T., and Kokufuta, E. (1999) New intelligent polymer gel: a self-oscillating gel with peacemaking and actuating functions. *J. Artif. Organs*, **2**, 135–140.
150. Andresen, T.L., Jensen, S.S., and Jorgensen, K. (2005) Advanced strategies in liposomal cancer therapy: problems and prospects of active and tumor specific drug release. *Prog. Lipid Res.*, **44**, 68–97.
151. Minelli, C., Lowe, S.B., and Stevens, M.M. (2010) Engineering nanocomposites materials for cancer therapy. *Small*, **6**, 2336–2357.
152. Amir, R.J., Zhong, S., Pochan, D.J., and Hawker, C.J. (2009) Enzymatically triggered self-assembly of block copolymers. *J. Am. Chem. Soc.*, **131**, 13949–13950.
153. Woodcock, J.W., Jiang, X.G., Wright, R.A.E., and Zhao, B. (2011) Enzyme-induced formation of thermoreversible micellar gels from aqueous solutions of multiresponsive hydrophilic ABA triblock copolymers. *Macromolecules*, **44**, 5764–5775.
154. Traitel, T., Cohen, Y., and Kost, J. (2000) Characterization of glucose sensitive insulin release systems in simulated in vivo conditions. *Biomaterials*, **21**, 1679–1687.
155. Albin, G., Horbett, T.A., and Ratner, B.D. (1985) Glucose sensitive membranes for controlled delivery of insulin: insulin transport studies. *J. Controlled Release*, **2**, 153–164.
156. Albin, G.W., Horbett, T.A., Miller, S.R., and Ricker, N.L. (1987) Theoretical and experimental studies of glucose sensitive membranes. *J. Controlled Release*, **6**, 267–291.
157. Cartier, S., Horbett, T.A., and Ratner, B.D. (1995) Glucose-sensitive coated porous filters for control of hydraulic permeability and insulin delivery from a pressurized reservoir. *J. Membr. Sci.*, **106**, 17–24.
158. You, L., Lu, F., Li, Z., Zhang, W., and Li, F. (2003) Glucose-sensitive aggregates formed by poly(ethylene oxide)-*block*-poly(2-glucosyl-oxyethyl acrylate) with concanavalin A in dilute aqueous medium. *Macromolecules*, **36**, 1–4.
159. Schattling, P., Jochuma, F.D., and Theato, P. (2014) Multi-stimuli responsive polymers – the all-in-one talents. *Polym. Chem.*, **5**, 25–36.
160. Cheng, R., Meng, F., Deng, C., Klok, H.-A., and Zhong, Z. (2013) Dual and multi-stimuli responsive polymeric

nanoparticles for programmed site-specific drug delivery. *Biomaterials*, **34**, 3647–3657.

161. (a) Mu, B. and Liu, P. (2012) Temperature and pH dual responsive crosslinked polymeric nanocapsules via surface-initiated atom transfer radical polymerization. *React. Funct. Polym.*, **72**, 983–989; (b) Schilli, C.M., Zhang, M., Rizzardo, E., Thang, S.H., Chong, Y.K., Edwards, K., Karlsson, G., and Müller, A.H.E. (2004) A new double-responsive block copolymer synthesized via RAFT polymerization: poly(*N*-isopropylacrylamide)- block -poly(acrylic acid). *Macromolecules*, **37**, 7861–7866; (c) Kulkarni, S., Schilli, C., Grin, B., Müller, A.H.E., Hoffman, A.S., and Stayton, P.S. (2006) Controlling the aggregation of conjugates of streptavidin with smart block copolymers prepared via the RAFT copolymerization technique. *Biomacromolecules*, **7**, 2736–2741.
162. Soppimath, K.S., Tan, D.C.W., and Yang, Y.Y. (2005) pH-triggered thermally responsive polymer core-shell nanoparticles for drug delivery. *Adv. Mater.*, **17** (3), 318–323.
163. Soppimath, K.S., Liu, L.H., Seow, W.Y., Liu, S.Q., Powell, R., Chan, P. *et al.* (2007) Multifunctional core/shell nanoparticles self-assembled from pH-induced thermosensitive polymers for targeted intracellular anticancer drug delivery. *Adv. Mater.*, **17** (3), 355–362.
164. Zhang, L.Y., Guo, R., Yang, M., Jiang, X.Q., and Liu, B.R. (2007) Thermo and pH dual-responsive nanoparticles for anti-cancer drug delivery. *Adv. Mater.*, **19** (19), 2988e92.
165. Chen, Y.C., Liao, L.C., Lu, P.L., Lo, C.L., Tsai, H.C., Huang, C.Y. *et al.* (2012) The accumulation of dual pH and temperature responsive micelles in tumors. *Biomaterials*, **33** (18), 4576–4588.
166. Lo, C.L., Lin, K.M., and Hsiue, G.H. (2005) Preparation and characterization of intelligent core-shell nanoparticles based on poly(D, L-lactide)-g-poly(*N*-isopropyl-acrylamide- co-methacrylic acid). *J. Controlled Release*, **104** (3), 477–488.
167. Cui, W., Lu, X.M., Cui, K., Niu, L., Wei, Y., and Lu, Q.H. (2012) Dual-responsive controlled drug delivery based on ionically assembled nanoparticles. *Langmuir*, **28** (25), 9413–9420.
168. Chiang, W.H., Ho, V.T., Huang, W.C., Huang, Y.F., Chern, C.S., and Chiu, H.C. (2012) Dual stimuliresponsive polymeric hollow nanogels designed as carriers for intracellular triggered drug release. *Langmuir*, **28** (42), 15056–15064.
169. Rapoport, N. (2007) Physical stimuli-responsive polymeric micelles for anti-cancer drug delivery. *Prog. Polym. Sci.*, **32** (8-9), 962–990.
170. Meng, F.H., Hennink, W.E., and Zhong, Z.Y. (2009) Reduction-sensitive polymers and bioconjugates for biomedical applications. *Biomaterials*, **30** (12), 2180–2198.
171. Zhang, J.C., Wu, L.L., Meng, F.H., Wang, Z.J., Deng, C., Liu, H.Y. *et al.* (2011) pH and reduction dual-bioresponsive polymersomes for efficient intracellular protein delivery. *Langmuir*, **28** (4), 2056–2065.
172. Pan, Y.J., Chen, Y.Y., Wang, D.R., Wei, C., Guo, J., Lu, D.R. *et al.* (2012) Redox/pH dual stimuliresponsive biodegradable nanohydrogels with varying responses to dithiothreitol and glutathione for controlled drug release. *Biomaterials*, **33** (27), 6570–6579.
173. Shu, S.J., Zhang, X.G., Wu, Z.M., Wang, Z., and Li, C.X. (2010) Gradient cross-linked biodegradable polyelectrolyte nanocapsules for intracellular protein drug delivery. *Biomaterials*, **31** (23), 6039–6049.
174. Guo, M., Yan, Y., Zhang, H.K., Yan, H.S., Cao, Y.J., Liu, K.L., Wan, S., Huang, J., and Yue, W. (2008) Magnetic and pH responsive nanocarriers with multilayer core-shell architecture for anticancer drug delivery. *J. Mater. Chem.*, **18** (42), 5104–5112.
175. Phillips, D.J. and Gibson, M.I. (2012) Degradable thermoresponsive polymers which display redox-responsive LCST behaviour. *Chem. Commun.*, **48**, 1054–1105.
176. Morimoto, N., Qiu, X.P., Winnik, F.M., and Akiyoshi, K. (2008) Dual

stimuli-responsive nanogels by self-assembly of polysaccharides lightly grafted with thiol-terminated poly(*N*-isopropylacrylamide) chains. *Macromolecules*, **41** (16), 5985–5987.

177. Lv, W.P., Liu, S.Q., Feng, W.Q., Qi, J.J., Zhang, G.L., Zhang, F.B. *et al.* (2011) Temperature- and redox-directed multiple self assembly of poly(*N*-isopropylacrylamide) grafted dextran nanogels. *Macromol. Rapid Commun.*, **32** (14), 1101–1107.
178. Tan, J.J., Kang, H.L., Liu, R.G., Wang, D.Q., Jin, X., Li, Q.M. *et al.* (2011) Dual-stimuli sensitive nanogels fabricated by self-association of thiolated hydroxypropyl cellulose. *Polym. Chem.*, **2** (3), 672–678.
179. Shubayev, V.I., Pisanic Ii, T.R., and Jin, S. (2009) Magnetic nanoparticles for theragnostics. *Adv. Drug Delivery Rev.*, **61** (6), 467–477.
180. Wang, S.H., Shi, X., VanAntwerp, M., Cao, Z., Swanson, S.D., Bi, X. *et al.* (2007) Dendrimer-functionalized iron oxide nanoparticles for specific targeting and imaging of cancer cells. *Adv. Funct. Mater.*, **17** (16), 3043–3050.
181. Hu, F.Q., Wei, L., Zhou, Z., Ran, Y.L., Li, Z., and Gao, M.Y. (2006) Preparation of biocompatible magnetite nanocrystals for in vivo magnetic resonance detection of cancer. *Adv. Mater.*, **18** (19), 2553–2556.
182. Guo, M., Que, C.L., Wang, C.H., Liu, X.Z., Yan, H.S., and Liu, K.L. (2011) Multifunctional superparamagnetic nanocarriers with folate-mediated and pH-responsive targeting properties for anticancer drug delivery. *Biomaterials*, **32** (1), 185–194.
183. Jochum, F.D., Zur Borg, L., Roth, P.J., and Theato, P. (2009) Thermo-and light-responsive polymers containing photoswitchable azobenzene end groups. *Macromolecules*, **42**, 7854–7862.
184. Kungwatchakun, D. and Irie, M. (1988) Photoresponsive polymers. Photocontrol of phase separation temperature of aqueous solutions of poly(*N*-isopropylacrylamide) with pendant azobenzene groups. *Makromol. Chem. Rapid Commun.*, **9**, 243–246.
185. Jochum, F.D. and Theato, P. (2009) Temperature and light sensitive copolymers containing azobenzene moieties prepared via a polymer analogous reaction. *Polymer*, **50**, 3079–3085.
186. (a) Kröger, R., Menzel, H., and Hallensleben, M.L. (1994) Light controlled solubility change of polymers copolymers of N, N dimethylacrylamide and 4-phenylazophenyl acrylate. *Macromol. Chem. Phys.*, **195**, 2291–2298; (b) Tao, X., Gao, Z., Satoh, T., Cui, Y., Kakuchi, T., and Duan, Q. (2011) Synthesis and characterization of well-defined thermo- and light responsive diblock copolymers by atom transfer radical polymerization and click chemistry. *Polym. Chem.*, **2**, 2068–2073; (c) Dirani, A., Laloyaux, X., Fernandes, A.E., Mathy, B., Schicke, O., Riant, O., Nystenand, B., and Jonas, A.M. (2012) Reversible photomodulation of the swelling of poly(oligo(ethylene glycol) methacrylate) thermoresponsive polymer brushes. *Macromolecules*, **45**, 9400–9408.
187. Tang, X., Liang, X., Gao, L., Fan, X., and Zhou, Q. (2010) Water-soluble triply-responsive homopolymers of N,N-dimethylaminoethyl methacrylate with a terminal azobenzene moiety. *J. Polym. Sci., Part A: Polym. Chem.*, **48**, 2564–2570.
188. Zhang, J., Liu, H.-J., Yuan, Y., Jiang, S., Yao, Y., and Chen, Y. (2013) Tunable and switchable dielectric constant in an amphidynamic crystal. *ACS Macro Lett.*, **2**, 67–71.
189. Schattling, P., Jochum, F.D., and Theato, P. (2011) Multi-responsive copolymers: using thermo-, light-and redox stimuli as three independent inputs towards polymeric information processing. *Chem. Commun.*, **47**, 8859.
190. Uchiyama, S., Kawai, N., de Silva, A.P., and Iwai, K. (2004) Fluorescent polymeric AND logic gate with temperature and pH as inputs. *J. Am. Chem. Soc.*, **126**, 3032–3033.
191. Klaikherd, A., Nagamani, C., and Thayumanavan, S. (2009) Multi-stimuli sensitive amphiphilic block copolymer assemblies. *J. Am. Chem. Soc.*, **131** (13), 4830–4838.

192. Qiao, Z.Y., Zhang, R., Du, F.S., Liang, D.H., and Li, Z.C. (2011) Multi-responsive nanogels containing motifs of ortho ester, oligo(ethylene glycol) and disulfide linkage as carriers of hydrophobic anti-cancer drugs. *J. Controlled Release*, **152** (1), 57–66.
193. Bilalis, P., Chatzipavlidis, A., Tziveleka, L.A., Boukos, N., and Kordas, G. (2012) Nano designed magnetic polymer containers for dual stimuli actuated drug controlled release and magnetic hyperthermia mediation. *J. Mater. Chem.*, **22** (27), 13451–13454.
194. Chang, B.S., Sha, X.Y., Guo, J., Jiao, Y.F., Wang, C.C., and Yang, W.L. (2011) Thermo and pH dual responsive, polymer shell coated, magnetic mesoporous silica nanoparticles for controlled drug release. *J. Mater. Chem.*, **21** (25), 9239–9247.

9
Stimuli-Responsive Polymers: Biomedical Applications

Raju Francis, Nidhin Joy, Anjaly Sivadas, Geethy P. Gopalan, and Deepa K. Baby

9.1
Introduction

The requirement for exact and noninvasive diagnostic devices is urgent for identifying particular and important analytes connected with disorders, of envisioning the area and dissemination of influenced cells, and of reporting the movement of a therapeutic agent. From nano- to supramolecular assemblies, polymeric frameworks are accessible in an assortment of structures and have their own applications in different fields. The intelligent, smart, and environmentally sensitive polymeric complexes have far-reaching applications in biomedical fields. These smart systems were valuable in image sensing (diagnosis), controlled medication conveyance, and regenerative solution (treatment), furthermore in gating valves, or transport, microfluidics, and bioseparation [1–6]. These responsive frameworks containing polymers can be composed either with a responsive polymer or by consolidating a polymer (templates/transporter) with a responsive compound. In most of the works related to biomedical applications, smart polymers are relevant to the first category.

Polymer sensors that react to pertinent biomolecules and anlaytes, and also to pH and temperature, may be very useful in the detection of diseases that are normally either by a noteworthy awkwardness in chemicals or varieties of physical variables in nature which is intended for diagnostic purposes. Since checking these progressions and slopes is crucial to the analysis of specific maladies, awesome endeavors have been made in the field of polymeric biosensors. With the use of imaging techniques, delivery of drugs or other micro- or macromolecules is possible at the targeted location with the help of a smart polymeric complex. Delivery systems include three main categories, namely, low molecular weight drugs, protein and enzyme delivery, and final gene delivery. This chapter focuses on smart complex materials, which may be nano- or supramolecular built of SR polymers that find use in numerous applications in the biomedical field (Figure 9.1).

One important feature of stimuli-responsive (SR) material is reversibility, that is, the ability to return to its initial state. In nature, basic SR biopolymers such as proteins and nucleic acids are stable over wide ranges of external variables

Biomedical Applications of Polymeric Materials and Composites, First Edition.
Edited by Raju Francis and Sakthi Kumar.

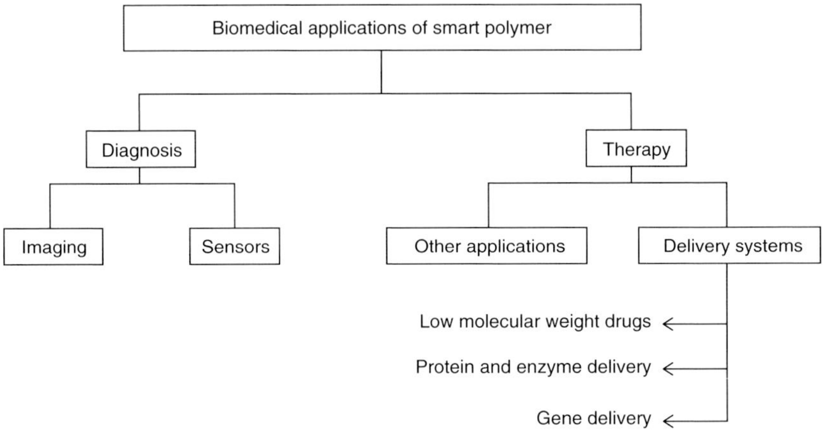

Figure 9.1 Classification of biomedical application of smart polymer.

but undergo drastic structural changes at given critical points [7]. Studies related to these natural polymers have led to the development of numerous synthetic biopolymers. James *et al.* explain the advantages and limitations of various SR polymers [8] (Table 9.1).

Table 9.1 Advantages and limitations of various stimuli-responsive polymers.

Stimulus	Advantage	Limitation
Temperature	Ease of incorporation of active moieties Simple manufacturing and formulation	Low mechanical strength, biocompatibility issues, instability of thermolabile drugs, injectability issues under application conditions
pH	Suitable for thermolabile drugs	Low mechanical strength, Lack of toxicity data
Light	Ease of controlling the trigger mechanism Accurate control over the stimulus	Chance of leaching out of noncovalently attached chromophores, Low mechanical strength of gel,
Electric field	Pulsative release with changes in electric current	Surgical implantation required; need of an additional equipment for external application of stimulus; difficulty in optimizing the magnitude of electric current
Ultrasound	Controllable protein release	Specialized equipment for controlling the release Surgical implantation required for nonbiodegradable delivery system
Mechanical stress	Possibility to achieve the drug release	Difficulty in controlling the release profile

9.2
Imaging

Imaging is indispensible for the diagnosis, treatment, and confirmation of therapy. Fluorescent polymeric sensors, for example, SR dendrimers are utilized as a part of imaging methods for the identification of sick tissues that show somewhat lifted temperatures or acidic pH. The fluorescent dyes sensitive to near infrared have superior depth penetration in tissue. These sensors allow for specific, rapid, and sensitive detection. Electrosensitive and light-sensitive polymers have been investigated extensively in medical imaging. Tumor tissues have a different refractive index from normal tissues; hence, this near-IR sensitive material can be used for imaging tumors.

Polymers have emerged as new PR materials because of their high efficiency, ease of synthesis, and low cost. A 100% diffraction efficiency was observed in guest–host PR polymer composites with 105 μm thick samples [9–11]. The composite consists of poly(*N*-vinylcarbazole) matrix, 2,4,7-trinitro-9-fluorenone (TNF) as the sensitizer, and *N*-ethylcarbazole as a plasticizer and can be used for imaging through scattering media, using a holographic time-gating technique at a wavelength that is compatible with the transparency of biological tissues and with the emission of low-cost semiconductor laser diodes [12]. This is because their high orientational birefringences provide a large dynamic range, large dipole moment, and high linear polarizability anisotropy.

Lee *et al.* prepared fluorescent pluronic triblock copolymers [13]. These (PEO–PPO–PEO) endcaps with a cyanine dye (Cy5.5) fluorescent thermosensor find application in biological and medical field because they are applicable in tissue imaging in the NIR region at different resolutions and depth penetrations with minimal tissue autofluorescence. Increases in temperature or concentration of pluronic can lead to a sol–gel transition by micelle packing. However, the impact of temperature is dependent on the composition and molecular weight of copolymers. Thus, it is possible to synthesize a thermosensor for monitoring a specific temperature range by using proper block copolymers. The sensitive quenching properties of polymeric sensors allow for the monitoring of temperature changes by visualized fluorescent images.

Yamamoto *et al.* synthesized an electrically powerless thermal and light-responsive poly(*N*-isopropylacrylamide) (PNIPAM) actuator in ambient air using a packaging technique [14]. In particular, this actuator can be activated by human body temperature as well as by sunlight without the need for another artificial power source. These nature-powered actuators are promising candidates for the development of a new class of ultimate low-power devices. This natural power source actuator can be used for a wearable device that wraps around a human body, a smart wall/curtain that opens and closes by sunlight, and so on (Figure 9.2).

Fluorinated poly(amidoamine) (PAMAM) starburst dendrimer was prepared by Criscione *et al.* [15]. The amphiphilic nature and easily modifiable surface of the PAMAM dendrimer make it an attractive vehicle for targeted drug delivery

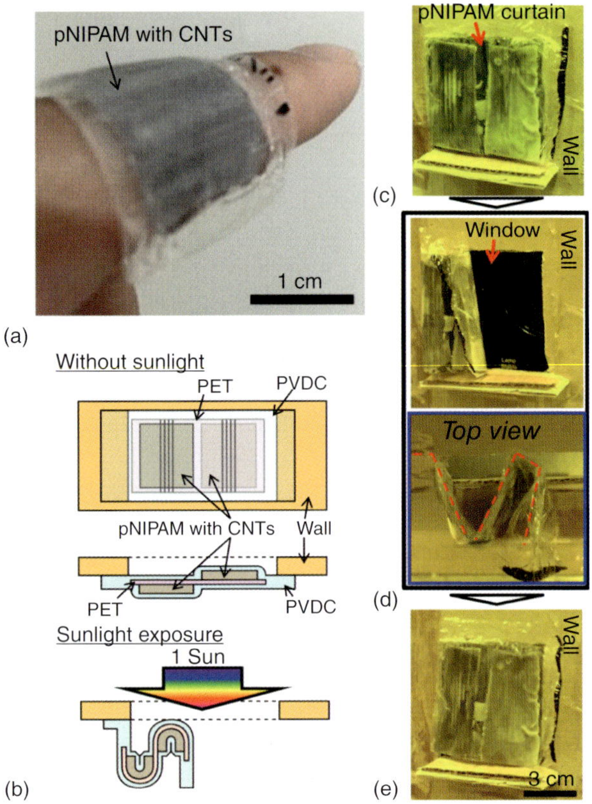

Figure 9.2 Demonstrations of the pNIPAM actuators stimulated by human skin temperature and sunlight. (a) Wearable sheet actuated by skin temperature wraps around a finger. (b) Schematic of the smart curtain design. Photos of (c) before sunlight exposure (closed), (d) after exposure for 15 min (open), and (e) after terminating sunlight exposure (closed). (Yamamoto 2015 [14]. Reproduced with permission from American Chemical Society.)

and molecular imaging. This system exhibits a stimulus-induced response to low external pH that enables controlled release of encapsulated agents. In addition, it offers a sufficiently high density of fluorine spins to enable detection of their site-specific accumulation *in vivo* by ^{19}F magnetic resonance imaging (^{19}f MRI). Due to changes in environmental pH, a shift in relaxation time was observed. Thus, the system can also be used as a powerful imaging technique for the localization of tumor, with acidic pH. Experiments with mice show that this dendrimer can be tracked with noninvasive imaging.

The overproduction of hydrogen peroxide creates numerous diseases, and there is currently great interest in developing contrast agents that can image hydrogen peroxide. *In vivo* imaging of hydrogen peroxide was done by Lee *et al.* using chemiluminescent nanoparticles formulated from peroxalate esters and fluorescent dyes [16]. The peroxalate nanoparticles have several attractive properties for *in vivo* imaging, such as tunable wavelength emission (460–630 nm) and excellent specificity for hydrogen peroxide over other reactive oxygen species. During a lipopolysaccharide-induced inflammatory response, the peroxalates were able to image hydrogen peroxide.

Various nanomaterials such as iron oxides and gold have been conjugated with nucleic acids for combined applications of imaging and gene delivery [17, 18]. In their study on gadolinium oxide core embedded in a polysiloxane shell, Bridot *et al.* observed that the inner part is functionalized by organic dyes and the outer part by poly(ethylene glycol) (PEG) [19]. This complex can be used in molecular imaging, because of their bioavailability and high relaxivity per particle, which provides a strong local contrast enhancement. ^{157}Gd has natural abundance around 20% and possesses a high neutron capture cross section. The interaction between the internalized biocompatible nanoparticles and a thermal neutron beam in neutron capture therapy destroys the hybrid Gd_2O_3 nanoparticles loaded tumor with energetic particles (Figure 9.3).

The biodegradable polymers with fusogenic properties (DNA delivery), pH-sensitive polymers with membrane permeation (oral biopharmaceutical delivery), and programmable gel-(drug delivery) incorporated light-sensitive polymers with

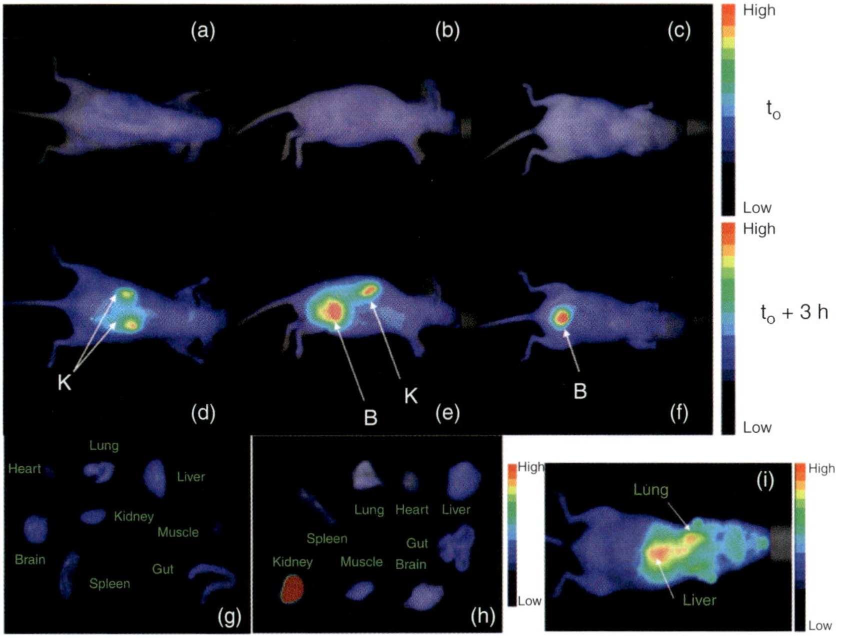

Figure 9.3 Fluorescence reflectance imaging of a nude mouse (a, b, c) before and (d, e, f) 3 h after the injection of GadoSiPEG2C (K, kidneys; B, bladder). Fluorescence reflectance imaging of some organs after dissection (g) of a control mouse (no particles injection) and (h) of the nude mouse visualized on pictures (a–f). (i) Fluorescence reflectance imaging of a nude mouse after the injection of GadoSi2C (particles without PEG). Each image is acquired with an exposure time of 200 ms. (Bridot 2007 [19]. Reproduced with permission from American Chemical Society.)

stimuli-sensitive properties have promising biomedical applications in cancer treatment and imaging of cancer [20].

9.3 Sensing

Nanoparticles or quantum dots (QDs) linked to responsive polymer were designed or synthesized for the development of polymeric sensors [21]. Localized surface plasmon resonance (LSPR) is generated around metal nanoparticles such as gold, silver, and copper. Negatively charged gold nanoparticles were adsorbed uniformly and selectively onto positively charged polymers [22]. Surface plasmon resonance spectroscopy (SPR) monitors the conformational changes of the polymer chains that induce a vertical motion to the nanoparticles. Mitsuishi *et al.* affirm that the detection of nanoscale optical changes is possible by the fabrication of hybrid nanoassemblies with PNIPAM brushes and Au nanoparticles [23]. These hybrid nanoassemblies will be applicable for use in nanosensor applications. Combining stimulus-responsive surfaces and semiconductor nanoparticles helps the formation of robust and cost-effective sensors for various applications. A poly(2-vinylpyridine) brush reversibly collapsing due to a pH switch from 2 to 5 is an example of pH nanosensor.

PNIPAM microgel particles offer good platforms for biosensing because of their large surface area, narrow size distribution and the versatility of functional groups on the surface. As an example, Ali *et al.* [24] achieved DNA manipulation on a PNIPAM microgel surface. 5′-Amine-modified DNA oligonucleotide (DNA1) was first coupled onto the microgel using EDC chemistry. Then the coupled DNA1 was ligated with a second DNA oligonucleotide (DNA2) in the presence of T4 DNA ligase and a template oligonucleotide. Rolling circle amplification (RCA) was carried out for signal amplification. Finally, hybridization with a fluorescent DNA probe (DNA3) allowed for signal detection. Paper strips immobilized with DNA oligonucleotide-modified microgels were further developed, which can be used to perform ligation/RCA-mediated amplification procedures for sensitive detection of DNA [25]. These DNA sensors have great promise in the identification of biological sources, such as specific pathogens.

We depict here a few illustrations utilizing the fluorescence resonance energy exchange method. Blends of responsive polymer with FRET produce temperature and pH sensors. Di-block copolymer of (PEG – PSDM) prepared with a FRET contributor as a linker between the two chains and a FRET acceptor as an end bunch on the PSDM chain is a case of this type [26]. At higher pH (more than 7.6), pH sensor emits the blue color that corresponds to the emission of the FRET donor, and at lower pH (less than 6.8), the pH sensor emits the green color that corresponds to the emission of the FRET acceptor. This indicates that lowering the pH from 7.6 to 6.8 induces the FRET due to the conformational change of polymeric linker from coil to globule. The PEGylated FRET sensor responds to a relatively small change in pH with well-defined on and off behavior and also has dispersion stability in aqueous media (Figure 9.4).

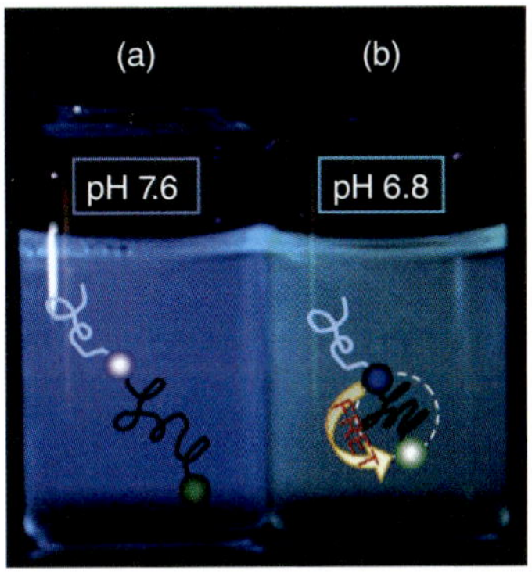

Figure 9.4 Fluorescence images of solutions containing **7** at (a) pH 7.6 and (b) pH 6.8 when the solutions are irradiated at 330 nm. (Hong 2006 [26]. Reproduced with permission from American Chemical Society.)

In the aforementioned examples, PNIPAM microgels only act as a platform. The most prominent property of the PNIPAM microgel is its sensitivity to external stimuli. Sensors can be designed if this property is coupled with a suitable reporting method. Compared with sensors based on bulky hydrogels, the microgel-based sensors have the benefit of responding much quicker. Thermosensitive properties of poly(*N*-isopropylacrylamide-co-Nile red)-coated magnetic nanostructures, upon passing through the lower critical solution temperature (LCST) of the polymer brush, help in correlation resulting in the formation of aggregates [27]. The nanoparticles displayed enhanced transverse (T2) NMR relaxometric behavior as the temperature was increased through the LCST. Moreover, incorporation of the environmentally sensitive Nile red dye into the copolymer leads to significant changes in fluorescence emission intensity upon aggregation, which present new possibilities for the remote fluorescence detection of aggregated structures. Combining a thermosensitive polymeric shell with a magnetic core paves the way for multistimuli-responsive nanoparticles, such as "smart" T2 contrast agents for magnetic resonance imaging (MRI) or materials that induce a biological response because of changes in brush structure around the magnetic core. (Figure 9.5).

Based on the glucose sensitivity of PBA-functionalized microgel, Wu *et al.* [28] designed an optical glucose sensor using fluorescent QDs as optical labels. The fluorescent CdS QDs were synthesized *in situ* in the interior of the copolymer microgels. The resultant hybrid microgel remains glucose sensitive, that is, it swells to a larger degree in the presence of glucose. The swelling of the microgel results in an increase in the number of emission quenching centers located on the polymer–CdS QD interface, which in turn results in the quenching of the fluorescence of the CdS QDs. Therefore, the optical detection of glucose can be achieved from the glucose-induced fluorescence quenching. This sensor was further improved by using a PBA with a low pK_a [29]. As a result, the sensor can detect glucose at physiological pH.

Peng *et al.* engineered a hydrogel using DNA duplexes as photoreversible cross-links [30]. This photosensitive dynamic hydrogel was prepared by grafting

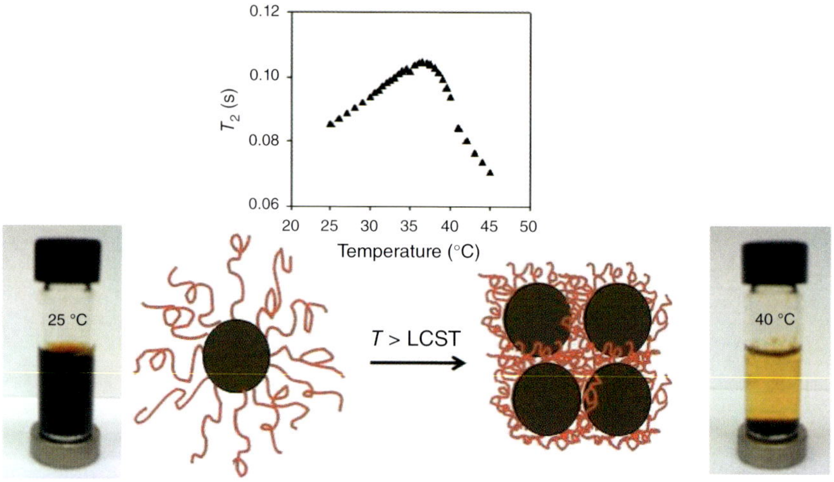

Figure 9.5 Dispersion–flocculation behavior of magnetite-PNIPAM nanoparticles, as a function of temperature and magnetic field (concentration = 20 mg ml^{-1}). (Balasubramaniam 2011 [27]. Reproduced with permission from American Chemical Society.)

azobenzene-tethered, single-stranded DNA and its cDNA to the hydrogel network so that the degree of cross-linking could be regulated by light. The macroscopic volume of the hydrogel can be manipulated through the photoreversible DNA hybridization controlled by alternate irradiation of UV and visible light (Figure 9.6).

Fluorescent polymeric sensors are another class of sensors that are obtained by combining stimuli-sensitive monomers and polymerizable fluorescent dyes. Changes in the fluorescence signal are the result of polymer chain hydrophilicity. PNIPAM-combined benzofurazan dye is an example of this type [31, 32]. Temperature is related to the fluorescence power varieties that are affected by neighborhood fixation inclinations and connected with sign to commotion proportion.

In another work, Wu *et al.* [33] designed a composite PNIPAM microgel that is both pH and H_2O_2 responsive. They used a copolymer microgel of [P(NIPAM-AAc-AAm)] as the template to direct the assembly of Calcon dye. It was found that the poly acrylamide segment in the microgels is crucial to direct the long-range ordered assembly of Calcon dye molecules on the microgel template, which acts as an optical identification code and an H_2O_2-sensitive component. While pH has no effect on the PL intensity of the free Calcon dye solution, the PL intensity of the P(NIPAM-AA-AAm)–Calcon composite microgel dispersions was dramatically enhanced with decreasing pH. The enhanced PL is due to the deswelling of the microgel, which may either cause a change in the local optical electric field around the Calcon domains or make the Calcon domains more closely packed. As H_2O_2 can break the azo bond in the Calcon dye, the PL intensity of the composite microgel decreases with time in the presence of H_2O_2. Compared with free Calcon dye solution, the H_2O_2 sensitivity of the

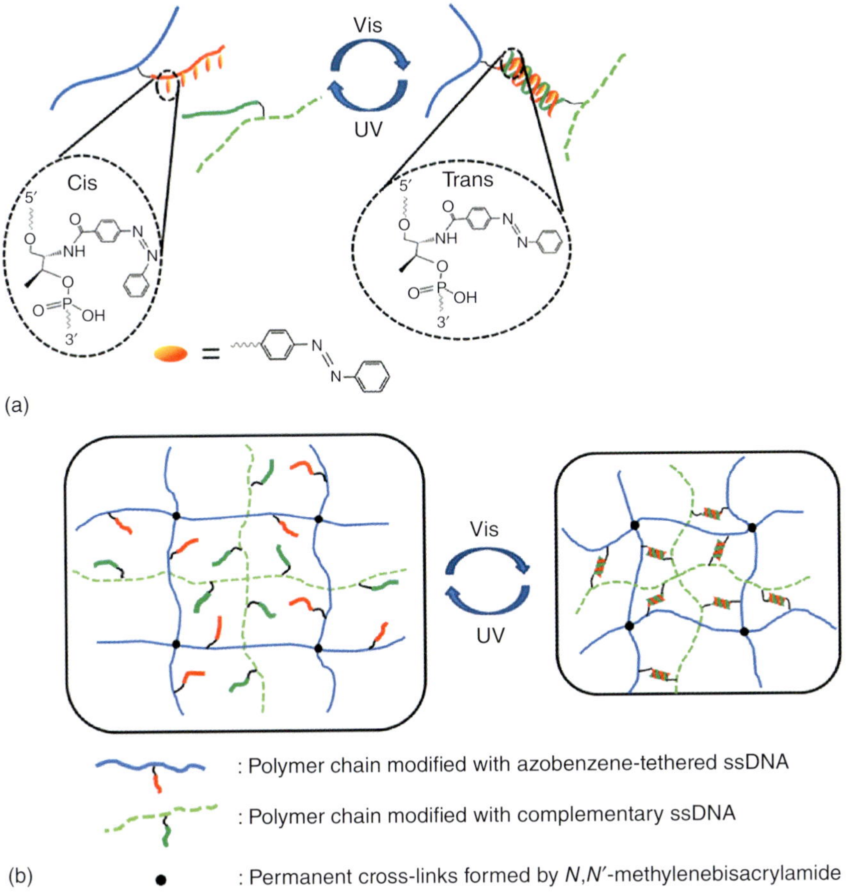

Figure 9.6 (a) Light-controlled formation of DNA duplex based on azobenzene isomerization in the hydrogel. (b) Reversible volume transition of the DNA-cross-linked hydrogel regulated by UV and visible light. (Peng 2012 [30]. Reproduced with permission from American Chemical Society.)

composite microgels is much higher. Therefore, this novel composite microgel can be developed as an optical pH and H_2O_2 sensor.

9.4
Delivery of Therapeutic Molecules

Delivery devices that allow remote, repeatable, and reliable switching of drug flux could have a marked impact on the treatment of a variety of medical conditions. An ideal device for on-demand drug delivery should safely contain a large quantity of drug, release little or no drug in the "off" state, and be repeatedly switchable to the "on" state without mechanically disrupting the device [34].

9.4.1
Low Molecular Weight Drug

Controlled delivery of drugs is a particularly important application that is caused by the reversible collapse and expansion of responsive polymers. Stimuli polymer hydrogels have potential use in a variety of drug loading and release formats, and their release characteristics can be tailored to suit a range of target environments. Although the detailed kinetics of drug release from these systems are complex [35–38] to a first approximation correlations between gel collapse point, matrix structure and drug release can be obtained. Appropriate synthesis then allows delivery systems to be prepared that will respond at a predesignated pH and/or temperature to release a therapeutic. For drug delivery applications, the polymer response should be nonlinear, that is, with distinct "on" and "off" states, and there is a drive to develop materials that display very sharp transitions for a small stimulus or change in environment. Natural therapeutics and pharmaceuticals are regularly constrained by short half-lives, poor bioavailability, and chemical and physical stability. Physical instability leads to denaturation, aggregation, and precipitation. Chemical instability of drugs leads to oxidation, deamidation, hydrolysis, and racemization. These types of polymers offer a medication conveyance stage that can be utilized to convey drugs at a controlled rate and in a stable and organically dynamic structure. DOX, paclitaxel (PAX), camptothecin, dexamethasone, cisplatin, indomethacin, and *N*-acetylcysteine are drugs in which DOX is the most widely studied anticancer hydrophobic drug [39–43].

Poly(*N*-isopropylacrylamide) is the most wildly used polymer in the construction of drug delivery systems. PNIPAM exhibits a LCST of 30 °C in water that is attributed to alterations in the hydrogen-bonding interactions of the amide group [44–47]. Poly(*N*-isopropylacrylamide)-incorporated cross-linked polymer used as a device for controlled delivery of drugs is a particularly important class because they exploit the thermally reversible collapse or shrinkage above the LCST.

Tumor tissues are characterized by some specific features: high hydrostatic pressure on the tumor, low oxygen concentration, high lactic acid concentration, and a consequent pH decrease to values between 6.0 and 7.4. These features help to separate the drug from the carrying polymer. Biodegradable pH-sensitive poly(β-amino ester) produces a PAX nanoparticles system, which is more effective in reducing the tumor cells [48]. Other biodegradable pH-sensitive polymeric systems used for anticancer drugs are PDMAEMA and 2-hydroxyethyl (methacrylate) [49], poly(histidine)-β-PEG and poly(L-lactic acid)-β-PEG [50], and PCL [51].

Hydrophilic and hydrophobic end group and changes in molecular weight of polymeric chain also affect the LCST. The LCST transitions and aqueous solution behavior of four-arm NIPAM star polymers and their hydrolyzed linear arms were synthesized using a RAFT agent pentaerythritoltetrakis(3-(*S*-benzyltrithiocarbonyl) propionate) (PTBTP) [52]. Star polymer LCST transitions were found to be significantly lowered either due to the tethering of PNIPAM chains to the RAFT agent star core or due to a combination of the core and benzyl end groups. The presence of a hydrophilic and hydrophobic end group on the opposite ends of the polymer chain is suggested to cause this effect.

The classic micellar structure is limited for the encapsulation of hydrophobic drugs in its core. Polymeric vesicles have an ability to encapsulate hydrophobic and hydrophilic therapeutic agents. Varieties of polymeric nanocarriers are available for delivering hydrophilic and hydrophobic drugs, proteins, genes, and enzymes. Other polymeric nanostructures used in nanomedicines are dendrimers, smart surfaces, and nanogels [53, 54]. The vast majority of the low atomic weight medications are hydrophobic that restricts their utilization because of solvency issues. For solving this, their pharmacodynamics and pharmacokinetics are greatly enhanced. Some of the examples are disused here for understanding the synthesis and application of drug delivery systems.

Well-defined AB_2, Y-shaped star copolymers of PNIPAM-*b*-$(PZLL)_2$, and PNIPAM-*b*-$(PLL)_2$ were synthesized through the combination of ATRP, ring-opening polymerization (ROP), and click chemistry [55]. Propargylamine was employed as the ROP initiator for the preparation of alkynyl-terminated PZLL. After the removal of the benzyloxycarbonyl group from PNIPAM-*b*-$(PZLL)_2$, water-soluble PNIPAM-*b*-$(PLL)_2$ was obtained. Shell-cross-linked (SCL) PNIPAM-*b*-$(PLL)_2$ micelles are considered to be excellent drug nanocarriers due to the following advantages. First, the structure of the nanocarrier is permanently stable due to the introduction of shell cross-linking. Second, as the SCL micelles possess temperature-responsive cores, the encapsulation and subsequent triggered release of drugs are possible. Finally, the permeability of the shell can also be controlled by the adjustment of the cross-linking degree (Figure 9.7).

The PNIPAM-based composite membrane consisted of ethyl cellulose (the membrane support), superparamagnetic magnetite nanoparticles (the triggering entity), and thermosensitive PNIPAM-based nanogels [56]. This membrane enabled rapid, repeatable, and tunable drug delivery upon the application of an external oscillating magnetic field. Membranes were prepared by coevaporation so that the nanogel and magnetite nanoparticles were entrapped in ethyl cellulose to form a disordered network. To assess the inducible drug-releasing properties *in vivo*, a membrane was excised after 45 days of implantation, the thin tissue capsule was removed, and the thermally triggered fluorescein flux was measured. No significant difference was observed in the flux differential between the "on" and "off" states suggesting that protein adsorption or biofilm formation *in vivo* does not significantly impact the functionality of the membrane. It can undergo a sharp, volume phase transition at $\geq 40\,°C$ and so can be switched from the "off" state at normal physiological temperature to the "on" state at a temperature where it would not typically be triggered by fever, local inflammation, and so on. The membrane could be switched on and off rapidly by the removal of an external oscillating magnetic field. At the applied magnetic frequency, the water inside the cell was heated from 37 to $42\,°C$ over the course of 10 min. Heat generated by magnetite induction heating was transferred to the adjacent thermosensitive

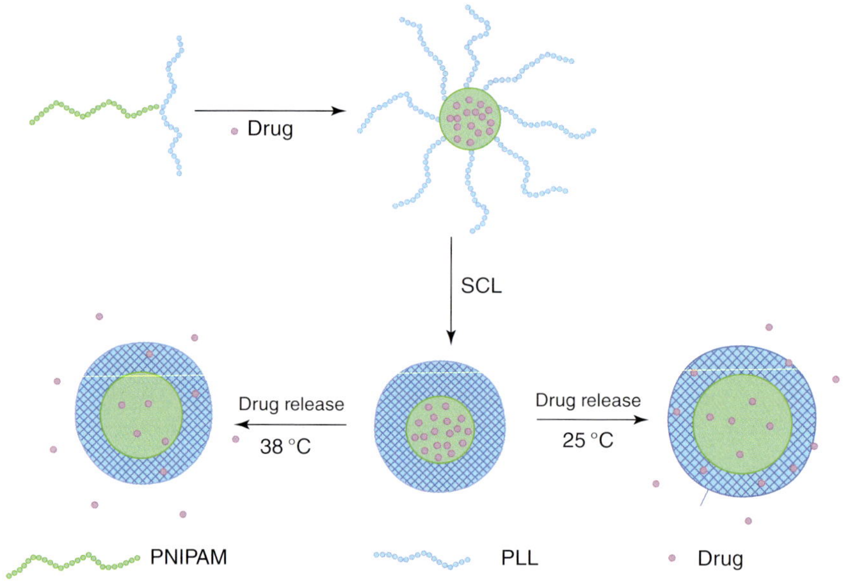

Figure 9.7 Cumulative drug releases from micelles at different temperatures. (Li 2010 [55]. Reproduced with permission from American Chemical Society.)

nanogels, causing the nanogels to shrink and permit drug diffusion out of the device (Figure 9.8).

Francis *et al.* synthesized a thermosensitive drug delivery hydrogel system composed of temperature-sensitive NIPAM and biocompatible and pH-sensitive maleic acid by sedimentation polymerization [57]. The morphological data of hydrogel revealed that the surface structure of this rigid hard biodegradable hydrogel was poriferous. Experiments on drug release from the cross-linked NIPAM-co-maleic acid hydrogel loaded with ibuprofen showed that the release rate depended on acidity or basicity (polarity) of the medium and the gel, and swelling ratio of the gel network was a function of the environmental pH and temperature. Here, the drug release study was extended to acidic and basic conditions because of the fact that pH varies from acidic to basic with respect to the stomach and intestine.

Li *et al.* observed that complex micelles with environmentally sensitive properties are useful in intelligent drug delivery [58]. pH-sensitive polyelectrolyte complex micelles were assembled from two oppositely charged graft copolymers (chitosan-(CS)-*g*-PNIPAM) and sodium alginate-*g*-poly(*N*-isopropylacrylamide-co-*N*-vinyl-pyrrolidone) [ALG-*g*-P(NIPAM-co-NVP)]. Glutaraldehyde, as a chemical cross-linking agent and the core, was formed by electrostatic interactions between positively charged CS and negatively charged ALG.

The drug-loaded micelles were prepared by using effective chemotherapeutic anticancer drugs 5-fluorouracil (5-FU) as a model drug [59, 60]. To improve the

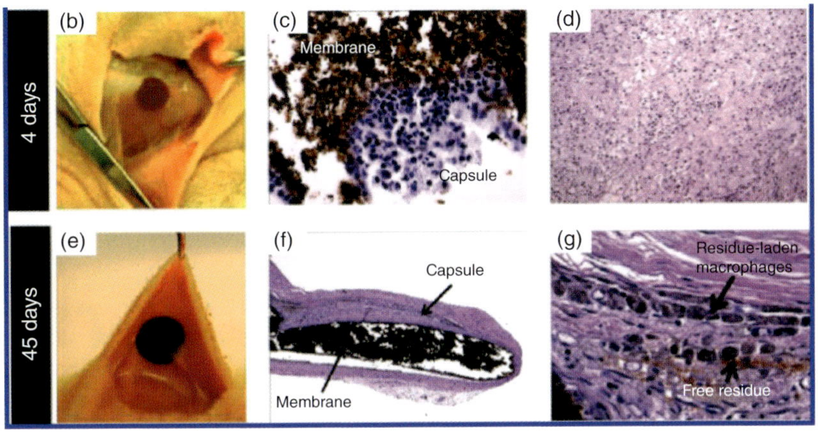

Figure 9.8 Biological testing of membranes: (b–g) tissue response to implanted nanogel-loaded membrane (25% nanogel, 27% ferrofluid) after 4 and 45 days of implantation: (b) top view, 4 days postimplantation; (c) histological section of membrane–tissue interface, 400× magnification; (d) histological section of capsule inflammatory response, 100× magnification; (e) top view, 45 days postimplantation; (f) histological section of membrane–tissue interface, 40× magnification; (g) histological section of capsule inflammatory response, 400× magnification. (Hoare 2009 [56]. Reproduced with permission from American Chemical Society.)

drug's bioavailability, reduce side effects, improve selective action, and increase therapeutic efficacy, polyelectrolyte complex micelles have been the preferred choice as drug delivery carriers [61]. 5-FU containing negative O, N, and F atoms may form hydrogen bondings with PEC micelles.

For PEC-GA micelles, the cumulative 5-FU release was 33.4%, 73.2%, and 98.8% at 25, 37, and 45 °C. The increased drug release at high temperatures may be due to micelles lost during hydrogen-bonding interactions with 5-FU [62, 63]. The amount of 5-FU released from PEC micelles was faster at pH 2.0 and 7.2 but slower at pH 5.6 at 37 °C. This could be explained by the observation that medium pH had no effect on the electrostatic complex micelles as well as on the interactions between drugs and micelles. Cytotoxicity assays showed that drug-loaded micelles retained high cell inhibition efficiency in HeLa cells. These polyelectrolyte complex micelles with environmentally sensitive properties can be used in the field of intelligent drug delivery.

Dendritic polyesters have significant advantages in the liberation of DOX over classic polymers, due to low polydispersity, specific morphology, and high density of functional groups [64]. This all around characterized engineering helps them to entangle drugs through embodiment, covalent connection (conjugation), and complexation (electrostatic cooperation) [65]. Drug polymer conjugates are more appealing than drug–dendrimer complexes due to its expanded stability and higher payloads. The arrival of medications from polymersomes by means of poration in the film impelled by pH-activated corruption of the PLA blocks and that their primary confinement is the somewhat moderate rate of poly(lactic corrosive) hydrolysis which is reported by Ahmed *et al.* in another work [66].

Kurtoglu *et al.* reported that PAMAM dendrimer–drug conjugates with disulfide linkages are used for intracellular drug delivery [67]. The PAMAM dendrimer–drug conjugates can deliver 60 w% of drug within 1 hour, whereas the conjugate did not release the drug at plasma glutathione (GSH) levels. This study establishes that PAMAM dendrimers can release high drug payloads in a short time intracellularly, through the use of a "small," natural biomolecule GSH.

The methodologies for the controlled drug delivery of proteins are the utilization of smart surfaces which is responsive to temperature, chemical stimuli, or electrical stimuli. The great possibility for drug delivery process is the grafting of polymer films on the surfaces, since they have high storage and high maintenance ability and can uptake and discharge biomacromolecules on interest [68]. An example of an electrically response framework is nerve development variable [69] or adenosine triphosphate [70] stacked on a polypyrrole conductive film and discharged upon electrical initiation. Yavuz *et al.* synthesized that PNIPAM covalently connected to gold nanocages by means of thiolate linkage can be utilized as an on on-off gate process [71]. The controlled release of DOX and lysozyme was also investigated. PNIPAM experienced reversible conformational changes bringing about an on-off gating of the pores by utilizing the photothermal effect of the gold nanocages.

Another class of SR polymeric material is *in situ* forming polymer gels that have great potential in drug delivery. An example is biodegradable pH/temperature-sensitive triblock copolymer hydrogels composed of PEG and PAEU [72]. Interactions (hydrogen bond and ionic bond) between copolymers and drug/protein molecules are enhanced by the presence of urethane and tertiary amine groups in the synthesized copolymers. The presence of a copolymer solution at low pH and temperature facilitates the formulation of a hydrogel precursor with therapeutic agents, while the transition to the gel state at the physiological conditions provides the potential application as a drug/protein carrier. This hydrogel system controlled the release of human growth hormone (HGH) for more than 5 days *in vitro* and 3 days *in vivo* without an initial burst.

Electrically controlled delivery systems are another type of drug delivery systems, in which hydrogels generally shrink or swell under the influence of an electric field. Sonophoresis, iontophoresis, and infusion pumps are the three main technologies in electrically controlled delivery systems. We infer that medication conveyance is the technique or procedure of managing a pharmaceutical compound to accomplish a helpful impact on people or creatures. The basic factors of this process are to deliver the drug to proper area, at the correct time and at the right concentration. Low solvency, ecological or enzymatic debasement, quick freedom rates from the body, nonspecific poisonous quality, and powerlessness to cross the natural boundaries are a portion of the difficulties to accomplishing fruitful medication conveyance [73–75].

9.4.2
Gene Delivery

Faulty or disordered genes are in charge of hereditary illnesses. In quality treatment, the very important thing is the conveyance of the proper remedial quality (DNA) into the cells that will supplant, repair, or direct the defective gene that causes the ailment. DNA is a contrarily charged hydrophilic particle, so its section through adversely charged hydrophobic cell layer is not practical. For this purpose, gene delivery carriers, also called *vectors* or *vehicles*, are used [76, 77]. Viruses are first used as vehicles and their main limitation is immune response, so nonviral carriers have been developed. Presently polymer-based nonviral bearers are utilized in light of the fact that polymers are less expensive, more secure than viruses, and furthermore simpler to tailor contrasted with other gene delivery transporters like liposomes [78–82].

Ward and Georgiou explain the following main steps in gene delivery in his review [83]:

- DNA and polymer complexation or DNA complexation.
- Addition of DNA/polymer complex (polyplex) onto cells for a period of time (transfection time) or complex traversing the cell membrane to the cytoplasm.
- Removal of complex from the cells via DNA release into the cytoplasm.
- DNA transfer into nucleus done by the cells is left to incubate for a time period (incubation time).

Lin *et al.* reported that liposome, micelle, and nanoparticles are used as drug delivery systems for drug and gene delivery [84] (Figures 9.9 and 9.10).

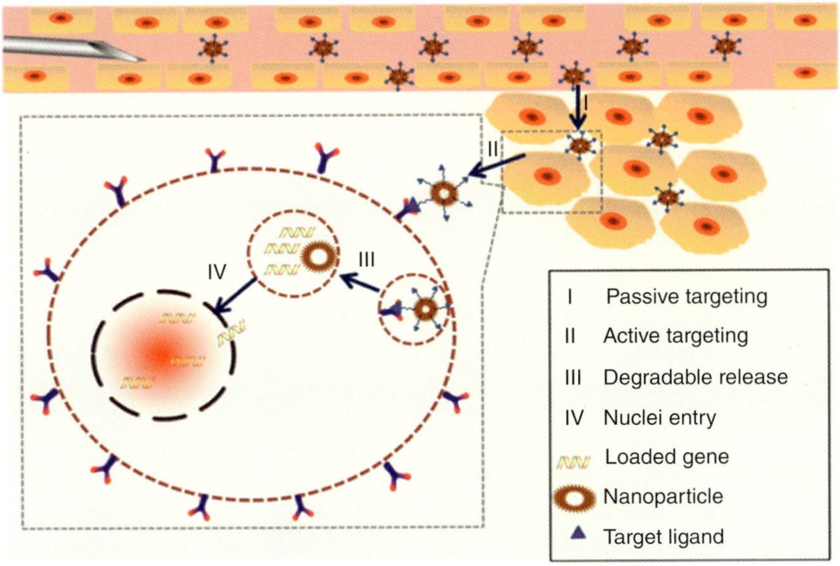

Figure 9.9 Targeting mechanism of gene delivery in nanoparticle systems. (Lin 2015 [84]. Reproduced with permission from American Chemical Society.)

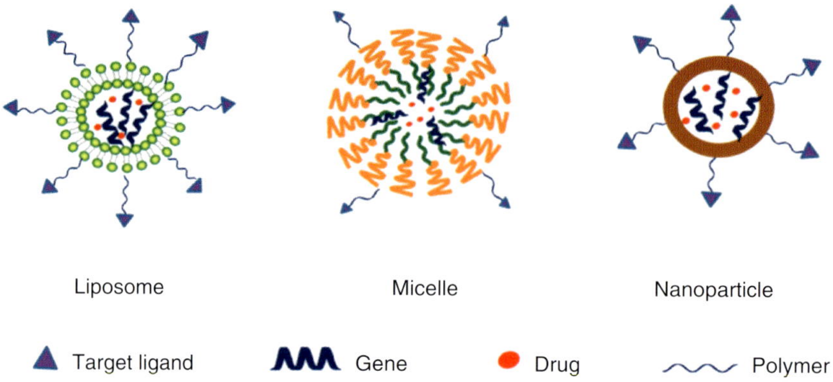

Figure 9.10 Various drug delivery systems for drug and gene delivery. (Lin 2015 [84]. Reproduced with permission from American Chemical Society.)

Thermoresponsive polymers, for example, PEI with joined PNIPAM [85], direct and expanded NIPAM, DMAEMA, and PEI polymers [86], and CS united with PNIPAM [87] have been utilized to upgrade the transfection proficiency by changing the temperature through the complexation and/or during the incubation or transfection period. In some cases, only the incubation or complexation temperature was varied [88–90], while in others both complexation and incubation temperature were varied [91].

Yang *et al.* synthesized thermoresponsive diblock copolymers, poly[2-(2-methoxyethoxy) ethyl methacrylate]-*b*-poly(2-hydroxyethyl methacrylate) ($PMEO_2MA$-*b*-PHEMA) by ATRP [92]. PEI was then grafted to the copolymer to fabricate PEIMH copolymer vectors. Variable temperature agarose retardation, zeta potential, and time-resolved fluorescence assays were performed to elucidate the temperature-sensitive DNA condensation. At a temperature above LCST, the collapsed $PMEO_2MA$ polymer chains squeezed the loosely bound ethidium bromide out of complex to become free species; thereby, DNA was more tightly packaged by PEIMH. Temporary cooling was shown to improve the transfection efficiency of PEIMH in COS-7 and HEK293 cell lines. The variable temperature protocol is more efficient in improving gene expression level in HEK293 cells. The transfection efficiency was superior, and cytotoxicity was lower at an optimal weight ratio of vector/DNA.

Zhou *et al.* reported a nonviral gene transfection method in which DNA complexes were kept in contact with a deposition surface [93]. They designed a star-shaped thermoresponsive copolymer with four chains for DNA deposition. Each chain has a cationic PDMAPAAm block that forms an inner domain for DNA binding and a thermoresponsive PNIPAM block that forms an outer domain for surface adsorption. A complex formed by simple mixing of luciferase-encoding plasmid DNA and copolymer and the polyplexes could deposit on the substrate by precipitation upon warming. COS-1 cells were cultured on the polyplex-deposited substrate in a culture medium, and the luciferase activity was enhanced with an increase in the charge ratio (surfactant/pDNA) with permissible cellular cytotoxicity.

9.4.3 Proteins and Enzymes Delivery

Biomacromolecules are often fragile and chargeable and, therefore, have to be shielded from potentially harmful species in the body. Either by reversible association with polyelectrolytes to frame PIC micelles or by means of exemplification in the lumen of polymeric vesicles, we can overcome the challenges in proteins and chemicals conveyance. Although there are many reports related to the encapsulation and subsequent release of functional proteins into responsive polymersomes [94–96], only few are available that are related to protein release with demonstrated biomedical applications [97, 98]. SR polymers trigger the separation of PIC micelles by means of the debasement of chemical bonds through pH or a diminishing condition, via temperature changes, or by means of charge transformation incited by the expansion of counter ions or pH change [99].

pH-responsive polymers covalently bound to the enzyme glucose oxidase were used for insulin delivery [100]. Glucuronic acid formed by the oxidation of glucose by glucose oxidase causes changes in the pH environment. Polycationic polymers are generally used for the synthesis of pH-sensitive hydrogel, which undergo phase transition and release insulin. For example, insulin delivery is possible by the ionization of poly(2-diethylaminoethyl methacrylate) (PDEAEMA) at lower pH in an acid environment, which increases the membrane permeability [101]. Various modified insulin delivery systems are now available; some of them are poly(acrylic acid)-*g*-poly(ethylene glycol), poly(methacrylic acid-*g*-ethylene glycol) [102], poly(*N*,*N*-dimethylaminoethyl methacrylate-*g*-2-hydroxyethyl (methacrylate)) [103], and so on. Glucuronic acid decreases the pH within the polymeric net, and that causes protonation of pH-responsive polymers. This causes the swelling of the hydrogel, increasing the electrostatic repulsion and the pore size. The increase in pore size causes the increase of insulin delivery from the polymeric matrix.

9.5 Other Applications

Tissue designing is an interdisciplinary field that uses the standards of both building and life sciences for enhancing the functions of tissues. It expects to recover or supplant organically harmed organs in an extensive variety of medicinal conditions, for example, spinal cord injury (SCI), heart diseases, osteoarthritis, cirrhosis, disfiguration, and diabetes [104–109]. In tissue engineering, the cells will be seeded in biocompatible scaffold/material and consequently tissue will mature; this is currently a fast growing research area. The material/framework is normally natural materials, for example, proteins or engineered polymers, with suitable 3D structures that will give adequate mechanical backing at the harm site and can pass on both supplements and development variables to the exemplified cells. Compared to natural products, synthetic polymers have numerous points of interest: their mimic functionalities are like those of native neuronal tissue such as extracellular framework (ECM), and their mechanical and compound properties are simple to tailor; notwithstanding, they ought to be nontoxic, enzymatically nondegradable, financially savvy, and promptly accessible [110, 111]. Cells in tissues develop in a fairly complex manner, encompassed by ECM, which evokes an extensive variety of natural flags and discharges different organic components, controlling both cell conduct and expansion (Figure 9.11) [112].

In tissue engineering, thermoresponsive polymers have two main applications:

1) As substrates that enable the cell growth and proliferation.
   Thermoresponsive polymer is used to regulate cells' attachment and detachment from a surface. To overcome the problems associated with scaffolds, Varghese *et al.* synthesized scaffold-free tissue multilayered constructs [113]. Thermoresponsive surfaces were prepared by coating tissue culture

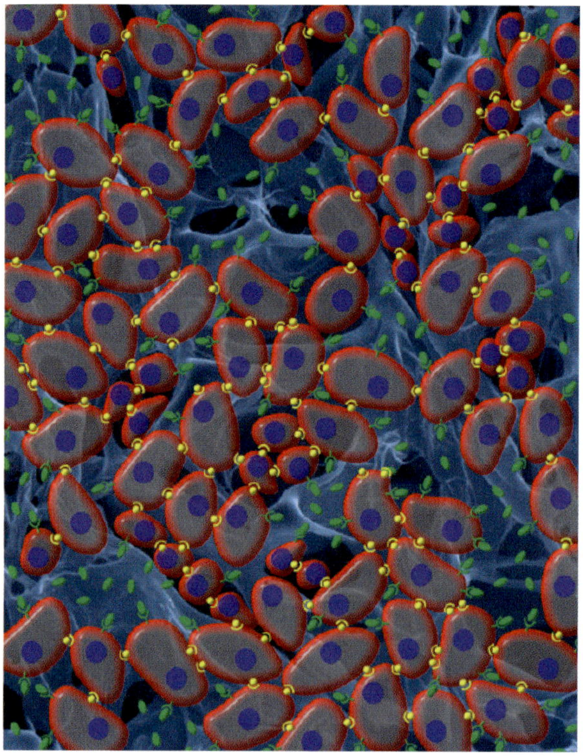

Figure 9.11 Cells (in red, with blue nuclei) interact with the tissue-engineered scaffold through chemical (green ovals) and mechanical stimuli and with each other (yellow circles). These interactions define the cell microenvironment and guide cellular function and differentiation. (Shoichet 2010 [112]. Reproduced with permission from American Chemical Society.)

polystyrene with the copolymer of NIPAM and methyl methacrylate solution in isopropanol. Its thermoresponsive nature with good cytocompatibility makes it a promising substrate for cell culture and tissue engineering applications associated with skin and cornea (Figure 9.12).

2) As injectable gels.

The second application includes the embodiment of cells in a 3D structure in the body. The *in situ* development of cell/scaffold contrast permits the conveyance of exemplified cells, supplements, and development variables to imperfections of any shape utilizing insignificantly obtrusive strategies as appeared in the figure. Thermoresponsive polymer is blended at room temperature with the cells and afterward infused into the body. Upon infusion, because of the temperature increment to 37 °C (over the polymer's LCST), the polymer frames a physical gel, and cells are embodied inside the 3D structure of the gel. As an example, thermoresponsive triblock copolymers synthesized with the highest content of the hydrophobic *N*-butyl methacrylate and lower content of 2-(dimethylamino)ethyl methacrylate (DMAEMA) and PEGMA form a stable physical gel [114]. Study of this gel architecture can facilitate the design and engineering of injectable copolymers for tissue engineering that could enable the *in situ* formation of physical gels at body temperature.

Comolli *et al.* propose to use PNIPAM–PEG as a minimally invasive, injectable scaffold platform for the repair of SCI [115]. PNIPAM–PEG injectable scaffold must maintain its mass and volume over time in physiological conditions. The release of both brain-derived neurotrophic factor (BDNF) and neurotrophin-3 (NT-3) was sustained for up to 4 weeks, with a minimal burst exhibited for both neurotrophins, and they are bioactivity after 4 weeks. PNIPAM–PEG scaffold is similar to native neuronal tissue and compatible with bone marrow stromal cells, allowing their survival and attachment for up to 31 days. These results indicate that PNIPAM–PEG is a promising candidate for the treatment of SCI.

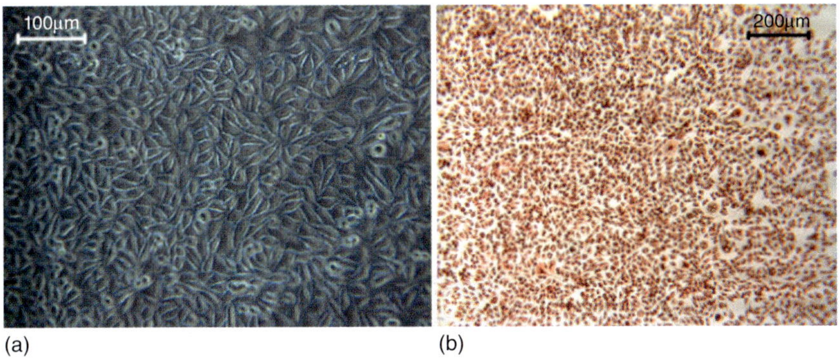

Figure 9.12 L929 cell culture on NIPAM–MMA copolymer. (a) Phase-contrast micrograph after 72 h and (b) neutral red-stained cells indicating their viability on copolymer. (Varghese 2010 [113]. Reproduced with permission from Springer.)

9.6 Conclusion

To conclude, SR polymers have discovered biomedical applications in numerous structures, from diagnosis (e.g., detecting and imaging) to treatment (e.g., tissue designing) and the conveyance of therapeutic particles (e.g., medications or genes). Tissue engineering and injectable implants are the other uses that enhance their application in biomedical or pharmaceutical field. Structural changes of polymer with respect to external environment like physical, chemical, and biological stimuli will have a definite impact in the medical field.

As compared to natural smart polymers such as elastin, synthetic biodegradable polymers have many applications due to their availability, low cost, ease of synthesis, and ability of modification. SR polymers have a great potential in the fields of chemistry, biology, pharmacy, and medicine, with an aim to fulfill the various needs in the biomedical field.

Abbreviations

AAc	acrylic acid
AAm	acrylamide
ATRP	atom transfer radical polymerization
CS	chitosan
DOX	doxorubicin
FU	fluorouracil
FRET	fluorescence resonance energy transfer
LCST	lower critical solution temperature
PAMAM	poly(amidoamine)
PAEU	poly(b-amino ester urethane)
PAX	paclitaxel
PCL	poly(ε-caprolactone)
PDMAEMA	poly(*N*,*N*-dimethylaminoethyl methacrylate)
PDMAPAAm	poly(*N*,*N*-dimethylaminopropyl acrylamide)
PEI	polyethylenimine
PR	photorefractive
PEO	poly(ethylene oxide)
PEG	poly(ethylene glycol)
PEGMA	poly(ethylene glycol)-methyl methacrylate
PLL	poly(L-lysine)
PPO	poly(propylene oxide)
PNIPAM	poly(*N*-isopropylacrylamide)
PSDM	poly(sulfadimethoxine)
PZLL	poly(ε-benzyloxycarbonyl-L-lysine)
QDs	quantum dots
SR	stimuli-responsive

References

1. Hoffman, A.S. (2013) Stimuli-responsive polymers: biomedical applications and challenges for clinical translation. *Adv. Drug Delivery Rev.*, **65**, 10–16.
2. de las Heras Alarcón, C., Pennadam, S., and Alexander, C. (2005) Stimuli responsive polymers for biomedical applications. *Chem. Soc. Rev.*, **34**, 276–285.
3. Stuart, M.A.C., Huck, W.T.S., Genzer, J., Müller, M., Ober, C., Stamm, M., Sukhorukov, G.B., Szleifer, I., Tsukruk, V.V., Urban, M., Winnik, F., Zauscher, S., Luzinov, I., and Minko, S. (2010) Emerging applications of stimuli-responsive polymer materials. *Nat. Mater.*, **9**, 100–113.
4. Bawa, P., Pillay, V., Choonara, Y.E., and du Toit, L.C. (2009) Stimuli-responsive polymers and their applications in drug delivery. *Biomed. Mater.*, **4**, 1–15.
5. Aguilar, M.R., Elvira, C., Gallardo, A., Vázquez, B., and Román, J.S. (2007) Smart polymers and their applications as biomaterials. *Smart Polym.*, **3**, 1–27.
6. Almeida, H., Amaral, M.H., and Lobão, P. (2012) Temperature and pH stimuli-responsive polymers and their applications in controlled and self regulated drug delivery. *J. Appl. Pharm. Sci.*, **2**, 1–10.
7. Kumar, A., Srivastava, A., Galaev, I.Y., and Mattiasson, B. (2007) Smart polymers: physical forms and bioengineering applications. *Prog. Polym. Sci.*, **32**, 1205–1237.
8. James, H.P., John, R., Alex, A., and Anoop, K.R. (2014) Smart polymers for the controlled delivery of drugs – a concise overview. *Acta Pharm. Sin. B*, **4**, 120–127.
9. Donckers, M.C.J.M., Silence, S.M., Walsh, C.A., Hache, F., Burland, D.M., Moerner, W.E., and Twieg, R.J. (1993) Net two-beam-coupling gain in a polymeric photorefractive material. *Opt. Lett.*, **18**, 1044–1046.
10. Liphardt, M., Goonesekera, A., Jonees, B.E., Ducharme, S., Takacs, J.M., and Zhang, L. (1994) High performance photorefractive polymers. *Science*, **263**, 367.
11. Meerholz, K., Volodin, B.L., Sandalphon, D., Kippelen, B., and Peyghambarian, N. (1994) A photorefractive polymer with high optical gain and diffraction efficiency near 100%. *Nature*, **371**, 497–500.
12. Kippelen, B., Marder, S.R., Hendrickx, E., Maldonado, J.L., Guillemet, G., Volodin, B.L., Steele, D.D., Enami, Y., Sandalphon, D., Yao, Y.J., Wang, J.F., Rockel, H., Erskine, L., and Peyghambarian, N. (1998) Infrared photorefractive polymers and their applications for imaging. *Science*, **279**, 54–57.
13. Lee, S.Y., Lee, S., Youn, I.C., Yi, D.K., Lim, Y.T., Chung, B.H., Leary, J.F., Kwon, I.C., Kim, K., and Choi, K. (2009) A near-infrared fluorescence-based optical thermosensor. *Chem. Eur. J.*, **15**, 6103–6106.
14. Yamamoto, Y., Kanao, K., Arie, T., Akita, S., and Takei, K. (2015) Air ambient-operated pNIPAM-based flexible actuators stimulated by human body temperature and sunlight. *ACS Appl. Mater. Interfaces*, **7**, 11002–11006.
15. Criscione, J.M., Le, B.L., Stern, E., Brennan, M., Rahner, C., Papademetris, X., and Fahmy, T.M. (2009) Self-assembly of pH-responsive fluorinated dendrimer-based particulates for drug delivery and noninvasive imaging. *Biomaterials*, **30**, 3946–3955.
16. Lee, D., Khaja, S., Velasquez-Castano, J.C., Dasari, M., Sun, C., Petros, J., Taylor, W.R., and Murthy, N. (2007) *In vivo* imaging of hydrogen peroxide with chemiluminescent nanoparticles. *Nat. Mater.*, **6**, 765–769.
17. Medarova, Z., Pham, W., Farrar, C., Petkova, V., and Moore, A. (2007) *In vivo* imaging of siRNA delivery and silencing in tumors. *Nat. Med.*, **13**, 372–377.
18. Lee, J.H., Lee, K., Moon, S.H., Lee, Y., Park, T.G., and Cheon, J. (2009) All in-one target-cell-specific magnetic

nanoparticles for simultaneous molecular imaging and siRNA delivery. *Angew. Chem. Int. Ed.*, **48**, 4174–4179.

19. Bridot, J.-L., Faure, A.-C., Laurent, S., Rivie, C., Billotey, C., Hiba, B., Janier, M., Josserand, V., Coll, J.-L., Elst, L.V., Muller, R., Roux, S., Perriat, P., and Tillement, O. (2007) Hybrid gadolinium oxide nanoparticles: multimodal contrast agents for *in vivo* imaging. *J. Am. Chem. Soc.*, **129**, 5076–5084.
20. Jeong, B. and Gutowska, A. (2002) Lessons from nature: stimuli- responsive polymers and their biomedical applications. *Trends Biotechnol.*, **20**, 305–311.
21. Westenhoff, S. and Kotov, N.A. (2002) Quantum dot on a rope. *J. Am. Chem. Soc.*, **124**, 2448–2449.
22. Tokareva, I., Minko, S., Fendler, J.H., and Hutter, E. (2004) Nanosensors based on responsive polymer brushes and gold nanoparticle enhanced transmission surface plasmon resonance spectroscopy. *J. Am. Chem. Soc.*, **126**, 15950–15951.
23. Mitsuishi, M., Koishikawa, Y., Tanaka, H., Sato, E., Mikayama, T., Matsui, J., and Miyashita, T. (2007) Nanoscale actuation of thermoreversible polymer brushes coupled with localized surface plasmon resonance of gold nanoparticles. *Langmuir*, **23**, 7472–7474.
24. Ali, M.M., Su, S., Filipe, C.D.M., Pelton, R., and Li, Y. (2007) Enzymatic manipulations of DNA oligonucleotides on microgel: towards development of DNA-microgel bioassays. *Chem. Commun.*, **43**, 4459–4461.
25. Ali, M.M., Aguirre, S.D., Xu, Y.Q., Filipe, C., Pelton, R., and Li, Y.F. (2009) Detection of DNA using bioactive paper strips. *Chem. Commun.*, **43**, 6640–6642.
26. Hong, S.W., Ahn, C.H., Huh, J., and Jo, W.H. (2006) Synthesis of a PEGylated polymeric pH sensor and its pH sensitivity by fluorescence resonance energy transfer. *Macromolecules*, **39**, 7694–7700.
27. Balasubramaniam, S., Pothayee, N., Lin, Y., House, M., Woodward, R.C., St. Pierre, T.G., Davis, R.M., and Riffle, J.S. (2011) Poly(N-isopropylacrylamide)-coated superparamagnetic iron oxide nanoparticles: relaxometric and fluorescence behavior correlate to temperature-dependent aggregation. *Chem. Mater.*, **23**, 3348–3356.
28. Wu, W., Zhou, T., Shen, J., and Zhou, S. (2009) Optical detection of glucose by CdS quantum dots immobilized in smart microgels. *Chem. Commun.*, **29**, 4390–4392.
29. Wu, W., Zhou, T., Aiello, M., and Zhou, S. (2010) Construction of optical glucose nanobiosensor with high sensitivity and selectivity at physiological pH on the basis of organic-inorganic hybrid microgels. *Biosens. Bioelectron.*, **25**, 2603–2610.
30. Peng, L., You, M., Yuan, Q., Wu, C., Han, D., Chen, Y., Zhong, Z., Xue, J., and Tan, W. (2012) Macroscopic volume change of dynamic hydrogels induced by reversible DNA hybridization. *J. Am. Chem. Soc.*, **134**, 12302–12307.
31. Uchiyama, S., Kawai, N., de Silva, A.P., and Iwai, K. (2004) Fluorescent polymeric AND logic gate with temperature and pH as inputs. *J. Am. Chem. Soc.*, **126**, 3032–3033.
32. Uchiyama, S., Matsumura, Y., de Silva, A.P., and Iwai, K. (2003) Fluorescent molecular thermometers based on polymers showing temperature-induced phase transitions and labeled with polarity-responsive benzofurazans. *Anal. Chem.*, **75**, 5926–5935.
33. Wu, W., Zhou, T., Aiello, M., and Zhou, S. (2009) Optically pH and H_2O_2 dual responsive composite colloids through the directed assembly of organic dyes on responsive microgels. *Chem. Mater.*, **21**, 4905–4913.
34. Cheng, R., Meng, F., Deng, C., Klok, H.-A., and Zhong, Z. (2013) Dual and multi-stimuli responsive polymeric nanoparticles for programmed site-specific drug delivery. *Biomaterials*, **34**, 3647–3657.
35. Kato, N., Sakai, Y., and Kanazawa, A. (2003) Deswelling kinetics of a porous poly(N isopropylacrylamide/methacrylic acid) gel prepared by freeze-drying. *Bull. Chem. Soc. Jpn.*, **76**, 543–544.

36. Gan, D.J. and Lyon, L.A. (2001) Tunable swelling kinetics in core-shell hydrogel nanoparticles. *J. Am. Chem. Soc.*, **123**, 7511–7517.
37. Kaneko, Y., Nakamura, S., Sakai, K., Kikuchi, A., Aoyagi, T., Sakurai, Y., and Okano, T. (1999) Synthesis and swelling-deswelling kinetics of poly(N-isopropylacrylamide) hydrogels grafted with LCST modulated polymers. *J. Biomater. Sci., Polym. Ed.*, **10**, 1079–1091.
38. Kaneko, Y., Yoshida, R., Sakai, K., Sakurai, Y., and Okano, T. (1995) Temperature-responsive shrinking kinetics of poly(N-isopropylacrylamide) copolymer gels with hydrophilic and hydrophobic comonomers. *J. Membr. Sci.*, **101**, 13–22.
39. Giacomelli, C., Schmidt, V., and Borsali, R. (2007) Nanocontainers formed by self-assembly of poly(ethylene oxide)-b-poly(glycerol monomethacrylate)—drug conjugates. *Macromolecules*, **40**, 2148–2157.
40. Bae, Y., Fukushima, S., Harada, A., and Kataoka, K. (2003) Design of environment-sensitive supramolecular assemblies for intracellular drug delivery: polymeric micelles that are responsive to intracellular pH change. *Angew. Chem. Int. Ed.*, **42**, 4640–4643.
41. Ponta, A. and Bae, Y. (2010) PEG-poly(amino acid) block copolymer micelles for tunable drug release. *Pharm. Res.*, **27**, 2330–2342.
42. Alani, A.W.G., Bae, Y., Rao, D.A., and Kwon, G.S. (2010) Polymeric micelles for the ph-dependent controlled, continuous low dose release of paclitaxel. *Biomaterials*, **31**, 1765–1772.
43. Xiong, X.B., Ma, Z., Lai, R., and Lavasanifar, A. (2010) The therapeutic response to multifunctional polymeric nano-conjugates in the targeted cellular and subcellular delivery of doxorubicin. *Biomaterials*, **31**, 757–768.
44. Francis, R., Joy, N., Aparna, E.P., and Vijayan, R. (2014) Polymer grafted inorganic nanoparticles, preparation, properties, and applications: a review. *Polym. Rev.*, **54**, 268–347.
45. Qi, M., Li, G., Yu, N., Meng, Y., and Liu, X. (2014) Synthesis of thermo-sensitive polyelectrolyte complex nanoparticles from CS-*g*-PNIPAM and SA-*g*-PNIPAM for controlled drug release. *Macromol. Res.*, **22**, 1004–1011.
46. Tan, L., Liu, J., Zhou, W., Wei, J., and Peng, Z. (2014) A novel thermal and pH responsive drug delivery system based on ZnO@PNIPAM hybrid nanoparticles. *Mater. Biol. Appl.*, **45**, 524–529.
47. Qasim, M., Baipaywad, P., Udomluck, N., Na, D., and Park, H. (2014) Enhanced therapeutic efficacy of lipophilic Amphotericin B against *Candida albicans* with amphiphilic poly(*N*-isopropylacrylamide) nanogels. *Macromol. Res.*, **22**, 1125–1131.
48. Shenoy, D., Little, S., Langer, R., and Amiji, M. (2005) Poly(ethylene oxide)-modified poly(β-amino ester) nanoparticles as a pH-sensitive system for tumor-targeted delivery of hydrophobic drugs: *in vitro* evaluations. *Mol. Pharm.*, **2**, 357–366.
49. You, J., Almeda, D., Ye, G.J.C., and Auguste, D.T. (2010) Bioresponsive matrices in drug delivery. *J. Biol. Eng.*, **4**, 1–12.
50. Macewan, S.R., Callahan, D.J., and Chilkoti, A. (2010) Stimulus-responsive macromolecules and nanoparticles for cancer drug delivery. *Nanomedicine (Lond.)*, **5**, 793–806.
51. Chawla, J.S. and Amiji, M.M. (2002) Biodegradable poly(ε-caprolactone) nanoparticles for tumor-targeted delivery of tamoxifen. *Int. J. Pharm.*, **249**, 127–138.
52. Plummer, R., Hill, D.J.T., and Whittaker, A.K. (2006) Solution properties of star and linear poly(N-isopropylacrylamide). *Macromolecules*, **39**, 8379–8388.
53. Onaca, O., Enea, R., Hughes, D.W., and Meier, W. (2009) Stimuli-responsive polymersomes as nanocarriers for drug and gene delivery. *Macromol. Biosci.*, **9**, 129–139.
54. MacEwan, S.R., Callahan, D.J., and Chilkoti, A. (2010) Stimulus-responsive macromolecules and nanoparticles for cancer drug delivery. *Nanomedicine*, **5**, 793–806.

55. Li, L.-Y., He, W.-D., Li, J., Zhang, B.-Y., Pan, T.-T., Sun, X.-L., and Ding, Z.-L. (2010) Shell-cross-linked micelles from PNIPAM-b-$(PLL)_2$ Y-shaped miktoarm star copolymer as drug carriers. *Biomacromolecules*, **11**, 1882–1890.
56. Hoare, T., Santamaria, J., Goya, G.F., Irusta, S., Lin, D., Lau, S., Padera, R., Langer, R., and Kohane, D.S. (2009) A magnetically triggered composite membrane for on-demand drug delivery. *Nano Lett.*, **9**, 3651–3657.
57. Francis, R., Baby, D.K., and Kumar, D.S. (2012) Poly(N-isopropylacrylamide) hydrogel: effect of hydrophilicity on controlled release of ibuprofen at different pH. *J. Appl. Polym. Sci.*, **124**, 5079–5088.
58. Li, G., Song, S., Zhang, T., Qi, M., and Liu, J. (2013) pH-sensitive polyelectrolyte complex micelles assembled from CS-g-PNIPAM and ALG-g-P(NIPAM-co-NVP) for drug delivery. *Int. J. Biol. Macromol.*, **62**, 203–210.
59. Rejinold, N.S., Chennazhi, K.P., Nair, S.V., Tamura, H., and Jayakumar, R. (2011) Biodegradable and thermo-sensitive chitosan-g-poly (N-vinylcaprolactam) nanoparticles as a 5-fluorouracil carrier. *Carbohydr. Polym.*, **83**, 776–786.
60. Xing, J., Deng, L., and Dong, A. (2010) Chitosan/alginate nanoparticles stabilized by poloxamer for the controlled release of 5-fluorouracil. *J. Appl. Polym. Sci.*, **117**, 2354–2359.
61. Zheng, Y., Yang, W., Wang, C., Hu, J., Fu, S., Dong, L., Wu, L., and Shen, X. (2007) Nanoparticles based on the complex of chitosan and polyaspartic acid sodium salt: preparation, characterization and the use for 5-fluorouracil delivery. *Eur. J. Pharm. Biopharm.*, **67**, 621–631.
62. Wang, M., Fang, Y., and Hu, D. (2001) Preparation and properties of chitosan/poly(N- isopropylacrylamide) full-IPN hydrogels. *React. Funct. Polym.*, **48**, 215–221.
63. Zhang, T., Li, G., Guo, L., and Chen, H. (2012) Synthesis of thermo-sensitive CS-g-PNIPAM/CMC complex nanoparticles for controlled release of 5-FU. *Int. J. Biol. Macromol.*, **51**, 1109–1115.
64. Lee, C.C., Gillies, E.R., Fox, M.E., Guillaudeu, S.J., Frechet, J.M., Dy, E.E., and Szoka, F.C. (2006) A single dose of doxorubicin-functionalized bow-tie dendrimer cures mice bearing C-26 colon carcinomas. *Proc. Natl. Acad. Sci. U.S.A.*, **103**, 16649–16654.
65. Astruc, D., Boisselier, E., and Ornelas, C. (2010) Dendrimers designed for functions: from physical, photophysical, and supramolecular properties to applications in sensing, catalysis, molecular electronics, photonics, and nanomedicine. *Chem. Rev.*, **110**, 1857–1959.
66. Ahmed, F., Pakunlu, R.I., Brannan, A., Bates, F., Minko, T., and Discher, D.E. (2006) Biodegradable polymersomes loaded with both paclitaxel and doxorubicin permeate and shrink tumors, inducing apoptosis in proportion to accumulated drug. *J. Controlled Release*, **116**, 150–158.
67. Kurtoglu, Y.E., Navath, R.S., Wang, B., Kannan, S., Romero, R., and Kannan, R.M. (2009) Poly(amidoamine) dendrimer–drug conjugates with disulfide linkages for intracellular drug delivery. *Biomaterials*, **30**, 2112–2121.
68. Mendes, P.M. (2008) Stimuli-responsive surfaces for bio-applications. *Chem. Soc. Rev.*, **37**, 2512–2529.
69. George, P.M., LaVan, D.A., Burdick, J.A., Chen, C.Y., Liang, E., and Langer, R. (2006) Electrically controlled drug delivery from biotin-doped conductive polypyrrole. *Adv. Mater.*, **18**, 577–581.
70. Pernaut, J.-M. and Reynolds, J.R. (2000) Use of conducting electroactive polymers for drug delivery and sensing of bioactive molecules. A redox chemistry approach. *J. Phys. Chem. B*, **104**, 4080–4090.
71. Yavuz, M.S., Cheng, Y., Chen, J., Cobley, C.M., Zhang, Q., Rycenga, M., Xie, J., Kim, C., Song, K.H., Schwartz, A.G., Wang, L.V., and Xia, Y. (2009) Gold nanocages covered by smart polymers for controlled release with near-infrared light. *Nat. Mater.*, **8**, 935–939.
72. Huynh, C.T., Kang, S.W., Li, Y., Kim, B.S., and Lee, D.S. (2011) Controlled release of human growth hormone

from a biodegradable pH/temperature-sensitive hydrogel system. *Soft Matter*, 7, 8984–8990.
73. Juillerat-Jeanneret, L. (2008) The targeted delivery of cancer drugs across the blood-brain barrier: chemical modifications of drugs or drug-nanoparticles? *Drug Discovery Today*, **13**, 1099–1106.
74. Goodman, T.T., Ng, C.P., and Pun, S.H. (2008) 3-D tissue culture systems for the evaluation and optimization of nanoparticle-based drug carriers. *Bioconjugate Chem.*, **19**, 1951–1959.
75. Ganta, S., Devalapally, H., Shahiwala, A., and Amiji, M. (2008) A review of stimuli-responsive nanocarriers for drug and gene delivery. *J. Controlled Release*, **126**, 187–204.
76. Merdan, T., Kopecek, J., and Kissel, T. (2002) Prospects for cationic polymers in gene and oligonucleotide therapy against cancer. *Adv. Drug Delivery Rev.*, **54**, 715–758.
77. Felgner, P.L. (1997) Nonviral strategies for gene therapy. *Sci. Am.*, **276**, 102–106.
78. Han, S., Mahato, R.I., Sung, Y.K., and Kim, S.W. (2000) Development of biomaterials for gene therapy. *Mol. Ther.*, **2**, 302–317.
79. Godbey, W.T. and Mikos, A.G. (2001) Recent progress in gene delivery using non-viral transfer complexes. *J. Controlled Release*, **72**, 115–125.
80. Crommelin, D.J.A., Storm, G., Jiskoot, W., Stenekes, R., Mastrobattista, E., and Hennink, W.E. (2003) Nanotechnological approaches for the delivery of macromolecules. *J. Controlled Release*, **87**, 81–88.
81. Jagur-Grodzinski, J. (2003) Biomedical applications of polymers 2001–2002. *E-Polymers*, **12**, 1–38.
82. Kabanov, A.V. (1999) Taking polycation gene delivery systems from *in vitro* to *in vivo*. *Pharm. Sci. Technol. Today*, **2**, 365–372.
83. Ward, M.A. and Georgiou, T.K. (2011) Thermoresponsive polymers for biomedical applications. *Polymers*, **3**, 1215–1242.
84. Lin, G., Zhang, H., and Huang, L. (2015) Smart polymeric nanoparticles for cancer gene delivery. *Mol. Pharm.*, **12**, 314–321.
85. Lavigne, M.D., Pennadam, S.S., Ellis, J., Alexander, C., and Gorecki, D.C. (2007) Enhanced gene expression through temperature profile-induced variations in molecular architecture of thermoresponsive polymer vectors. *J. Gene Med.*, **9**, 44–54.
86. Twaites, B.R., Alarcon, C.D.H., Lavigne, M., Saulnier, A., Pennadam, S.S., Cunliffe, D., Gorecki, D.C., and Alexander, C. (2005) Thermoresponsive polymers as gene delivery vectors: cell viability, DNA transport and transfection studies. *J. Controlled Release*, **108**, 472–483.
87. Mao, Z.W., Ma, L., Yan, J., Yan, M., Gao, C.Y., and Shen, J.C. (2007) The gene transfection efficiency of thermoresponsive N,N,N-trimethyl chitosan chloride-*g*-poly(N-isopropylacrylamide) copolymer. *Biomaterials*, **28**, 4488–4500.
88. Kurisawa, M., Yokoyama, M., and Okano, T. (2000) Gene expression control by temperature with thermo-responsive polymeric gene carriers. *J. Controlled Release*, **69**, 127–137.
89. Takeda, N., Nakamura, E., Yokoyama, M., and Okano, T. (2004) Temperature-responsive polymeric carriers incorporating hydrophobic monomers for effective transfection in small doses. *J. Controlled Release*, **95**, 343–355.
90. Twaites, B.R., Alarcon, C.D., Cunliffe, D., Lavigne, M., Pennadam, S., Smith, J.R., Gorecki, D.C., and Alexander, C. (2004) Thermo and pH responsive polymers as gene delivery vectors: effect of polymer architecture on DNA complexation *in vitro*. *J. Controlled Release*, **97**, 551–566.
91. Cheng, N., Liu, W.G., Cao, Z.Q., Ji, W.H., Liang, D.C., Guo, G., and Zhang, J.Y. (2006) A study of thermoresponsive poly(N-isopropylacrylamide)/polyarginine bioconjugate non-viral transgene vectors. *Biomaterials*, **27**, 4984–4992.
92. Yang, J.H., Zhang, P., Tang, L., Sun, P., Liu, W.G., Zuo, A.J., and Liang, D.C. (2010) Temperature-tuned DNA

condensation and gene transfection by pei-*g*-(pmeo(2)ma-*b*-phema) copolymer-based nonviral vectors. *Biomaterials*, **31**, 144–155.
93. Zhou, Y.M., Ishikawa, A., Okahashi, R., Uchida, K., Nemoto, Y., Nakayama, M., and Nakayama, Y. (2007) Deposition transfection technology using a DNA complex with a thermoresponsive cationic star polymer. *J. Controlled Release*, **123**, 239–246.
94. Napoli, A., Boerakker, M.J., Tirelli, N., Nolte, R.J.M., Sommerdijk, N.A.J.M., and Hubbell, J.A. (2004) Glucose-oxidase based self-destructing polymeric vesicles. *Langmuir*, **20**, 3487–3491.
95. Lee, J.C.M., Bermudez, H., Discher, B.M., Sheehan, M.A., Won, Y.-Y., Bates, F.S., and Discher, D.E. (2001) Preparation, stability, and *in vitro* performance of vesicles made with diblock copolymers. *Biotechnol. Bioeng.*, **73**, 135–145.
96. Cabane, E., Malinova, V., Menon, S., Palivan, C.G., and Meier, W. (2011) Photoresponsive polymersomes as smart, triggerable nanocarriers. *Soft Matter*, 7, 9167–9176.
97. Christian, D.A., Cai, S., Bowen, D.M., Kim, Y., Pajerowski, J.D., and Discher, D.E. (2009) Polymersome carriers: from self-assembly to siRNA and protein therapeutics. *Eur. J. Pharm. Biopharm.*, **71**, 463–474.
98. Cabane, E., Zhang, X., Langowska, K., Palivan, C.G., and Meier, W. (2012) Stimuli-responsive polymers and their applications in nanomedicine. *Biointerphases*, 7, 1–27.
99. Lee, Y. and Kataoka, K. (2009) Biosignal-sensitive polyion complex micelles for the delivery of biopharmaceuticals. *Soft Matter*, **5**, 3810–3817.
100. Kulkarni, S.S. and Aloorkar, N.H. (2010) Smart polymers in drug delivery: an overview. *J. Pharm. Res.*, **3**, 100–108.
101. Fogueri, L.R. and Singh, S. (2009) Smart polymers for controlled delivery of proteins and peptides: a review of patents. *Recent Pat. Drug Delivery Formul.*, **3**, 40–48.
102. Foss, A.C., Goto, T., Morishita, M., and Pepas, N.A. (2004) Development of acrylic-based copolymers for oral insulin delivery. *Eur. J. Pharm. Biopharm.*, **57**, 163–169.
103. Gil, E.S. and Hudson, S.M. (2004) Stimuli-responsive polymers and their bioconjugates. *Prog. Polym. Sci.*, **29**, 1173–1222.
104. Klouda, L. and Mikos, A.G. (2008) Thermoresponsive hydrogels in biomedical applications. *Eur. J. Pharm. Biopharm.*, **68**, 34–45.
105. Yoon, D.M. and Fisher, J.P. (2007) Polymeric scaffolds for tissue engineering applications, in *Tissue Engineering* (ed. J.P. Fisher), Taylor & Francis, Boca Raton, FL.
106. Kretlow, J.D., Klouda, L., and Mikos, A.G. (2007) Injectable matrices and scaffolds for drug delivery in tissue engineering. *Adv. Drug Delivery Rev.*, **59**, 263–273.
107. Reddi, A.H. (2007) Growth factors and morphogens: signals for tissue engineering, in *Tissue Engineering* (ed. J.P. Fisher), Taylor & Francis, Boca Raton, FL.
108. Vert, M. (2007) Polymeric biomaterials: strategies of the past *vs.* Strategies of the future. *Prog. Polym. Sci.*, **32**, 755–761.
109. Salem, A.K. and Leong, K.W. (2005) Scaffolds for delivery and regenerative medicine, in *Scaffolding in Tissue Engineering* (eds P.X. Ma and J.H. Elisseeff), Taylor & Francis, Boca Raton, FL.
110. Girgorescu, G. and Hunkelerm, D. (2003) Cell encapsulation: generalities, methods, applications and bioartificial pancreas case study, in *Synthetic Polymers for Biotechnology and Medicine* (ed. R. Freitag), Eurekah.com/Landes Bioscience, Georgetown, TX.
111. Place, E.S., George, J.H., Williams, C.K., and Stevens, M.M. (2009) Synthetic polymer scaffolds for tissue engineering. *Chem. Soc. Rev.*, **38**, 1139–1151.
112. Molly, S. (2010) Shoichet, polymer scaffolds for biomaterials applications. *Macromolecules*, **43**, 581–591.
113. Varghese, V.M., Raj, V., Sreenivasan, K., and Kumary, T.V. (2010) *In vitro* cytocompatibility evaluation of a

thermoresponsive nipaam-mma copolymeric surface using l929 cells. *J. Mater. Sci. - Mater. Med.*, **21**, 1631–1639.

114. Ward, M.A. and Georgiou, T.K. (2010) Thermoresponsive terpolymers based on methacrylate monomers: effect of architecture and composition. *J. Polym. Sci., Part A: Polym. Chem.*, **48**, 775–783.

115. Comolli, N., Neuhuber, B., Fischer, I., and Lowman, A. (2009) *In vitro* analysis of PNIPAAm–PEG, a novel, injectable scaffold for spinal cord repair. *Acta Biomater.*, **5**, 1046–1055.

10
Functionally Engineered Sol–Gel Derived Inorganic Gels and Hybrid Nanoarchitectures for Biomedical Applications

Vazhayal Linsha, Kallyadan Veettil Mahesh, and Solaiappan Ananthakumar

10.1
Introduction

> GELS!!! What is gel? … … 'If it looks like a gel, feels like a gel and responds like a gel, it must be a gel (???)' … … … 'It is a state to reorganize than to define' (Dorothy Jordan) … … 'A gel is a gel, as long as one cannot prove that it is not a gel' (K. te Nijenhuis) … … … …

In our daily life, most of us encounter gels often without even realizing it. It is found in a variety of materials including toothpastes, soap, hair gel, gel pens, food products, medicines, electronic machinery, and so on. These gels are composed of either organic or inorganic components. Many of these materials are produced as a result of activities that are conducted in the research field. Thus, research in functional gels is being a hot topic of interest to chemists, physicists, biologists, and materials scientists who aim to fully exploit the prospect of creating new materials to benefit from the best of the three domains: inorganic, organic, and biological. This leads us to focus the present chapter on the illustration of functional gels, specifically sol–gel derived gels and nanoarchitectures, and to elucidate some of the recent advances of such materials in the biomedical field.

From a scientific point of view, gels have long been a topic of debate. Scientists have defined gels in various ways since the time of their recognition. Long back in the year 1861, Graham defined "gels" as [1]: *while the rigidity of the crystalline structure shuts out external expressions, the softness of the gelatinous colloid partakes of fluidity and enables the colloid to become a medium for liquid diffusion, like water itself.*

Later in the same year 1861, Jordan Lloyd defined "gel" as [2]: *only one rule seems to hold for all gels and that is that they must be built up from two components, one which is a liquid at the temperature under consideration and the other which, the gelling substance proper, often spoken of as the gelators, is a solid. The gel itself has the mechanical properties of a solid, i.e. it can maintain its form under stress of its own weight and under any mechanical stress it shows the phenomenon of strain.*

Biomedical Applications of Polymeric Materials and Composites, First Edition.
Edited by Raju Francis and Sakthi Kumar.

Gels are the intermediate state of matter containing both solid and liquid components. The three-dimensional gel network composed of either organic macromolecules (primarily polymers) or inorganic particles are immobilized in liquid as continuous phases. Gels can be classified based on the nature of the solvent immobilized, their physical nature and the drying technique that is adopted to form the solid gel mass. The classification of various gel forms is illustrated in Figure 10.1.

Gels are majorly classified as non-reversible gels and reversible gels [3, 4]. When gels are made of covalently formed cross-links, they are called *non-reversible gels/chemical gels*. If non-covalent interactions such as hydrogen bonds, ionic bonds, or solvophobic interactions are involved in their formation, they are called *reversible gels/physical gels*. Both polymeric and certain inorganic oxides can form three-dimensional gel networks by chemical bonding. For example, polymeric resins such as epoxy resin and a hardener are mixed to form a three-dimensional network, which on curing forms a stiff chemical gel. Similarly, inorganic oxides, especially certain metal-alkoxides such as silicon-alkoxide, undergo hydrolysis and condensation in the presence of water or an organic solvent to form a chemically cross-linked non-reversible chemical gel network of metal-oxo-metal clusters.

Formation of physical/reversible gels is well known in biological and organic systems, but has been less studied and reported in inorganic systems. Organogels/low molecular weight organic gelators (LMWGs) [5–7], natural/biopolymeric gels (e.g., cellulose derivatives, gelatin, polysaccharides, gellan

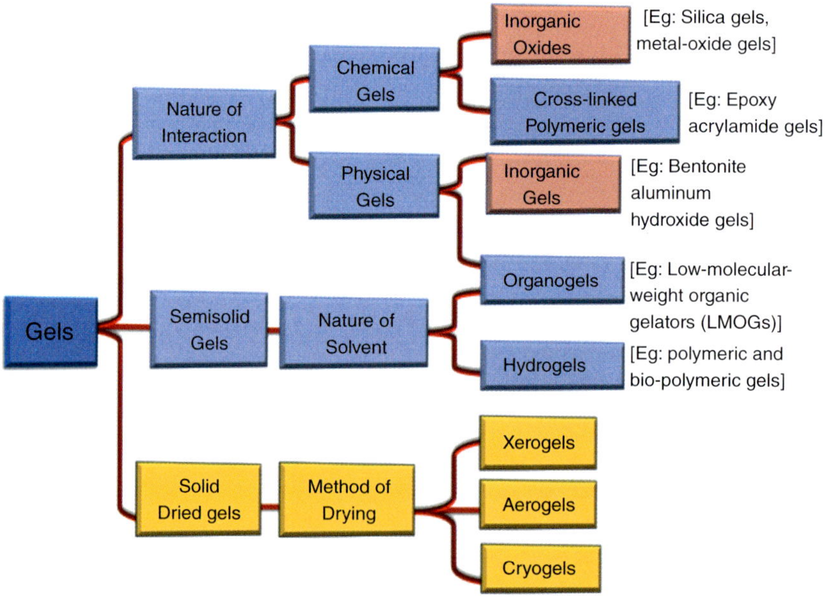

Figure 10.1 Classification of various types of gels.

gum, proteins), synthetic polymeric gels (e.g., polystyrene and polyethylene oxide and pluronic triblock copolymers such as poly-(ethylene glycol)-poly-(propylene glycol)-poly(ethylene glycol) (PEG-PPG-PEG) etc.) have been widely investigated as stimuli-responsive physical gels [8–10]. These networks are broken down easily by an external stimulus, such as heat, mechanical stress, electric and magnetic field, acid or base, and electrochemical reactions [9–12]. They undergo formation and degradation when specific changes in the conditions (external stimulus) are induced.

The gels can be dried and obtained in various solid forms. Depending upon the method of drying, gels may be classified as xerogel (obtained by using the conventional drying method), cryogel (obtained by the freeze drying process), and aerogel (formed by replacing the liquid phase with air by the supercritical drying method).

10.2 Some of the Useful Definitions of Various Gel Forms

10.2.1 Based on the Nature of the Solvent, Entrapped Gels are Classified as Hydrogels and Organogels (Figure 10.2)

10.2.1.1 Hydrogels/Aquagels (Water-Based Gels)

These are gels that contain water as their continuous liquid phase (i.e., they can contain over 99.9% of water). Inorganic gels (e.g., aluminum hydroxide and silicone hydrogel) and polymeric gels (gelatin, cellulose, and poloxamer) are some of the common hydrogels.

10.2.1.2 Organogels (Gels with a Non-Aqueous Solvent)

Gels of this type contain any kind of organic solvent or oil as their continuous liquid phase. Polymeric gels (e.g., polyethylene glycol, polylactic acid, polycarbonate, and polyalkylene) and LMWGs (e.g., fatty acids, amino acids, and *n*-alkanes) are some of the common organogels.

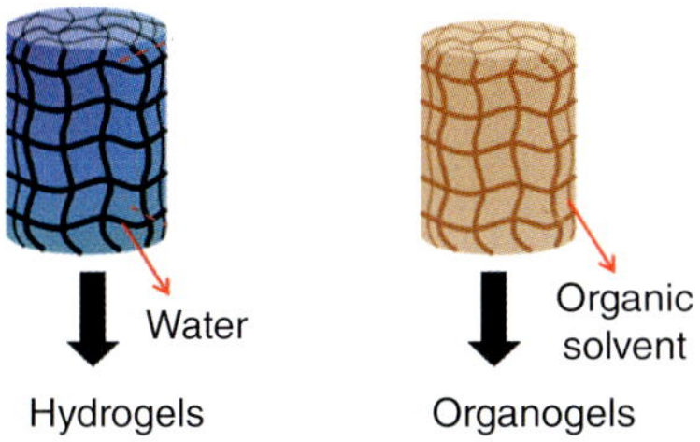

Figure 10.2 Classification of gels based on nature of solvent.

10.2.2 Based on Physical Nature, Gels are Classified as Elastic and Rigid Gels (Figure 10.3)

10.2.2.1 Elastic Gels (Physical Gels)

These gels are formed by some physical aggregation or temporary cross-linking interactions. Agar gel, cellulose, guar gum, and alginates exhibit an elastic behavior. The fibrous polymeric network is cross-linked at the point of junction by relatively weak bonds such as hydrogen bonds and by dipole attraction. On dehydration it can be changed to a solid structure and can be reverted to its original form by absorbing water; this phenomenon is called *imbibition*.

10.2.2.2 Rigid Gels (Chemical Gels)

These are formed by strong chemical cross-linking. In silica gel, molecules are held by strong siloxane (Si–O–Si) linkage to give a polymer structure possessing a network of pores. They neither change back to their original form nor do they show imbibition. Some other examples are alumina, titania- and ferric oxide-based metal-oxide gels, and so on.

10.2.3 Based on Drying Techniques, Gels are Classified as Xerogels, Aerogels, and Cryogels (Figure 10.4)

10.2.3.1 Xerogels

Solid gels with no solvent concentration are known as *xerogels*, which are formed after evaporation of the solvent in a hydrogel or an organogel by drying at ambient conditions. Xerogels usually retain less porosity (15–50%) and surface area ($100–900\ m^2\ g^{-1}$), in addition to having very small pore size (1–10 nm).

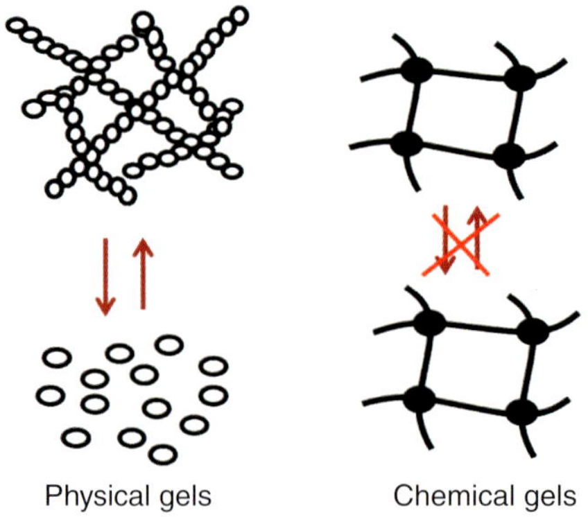

Figure 10.3 Classification of gels based on physical interactions.

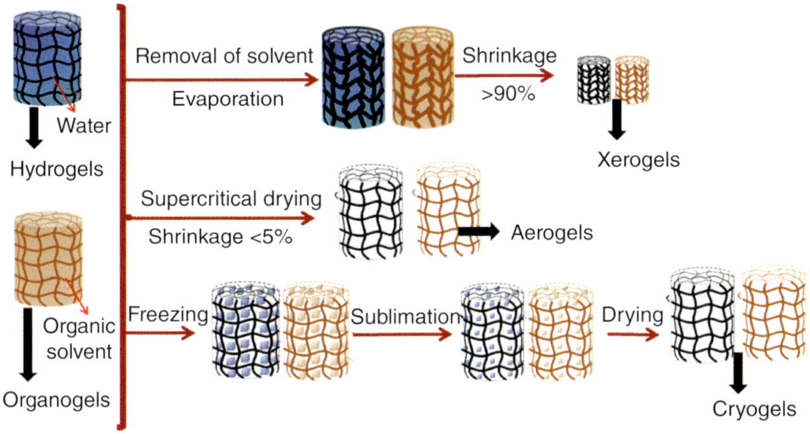

Figure 10.4 Classification of gels based on drying techniques.

10.2.3.2 Cryogels

This is another solid gel mass obtained by the drying technique in which the liquid in the gel is frozen into a solid and then sublimed. The vapor can be removed by vacuum pumping, and the resultant gel is called *cryogel* since cryogenic conditions are typically involved in drying.

10.2.3.3 Aerogel

These solid gels are formed when the solvent removal occurs under supercritical conditions; the network does not shrink and a highly porous, low-density material is produced. Aerogels are materials with exceptional properties including very low density, enormous high specific surface areas, and excellent thermal insulation. Silica aerogel (the first known inorganic aerogels), organic or carbon aerogels, and graphene aerogels are some of the common aerogels known. Interestingly, as of 2013, graphene is recorded as the world's lightest material.

10.2.4 Based on Rheological Properties, Gels are Classified as Plastic Gels, Pseudoplastic Gels, and Thixotropic Gels (Figure 10.5)

Based on the flow and deformation, viscoelastic materials are categorized as Newtonian or non-Newtonian material [13]. For a Newtonian material, a direct proportionality exists between shear rate and shear stress; that is, the viscosity remains constant with respect to the time of shearing. If no direct relationship exists between shear stress and shear rate, such a material is called *non-Newtonian material*. Non-Newtonian material shows both time-independent properties (plasticity, pseudoplasticity, and dilatancy) and time-dependent properties (thixotropy and rheopexy) [13–15]. In rheological studies, a flow curve represents the relationship between shear stress (τ) and shear rate (γ) and a viscosity curve represents the relationship between viscosity (η) and shear rate (γ) or shear

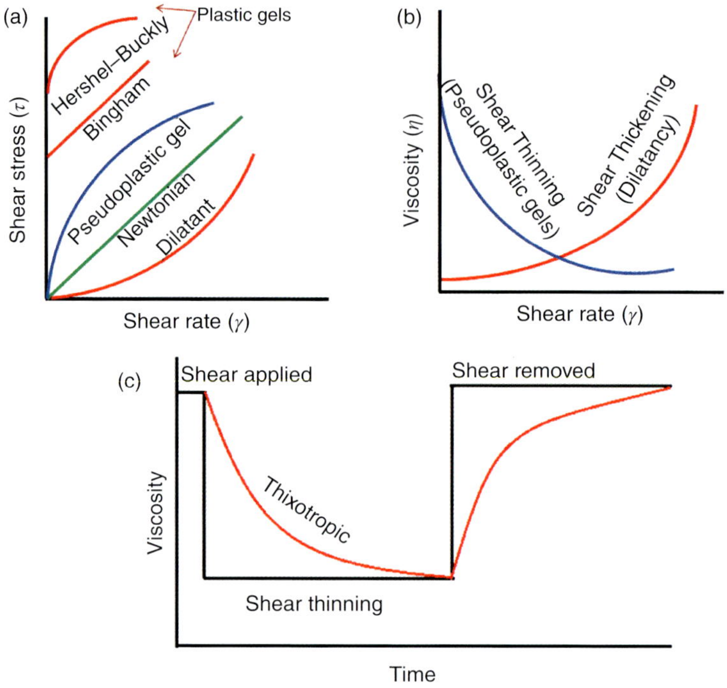

Figure 10.5 (a) Flow curve representing various types of rheological behavior. (b) Viscosity curve of a pseudoplastic and dilatant gel. (c) Viscosity–time curve of thixotropic gels.

stress (τ). Major types of rheological properties exhibited by gels are their plastic, pseudoplastic, and thixotropic behavior.

10.2.4.1 Plastic Gels

These are gels that require a finite yield stress or yield point, to make them flow. The gels are not deformed below the yield point, but get deformed above the yield point. Bingham and Herschel–Bulkley models represent the viscoplasticity of the material. Flocculated aluminum hydroxide gel and polymeric PVC gel exhibit a plastic flow and the plot of the flow curve gives the yield stress of the gels above which the gel deforms and begins to flow.

10.2.4.2 Pseudoplastic Gels

These gels exhibit a decrease in viscosity with increase in shear stress, with no yield value; such gels are also called as *shear thinning gels*. Sodium alginate and most of the cellulosic gels exhibit pseudoplastic flow.

10.2.4.3 Dilatant Gels

These gels exhibit an increase in viscosity with increase in shear stress. Dilatancy is also known as *shear thickening* behavior. Suspensions of starch in water, aqueous glycerin, and concentration of inorganic pigments in water are all examples that exhibit dilatancy.

10.2.4.4 Thixotropic Gels

These gels exhibit a property wherein they dissolve when stirred or shaken and return to the gel state upon resting. The bonds between the particles in these gels are very weak and can be broken down by mechanical stress. The resulting solution will revert back to the gel state by subsequent rest phase due to the clustering of the particles or by physical cross-linking. Agar gels, gelatin gels, iron oxide gels, and certain clays such as kaolin and bentonite, exhibit thixotropic property.

Until now, we have very briefly elucidated the structural properties of various kinds of gels, and key terminologies have been used to define such gels. Now, in the coming section we will be discussing the various inorganic metal oxide gels and hybrid inorganic–organic nanostructures derived from the sol–gel synthetic route. Furthermore, we aim to illustrate the versatility of this material by focusing on the recent applications in the biomedical field.

10.3 Inorganic Metal-Oxide Gels and Hybrid Nanoarchitectures

Inorganic metal-oxide gels have been known since the early developments in sol–gel chemistry. The first inorganic gel reported in 1846 by Ebelmen was the silica gel derived from silicon-alkoxide [16]. The first alumina gel was synthesized in 1870 by Cossa [17]. Since then, sol–gel synthetic chemistry has experienced tremendous advancement in the development of inorganic metal-oxide gels. Many types of metal-oxide gels such as silicon dioxide (silica), aluminum oxide (alumina), titanium dioxide (titania), zirconium dioxide (zirconia), and aluminosilicate gels are derived from metal salt and metal-alkoxide precursors [17, 18]. Apart from this, sol–gel processing is a versatile technology for the synthesis of hybrid materials with diverse properties, which has now turned out to be a fascinating field of research in materials chemistry. Thus, in the coming section we have first very briefly described the chemistry of sol–gel processing of inorganic metal-oxide gels, and followed it by emphasizing on inorganic–organic hybrid nanostructured material obtained by the sol–gel processing route. Since the chapter focuses on biomedical applications, emphasis is given on sol–gel derived inorganic gels and nanostructured materials that are exceedingly explored for bio-application.

10.4 Sol–Gel Synthesis of Inorganic Metal-Oxide Gels

The sol–gel method is an important technique for processing metal-oxide gels at low temperature, which has been practiced for the past two centuries. The detailed physics and chemistry involved in the sol–gel processing has been reviewed in many books and journal publications [17–19]. Sol–gel process may be simply described as: *Formation of an oxide gel network through poly-condensation reactions of a molecular precursor in a liquid at low temperature.*

Generally, a sol–gel reaction involves two different systems of gelation routes: one follows condensation of colloidal particles and cluster growth, and the other follows cross-linking of polymeric molecules (Figure 10.6).

Colloidal gels are generally formed from metal salts such as chlorides, nitrates, and sulfates. In a colloidal pathway, first the nanoparticles (NPs) with a size below a micrometer are synthesized, which is found to be in a dispersed state in the solvent, and the suspension is termed a *colloidal sol*. In the second step, discrete colloidal particles cross-link with each other by hydrogen bonding or by electrostatic attraction so as to build a three-dimensional gel network. The transformation of a sol to a gel constitutes the gelation process, and the gels that are obtained are termed *colloidal gels* [20]. Here, the electrolytic and steric effects of the particles of the colloidal sol induce the gel formation mechanism. On the other hand, in polymeric gels, chemical reaction is the driving force for gelation. Here, linear polymeric chains are formed without the intermediate formation of individual particles. When this occurs, suspensions of highly branched three-dimensional gel structure are obtained, and they are termed *polymeric gels* [20]. Metal-alkoxides are most widely used precursors for polymeric gel formation. In the case of sol–gel synthesis of silica gels, depending upon the conditions, such as pH, water to alkoxide molar ratio and dilution, either colloidal or polymeric gels can be obtained [20]. Silica sol derived from alkoxide solution, forms linear polymeric species at low pH (i.e., pH >2.5) and lower water to alkoxide ratio and, hence, results in the formation of polymeric gel whereas, at higher pH (pH >2.5), weakly cross-linked silica clusters are formed regardless of water to alkoxide molar ratio, and thus form colloidal silica gels.

At the advent of sol–gel technology, metallic salts were commonly used as the precursors for the synthesis of inorganic metal-oxide gels. But now, metal-alkoxides are largely used for the synthesis. The major steps involved in the

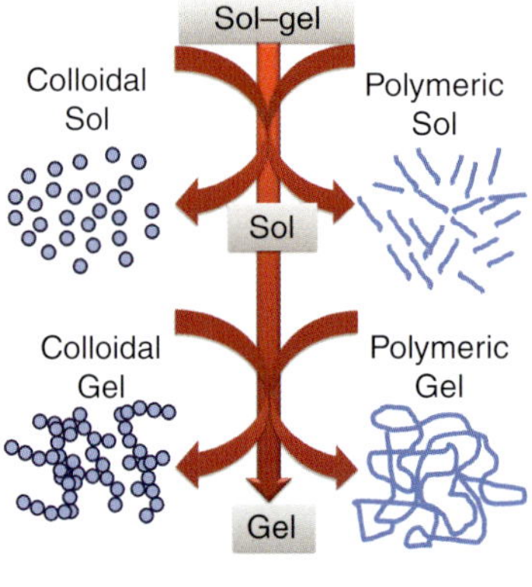

Figure 10.6 The two main types inorganic gels derived from sol–gel technique are colloidal and polymeric gel.

sol–gel process when metal-alkoxide is used as the precursor are:

$$M - OR + H_2O \rightarrow M - OH + HO - R \rightarrow \text{Hydrolysis}$$
$$M - OR + HO - M \rightarrow M - O - M + HO - R \rightarrow \text{Condensation (alcoxolation)}$$
$$M - OH + HO - M \rightarrow M - O - M + H_2O \rightarrow \text{Condensation (oxolation)}$$

where M stand for metal and R stands for alkyl groups. Basically, the transition from a sol to a gel relies on the hydrolysis and condensation reactions. The alkoxy group of metal-alkoxide reacts with the water to form a hydroxyl group, which is called *hydrolysis*. After the alkoxide is partly hydrolyzed, condensation occurs. Different metal atoms are bridged by an oxygen atom via an alcoxolation reaction between a hydroxyl group and an alkoxy group or an oxolation reaction between two separated hydroxyl groups. As a result, a stable dispersion of metal-oxide sol covered with an active group such as the hydroxyl is formed in the solvent. These are cross-linked via the condensations of surface active groups resulting in the formation of metal-oxide gels. Process parameters such as pH, solvent, catalyst, precursor's concentrations, temperature, and so on, can significantly affect the final gel properties. These fundamental investigations have been intensively explored by different researchers [21–23]. However, in the final step, most of the inorganic metal-oxide gels are dried using various techniques, which produce so-called xerogels and aerogels. Other than silica, alumina, zirconia, titania, and so on are some of the well-known and widely studied inorganic metal-oxide gels [21–25].

Inorganic metal-oxide aerogels and xerogels are classic nanoporous materials derived out of sol–gel metal-oxide gels. Given the importance of metal-oxide aerogels, we will discuss it in detail. The basic research scheme involved in the synthesis of metal-oxide aerogels is shown in Figure 10.7.

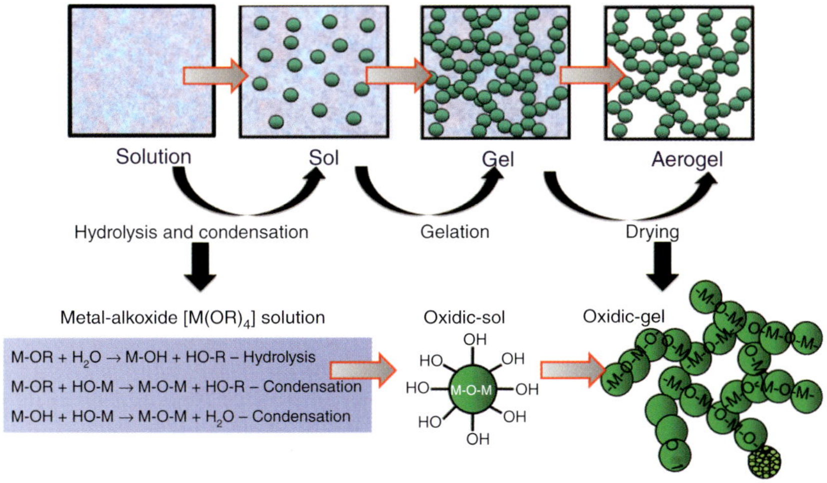

Figure 10.7 Basic synthesis scheme for the metal-oxide aerogels.

Metal-alkoxides are well-known precursors for the synthesis of metal-oxide aerogels [26]. As per the sol–gel synthetic route metal-alkoxides are subjected to hydrolysis and condensation reactions. The sols derived from the metal-alkoxide are generally more stable and well dispersed in the solvent. It is composed of nanoscale oxidic particles covered with active hydroxyl groups. When these nanooxidic particles are cross-linked by condensation of surface active hydroxyl groups, it results in gelation to form a metal-oxo-metal gel network. When solvent molecules are removed, without disturbing the three-dimensional gel frameworks by supercritical drying, metal-oxidic aerogels are formed. Drying of the wet gels is one of the critical steps involved in aerogel synthesis [26, 27]. Shrinkage of the gel has to be minimized during the drying step. Hence, during the supercritical drying process, the solvent in the wet gel is removed above the critical temperature and critical pressure of the concerned solvent is locked in the wet gel. Thus, there will be no liquid–vapor interface in the pores during drying. As a consequence, aerogels with no shrinkage is obtained. Similarly, other methods such as freeze drying can be adopted to obtain aerogels [26], wherein pore liquid is frozen and sublimed under vacuum, to avoid liquid–vapor interface during drying.

Remarkable properties of these materials showed great potential for a wide range of applications. Particularly, metal-oxide aerogels gained more importance because of their very low density, outstanding textural properties, large surface area, low thermal conductivity, refractive index, and dielectric constant [26–28]. Silica was the first reported aerogel by Kistler in the early 1930s, which was produced by making use of the sol–gel reaction of silica-alkoxides [29]. Soon after that, wide varieties of inorganic-oxide aerogels such as alumina [30], titania [31], zirconia [32], iron oxide [33] and many others; non-oxides such as chalcogenides [34]; and organic aerogels such as carbon and polymeric aerogels [35, 36] were developed.

In addition to various single component aerogels, binary and ternary oxide aerogels were developed. In such multicomponent or mixed-oxide aerogels, because of the large difference in reaction rate of mixed-oxide precursors, phase separation and heterogeneous structure are largely formed. To control the sol–gel reaction rate of mixed-oxide gels, bidentate ligands are often used [30]. Similarly, to improve the existing properties of aerogels, such as high surface area, hydrophobicity, flexibility, and transparency, organic modification were carried out to obtain hybrid aerogels [36–40]. Because of their exceptional characteristics and diverse chemical compositions, aerogels, especially metal-oxide aerogels, have significant prospects in new fields of functional materials.

The sol–gel process is one of the fastest growing technologies in modern chemistry and is expected to provide a versatile solution for processing advanced functional materials. The main advantages of this process are ensuring better homogeneity and purity of the obtained material, requiring low processing temperature thereby saving energy, and resulting in special properties that improve material quality. It offers the possibility of fabricating advanced materials in

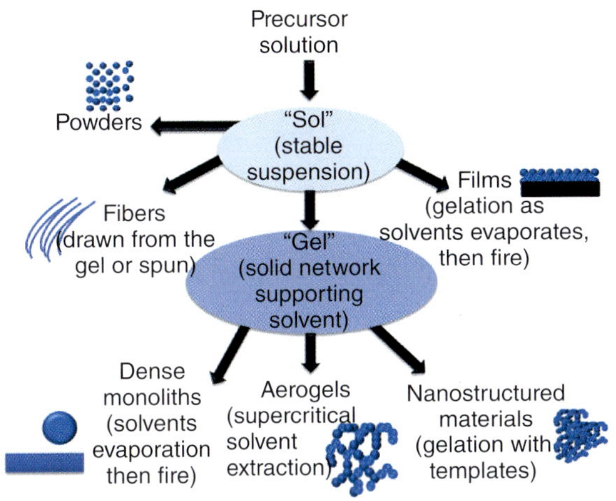

Figure 10.8 Various materials obtained by sol–gel technology and its processing route.

various structures: ultra-fine or spherical powders, fibers, dense monoliths, aerogels, thin films, and diverse nanostructured materials. Various sol–gel materials obtained and their processing route are shown schematically in Figure 10.8. The flexibility of sol–gel technology facilitates in controlling the characteristics of the material required for functional applications. We will highlight the use of sol–gel derived materials in biomedical applications in the later section of this chapter.

10.5 Physically Cross-Linked Inorganic and Hybrid Gel

So far, we have addressed the covalently linked inorganic gel system. Non-covalently associated inorganic gels by weak supramolecular interactions or stimuli-responsive behavior are very rarely studied and reported in a sol–gel system. In this section, we will be discussing some of the rare reports on physically cross-linked inorganic and hybrid inorganic–organic gels.

Physically cross-linked self-assembling gels are capable of delivering responsive functions upon sensing any external stimuli (Figure 10.9). They have received considerable attention in recent time in the designing of advanced functional soft biomaterials [10, 41, 42]. Since physically cross-linked gels show stimuli-responsive, smart function, plentiful interest has been triggered in designing soft gels out of natural/synthetic polymers, biomolecules of amino acids and peptide chains, low molecular weight organo gelators (LMOGs) and inorganic–organic hybrids, via supramolecular association. So far, a comprehensive research effort has been made to form three-dimensional (3D) gel assembly through different physical and chemical cross-linking strategies. Such molecularly engineered organo/hydro gels display fascinating reversible nature where the gels revert to their original state after a physical or chemical disturbance. Switching of

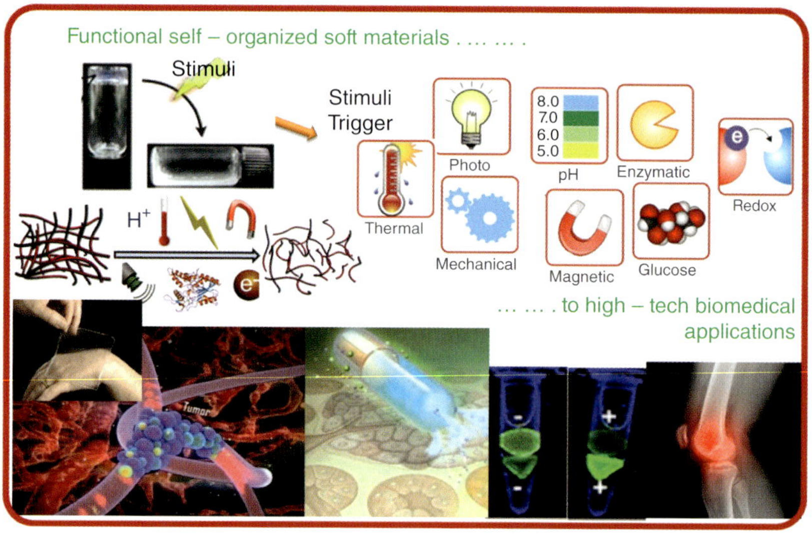

Figure 10.9 An overview of various external stimuli-triggered formation of soft gel for designing functional soft biomaterial.

reversibility has been recorded in response to factors such as change in temperature, pH, electric or magnetic fields, ionic strength, solvent polarity, and mechanical stimulation (Figure 10.9) [5–7, 10, 11, 41–44].

Studies indicate that this kind of remarkable functioning of synthetic soft gels finds applications in tissue engineering, cell culture, bio-adhesion mediators, drug delivery systems, wound healing, injectable therapies, and so on. Usually, in the inorganic system, the formation of covalent bonds allows an irreversible sol–gel transition, or else such systems deliberately require chemical anchoring from organo/polymeric molecules to aid stimuli-responsive gel assembly [7, 10, 11]. Reviewing the literature reports on various types of physically cross-linked gels, major reports were based on stimuli-responsive organic and polymeric gels; reports were scanty in self-association of inorganic nanoparticles as a main node in forming transient 3D gel network.

Normally, colloidal metal-oxide gels formed in the intermediate stage of sol–gel synthesis exhibit a solid-like linear viscoelastic rheological property. Due to its rigid siloxane networking, silica forms a chemical gel, in which bond destruction is irreversible, whereas, some of the investigations on alumina-based colloidal system, especially aluminum oxy hydroxide (boehmite), reported the formation of a physical gel [13–15, 45]. Both colloidal and polymeric alumina gels can form weak gel assemblies. Gelation studies in boehmite gels also reported "thixotropic gelation" in which destruction–reconstruction of a gel network is possible. Thixotropy is a time-dependent rheological property showing shear-thinning behavior, with reversible mechano-responsive property [13, 14]. Other than boehmite, metal-oxides such as ferric-oxide and alumino-silicate gels also show thixotropic properties [15, 46, 47]. In some of the studies, metal-oxides are made

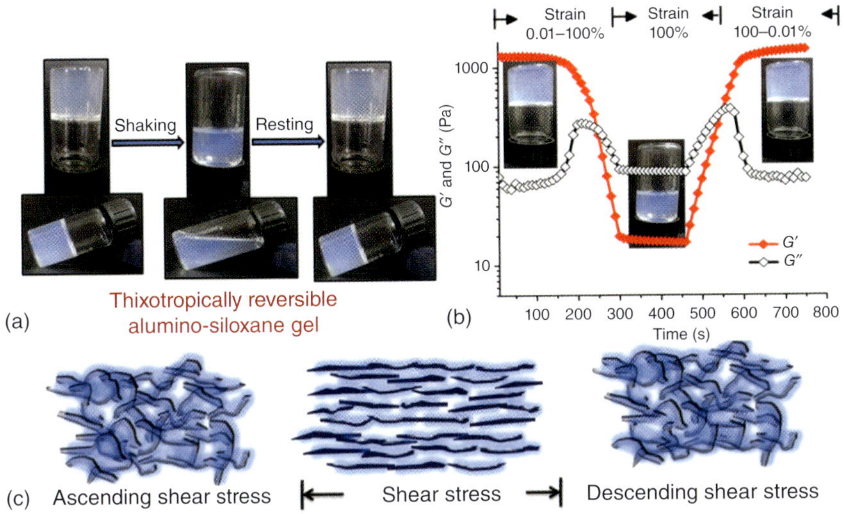

Figure 10.10 (a) Photograph of thixotropically reversible alumino-siloxane gel. (b) Step-strain time dependent rheological analysis of the alumino-siloxane gel. (c) Schematic representation of possible structural changes in aquagel subjected to shear flow. (Linsha 2015 [47]. Reproduced with permission of The Royal Society of Chemistry.)

to cross-link with (bio) a polymeric organic network to induce stimuli-responsive behavior with physically weak gel networking [7, 48]. Our group reported the formation of physically weak assembly of inorganic alumino-siloxane gels at room temperature without the addition of any external gelators or monomer molecules as shown in Figure 10.10 [47]. The alumino-siloxane gels obtained by sol–gel synthesis showed a unique thixotropic (mechano-responsive) property with an impressive recovery rate (Figure 10.10b). It was identified to be a mechanically stable, injectable, and non-cytotoxic medium for drug delivery applications.

10.6 Sol–Gel Derived Hybrid Metal-Oxides Nanostructures

Basically, the conventional division between inorganic and organic chemistry has been such that, for a long time these two fields of science were addressed by quite different groups of chemists, with practically no contact between them. More recently, these two fields of chemistry have begun to amalgamate with the development of hybrid inorganic–organic material. Synthesis of hybrid materials can be achieved via a modification of inorganic structure with organic components. Various synthetic strategies were adopted for the design of new hybrid materials. Sol–gel chemistry is considered to be a significant tool for the incorporation of organic (bio) components into the inorganic network, allowing the preparation of a variety of hybrid architectures. In the coming section, we will briefly discuss hybrid metal-oxide nano structured materials derived from the sol–gel synthetic route.

Sol–gel polymerization coupled with self-assembly of amphiphilic molecules (surfactant templates), results in a supramolecular association of organic molecules within inorganic matrices. The templating effect of supramolecular systems in the inorganic matrix leads to the formation of a mesostructured hybrid phase (Figure 10.11A). The synthesis can be performed in either acidic or basic medium. The most well-known representatives of this class of materials are silica-based mesoporous inorganic–organic hybrids. Synthesis of mesostructured silica has proved to be a major breakthrough for materials science in the past decades [49–53]. Here, we can have a very brief overview of inorganic–organic hybrid mesostructured sol–gel material.

Mesoporous silica (MSN) comprises an amazing family of porous materials that show ordered arrangements of pores as channels and cavities with different geometries. The source of silica can be fumed silica, sodium silicate, or a tetra alkyl ortho-silicate, and organosilane. The synthesis of MSN was first reported in the early 1990s. Since then, a variety of highly ordered MSN materials such as MCM-41[50], MCM-48 [51], SBA-15 [52], MSU [53], FDU [53], HMS [54], KIT [55], and so on have been successfully synthesized using different synthesis

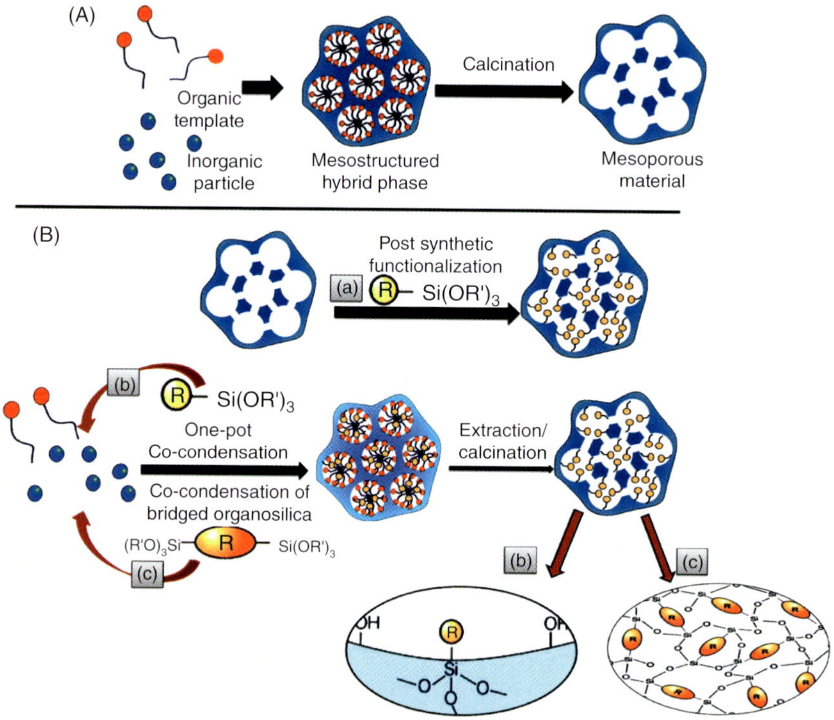

Figure 10.11 General synthetic pathway for (A) mesoporous silica (B) mesoporous inorganic–organic hybrid silica.

conditions and types of templating agents. These materials showed exceptional properties such as high surface area (*ca.* 1000 $m^2 g^{-1}$), large pore volume (*ca.* 1 $cm^3 g^{-1}$), and tunable pore diameters (*ca.* 2–10 nm) which are well organized in the 3D- and 2D-mesostructures [48–54]. The textural and structural properties of these sol–gel nanostructured materials were attained by properly tuning the synthetic parameters such as surfactant/precursor ratio, pH, solvent, and so on. A series of investigations were carried out and reported by many researches, for designing new hybrid MSN nanostructures by the above-mentioned synthetic route [56–58].

Modification of mesoporous walls of the silica framework with organic functional groups lead to hybrid mesoporous materials [58]. The functionalization of the MSN is necessary for different reasons, such as to improve surface properties, to modify the textural and structural features, and so on . Extensive efforts have been undertaken to incorporate organic components within an inorganic framework to achieve synergetic properties of both organic and inorganic components. Normally, organic functionalization can be achieved by: (i) grafting of organic components on the surface of pure silica matrix (via. post-functionalization method) (ii) one-pot co-condensation of silica with organo-silylating agents, and (iii) use of bridged organic precursors to form periodic mesoporous materials (Figure 10.11B).

When mesoporous structure is functionalized via the post-synthetic grafting method, organic functional groups are found to be located on the exterior surface. This method shows its own drawback, namely, blocking the interior mesochannels of porous structure, and can also lead to a heterogeneous surface coverage. While, in a co-condensation method, the organic molecules can be homogeneously distributed in the system, with a better control over the functionalization procedure. Similarly, multifunctionality can also be induced in the system by introducing bridged organic precursors.

In addition, key properties of the material can be well adjusted by incorporation of molecular functionality in a controlled way, which are crucial for various applications. Thus, selective functionalization of sol–gel derived mesoporous material becomes a point of interest when designing more sophisticated materials with multifunctionality [59–61]. Thus, the emerging area of chemistry and life sciences opens up great opportunities for researchers to exploit this material for designing controllable drug delivery systems and targeted theranostics functions in biology and medicine. This will be discussed in detail in the following section.

10.7
Biomedical Applications of Sol–Gel Derived Inorganic and Hybrid Nanoarchitectures for Both Therapeutic and Diagnostic (Theranostics) Functions

In the past few decades "soft organic materials" such as lipid-based and (bio) polymeric materials dominated the field of biomedical applications for therapeutic and diagnostic functions. With the burgeoning of nanotechnology, a great deal of interest in inorganic and inorganic–organic hybrid materials for theranostic functions has been shown. Indeed, these materials have extraordinary properties that can resolve many of the medical problems when compared to polymeric pulpits. The new group of materials representing sol–gel derived inorganic gels and hybrid nanoarchitectures, show good potential for fulfilling the current requirements and challenges in the biomedical field. In this section we will focus on sol–gel derived matrixes, especially inorganic metal-oxide gels and hybrid nanomaterial, and explore their potential for theranostic functions.

10.8 Sol–Gel Matrices for Controlled Drug Delivery

10.8.1 Metal-Oxide Xerogels

The use of silica-based metal-oxides gels, as matrices for controlled drug release, has been largely demonstrated in various research reports [62–69]. Silica xerogels were investigated as a potential biomaterial for the extended and controlled release of different kinds of biologically active agents [62, 63]. Kortesuo and coworkers reported that silica xerogel could be impregnated with tritium-labeled toremifene citrate for controlled drug release [64]. The study established that silica xerogel is a biocompatible, biodegradable, and controllably resorbable material and hence it is a promising matrix for use in the sustained delivery of drugs. Bottcher and coworkers [66] performed a detailed analysis of drug release behavior from silica xerogels by incorporating nifedipine into a silica matrix using the sol–gel technique. Similarly, Maver and collaborators [68] incorporated the same nifedipine drug in a hybrid silica xerogels matrix. This study focused on the importance of the physical state of nifedipine in a silica matrix and concluded that the solid matrix may contain the drug in the amorphous form rather than in the crystalline state. In general, the amorphous form of drugs shows a faster dissolution and higher solubility when compared with the crystalline form. Roveri *et al.* [69] investigated the effect of release kinetics of heparins from sol–gel derived silica xerogel matrix. Here, the authors concluded that drug release kinetics depends on the specific surface area of the xerogel matrix, which could be modified by varying the catalyst/alkoxide molar ratio. The release kinetics of heparin from xerogels matrix depended on the molecular mass of the heparin; in this study, release kinetics mostly fitted with the Higuchi diffusion model, but in the case of matrices with lower surface areas, zero-order kinetics was observed. In many of the studies, various xerogel synthesis parameters (such as pH, water/alkoxide ratio, temperature, type or concentration of the catalyst, and drying and heating conditions) were evaluated for their effects on the embedded drug release properties [66–69]. All these studies concluded that the drug release pattern strongly depends on the physical, chemical, structural, and textural features of the sol–gel matrix.

10.8.2 Metal-Oxide Aerogels

Currently, research is being focused on improving the pharmacokinetics and pharmacodynamics of the controlled drug delivery system. Because of high surface area, porosities, and open porous framework, inorganic aerogels represent a promising class of material for drug delivery [70–73]. Apart from such unique properties, flexibility of sol–gel chemistry plays an important role in designing an aerogel-based drug delivery system.

Drug molecules can be loaded in an aerogel matrix by various routes. Three different methods that are generally adopted for drug loading in an aerogel matrix, are well illustrated in Figure 10.12 [71]. Although loading of drug before the gelation process (Figure 10.12a) can be considered to be a simplified process, there is a chance of leaching out of drug molecules at the time of solvent exchange and aging process. Drug can also be loaded, through solvent exchange and aging process (Figure 10.12b). This method requires an extended time, and care has to be taken to ensure that the solvent and the drug molecules are compatible. In another approach, drugs are loaded directly into a pure aerogel matrix (Figure 10.12c). In such cases, the structure of the aerogel matrix collapses when immersed in the drug solution (especially in case of fragile silica aerogels). Hence, recently, new techniques have been adopted for drug loading. One such method is loading the drug from the supercritical phase. Here, drugs are necessary to be soluble in supercritical fluids such as CO_2, and offer various advantages such as non-toxicity, easy removability, control over thermodynamics of adsorption

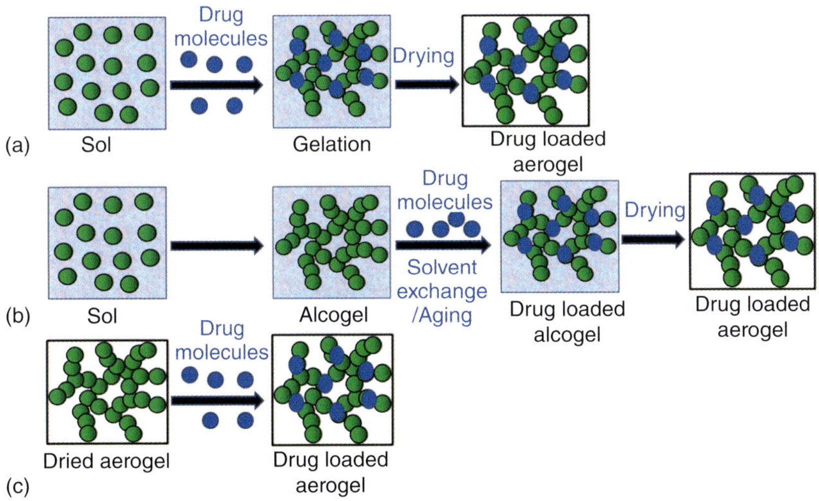

Figure 10.12 Different methods adopted for drug loading in aerogel matrix. (a) Addition of drug before gelation in sol–gel synthesis. (b) Addition of drug during aging process in sol–gel process. (c) Addition of drugs in pure (dried) aerogels obtained after sol–gel synthesis.

process [72, 73]. Various studies showed that it was one of the effective methods used in drug loading [72–75].

Among various inorganic metal-oxide aerogels that were investigated for drug delivery, silica-based materials were shown to be chemically inert and biocompatible with the human body [70]. Schwertfeger *et al.* [70] first reported the use of both hydrophilic and hydrophobic aerogels (e.g., silica, alumina, titania, zirconia, or mixtures) as a potential carrier material for several pharmaceutically active compounds (PhACs). They have demonstrated that hydrophilic aerogels are suitable for the incorporation of hydrophobic drugs and hydrophobic aerogels are suitable for hydrophilic drugs. Similarly, Smirnova and coworkers [72–76] conducted numerous experiments using silica aerogels for drug delivery applications. Instead of adsorption of drugs directly on the surface of pure aerogel matrix, this group studied the adsorption of drugs by dissolving in supercritical-CO_2. This could improve the solubility of poorly soluble active drugs such as furosemide-sodium [70], griseofulvin [72, 73], ketoprofen [72, 74], penbutulol hemisulfate [70], methylprednisolone [70], miconazole [74], and so on. The same group demonstrated that large amount of drugs can be loaded in an aerogel matrix by adsorption from supercritical-CO_2 [73]. They have concluded that loading mainly depends on the molecular size of drug molecules, and their release rate can be improved to four to five times higher than their crystalline form. Similarly, in another study they have demonstrated the thermodynamic of adsorption isotherm of various types of drugs such as ketoprofen, griseofulvin, miconazole, flurbiprofen, and dithranol [72, 73] from supercritical-CO_2. In most of the cases, the adsorption isotherm fitted into Langmuir model, which signifies that loading can be increased until it reaches the saturation point of aerogel matrix. If the solubility of drugs in supercritical-CO_2 is found to be lower, it was observed that the drug adsorbed in the matrix remain low and do not reach the saturation point. Similarly, solubility of the drug in supercritical-CO_2 not only depends on the chemical nature of the drug but also on temperature, pressure, and density of the supercritical phase. In addition to silica aerogels other inorganic aerogels such as titania, alumina, dysprosia, and inorganic–organic hybrid aerogels [77–81] were recently studied for their roles in drug delivery applications.

10.8.3 Physically Cross-Linked Inorganic and Hybrid Gel

Stimuli-responsive physical gels find applications in tissue engineering, cell culture, bio-adhesion mediators, drug delivery systems, wound healing, injectable therapies, and so on. Physically cross-linked and stimuli-responsive behavior are generally reported in a polymeric gel system. Polymer-based physical gels are explored widely for biomedical applications. Now, physically cross-linked sol–gel derived metal-oxide gels and their hybrids obtained by cross-linking with organic components are emerging as new materials for biomedical applications.

Physically cross-linked gels are always preferred for injection therapies and topical drug delivery applications. Sol–gel derived silica has proved to be an excellent material for controlled drug delivery system; however, it has shown to be incapable for use in injection therapies and topical drug delivery applications. On the other hand, sol–gel alumina-based metal-oxides were considered to be an excellent candidate for injection therapy and wound healing [47, 82–85] applications. This is because, sol–gel silica mostly forms chemical gels, while sol–gel alumina can form physically cross-linked gel structures. Alumina gel is the only sol–gel material approved by the FDA and EMA as a common immunologic adjuvant [86, 87], although sol–gel alumina is much less developed when compared to sol–gel silica for biomedical applications. Recently, Vinogradov and coworkers [82] reported sol–gel alumina with encapsulated protein as injectable carriers for bioactive molecules. Protein entrapped in sol–gel alumina was found to show high thermal stability and chemical activity. The same group extended the work with various other proteins, and demonstrated a remarkable stability with no loss of activity of protein from the sol–gel matrix [88–90]. Similarly, in another work they have studied the wound healing capability of a sol–gel alumina biocomposite and evaluated the material for wound dressing applications [84]. Thus, they have concluded that sol–gel alumina is an effective material for the treatment of infectious and chronic wounds. Recently, our group reported alumino-siloxane-based thixotropic gels for topical and injectable drug delivery applications [47]. In this study, we have used alumino-siloxane-based hybrid gels for encapsulation and sustained release of fluconazole, an antifungal drug. From rheological analysis we could well demonstrate the mechano-responsive behavior (thixotropic property) of alumino-siloxane gels (Figure 10.13a). The gel showed excellent structural and mechanical stability, non-cytotoxicity, and biocompatibility. The thixotropic property of the alumino-siloxane gel was successfully used for encapsulation,

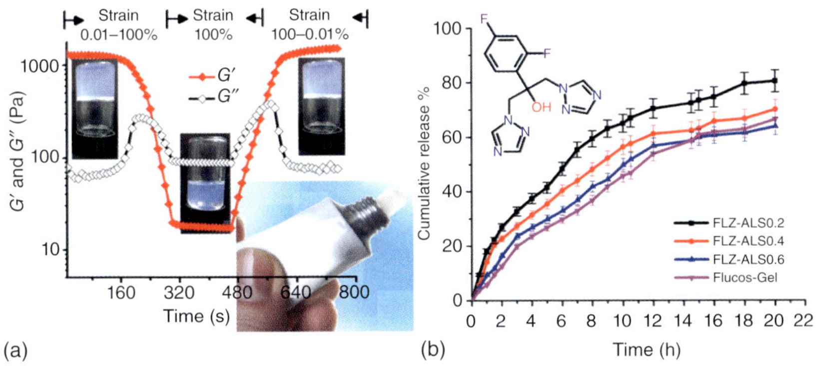

Figure 10.13 (a) Step-strain time-dependent rheological analysis demonstrating the mechano-responsive (thixotropic) behavior of alumino-siloxane gels. (b) *In vitro* release profile of fluconazole from various alumino-siloxane gels formulations and marketed Flucos gel, with 0.5% (w/w) fluconazole loading, at physiological pH 7.4 and temperature 37 ± 1 °C. (Linsha 2015 [47]. Reproduced with permission of The Royal Society of Chemistry.)

followed by controlled release of the drug fluconazole (Figure 10.13b). Thus, from all these recent reports we can conclude that physically cross-linked inorganic soft metal-oxide gels open a new platform for biomedical applications.

10.8.4 Silica-Based Hybrids and Ordered Mesoporous Materials

Of all the sol–gel derived materials one of the well-established category of materials for biomedical applications is the silica-based ordered mesoporous material [91–97]. When compared to metal-oxide xerogels and aerogels, ordered mesoporous material posses more homogeneous structural features, which are suitable for adsorption and release of therapeutic and diagnostic agents in pharma applications. The unique features such as ordered pore network, high pore volume, high surface area make MSN a special candidate for use in controlled drug delivery systems. Silica-based ordered mesoporous material (MCM 41) was first reported in 2001, by Regi, for drug delivery application [91]. Since then, intensive research has been carried out with silica-based mesoporous materials such as MCM-41, SBA-15, FDU-5, and MCF for the design of controlled drug delivery systems [91–95]. The controlled release of drugs molecules from these materials were strongly dependent on their structural and textural features. Regi and coworkers [94] studied the effect of pore size in loading and release of drug from MCM 41 using ibuprofen as the model drug. When ibuprofen was loaded in MCM-41 having a pore size in the range of 2.5 and 3.6 nm, a gradual increase in release rate with pore size was observed. Similarly, Andersson *et al.* [96] reported that drug release kinetics depends not only on pore size but also on pore connectivity and pore geometry of the mesoporous structure. Apart from the pore features, the surface area of the material also plays a key role in both drug release and drug loading capacity. Regi *et al.* [97] studied the loading of alendronate in mesoporous materials MCM 41 and SBA 15 having a surface area of 1157 and 719 $m^2 g^{-1}$, respectively. Loading efficiency of MCM 41 was 139 $m^2 g^{-1}$ whereas, for SBA 15 it was 83 $mg g^{-1}$. Hence, many of the studies in this regard concluded that surface area and pore size of the mesoporous material plays a crucial role in drug adsorption and release kinetics [94–99].

MSN garnered much more attention in the biomedical field when organically functionalized hybrid mesoporous materials were explored for controlled drug delivery properties [100–102]. Drug release could be very effectively controlled by functionalization of mesopore walls with suitable organic groups. Furthermore, it could improve the penetration of certain hydrophobic drugs, which was considered to be a great challenge until then [103]. Several research groups have reported that organic modification could fine tune the surface properties such as acid–base property, dissolution property, physiochemical activity [103–107]. Organosilanes, especially aminopropyl silane were identified to be one of the best functionalizing agents for regulating the controlled drug release property of the mesoporous matrix [105–107]. Consequently, organically functionalized MSN can be loaded with a large number of anti-inflammatory, antibiotics, anti-tumor drugs etc. having different molecular size and shapes, which could release in controlled manner form human body (Figure 10.14a). The ordered MSN surface is not only useful for the local drug delivery system, but can also react with physiological fluids, leading to the formation of nanoapatite-like layers that are similar to natural bone [97] (Figure 10.14b). *In vitro* bio-activity studies of various nanostructured mesoporous materials (MCM-41, SBA-15, and MCM-48) carried out by soaking in simulated body fluid (SBF), revealed the formation of a nanoapatite-like layer on the surface of the material within 30–60 days. It can also act as cellular scaffolds with embedded proteins, peptides, or growth factors that would be released to the medium promoting cell proliferation and differentiation. Thus, the property of controlled release and the inherent bioactivity of these materials both open new opportunities in biomedical application especially for bone regeneration and tissue engineering.

Immense improvement in the research of sol–gel derived inorganic–organic hybrids led to the discovery of "smart materials", which provided remarkable contribution to the biomedical field. Among them, stimuli-triggered materials for drug delivery application received huge attention. This kind of hybrid matrix for drug delivery is discussed in the following section.

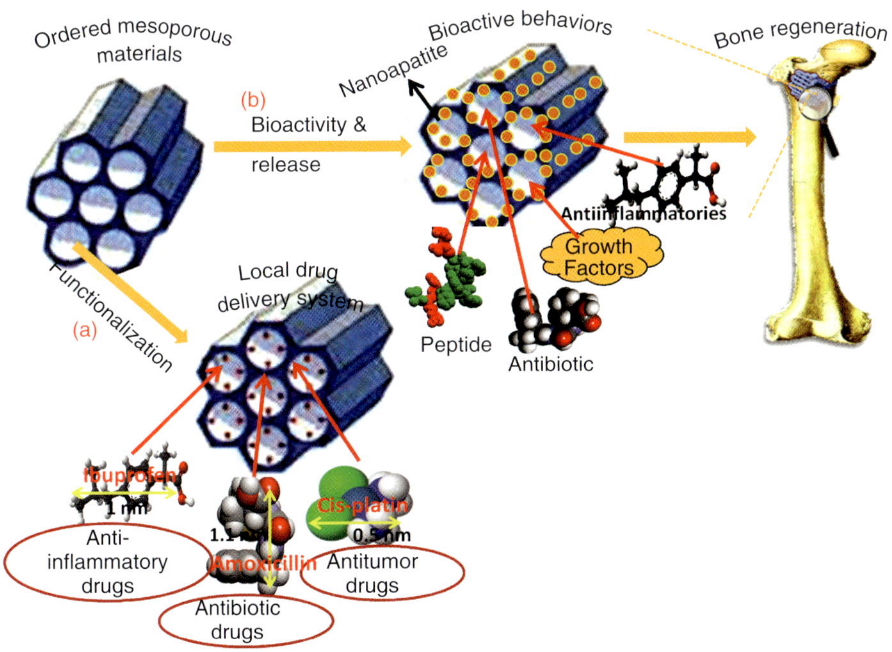

Figure 10.14 (a) Ordered mesoporous materials new perspective for controlled drug delivery systems and (b) bone regeneration for tissue engineering.

10.9
Stimuli-Responsive Drug Delivery Systems

Various types of material, especially sol–gel silica, have been explored for stimuli-responsive drug release systems. In stimuli-responsive systems, drugs are mostly encapsulated in the matrix and released when desired in the presence of different external and internal triggers (stimuli) [108–112]. There are several stimuli, such as chemicals, temperature, pH, light irradiation, ultrasound, and even electric or magnet fields (Figure 10.15) that can activate encapsulated guest molecules [110–114]. Hence, these stimuli-responsive systems are considered to be a "smart" drug delivery system. Because of the variety of pH gradients in the human body, one of the most investigated stimuli is pH-responsive drug delivery [108–111].

Our group demonstrated the stimuli-responsive behavior of sol–gel derived alumino-siloxane aerogels for controlled drug release [81]. Meso-channeled alumino-siloxane aerogels showed higher drug loading capacity and pH-responsive drug releasing capability. Sol–gel derived MSN is one of the major stimuli-responsive drug delivery material investigated by many researches [111–122]. Yang and coworkers [115] modified the surface of SBA-15 with ionized carboxylic acid group (COO−) and polycations by weak ionic interaction, which sealed the mesopore channels, after loading with vancomycin drug. When pH was altered to the acidic range, ionized carboxylic acid gets protonated and polycations move away, leading to the opening of pores followed by releasing of vancomycin. Similarly, Zink and coworkers [113, 116, 117] designed "nanovalves" at the opening of mesoporous MCM-41, using supramolecules such as rotaxanes,

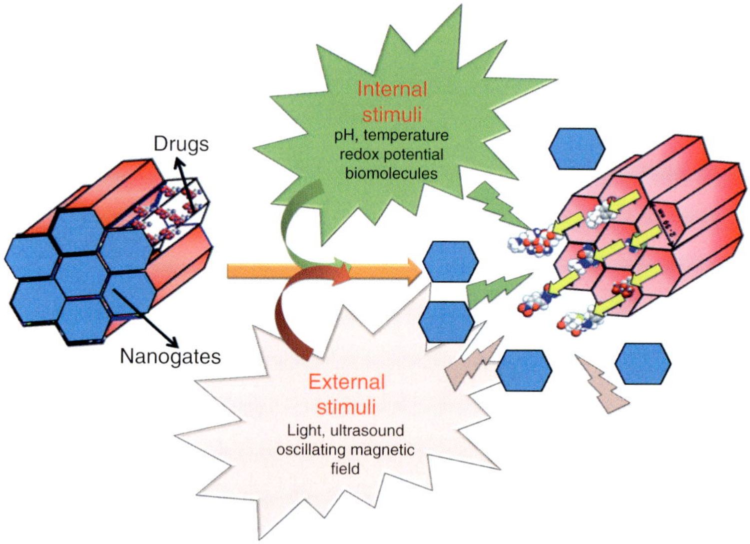

Figure 10.15 Various external and internal stimuli suitable for a smart drug delivery system from sol–gel mesoporous silica.

alpha-cyclodextrine, and other analogues. These nanovalves "open" and "close" in the presence of stimuli. Consequently, they could successfully demonstrate the pH-responsive behavior of MSN.

Some of the studies also demonstrated the influence of the thermo-responsive nature of sol–gel derived, organically functionalized MSN in controlled drug release [118, 119]. Recently it was revealed that the local temperature of many of the cancer cells is somewhat higher than normal body temperature. So, designing various types of thermo-responsive drug delivery systems has attracted huge research interest for cancer targeted therapy. Temperature-sensitive polymers such as poly(*N*-isopropylacrylamide) (PNIPAM) were commonly used to modify the mesoporous surface. The PNIPAM can change their molecular conformation in response to temperature. In an aqueous environment, PNIPAM are hydrated, below the lower critical solution temperature of 32 °C, resulting in an extended polymeric conformation, thereby preventing the removal of loaded guest molecules. When the surrounding temperature increases above the critical solution temperature, dehydrated polymers are formed with disintegrated conformation. This leads to the opening of the mesopore and the successive release of loaded gusted molecules. Such polymer encapsulated MSN has the capability to release the drug depending on the surrounding temperature.

Similarly, MSN responds to the external magnetic field, by encapsulating magnetic nanoparticles, especially, magnetically active iron-oxide nanoparticles [118, 120] within the mesoporous structure. Giri *et al.* [120] reported that, MSN when synthesized by co-condensation with mercaptopropyl silanes and subsequent modification with carboxyethyl-2-pyridyl disulfide, leads to the formation of acid-functionalized mesoporous nanostructures. This acid-functionalized silica is loaded with drug molecules that are smaller than 3 nm, such as fluorescein, and capped with super-paramagnetic iron-oxide nanoparticles. It was observed that in the presence of an adequate external magnetic field, capped magnetic nanoparticles are removed to release entrapped drug molecules as shown in Figure 10.16.

Apart from this, when mesoporous entrance is modified with certain organic or inorganic functionalities, it responds to chemical signals. Lin and coworkers [121] loaded vancomycin and adenosine triphosphate in MCM-41 and modified the mesochannels with CdS nanoparticles. In the presence of disulfide bond-reducing molecules (such as dithiothreitol or mercaptoethanol), capped CdS nanoparticles are removed from the channel ends. This results in the controlled release of loaded drug molecules, as shown in the schematic illustration of Figure 10.17.

Similarly, redox-triggered release studies were also conducted by capping mesopores with pseudorotaxane [122–124]. Here, rotaxane molecules act as nanovalves that open and close with selective redox process. Zink and coworkers [124] fabricated redox-controlled nanovalves on MSN using two bistable [2] rotaxanes as the gatekeepers. Such nanovalves have IN or OUT locations based on the position of used rotaxanes with respect to the entrances of the mesoporous channels. Therefore, such finely tuned nanovalves are essential to

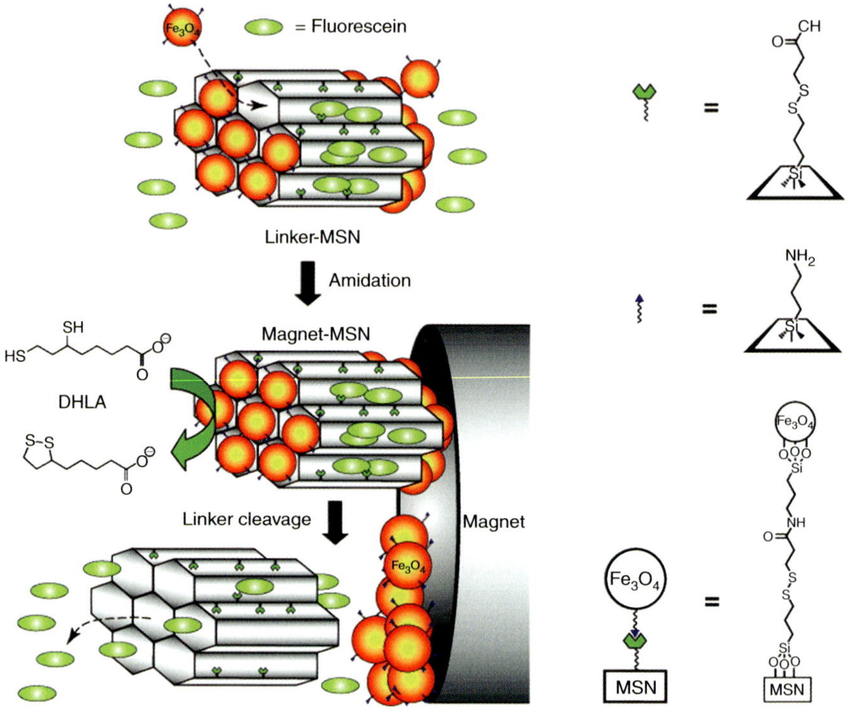

Figure 10.16 Schematic of the stimuli-responsive delivery system (magnet-MSN) based on mesoporous silica nanorods capped with superparamagnetic iron oxide nanoparticles. The controlled release mechanism of the system is based on reduction of the disulfide linkage between the Fe_3O_4 nanoparticle caps and the linker-MSN hosts by reducing agents such as DHLA. (Giri 2005 [120]. Reproduced with permission of Wiley.)

the future design of drug delivery systems that can release drugs with different structural dimensions.

In addition to these stimulis light and sound can trigger the drug release mechanism from mesoporous channels. Light of suitable wavelength can act as stimuli to trigger the release of drug from the mesochannels. Fujiwara and coworkers reported photo-controlled drug delivery, by modifying the mesopore surface with a coumarin group [102]. Coumarin can undergo reversible dimerization in the presence of UV light above wavelength 310 nm and can return to monomer below 210 nm. These processes stimulate the release of drug from the pore channels. Many of the groups [125, 126] demonstrated the release of drug by modifying with photosensitive azo-benzene derivatives. When drug molecules are loaded within azo-benzene-modified mesochannels, they could retain the drug in the pores in the absence of light and release it in the presence of light. These types of modifications are also found to be much effective for cancer targeted drug delivery [126]. Similarly, ultrasounds can be used as stimuli for pulsed delivery of certain drug

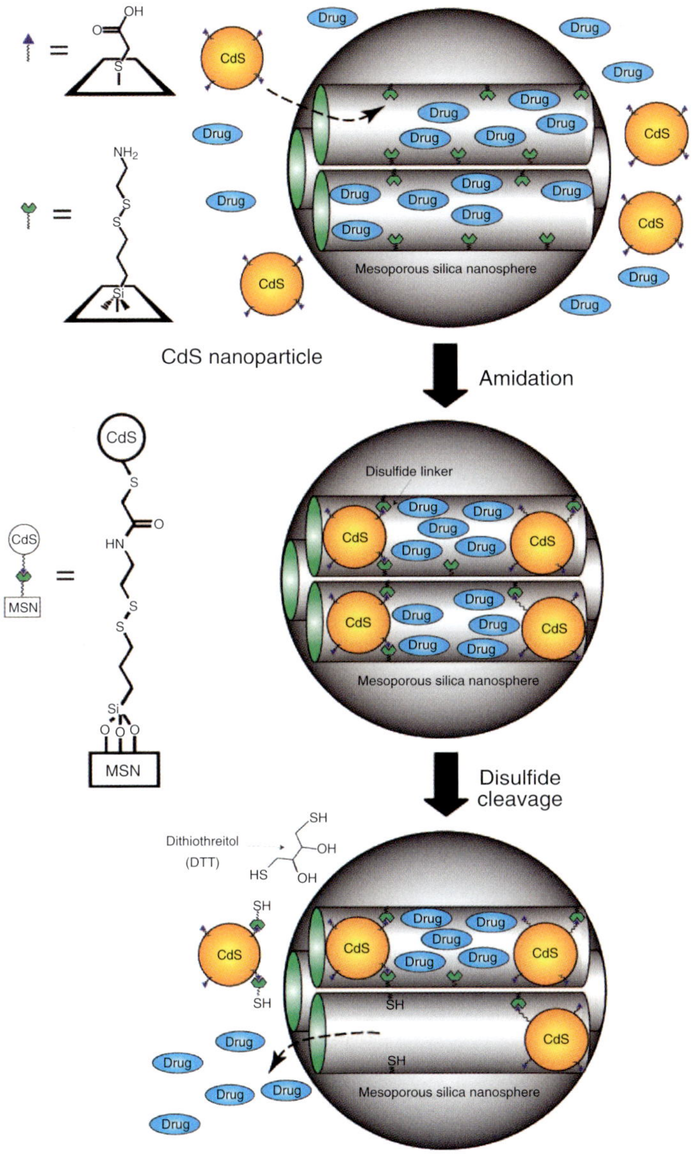

Figure 10.17 Schematic representation of the CdS nanoparticle-capped mesoporous silica-based drug/neurotransmitter delivery system. The controlled release mechanism of the system is based on chemical reduction of the disulfide linkage between the CdS caps and the mesoporous silica-hosts. (Lai 2003 [121]. Reproduced with permission of American Chemical Society.)

molecules. In such cases, mesopores were modified with organic moieties such as poly (dimethylsiloxane) [127] for the release of drugs.

Design and development of various stimuli-responsive drug delivery systems based on sol–gel derived MSN can be considered to be a good competitor for polymer-based stimuli-responsive gels. As the research is exceptionally well progressing in new aspects of “mesoporous materials for nanomedicine”. Consequently, sol–gel derived MSN nanoparticles offer great possibilities for targeted therapy or chemotherapeutics and imaging applications.

10.10 Sol–Gel Matrix Targeted Cancer Therapy

Currently, one of the big challenges in the biomedical field is the design of novel materials for cancer targeted therapy or “chemotherapeutics” as, anti-cancer drugs can generally cause serious side-effects to normal or healthy cells. Cell targeting is one relevant criterion that needs to be satisfied by such therapeutic agents. For more effective cellular targeting, it is necessary to have in-depth knowledge about the receptors that can over-express on the tumor cells [128–130]. The ability of these receptors to selectively bind the cancerous cells with the aid of molecular recognition or receptor-mediated endocytosis makes it promising for use in targeted treatment [129].Various targeting agents such as peptides and antibodies, or simple molecules, such as folic acid or mannose are used for cell targeting. All the above mentioned targeting agents have the ability to over-express cellular receptors on the cancer cell and act according to the metabolic and nutritional demands of cancer cells. Since folic acid receptors can over-express on most of the cancer cells, such as endometrial, ovarian, renal cell, breast, and brain cells, they have emerged as an attractive targeting ligand for cancer therapy [129–131].

So far, many studies have been carried out by binding various receptors on MSN to trigger receptor-mediated endocytosis. Guo *et al.* studied the functionalization of MSN with folic acid receptors acting as both capping agents and targeting agents. They have established that folic acid on the meso-channels not only improved the internalization efficiency but also effectively capped the mesoporous channels for controlled drug release by selective targeting of human epithelial cells [131]. Similarly, selective targeting of breast cancer cells was studied using monoclonal antibody when functionalized on the surface of MSN [132]. A schematic representation of the administrative route of functionalized mesoporous nanostructured silica developed for cancer targeted therapy is shown in Figure 10.18 [128].

Linden and coworkers [133] studied the targeting efficiency of hybrid MSN functionalized with hyperbranched polymer, poly(ethyleneimine). The hybrid system was further modified with fluorescent molecule (fluorescein isothiocyanate) and folic acid receptors. The internalization of this hybrid material was studied in

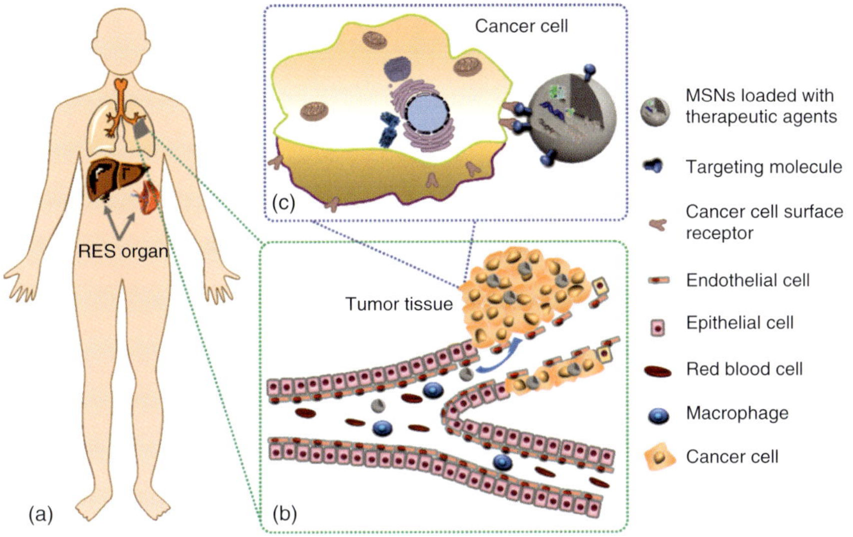

Figure 10.18 Schematic representations of administrative route followed by mesoporous nanostructured material developed for cancer targeted therapy. (Tang 2012 [128]. Reproduced with permission of Wiley.)

the cell line expressing folate receptors. A significantly higher internalization was shown by cancer cells when compared to normal healthy cells.

Various other types of functionalization such as decoration with magnetic nanoparticle, luminescent labeling with organic dyes, and multi-functionalization using both magnetic and luminescent particles have been carried on the surface of mesoporous material [134, 135] by aiming targeted cancer therapy. Iron oxide-based magnetic nanoparticle, for example, Fe_2O_3 and Fe_3O_4 were commonly used for functionalization of MSN for cancer targeted therapy [134, 136]. Chen *et al.* [137] designed magnetic-responsive rattle-type hollow structure of $Fe_2O_3@SiO_2@mSiO_2$ and $Fe_2O_3@mSiO_2$ hollow nanocapsules. Higher loading efficiency of the anti-cancer drug doxorubicin was observed in rattle-type hollow structure. It was also proved to be a wonderful anticancer drug carrier by showing good cytotoxicity against MCF-7 cell line.

Similarly, luminescent organic dyes such as fluorescein isothiocyanates, rhodamine, and cyanine dyes were labeled within a sol–gel matrix of MSN to deliver it to cancerous sites for stimulating apoptosis [135, 138]. Silica matrix prevents photobleaching and quenching of organic dye when exposed to the harsh environment. Multi-stimuli-responsive behavior was also studied to control the drug release from MSN, by suitable functionalization [139, 140]. Chang *et al.* [140] reported the pH and thermo-responsive MSN for drug release. Similarly, Liu and coworkers [139] reported multi-stimuli-responsive polymer functionalized MSN capped with β-cyclodextrin and a cross-linker of the diazo group over the meso channels of the silica surface (Figure 10.19). In the presence of three different

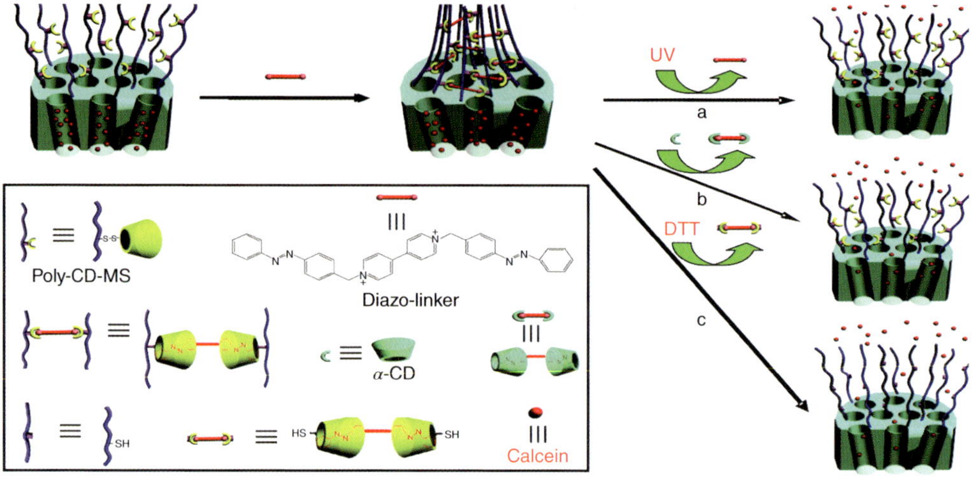

Figure 10.19 Schematic illustration of a multi-responsive nanogated ensemble based on supramolecular polymeric network-capped mesoporous silica. (Liu 2009 [139]. Reproduced with permission of American Chemical Society.)

stimuli, the encapsulated drug molecules release: (i) UV light that causes isomeric transformation of azo-benzene groups, (ii) α-cyclodextrin competitive binding to displace β-cyclodextrin, (iii) addition of disulfide reducing agents (dithiothreitol) to cleave the disulphide (S–S) bond between β-cyclodextrin and polymeric main chain.

Varieties of active and passive release behavior were demonstrated for tumor targeted drug delivery. Still serious efforts are required for *in vivo* studies, to overcome the biological barriers, to reach these nanostructured carrier materials to tumor cells and release therapeutic agents at targeted cells.

10.11 Sol–Gel Matrices for Imaging and Radiotherapy (Radiolabeling)

Cancer treatments involve surgery, radiotherapy, chemotherapy, immunotherapy, hormone therapy, gene therapy, and so on, of which radiotherapy is one of the crucial diagnostic techniques. Recently, research efforts were put forward to use sol–gel materials for cancer theranostic applications [128]. Since sol–gel synthesized material was found to possess a surface active group, which improves the surface functionalization ability of the material. Various strategies were adopted to synthesize sol–gel material with modified surface active groups, for diagnostics applications in modern medicine. Such surface active groups not only improve the dispersibility of the sol–gel particles but also provide a site of attachment for drugs, organic luminescent moieties, radioisotopes, and so on used in imaging and therapeutic applications [141–144]. Out of various types of sol–gel derived materials, MSN nanostructures are investigated largely for cancer diagnostic and imaging applications [144–150]. The major imaging techniques for which sol–gel mesoporous nanoparticles have been more explored are, magnetic resonance imaging (MRI), photodynamic therapy (PDT), positron emission tomography imaging (PET), and single-photon emission computed tomography (SPECT), and so on.

10.11.1 Magnetic Resonance Imaging (MRI)

MRI is one of the medical diagnostic techniques with high spatial resolution (50 to 250 mm) and excellent tissue contrast. Studies were conducted by immobilizing highly luminescent species (MRI contrast agents) such as fluorescent NPs (organic dye, quantum dots) and metal NPs (europium Eu^{3+}, gadolinium Gd^{3+}) into sol-gel nanostructures for specific targeting, imaging and detection of cancer cells. Delville and coworkers [144] designed high-spin paramagnetic Gd^{3+} chelates, that is, Gd^{3+}-DTPA on metal oxide such as silica and alumina. DTPA stands for diethyl-enetriamine pentaacetic acid and it is considered to be the first FDA-approved contrast agent in clinical use [145]. The results indicated that, Gd^{3+}-DTPA based new contrast agents lead to a huge reconcentration of Gd^{3+} paramagnetic species inside chemoattracted microglial, brain tumors cells. This reconcentration phenomenon gives rise to high signal-to-noise ratios on MRI images of cells after particle internalization, which gave a new insight into MR cell tracking. Tagaya and coworkers [146] synthesized luminescent Eu^{3+} doped nanoporous silica (Eu:NPS) sphere by covalently functionalizing with folic-acid (FA) by cross-linking with 3-aminopropyltriethoxysilane (APTES) (Figure 10.20). In this study they have concluded that, the FA-functionalized Eu:NPS nanospheres showed high cytocompatibility for HeLa cancer cells and NIH3T3 fibroblasts, and proving to be a good material for specific targeting and imaging of cancer cells.

Since MSN possesses large surface areas, high accessible pore volumes, ease of chemical modification and excellent biocompatibility, it offers great possibility of encapsulating and delivering large quantities of biogenic molecules and MIR contrast agents. Many studies were reported by loading MIR contrast agents such as paramagnetic complexes, super paramagnetic iron oxide nanoparticles in mesoporous structure [147–149] for cell imaging. Kim and coworkers [149] investigated the *in vitro* cytotoxicity of human mesenchymal cells, labeled with silica-coated magnetic nanoparticles by incorporating rhodamine dye. The optical and MRI images were successfully tracked in NOD-SCID mice, which demonstrated the retention capacity of silica-coated support in mesenchymal cells.

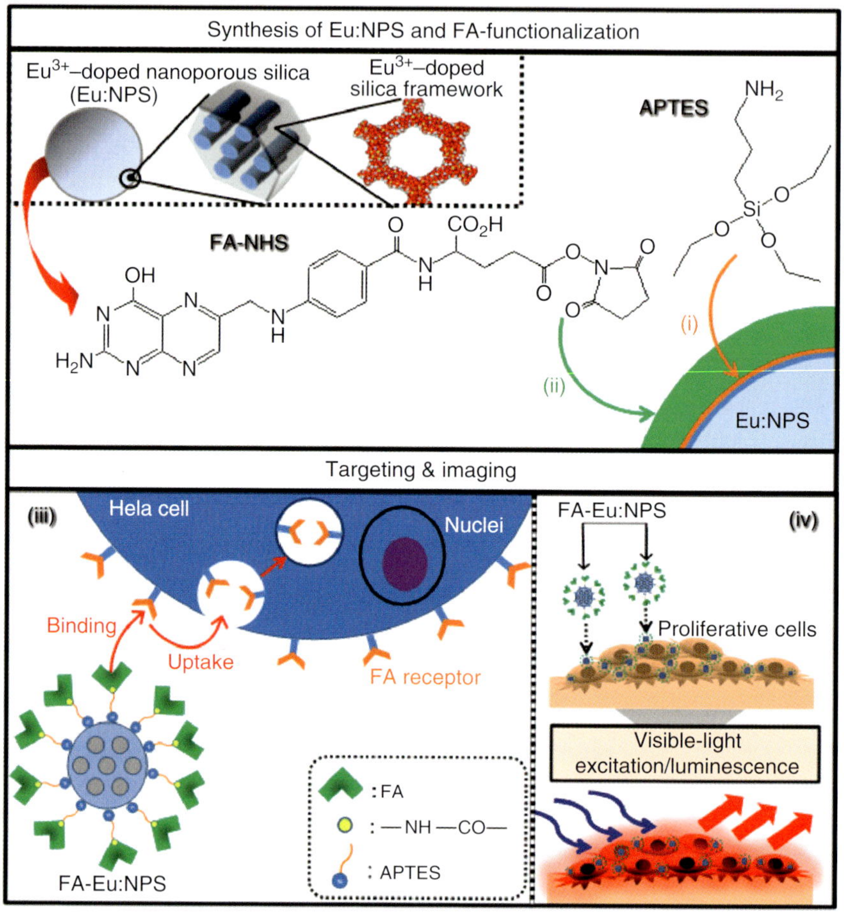

Figure 10.20 Schemes of the immobilizations of (i) APTES and (ii) FA-NHS molecules on the luminescent Eu:NPS surfaces and (iii) targeting and (iv) imaging of the proliferated HeLa cells by visible-light excitation and luminescence. (Tagaya 2014 [146]. Reproduced with permission of American Chemical Society.)

10.11.2 Photodynamic Therapy (PDT)

PDT is another well-established technique for cancer treatment. In this technique, photosensitizers (PSs) are delivered to target cells or tissues either passively or actively when irradiated with a laser light. Upon irradiation, the activated PSs transfer the energy from their triplet state to ground state oxygen to generate reactive oxygen species (ROS) that can destroy the surrounding cancer cells. Sol–gel derived MSN has been demonstrated to be an effective vehicle for the PSs and improved the efficacy of PDT, [143, 150]. The mesoporous structure of silica not only permits the accommodation of a large amount of PSs, but also helps to enhance the permeability of oxygen and generate singlet oxygen, which is essential for PDT [151, 152]. Efficiency of various types of PSs such as methylene blue, 2-devinyl-2-(1 hexyloxyethyl) pyropheophorbide, hypocrellin A, fullerene (C_{60}), tetra-substituted carboxyl aluminum phthalocyanine, protoporphyrin IX, and meta-tetra(hydroxyphenyl)chlorin [143, 150–154] were studied by encapsulating in sol–gel silica matrix. Prasad and Kopelman have carried out some of the pioneering work using sol–gel silica nanoparticles for PDT [152–154].

10.11.3
Positron Emission Tomography Imaging (PET)

PET is one of the radionuclide based imaging techniques that detects pairs of gamma rays emitted indirectly by a positron emitting radionuclide (tracer) with spatial resolution of 1 to 2 mm. Some of the radionuclides that are explored and studied for wide varieties of applications in nuclear medicine, are ^{131}I, ^{67}Ga, ^{123}I, ^{131}In, ^{99m}Tc, ^{881}Re, and so on, (gamma ray emitting tracers) and ^{18}F and ^{64}Cu (positron emitting tracers). Interesting research was carried out using sol–gel derived silica nanoparticles as a carrier for radionuclide for biomedical applications [155–157]. Prasad and coworkers [155] studied the efficiency of organically modified MSN when conjugated with fluorophores and radiolabeled with ^{124}I for PET imaging. They have demonstrated good biodistribution and potentiality of modified MSN for *in vivo* imaging.

Smith and coworkers [157] in 2013, reported amine functionalized silica, prepared by sol–gel processing for radio-labeling applications. Amine functionalized silica was initially conjugated with SarAr-isothiocyanate (SarAr-NCS) ligand, with tracer $^{57}Co^{2+}$ ($t_{1/2} = 271.8$ days) and its imaging efficacy was explored. Followed by this in the same year, Chen *et al.* [158] successfully demonstrated the effect of functionalized MSN for targeted PET imaging and image guided drug delivery. The main strategy they have adopted for the synthesis is shown in Figure 10.21A. The study involves the following steps: surface functionalization of MSN with thiol groups, PEGylation and conjugation with TRC105 antibody, and finally ^{64}Cu labeling to obtain ^{64}Cu-NOTA-mSiO_2-PEG-TRC105. Various *in vitro, in vivo, and ex vivo* experimental studies demonstrated that ^{64}Cu-NOTA-mSiO_2-PEG-TRC105 has an excellent bio-stability and target specificity. Coronal PET imaging of 4T1 tumor-bearing mice is shown in Figure 10.21B. The results displayed that ^{64}Cu-NOTA-mSiO_2-PEG-TRC105, may well accumulate at the 4T1 tumor-bearing site via both the enhanced permeability and retention effect. They could also successfully demonstrate the enhanced tumor targeted delivery of doxorubicin (DOX) after intravenous injection in 4T1 tumor-bearing mice using TRC105 as the targeting ligand and MSN as the drug carrier. Hence, they have concluded that ^{64}Cu-NOTA-mSiO_2-PEG-TRC105 will be a competent material for biomedical imaging/radiotherapy and cancer targeted drug delivery.

Similarly, Linden and coworkers in 2014 [159] studied the application of sol–gel derived MSN coupled with p-isothiocyanatobenzyldesferrioxamine (DFO) by labeling with ^{89}Zr, i.e.; ^{89}Zr-DFO-MSNs for PET imaging. Figure 10.22a,b shows

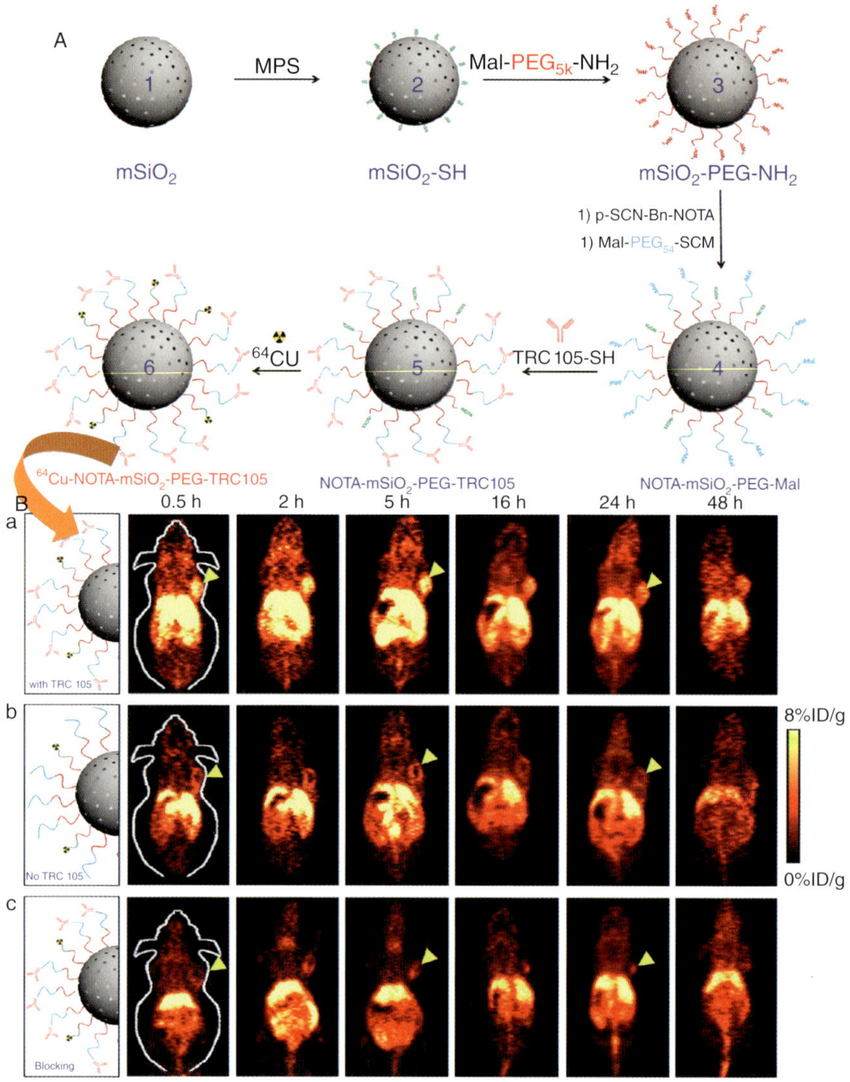

Figure 10.21 (A) A schematic illustration of the synthesis of 64Cu-NOTA-mSiO_2-PEG-TRC105. Uniform mSiO_2 nanoparticles (1) were first modified with –SH groups to form mSiO_2-SH (2). mSiO_2-SH was PEGylated with Mal-PEG5k-NH_2 to form mSiO_2-PEG-NH_2 (3), which was subjected to NOTA conjugation and subsequent PEGylation to yield NOTA-mSiO_2-PEG-Mal (4). NOTA-mSiO_2-PEGTRC105 (5) could be obtained by reacting TRC105-SH with (4) ^{64}Cu-labelingwasperformed in the last step to generate ^{64}Cu-NOTAmSiO_2-PEG-TRC105. (B) Serial coronal PET images of 4T1 tumor-bearing mice at different time points post injection of (a) ^{64}Cu-NOTA-mSiO_2-PEG-TRC105, (b) ^{64}Cu-NOTA-mSiO_2-PEG, or (c) ^{64}Cu-NOTA-mSiO_2-PEG-TRC105 with a blocking dose of TRC105. Tumors were indicated by yellow arrowheads. (Chen 2013 [158]. Reproduced with permission of American Chemical Society.)

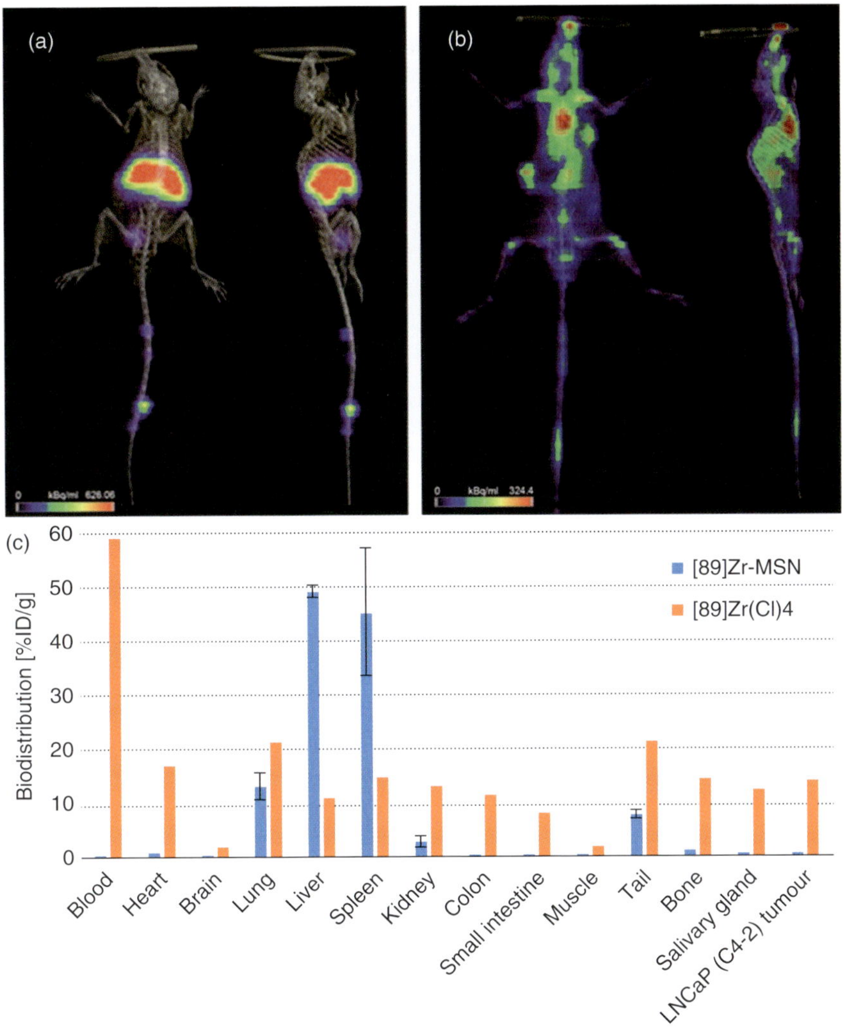

Figure 10.22 (a) PET image co-registered with the corresponding CT image of mice taken 1 h after injection ^{89}Zr-DFO-MSNs (b) ^{89}ZrCl4 solution into the tail vein. (c) Biodistribution curve of ^{89}Zr-DFO-MSNs as compared to ^{89}ZrCl4 in salt form. (Miller 2014 [159]. Reproduced with permission of The Royal Society of Chemistry.)

PET-CT images obtained by injecting ^{89}Zr-DFO-MSNs and free $^{89}ZrCl_4$ free salt solution into the tail vein of mice bearing a prostate cancer tumor (LNCaP C4-2). It was observed that, ^{89}Zr-DFO-MSNs accumulated in the heart, liver, and spleen whereas, $^{89}ZrCl_4$ was distributed throughout the body. Therefore, an excellent *in vivo* biodistribution was observed for ^{89}Zr-DFO-MSNs when compared to free $^{89}ZrCl_4$. The quantified biodistribution pattern of ^{89}Zr in both cases is shown in Figure 10.22c.

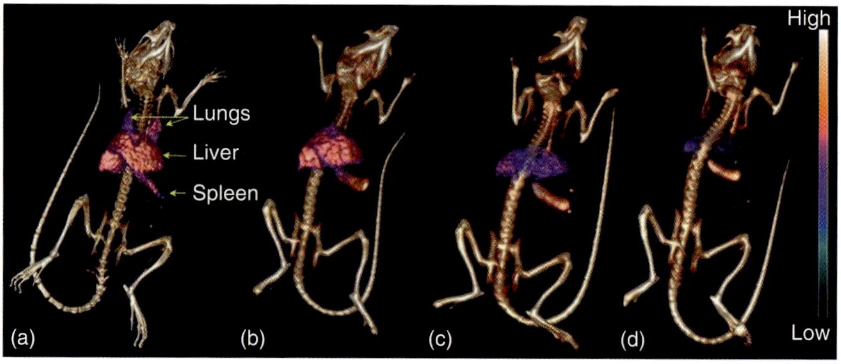

Figure 10.23 *In vivo* SPECT/CT imaging of a nude mouse injected with DT10 141Ce-rCONPs, at (a) 2 h, (b) 24 h, (c) 72 h, and (d) 144 h post injection. Images shown here were obtained from volume renderings that were adjusted to a uniform scale. (Yang 2013 [161]. Reproduced with permission of The Royal Society of Chemistry.)

Various other sol–gel derived metal-oxides such as aluminum oxide [160], cerium oxide [161], and zirconium oxide [162] were also recently exploited for radiolabeling applications. Recently, Yang *et al.* [161] demonstrated intrinsic radiolabeling of cerium oxide nanoparticles, by incorporating radionuclides such as ^{141}Ce, ^{111}In, and ^{65}Zn into the cerium oxide matrix. Radiolabeled cerium oxide was modified with biocompatible polymers dextran (DT10), which could improve the bio-stability, bio-compatibility, and intracellular internalization of radiolabeled cerium oxide (DT10-^{141}Ce-rCONPs). SPECT/CT image (Figure 10.23) of nude-mouse injected with (DT10 ^{141}Ce-rCONPs) expressed excellent *in vivo* biodistribution and demonstrated the mechanisms of radio protective properties of DT10 ^{141}Ce-rCONPs for biomedical imaging and theranostic applications. Similarly, ^{99m}Tc labeled zirconia nanoparticles capped ursolic acid [162] also showed better future for drug delivery and topical radiotherapy applications.

10.12
Concluding Remarks and Future Perspectives

Sol–gel chemistry was initially known for the processing of glass and ceramics. However, over the past two decades tremendous advance in sol–gel technology has opened new possibilities in material science. They have offered tremendous potential in the synthesis of hybrid sol–gel materials for innovative applications. Recently, functionally engineered sol–gel derived inorganic gels (including hydrogels, xerogels, and aerogels) and hybrid nanoarchitectures have gained immense attention of chemists, biologists, and material scientists, and are now emerging as a new platform in interdisciplinary research scenarios. These materials are currently transferring their possibilities among materials science and biomedical research fields. Thus, in this chapter, we have very briefly discussed the state of the art in the synthesis of functionally engineered sol–gel derived materials as well as their application in the biomedical field.

Sol–gel derived inorganic gels, and hybrid nanomaterials are now receiving significant attention in the biomedical field due to advantages such as good chemical stability, high mechanical strength, and relatively high biocompatibility when compared to conventional polymeric materials. It can also efficiently protect the encapsulated guest molecules from microbial attack and enzymatic degradation induced by pH, temperature, and so on and will not show any swelling and porosity changes, which are often encountered in (bio) polymeric systems. Unique properties such as flexibility, transparency, hydrophobicity, hydrophilicity, and thermal and chemical stability can be brought into sol–gel derived materials by suitable functionalization and consequently tune the material for hi-tech bio-applications.

Sol–gel metal-oxide gels, especially silica aerogels and xerogels, are deeply explored in drug delivery applications in the biomedical field. The major studies carried out so far showed that these materials have high capacity for loading drugs, excellent ability for controlled drug delivery, and the capacity to improve the stability of low-soluble drugs. Still, there exist several issues related to metal-oxide gels; rare reports are found to prove their biocompatibility/toxicity. Similarly, systematic investigations have not been carried out to spot the drug–matrix interactions. Another area that has hardly been investigated in inorganic gels is the targeted therapy and imaging in the biomedical field.

Hybrid MSN is another sol–gel derived nanomaterial, which has created a major breakthrough in the field of nanomedicine in the current era. This material has attracted more and more attention to their potential for both therapeutic and diagnostic applications. The main reason this material has shown such progress in this field is because it can be finely tailored with reference to size, surface chemistry, shape, and porous structure. As a drug delivery system it has amazingly high drug loading capacity, sustained and stimuli-responsive controlled drug releasing ability, and relatively high cyto/biocompatibility. The functionalization ability of the sol–gel mesoporous nanomaterial allows to incorporate the magnetic, photothermal, and luminescent properties to the material for therapeutic functions.

In addition to this, mesoporous nanosilica has emerged as a versatile material for cancer therapy. It has got various advantageous when compared to other polymeric and organic nanocarriers. The over dosage of anti-cancer drugs is considered to induce toxicity in the cells and cause severe adverse side effects. For this reason, chemotherapy deals with various unmanageable risk factors. Hence, mesoporous nanomaterials are intelligently designed, as a targeting drug delivery vehicle with stimuli-responsive release behavior. Different gatekeepers (stimuli-responsive agents) are created at the entrance of meso-channels to uncap and trigger the departure of drug molecules in the presence of various external stimuli. For the past few years, a wide range of *in vitro* studies has been carried out for targeted drug delivery applications [102, 108–139]. Some of the *in vivo* studies are also encouraging to move this material for use in clinical trials. But, still some challenges exist which have to be resolved. Interaction of silica nanoparticle with targeting ligand and its binding efficiency specifically to tumor sites needs to be further explored. Great effort has to be taken from biologists, toxicologists, and pathologists to completely understand the toxicity profile of sol–gel MSN.

Sol–gel derived MSN nanoparticles are also emerging as promising material for diagnostic and intracellular imaging applications. Recent studies regarding this topic revealed that this material has immense potential in chemo- and radiotherapy especially in the treatment of cancer. In 2011, by human clinical trials, US Food and Drug Administration (FDA) approved ultra-small sol–gel derived silica nanoparticles for targeted molecular imaging of cancer [163]. Radiolabeling of sol–gel derived inorganic nanoparticles in combination with photo-thermal and optical properties probes new opportunities in imaging applications. In the near future, more and more clinical trials have to be carried out with radiolabeled nanosilica for making it a powerful tool in diagnostics and imaging applications. It is also possible to improve the traditional concept of separate diagnosis and treatment by designing novel radiolabeled inorganic materials by inducing multifunctionality, which offers great possibilities for simultaneous detection, imaging, and therapy, that is, "theranostic functions" in the biomedical field.

Acknowledgment

The authors gratefully acknowledge the general support from the colleagues at Functional Materials Section, Materials Science and Technology Division, CSIR-NIIST, Thiruvananthapuram. The authors thank Mrs K.B. Babitha for the general help rendered for the completion of this chapter.

Abbreviations

APTES	3-aminopropyltriethoxysilane
DTPA	diethyl-enetriamine pentaacetic acid
DOX	doxorubicin
FA	folic-acid
FDA	Food and Drug Administration
LMWGs	low molecular weight organic gelators
MRI	magnetic resonance imaging
MSNs	mesoporous silica
NPs	nanoparticles
PDT	photodynamic therapy
DFO	p-isothiocyanatobenzyl-desferrioxamine
PEG-PPG-PEG	poly-(ethylene glycol)-poly-(propylene glycol)-poly(ethylene glycol)
PNIPAM	poly(*N*-isopropylacrylamide)
PET	positron emission tomography imaging
ROS	reactive oxygen species

SBF	simulated body fluid
SPECT	single-photon emission computed tomography
SarAr-NCS	SarAr-isothiocyanate

References

1. Graham, T. (1861) *Philos. Trans. R. Soc. London*, **151**, 183–224.
2. Jordan Lloyd, D. (1926) in *Colloid Chemistry*, vol. 1 (ed. J. Alexander), The Chemical Catalog Co, New York, pp. 767–782.
3. Jones, R.A.L. (2002) *Soft Condensed Matter*, Oxford University Press, 20.06.2002-195 Seiten.
4. Vlierberghe, S.V., Dubruel, P., and Schacht, E. (2011) *Biomacromolecules*, **12**, 1387–1408.
5. Weiss, R.G. (2014) *J. Am. Chem. Soc.*, **136**, 7519–7530.
6. Beck, J.B. and Rowan, S.J. (2003) *J. Am. Chem. Soc.*, **125**, 13922–13923.
7. Raeburn, J., Cardoso, A.Z., and Adams, D.J. (2013) *Chem. Soc. Rev.*, **42**, 5143–5156.
8. Oshaben, K.M. and Horne, W.S. (2014) *Biomacromolecules*, **15**, 1436–1442.
9. Liu, Z.X., Feng, Y., Yan, Z.C., He, Y.M., Liu, C.Y., and Fan, Q.H. (2012) *Chem. Mater.*, **24**, 3751–3757.
10. Yu, X., Cao, X., Chen, L., Lan, H., Liu, B., and Yi, T. (2012) *Soft Matter*, **8**, 3329–3334.
11. Narasimha, K. and Jayakannan, M. (2014) *ACS Appl. Mater. Interfaces*, **6**, 19385–19396.
12. Wang, Y., Li, W., and Wu, L. (2009) *Langmuir*, **25**, 13194–13200.
13. Bauer, W.H., Collins, E.A., and Eirich, F.R. (1967) *Rheology: Theory and Applications*, vol. 4, Chapter 8, Academic Press, New York.
14. Chhabra, R.P. and Richardson, J.F. (2008) *Non-Newtonian Flow and Applied Rheology*, 2nd edn, Butterworth-Heinemann, Oxford.
15. Barnes, H.A. (1997) *J. Non-Newtonian Fluid Mech.*, **70**, 1–33.
16. Ebelmen, M. (1846) *Ann. Chim. Phys.*, **16**, 129.
17. Cossa, A. (1870) *Il Nuova Cemento 3*, **3**, 228–230.
18. Pierre, A.C. (1998) *Introduction to Sol-Gel Processing*, Kluwer, Boston, MA.
19. Brinker, C.J. and Scherer, G.W. (1990) *Sol-Gel Science, the Physics and Chemistry of Sol-Gel Processing*, Academic Press, New York.
20. Zelinski, B.J.J. and Uhlmann, D.R. (1984) *J. Phys. Chem. Solids*, **45**, 1069–1090.
21. Mukherjee, S.P. (1980) *J. Non-Cryst. Solids*, **42**, 447–488.
22. Sakka, S. and Kamiya, K. (1982) *J. Non-Cryst. Solids*, **48**, 31–36.
23. Ulku, S., Balkose, D., and Baltacboglu, H. (1993) *Colloid. Polym. Sci.*, **271**, 709–713.
24. Acosta, S., Corriu, R.J.P., Leclercq, D., Lefevre, P., Mutin, P.H., and Vioux, A. (1994) *J. Non-Cryst. Solids*, **170**, 234–242.
25. Hay, J.N. and Raval, H.M. (1998) *J. Sol-Gel Sci. Technol.*, **13**, 109–112.
26. Fricke, J. (1988) *J. Non-Cryst. Solids*, **100**, 169–173.
27. Fricke, J. and Emmerling, A. (1998) *J. Sol-Gel Sci. Technol.*, **13**, 299–303.
28. Pierre, A.C. and Pajonk, G.M. (2002) *Chem. Rev.*, **102**, 4243–4265.
29. Kistler, S.S. (1931) *Nature*, **127**, 741.
30. Baumann, T.F., Gash, A.E., Chinn, S.C., Sawvel, A.M., Maxwell, R.S., and Satcher, J.H. (2005) *Chem. Mater.*, **17**, 395–401.
31. Husing, N. and Schubert, U. (1998) *Angew. Chem. Int. Ed. Engl.*, **37**, 23–45.
32. Chervin, C.N., Clapsaddle, B.J., Chiu, H.W., Gash, A.E., Satcher, J.H., and Kauzlarich, S.M. (2005) *Chem. Mater.*, **17**, 3345–3351.
33. Gan, L.H., Yue, T.Y., Chen, L.W., Li, G.M., and Zhou, B. (1997) *Acta Phys. Chim. Sin.*, **13**, 48–51.
34. Bag, S., Trikalitis, P.N., Chupas, P.J., Armatas, G.S., and Kanatzidis, M.G. (2007) *Science*, **317**, 490–493.

35. Pekala, R., Alviso, C., Lu, X., Gross, J., and Fricke, J. (1995) *J. Non-Cryst. Solids*, **188**, 34–40.
36. Tan, C.B., Fung, B.M., Newman, J.K., and Vu, C. (2001) *Adv. Mater.*, **13**, 644–646.
37. Kettunen, M., Silvennoinen, R.J., Houbenov, N., Nykanen, A., Ruokolainen, J., Sainio, J., Pore, V., Kemell, M., Ankerfors, M., and Lindstrom, T. (2011) *Adv. Funct. Mater.*, **21**, 510–517.
38. Xu, J., Liu, Y.M., Xue, B., Li, Y.X., Cao, Y., and Fan, K.N. (2011) *Phys. Chem. Chem. Phys.*, **13**, 10111–10118.
39. Ilhan, U.F., Fabrizio, E.F., McCorkle, L., Scheiman, D.A., Dass, A., Palczer, A., Meador, M.B., Johnston, J.C., and Leventis, N. (2006) *J. Mater. Chem.*, **16**, 3046–3054.
40. Chien, H.C., Cheng, W.Y., Wang, Y.H., and Lu, S.Y. (2012) *Adv. Funct. Mater.*, **22**, 5038–5043.
41. Nanda, J., Biswas, A., and Banerjee, A. (2013) *Soft Matter*, **9**, 4198–4208.
42. Nagahama, K., Ouchi, T., and Ohya, Y. (2008) *Adv. Funct. Mater.*, **18**, 1220–1231.
43. Ahn, S.-K., Kasi, R.M., Kim, S.-C., Sharma, N., and Zhoub, Y. (2008) *Soft Matter*, **4**, 1151–1157.
44. Pek, Y.S., Wan, A.C.A., Shekaran, A., Zhuo, L., and Ying, J.Y. (2008) *Nat. Nanotechnol.*, **3**, 671–675.
45. Freunlich, H. (1935) *Thixotropie*, Hermann, Paris.
46. Schalek, E. and Szegvari, A. (1923) *Kolloid Z.*, **33**, 326, English translation given in Bauer and Collins in [13].
47. Linsha, V., Nishanth, K.S., Sindhoor, T., Dileep, B.S.K., and Ananthakumar, S. (2015) *J. Mater. Chem. B*, **3**, 5978–5991.
48. Lemmers, M., Spruijt, E., Akerboom, S., Voets, I.K., van Aelst, A.C., Stuart, M.A.C., and van der Gucht, J. (2012) *Langmuir*, **28**, 12311–12318.
49. Kresge, C.T., Leonowicz, M.E., Roth, W.J., Vartuli, J.C., and Beck, J.S. (1992) *Nature*, **359**, 710–712.
50. Zhao, D., Feng, F., Huo, Q., Melosh, N., Fredrickson, G.H., Chmelka, B.F., and Stuky, G.D. (1998) *Science*, **279**, 548–552.
51. Beck, J.S., Chu, C.T., Johnson, I.D., Kresge, C.T., Leonowicz, M.E., Roth, W.J., and Vartuli, J.C. (1992) Synthesis of mesoporous crystalline material. US Patent 5,108,725 to Mobil Oil Corporation.
52. Beck, J.S., Vartul, J.C., Roth, W.J., Leonowicz, M.E., Kresge, C.T., Schmitt, K.D., Chu, C.T.W., Olsen, D.H., Sheppard, E.W., McCullen, S.B., Higgins, J.B., and Schlenker, J.L. (1992) *J. Am. Chem. Soc.*, **114**, 10834–10843.
53. Bagshaw, S.A., Prouzet, E., and Pinnavaia, T.J. (1995) *Science*, **269**, 1242–1244.
54. Tanev, P.T. and Pinnavaia, T.J. (1995) *Science*, **267**, 865–867.
55. Kleitz, F., Choi, S.H., and Ryoo, R. (2003) *Chem. Commun.*, **17**, 2136–2137.
56. de Juan, F. and Ruiz-Hitzky, E. (2000) *Adv. Mater.*, **12**, 430–432.
57. Ogawa, M., Kuroda, K., and Nakamura, T. (2002) *Chem. Lett.*, **31**, 632–633.
58. Feng, X., Fryxell, G.E., Wang, L.Q., Kim, A.Y., Liu, J., and Kemner, K.M. (1997) *Science*, **276**, 923–926.
59. Kickelbick, G. (2007) Hybrid Materials: Synthesis, Characterization, and Applications, Wiley-VCH Verlag GmbH, Weinheim.
60. Gomez-Romero, P. and Sanchez, C. (2004) Functional Hybrid Materials, Wiley-VCH Verlag GmbH, Weinheim.
61. Ruiz-Hitzky, E., Darder, M., Aranda, P., and Ariga, K. (2010) *Adv. Mater.*, **22**, 323–336.
62. Tao, S.L. and Desai, T.A. (2003) *Adv. Drug Delivery Rev.*, **55**, 315–328.
63. Guerrero, D.Q., Quintanar, A.G., Arzaluz, M.G.N., and Segundo, E.P. (2009) *Expert Opin. Drug Delivery*, **6**, 485–498.
64. Kortesuo, P., Ahola, M., and Karlsson, S. (2000) *Biomaterials*, **23**, 2795–2801.
65. Fuller, J.E., Zugates, G.T., Ferreira, L.S., Ow, H.S., Nguyen, N.N., Wiesner, U.B., and Langer, R.S. (2008) *Biomaterials*, **29**, 1526–1532.
66. Bottcher, H., Slowik, P., and Suss, W. (1998) *J. Sol-Gel Sci. Technol.*, **13**, 277–281.

67. Ahola, M., Kortesuo, P., and Kangasniemi, I. (2000) *Int. J. Pharm.*, **195**, 219–227.
68. Maver, U., Godec, A., and Bele, M. (2007) *Int. J. Pharm.*, **330**, 164–174.
69. Roveri, N., Morpurgo, M., and Palazzo, B. (2005) *Anal. Bioanal. Chem.*, **381**, 601–606.
70. Schwertfeger, F., Griesheim, F.A.Z., Krempel, H., and Jugenheim, S. (2001) Use of inorganic aerogels in pharmacy. Patent US006280744B1.
71. Aegerter, M.A., Leventis, N., and Koebel, M.M. (2011) in *Aerogel Handbook*, Advances in Sol–Gel Derived Materials and Technologies (eds M.A. Aegerter and M. Prassas), Springer, New York.
72. Smirnova, I., Suttiruengwong, S., Seiler, M., and Arlt, W. (2004) *Pharm. Dev. Technol.*, **9**, 443–452.
73. Smirnova, I., Turk, M., Wischumerski, R., and Wahl, M. .A. (2005) *Eng. Life Sci.*, **5**, 277–280.
74. Smirnova, I., Mamic, J., and Arlt, W. (2003) *Langmuir*, **19**, 8521–8525.
75. Smirnova, I., Suttiruengwong, S., and Arlt, W. (2004) *J. Non-Cryst. Solids*, **350**, 54–60.
76. Alnaief, M. and Smirnova, I. (2010) *J. Non-Cryst. Solids*, **356**, 1644–1649.
77. Wu, K.C.W., Yamauchi, Y., Hong, C.Y., Yang, Y.H., Liang, Y.H., Funatsu, T., and Tsunoda, M. (2011) *Chem. Commun.*, **47**, 5232–5234.
78. Avnir, D., Coradin, T., Lev, O., and Livage, J. (2006) *J. Mater. Chem.*, **16**, 1013–1030.
79. Bang, A., Sadekar, A.G., Buback, C., Curtin, B., Acar, S., Kolasinac, D., Yin, W., Rubenstein, D.A., Lu, H., Leventis, N., and Leventis, C.S. (2014) *ACS Appl. Mater. Interfaces*, **6**, 4891–4902.
80. Ulker, Z. and Erkey, C. (2014) *J. Controlled Release*, **177**, 51–63.
81. Linsha, V., Sindhoor, T., Mohamed, A.P., and Ananthakumar, S. (2014) *ACS Appl. Mater. Interfaces*, **6**, 15564–15574.
82. Rutenberg, A., Vinogradov, V.V., and Avnir, D. (2013) *Chem. Commun.*, **49**, 5636–5638.
83. Vinogradov, V.V., Vinogradov, A., Sobolev, V.E., Dudanov, I.P., and Vinogradov, V.V. (2015) *J. Sol-Gel Sci. Technol.*, **73**, 501–505.
84. Volodina, K.V., Soloveva, N.L., Vinogradov, V.V., Sobolev, V.E., Alexander, V.V., and Vladimir, V. (2014) *RSC Adv.*, **4**, 60445–60450.
85. Vinogradov, V.V., Komova, Y.M., Vinogradov, A., and Vinogradov, V. (2014) *Nanotechnol. Russ.*, **9**, 87–92.
86. World Health Organization (1976) Immunological Adjuvants. Technical Report Series 595, World Health Organization, Geneva.
87. Edelman, R. (1980) *Rev. Infect. Dis.*, **2**, 370–383.
88. Vinogradov, A.V., Ermakova, A.V., Butman, M.F., Hawkins, E.H., and Vinogradov, V.V. (2014) *Phys. Chem. Chem. Phys.*, **16**, 10614.
89. Vinogradov, V.V. and Avnir, D. (2014) *J. Mater. Chem. B*, **2**, 2868–2873.
90. Vinogradov, V.V. and Avnir, D. (2015) *RSC Adv.*, **5**, 10862–10868.
91. Regi, M.V., Ramila, A., del Real, R.P., and Pariente, J.P. (2001) *Chem. Mater.*, **13**, 308–311.
92. Regi, M.V. (2006) *Chem. Eur. J.*, **12**, 5934–5943.
93. Colilla, M., Barba, I.I., and Regi, M.V. (2008) *Expert Opin. Ther. Pat.*, **18**, 639–656.
94. Manzano, M. and Regi, M.V. (2010) *J. Mater. Chem.*, **20**, 5593–5604.
95. Chia, S., Urano, J., Tamanoi, F., Dunn, B., and Zink, J.I. (2000) *J. Am. Chem. Soc.*, **122**, 6488–6489.
96. Andersson, J., Rosenholm, J., Areva, S., and Linden, M. (2004) *Chem. Mater.*, **16**, 4160–4167.
97. Vallet-Regi, M., Balas, F., Colilla, M., and Manzano, M. (2007) *Drug Metab. Lett.*, **1**, 37–40.
98. Radin, S., Bassyouni, G.E., Vresilovic, E.J., Schepers, E., and Ducheyne, P. (2005) *Biomaterials*, **26**, 1043–1052.
99. Horcajada, P., Ramila, A., Pariente, J.P., and Regi, M.V. (2004) *Microporous Mesoporous Mater.*, **68**, 105–109.
100. Regi, M.V. (2006) *Dalton Trans.*, **44**, 5211–5220.
101. Hoffmann, F., Cornelius, M., Morell, J., and FrVba, M. (2006) *Angew. Chem. Int. Ed.*, **45**, 3216–3251.

102. Mal, N.K., Fujiwara, M., and Tanaka, Y. (2003) *Nature*, **421**, 350–353.

103. Doadrio, J.C., Sousa, E.M.B., Barba, I.I., Doadrio, A.L., Pariente, J.P., and Regi, M.V. (2006) *J. Mater. Chem.*, **16**, 462–467.

104. Zeng, W., Qian, X.F., Zhang, Y.B., Yin, J., and Zhu, Z.K. (2005) *Mater. Res. Bull.*, **40**, 766–772.

105. Balas, F., Manzano, M., Horcajada, P., and Regi, M.V. (2006) *J. Am. Chem. Soc.*, **128**, 8116–8117.

106. Tang, Q., Xu, Y., Wu, D., and Sun, Y. (2006) *Chem. Lett.*, **35**, 474–475.

107. Qu, F., Zhu, G., Huang, S., Li, S., and Qiu, S. (2006) *Chem. Phys. Chem.*, **7**, 400–406.

108. Zhu, Y., Shi, J., Shen, W., Dong, X., Feng, J., Ruan, M., and Li, Y. (2005) *Angew. Chem. Int. Ed.*, **44**, 5083–5087.

109. Park, C., Oh, K., Lee, S.C., and Kim, C. (2007) *Angew. Chem. Int. Ed.*, **46**, 1455–1457.

110. Zhou, Z., Zhu, S., and Zhang, D. (2007) *J. Mater. Chem.*, **17**, 2377–2468.

111. Tian, B.S. and Yang, C. (2009) *J. Phys. Chem. C*, **113**, 4925–4931.

112. You, Y.Z., Kalebaila, K.K., Brock, S.L., and Oupicky, D. (2008) *Chem. Mater.*, **20**, 3354–3359.

113. Nguyen, T.D., Leung, K.C.F., Liong, M., Liu, Y., Stoddart, J.F., and Zink, J.I. (2007) *Adv. Funct. Mater.*, **17**, 2101–2110.

114. Park, C., Lee, K., and Kim, C. (2009) *Angew. Chem. Int. Ed.*, **48**, 1275–1278.

115. Yang, Q., Wang, S., Fan, P., Wang, L., Di, Y., Lin, K., and Xiao, F.-S. (2005) *Chem. Mater.*, **17**, 5999–6003.

116. Leung, K.C.F., Nguyen, T.D., Stoddart, J.F., and Zink, J.I. (2006) *Chem. Mater.*, **18**, 5919.

117. Angelos, S., Yang, Y.-W., Patel, K., Stoddart, J.F., and Zink, J.I. (2008) *Angew. Chem. Int. Ed.*, **47**, 2222–2226.

118. Chang, J.H., Shim, C.H., Kim, B.J., Shin, Y., Exarhos, G.J., and Kim, K.J. (2005) *Adv. Mater.*, **17**, 634–637.

119. Aznar, E., Mondragon, L., and Ros-Lis, J.V. (2011) *Angew. Chem. Int. Ed.*, **50**, 11172–11175.

120. Giri, S., Trewyn, B.G., Stellmaker, M.P., and Lin, V.S.Y. (2005) *Angew. Chem. Int. Ed.*, **44**, 5038–5044.

121. Lai, C.Y., Trewyn, B.G., Jeftinija, D.M., Jeftinija, K., Xu, S., Jeftinija, S., and Lin, V.S.Y. (2003) *J. Am. Chem. Soc.*, **125**, 4451–4459.

122. Hernandez, R., Tseng, H.R., Wong, J.W., Stoddart, J.F., and Zink, J.I. (2004) *J. Am. Chem. Soc.*, **126**, 3370–3371.

123. Nguyen, T.D., Tseng, H.R., Celestre, P.C., Flood, A.H., Liu, Y., Stoddart, J.F., and Zink, J.I. (2005) *Proc. Natl. Acad. Sci. U.S.A.*, **102**, 10029–10034.

124. Nguyen, T.D., Liu, Y., Saha, S., Leung, K.C.F., Stoddart, J.F., and Zink, J.I. (2007) *J. Am. Chem. Soc.*, **129**, 626–634.

125. Ferris, D.P., Zhao, Y.L., Khashab, N.M., Khatib, H.A., Stoddart, J.F., and Zink, J.I. (2009) *J. Am. Chem. Soc.*, **131**, 1686–1688.

126. Lu, J., Choi, E., Tamanoi, F., and Zink, J.I. (2008) *Small*, **4**, 421–426.

127. Kim, H.J., Matsuda, H., Zhou, H.S., and Honma, I. (2006) *Adv. Mater.*, **18**, 3083–3088.

128. Tang, F., Li, L., and Chen, D. (2012) *Adv. Mater.*, **24**, 1504–1534.

129. Allen, T.M. (2002) *Nat. Rev. Cancer*, **2**, 750–763.

130. Sudimack, J. and Lee, R.J. (2000) *Adv. Drug Delivery Rev.*, **41**, 147–162.

131. Guo, R., Li, L.L., Zhao, W.H., Chen, Y.X., Wang, X.Z., Fang, C.J., Feng, W., Zhang, T.L., Ma, X., Lu, M., Peng, S.Q., and Yan, C.H. (2012) *Nanoscale*, **4**, 3577.

132. Tsai, C.P., Chen, C.Y., Hung, Y., Chang, F.H., and Mou, C.Y. (2009) *J. Mater. Chem.*, **19**, 5737–5743.

133. Rosenholm, J.M., Meinander, A., Peuhu, E., Niemi, R., Eriksson, J.E., Sahlgren, C., and Linden, M. (2009) *ACS Nano*, **3**, 197–206.

134. Ruız-Hernandez, E., Lopez-Noriega, A., Arcos, D., Izquierdo-Barba, I., Terasaki, O., and Vallet-Regi, M. (2007) *Chem. Mater.*, **19**, 3455–3463.

135. Insin, N., Tracy, J.B., Lee, H., Zimmer, J.P., Westervelt, R.M., and Bawendi, M.G. (2008) *ACS Nano*, **2**, 197–202.

136. Zhou, J., Wu, W., Caruntu, D., Yu, M.H., Martin, A., Chen, J.F., O'Connor, C.J., and Zhou, W.L. (2007) *J. Phys. Chem. C*, **111**, 17473–17477.

137. Chen, Y., Chen, H., Ma, M., Chen, F., Guo, L., Zhang, L., and Shi, J. (2011) *J. Mater. Chem.*, **21**, 5290–5298.
138. Wang, F., Tan, W.B., Zhang, Y., Fan, X., and Wang, M. (2006) *Nanotechnology*, **17**, R1.
139. Liu, R., Zhang, Y., and Feng, P. (2009) *J. Am. Chem. Soc.*, **131**, 15128–15129.
140. Chang, B., Sha, X., Guo, J., Jiao, Y., Wang, C., and Yang, W. (2011) *J. Mater. Chem.*, **21**, 9239–9247.
141. Lin, Y.S., Tsai, C.P., Huang, H.Y., Kuo, C.T., Hung, Y., Huang, D.M., Chen, Y.C., and Mou, C.Y. (2005) *Chem. Mater.*, **17**, 4570–4573.
142. Liu, H.M., Wu, S.H., Lu, C.W., Yao, M., Hsiao, J.K., Hung, Y., Lin, Y.S., Mou, C.Y., Yang, C.S., Huang, D.M., and Chen, Y.C. (2008) *Small*, **4**, 619–626.
143. Cheng, S.H., Lee, C.-H., Chen, M.C., Souris, J.S., Tseng, F.G., Yang, C.S., Mou, C.Y., Chen, C.-T., and Lo, L.W. (2010) *J. Mater. Chem.*, **20**, 6149–6157.
144. Voisin, P., Ribot, E.J., Miraux, S., Bouzier-Sore, A.K., Lahitte, J.F., Bouchaud, V., Mornet, S., Thiaudiere, E., Franconi, J.M., Raison, L., Labrugere, C., and Delville, M.H. (2007) *Bioconjugate Chem.*, **18**, 1053–1063.
145. Runge, V.M. (2000) *J. Magn. Reson. Imaging*, **12**, 205–213.
146. Tagaya, M., Ikoma, T., Xu, Z., and Tanaka, J. (2014) *Inorg. Chem.*, **53**, 6817–6827.
147. Ji, X.J., Shao, R.P., Elliott, A.M., Stafford, R.J., Esparza-Coss, E., Bankson, J.A., Liang, G., Luo, Z.P., Park, K., Markert, J.T., and Li, C. (2007) *J. Phys. Chem. C*, **111**, 6245–6251.
148. Cho, Y.S., Yoon, T.J., Jang, E.S., Hong, K.S., Lee, S.Y., Kim, O.R., Park, C., Kim, Y.J., Yi, G.C., and Chang, K. (2010) *Cancer Lett.*, **299**, 63–71.
149. Park, K.S., Tae, J., Choi, B., Kim, Y.-S., Moon, C., Kim, S.-H., Lee, H.-S., Kim, J., Kim, J., Park, J., Lee, J.-H., Lee, J.E., Joh, J.-W., and Kim, S. (2010) *Nanomed. Nanotechnol. Biol. Med.*, **6**, 263–276.
150. Qian, H.S., Guo, H.C., Ho, P.C.L., Mahendran, R., and Zhang, Y. (2009) *Small*, **5**, 2285.
151. Couleaud, P., Morosini, V., Frochot, C., Richeter, S., Raehm, L., and Durand, J.O. (2010) *Nanoscale*, **2**, 1083–1095.
152. Yan, F. and Kopelman, R. (2003) *Photochem. Photobiol.*, **78**, 587–591.
153. Kim, S., Ohulchanskyy, T.Y., Pudavar, H.E., Pandey, R.K., and Prasad, P.N. (2007) *J. Am. Chem. Soc.*, **129**, 2669–2675.
154. Roy, I., Ohulchanskyy, T.Y., Pudavar, H.E., Bergey, E.J., Oseroff, A.R., Morgan, J., Dougherty, T.J., and Prasad, P.N. (2003) *J. Am. Chem. Soc.*, **125**, 7860–7865.
155. Kumar, R., Roy, I., Ohulchanskky, T.Y., Vathy, L.A., Bergey, E.J., Sajjad, M., and Prasad, P.N. (2010) *ACS Nano*, **4**, 699–708.
156. Cloarec, J.P., Deligianis, N., Martin, J.R., Lawrence, I., Souteyrand, E., Polychronakos, C., and Lawrence, M.F. (2002) *Biosens. Bioelectron.*, **17**, 405–441.
157. Kong, L., Mume, E., Trianiand, G., and Smith, S.V. (2013) *Langmuir*, **29**, 5609–5616.
158. Chen, F., Hong, H., Zhang, Y., Valdovinos, H.F., Shi, S., Kwon, G.S., Theuer, C.P., Barnhart, T.E., and Cai, W. (2013) *ACS Nano*, **7**, 9027–9039.
159. Miller, L., Winter, G., Baur, B., Witulla, B., Solbach, C., Reske, S., and Linden, M. (2014) *Nanoscale*, **6**, 4928–4935.
160. Chakravarty, R., Shukla, R., Ram, R., Venkatesh, M., Tyagi, A.K., and Dash, A. (2011) *Anal. Chem.*, **83**, 6342–6348.
161. Yang, L., Sundaresan, G., Sun, M., Jose, P., Hoffman, D., McDonagh, P.R., Lamichhane, N., Cutler, C.S., Perez, J.M., and Zweit, J. (2013) *J. Mater. Chem. B*, **1**, 1421–1431.
162. Nagy, L.N., Mihaly, J., Polyak, A., Debreczeni, B., Csaszar, B., Szigyarto, I.C., Wacha, A., Czegeny, Z., Jakab, E., Klebert, S., Drotar, E., Dabasi, G., Bota, A., Balogh, L., and Kissc, E. (2015) *J. Mater. Chem. B*, **3**, 7529–7537.
163. Bradbury, M.S., Phillips, E., Montero, P.H., Cheal, S.M., Stam-buk, H., Durack, J.C., Sofocleous, C.T., Meester, R.J.C., Wiesner, U., and Patel, S. (2013) *Integr. Biol.*, **5**, 74–86.

11
Relevance of Natural Degradable Polymers in the Biomedical Field

Raju Francis, Nidhin Joy, and Anjaly Sivadas

11.1
Introduction

Biodegradable polymers are recently emerged polymers. Biodegradable polymers offer possible solutions to waste-disposal problems that are associated with traditional petroleum-derived plastics. Biopolymers are also referred to as natural polymers because they are formed in nature during the growth cycles of all organisms. They are generally water-soluble gums [1] that have novel and unique physical properties. Because of their wide diversity in structure and physical characteristics, these polysaccharides have found a wide range of applications in the food, pharmaceutical, and other industries. Biodegradation is a natural process by which organic chemicals in the environment are converted to simpler compounds, mineralized, and redistributed through elemental cycles such as the carbon, nitrogen, and sulfur cycles. Biodegradation can only occur within the biosphere as microorganisms play a central role in the biodegradation process. Some microorganisms and enzymes capable of degrading a vast number of synthetic biodegradable polymers have been recently identified. Polymers are used in drug delivery applications because they offer unique properties, which so far have not been attained by any other materials. Various natural gums and mucilages have been examined for their role as potential polymers for use in controlled and sustained drug release, in the past few decades. Natural polymers remain attractive compared with synthetic polymers primarily because they are commercial, readily available, capable of a multitude of chemical modifications, potentially degradable, and compatible due to their origin. Biodegradable polymers can degrade in biological fluids with progressive release of a dissolved or dispersed drug. Biosafety and biocompatibility are two important characteristics needed for the use of polymers in the field of pharmaceutical formulation and in novel drug delivery approaches. Biodegradable polymers degrade within the body due to natural biological processes, eliminating the need to remove a drug delivery system after release of the active agent. Most biodegradable polymers are designed to degrade because hydrolysis of the polymer chains result in

Biomedical Applications of Polymeric Materials and Composites, First Edition.
Edited by Raju Francis and Sakthi Kumar.

biologically acceptable, and progressively smaller, compounds. Degradation may take place through bulk hydrolysis, in which the polymer degrades in a fairly uniform manner throughout the matrix [2].

11.2 Natural Biopolymers and Its Application

Polymers have been used to control the rate of drug release, prevent toxicity, protect drugs from degradation before delivery, target drugs to the site of action, as well as improve absorption, bioavailability, and therapeutic efficacy. Although synthetic polymers can be tailor-made, natural polymers exhibit the advantages of excellent biodegradability, biocompatibility, cost-effectiveness, and environmental friendliness [3].

11.2.1 Chitosan

Chitosan derived from chitin is a natural biopolymer found in the marine environment and originates from crustaceans and the cell wall of fungi. It is known as linear polysaccharide and is composed of a glucosamine and *N*-acetylglucosamine ratio referred to as the degree of deacetylation. Depending on the source and the processing method, its molecular weight may range from 300 to 1000 kDa. Chitosan is normally insoluble in water and aqueous solutions above pH 7, but, in diluted acid with a pH less than 6, the protonated free amino group on glucosamine facilitates the solubility of that molecule [4–6]. Chitosan is nontoxic after oral administration in humans and is approved by the FDA. Chitosanase, lysozyme, and papain enzymes degrade CHI *in vitro*. *In vivo* degradation results from the lysozyme and occurs through the hydrolysis of the acetylated residues. The rate of degradation of chitosan inversely affects the degree of acetylation and crystallinity of the polymer. The highly deacetylated form demonstrates the lowest degradation rates and may last for several months *in vivo*. Chemical modification of chitosan can significantly affect its solubility and degradation rate [7]. Chitosan is biocompatible and biodegradable, and can be molded into porous structures (allows osteoconduction) [8]. Several studies have focused on the use of chitosan/calcium phosphate composite for this purpose. Chitosan /nanocrystalline calcium phosphate scaffolds characterized by a relatively rough surface and approximately 20 times greater area/unit mass than chitosan scaffolds indicate increased adsorption and improved cell attachment for bone regeneration [9]. In the development of chitosan/nano-HA scaffold conducted by Thein-Han and his coworkers [10], high molecular weight chitosan scaffolds were observed to have superior mechanical properties compared with medium molecular weight chitosan scaffolds. In addition, the significant increase in compression modulus of the nano-HA/chitosan composite was attributed to the good dispersion of nano-HA and the strong interaction between chitosan and nano-HA to form a composite. In the nanocomposite scaffold, the organic chitosan network uniformly covered the HA nanoparticles; interactions may have occurred similar to those occurring components of bone. Possible interactions involve Ca^{2+} and $PO4^{3-}$ charged species of HA with NH^{3+} of chitosan. However, the mechanical properties of the composites obtained were inadequate for bone regeneration. Chitosan with incorporation of collagen (CCS) composite microgranules were fabricated as bone substitutes for the purpose of obtaining high bone-forming efficacy. The microgranules have the flexibility to fill various types of defect sites with closer packing. The interconnected pores form spaces between the microgranules, which allow new bone ingrowth and vascularization [11]. Like any other biodegradable polymers, the mechanical strength of CCS significantly improved after adding HA or other calcium phosphate components [12]. Other than composite scaffold, chitosan also appeared in the form of membrane, which was fabricated with silica xerogel [13]. Their potential applications in guided bone regeneration (GBR) were investigated with regard to bone regeneration ability. The *in vivo* study in a rat calvarial model demonstrated significantly enhanced bone regeneration when using the chitosan/xerogel membrane compared to when using the pure chitosan one. Histomorphometric analysis performed 3 weeks after implantation revealed a fully closed defect in the hybrid membrane, whereas there was only 57% defect closure in the chitosan membrane. Another scientific study was conducted on modified chitosan structure with varied sulfate groups (structure is shown in Figure 11.1) [14]; the molecular weight and sulfur content were tailored to investigate the effects on the bioactivity of BMP-2. Low dose of synthetic sulfated chitosan (structure shown in Figure 11.1)

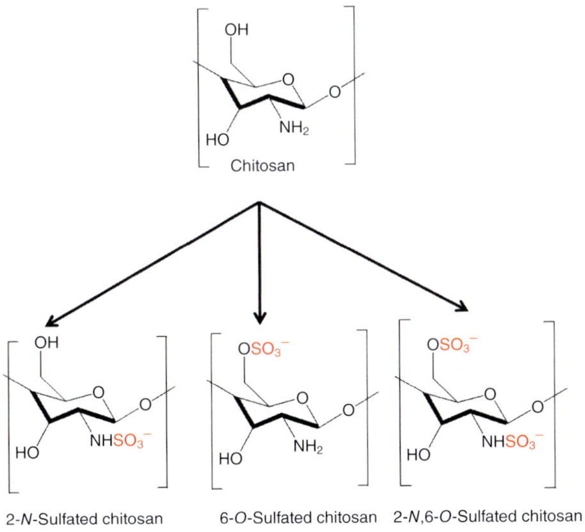

Figure 11.1 Chemical structures of chitosan modified with different sulfate groups. 2-*N*-Sulfated chitosan, 2SCS;6-*O*-Sulfated chitosan, 6SCS; 2-*N*, 6-*O*-Sulfated chitosan, 26SCS [14].

stimulated osteoblast differentiation induced by BMP-2 *in vitro* and ectopic bone formation *in vivo*. Another requirement of chitosan modification is to allow water solubility in a chitosan matrix, as observed by D'Ayala and coworkers [15].

11.2.2 Cellulose

Cellulose is the most abundant polysaccharide found in nature. Its value has been recognized in numerous traditional industries, such as construction, pulp and papermaking, and textile industries. Oxidation of cellulose is one of the most important modification methods to prepare value-added cellulose derivatives for further applications. Oxidized cellulose and regenerated cellulose are widely used as excellent hemostatic materials in various surgical operations and postsurgical adhesion prevention layers. Ascribed to its gelling properties, biodegradability, biocompatibility, and bioactivity of TEMPO-oxidized NFC, its structured hydrogel and aerogel materials have been used for biomedical applications such as in scaffolds for wound healing and three-dimensional (3D) cell culture, drug carrier and controlled release, cosmetic applications such as thickeners and water-retaining agents, and other applications [16, 17].

11.2.3 Proteins and Poly(amino acids)

Proteins are the most important classes of biomolecules. They are the major structural units of many tissues in which amino acid polymers are arranged in a 3D structure. It is an important biomaterial as it is a major component of natural tissues and is applied in hemostatic agents, scaffolds for tissue engineering, drug delivery vehicles, and sutures. Controlled degradation process happens in protein-based biomaterials [18]. The human body is able to synthesize a wide range of proteins in which the precursor molecules pass through four major stages prior to becoming functional proteins. Formation of the primary structure where a linear sequence of various amino acids is held together by peptide bonds occurs in the first stage. The constituent amino acids then participate in hydrogen bonding to form the secondary structure of protein. The linear primary structure arranges itself in the most stable structures as α-helices or -pleated ß sheets. These secondary structures then join together to form 3D tertiary structures, which in turn interact with other protein chains to form the more refined 3D quaternary structure of a multiunit protein [19].

11.2.4 Collagen

Collagen is the most abundant protein in mammals accounting for 30% of the protein content in the human body and forms a major component of skin and bone [20, 21]. It is a road-type polymer with a length of 300 nm and a molecular weight of 300,000. Its helical structure and its predictable mechanical properties are due to its repeating sequence [22]. It undergoes enzymatic degradation within the body via enzymes. It has been extensively investigated for biomedical applications due to the enzymatic degradability and physicochemical, mechanical, and biological properties. Collagen is mostly soluble in acidic aqueous solutions. It can be processed into different forms such as sheets, tubes, sponges, foams, nanofibrous matrices, powders, injectable viscous solutions, and dispersions. The degradation rate of collagen can be significantly altered by enzymatic pretreatment or cross-linking in biomedical applications. By increasing the cross-links, one could (i) increase the biodegradation time, making collagen less susceptible to enzymatic degradation; (ii) decrease the capacity of collagen to absorb water; (iii) decrease its solubility; and (iv) increase the tensile strength of collagen. As a biomaterial, collagen is biocompatible, biodegradable, and osteoconductive [23]. The composition of human bone is a well-known mineral/organic hybrid consisting of HA and mainly organic collagen constituents. Calcium phosphate/collagen composites are probably the most preferred for biomimetic constructs for osseous replacement or bone regeneration [24]. When associated with calcium phosphate particles or any other filler forming composite, collagen prevents filler dispersion in implants, resulting in an easily molded biomaterial [25]. In order to investigate the vicinity between collagen and calcium phosphate in bone substitute biomaterial, composites constituted of collagen and calcium phosphate doped by europium were synthesized by a precipitation method [26]. Interaction checked by Förster resonance energy transfer (FRET) devices showed a good yield from the composites, thereby promising to be a favorable bone substitute. Collagen coatings are known to enhance early cell adhesion and proliferation on calcium phosphate, increasing the *in vivo* osteointegration, osteoconduction, and osteoregenerative capacity of these materials [27, 28]. For these reasons, composite materials containing calcium phosphate and collagen have been developed [29] using methods such as particle–gel mixing and powder compression [30]. One scientific study regarding the effect of collagen/citric acid on the setting reaction of brushite found out that collagen has the ability to speed up the cement setting reaction and had compressive strength similar to that of spongious bone (48.9 MPa) [31]. When combined with citric acid, it helped to shorten the setting time, increase injectability, reduce viscosity, and improve the mechanical strength of the composite [32]. Citric acid also enables the mixing of a high collagen content gel (3 wt%) with the cement powder to form a brushite–collagen composite that was easy to work with. The effect of cross-linking on brushite–collagen composites was also studied by immersing the composite into a 2% glutaraldehyde solution in wet condition; the addition of neither collagen nor glutaraldehyde cross-linked collagen seemed to increase the compressive strength of the composite after storage in wet condition [33].

11.2.5 Carrageenans

Carrageenans are water-soluble polymers extracted from red algae. They are used in food and pharmaceutical industries as gelling and stabilizing agents, in microencapsulation, and in immobilization of drugs and enzymes. Carrageenans consist of alternating copolymers of a-(133)-D-galactose and *b*-(134)-3,6-anhydro-D- or L-galactose. Several isomers of carrageenan are known as *k*-, *λ*-, and *ι*-carrageenan, and they differ in the number and position of the ester sulfate groups on the repeating galactose units. *k*-Carrageenan has only one negative charge per disaccharide with a tendency to form a strong and rigid gel. *ι*-Carrageenan has two and *λ*-carrageenan bears on an average 2.7 charges per disaccharide unit. The gelling power of *λ*- and *ι*-carrageenans imparts excellent film-forming properties.

11.2.6 Elastin

Tropoelastin molecules are covalently bonded in elastin and are highly cross-linked insoluble polymer. Elastin is a major protein component of vascular and lung tissues. Unusual elastic properties of elastin make it reliable. Smooth muscle cells (SMCs) and fibroblasts intracellularly produced the tropoelastin molecules and are cross-linked extracellularly to form a secondary structure with b-turns. The pentapeptide VPGVG, the hexapeptide APGVGV, the nonapeptide VPGFGVGAG, and the tetrapeptide VPGG are the repeating sequences of tropoelastin. In this the pentapeptide VPGVG recurs up to 50 times in a single molecule. Results show from the *in vivo* biocompatibility studies that elastin elicits immune response to the same extent as do collagen implants. But the insolubility of native elastin limits its biomedical applications [34]. Elastin is used in biological coatings for synthetic vascular grafts [35] due to its minimal interaction with platelets. Synthetic elastin has been developed from recombinant human tropoelastin [36] to overcome the insolubility of elastin. Good mechanical and biological properties make them useful as elastic biomaterials for appropriate applications. When the temperature is increased above 25 °C, tropoelastin will undergo folding due to its transition from a disordered form to an ordered form at higher temperature called inverse temperature transition (ITT). Tropoelastin and its synthetic analogs are extensively investigated due to its unique thermal transition properties [37].

11.2.7 Elastin-Like Peptides

Artificial polypeptides composed of the pentapeptide repeats (VPGXG) n of human tropoelastin except the fourth amino acid are referred to as elastin-like polypeptides (ELPs) where X in ELP stands for a guest residue that can be any amino acid except proline and "n" represents number of pentapeptide repeats in the ELP. Elastin is the source of ELPs. ELPs have excellent biocompatibility and nonimmunogenic property, and degradation products are composed of natural amino acids that are nontoxic. They exhibit a reversible ITT.

ELPs will respond to stimuli such as pH, ionic strength, and light by the incorporation of appropriate guest residues in the molecule at the fourth position [38].

With advanced molecular biology, these molecules can be bioproduced using genetic engineering techniques. Monodisperse polymers of ELPs can be recombinantly synthesized with *E. coli* by the overexpression of a synthetic gene. Under mild conditions where ELPs are injectable, they will undergo phase transition. They can be used as a drug carrier vehicle and in cartilage tissue engineering [39]. Normal cartilage and cross-linked ELP show similar shear modulus. The dynamic shear modulus of the gel increased from 0.28 to 1.7 kPa after seeding with chondrocyte for 4 weeks in culture. So this result shows the feasibility of remodeling ELP matrices by the deposition of functional cartilage extracellular matrix (ECM) components [40]. Specific substrates can be developed for engineering various tissues by the incorporation of specific cell binding epitopes in ELPs due to its synthetic versatility [41]. Consequently the incorporation of RGD peptide into an ELP has significantly enhanced cell adhesion and spreading on ELP hydrogel matrices.

11.2.8
Albumin

Human blood plasma contains almost 50% of albumin protein, a water-soluble polymer with a molecular weight of 66 kDa. The function of albumin is to carry hydrophobic fatty acid molecules around the bloodstream and maintain blood pH. In the liver preproalbumins are synthesized, and they undergo further processing before getting released into the circulatory system. High content of cystine and charged amino acids such as aspartic and glutamic acids, lysine, and arginine and low content of tryptophan and methionine are among the characteristics of the composition of albumin. Albumin is a highly preferred degradable biopolymer for medical applications [42] because almost all tissues in the human body have the ability to degrade albumin. Due to the presence of functional groups along the polymer chain and its solubility, albumin is very easily processed to various shapes and forms such as membranes, microspheres, nanofibers, and nanospheres. Albumin is used as a carrier vehicle for intravenous drug/gene delivery [43] due to its excellent blood compatibility. It has also been investigated for its use in cardiovascular devices [44]. Albumin-based surgical adhesives have also been approved by the FDA for reapproximating the layers of large vessels, such as femoral, aorta, and carotid arteries (CryoLife Inc.), and are composed of glutaraldehyde, gelatin, and bovine serum albumin (BSA).

11.2.9
Fibrin

Fibrin is a biopolymer involved in the natural blood-clotting process. It is derived from fibrinogen, which has a molecular weight of 360 kDa. It is composed of three pairs of polypeptide chains. There are three major sections of the structure which consist of a central domain composed of fibrinopeptide E with two pairs of fibrinopeptides A and B molecules and two terminal domains of fibrinopeptide D.

Due to the cleavage of fibrinopeptides A and B, a linear fibril forms upon spontaneous fibrillogenesis in the presence of thrombin. The lateral association of these fibers leads to fibers with varying diameters ranging from 10 to 200 nm depending on the environmental conditions. Fibrinolysis occurs in the body due to the degradation of fibrin clot. It is initiated by a complex cascade of enzymes present in the human body [45]. With excellent biodegradability, injectability, and biocompatibility properties and the presence of several ECM proteins that favorably affects cell adhesion and proliferation, fibrin has become one of the biopolymers used as biomaterials: fibrin sealant was among the first products developed from fibrin. In various surgical procedures hemostasis and tissue sealing applications are done clinically worldwide with the help of different fibrin sealant products. Fibrin has also been investigated as a carrier vehicle for bioactive molecules due to its injectability and biodegradability. Certain growth factors (GFs) have a strong interaction with fibrin matrices [46] demonstrating that proteins can interact differently with fibrin clots. Various cross-linking techniques are currently under investigation to control the release profile of bioactive molecules from the fibrin matrix. It is found that fibrin matrices are excellent cell carrier vehicles. Bioseeds are applied in chronic wounds, and they are prepared by mixing keratinocytes with fibrin. Optimization of matrix properties is needed for each different cell type [47].

11.2.10 Hyaluronic Acid

Hyaluronic acid (HA) is a linear polysaccharide consisting of alternating units of *N*-acetyl-D-aglucosamine and glucuronic acid. It is a member of the glycosaminoglycan family. It is found in virtually every tissue in vertebrates. Rooster combs and bovine vitreous humor are the traditional sources for HA isolation. HA can undergo degradation within the body by free radicals, such as nitric oxide and MMPs found in the ECM. After degradation follows endocytosis. Lysosomal digestion of HA forms mono- and disaccharides, which are again converted into ammonia, carbon dioxide, and water via the Krebs cycle [48]. HA is very actively involved in many biological processes such as modulating cell migration and differentiation during embryogenesis, regulating ECM organization and metabolism, as well as playing important roles in metastasis, wound healing, and inflammation. HA polymer has been extensively investigated for wound dressing applications. Other properties of HA include its ability to promote angiogenesis and to be recognized by receptors on a variety of cells associated with tissue repair [49]. HA also improves collagen deposition and angiogenesis through mesenchymal and epithelial cell migration and differentiation, thus playing an important role in tissue repair. This leads HA to be an ideal biomaterial for tissue engineering and drug delivery applications. With HA's aqueous solubility, it can be fabricated into different types of porous and 3D structures. HA is used in clinical trials with a viscous formulation containing fibroblast growth factor (OSSIGELs) and is used as a synthetic bone graft to accelerate bone fracture healing. HYAFF11 is currently being used as a carrier vehicle for a variety of GFs and morphogens as well as bone marrow stromal cells. Studies show that better healing response is obtained with Hyaffs11 carrier compared to collagen [50]. Collagen-based materials as injectable soft tissue fillers [51] are being replaced with HA-based materials. To protect the sensitive eye tissue during cataract extraction, corneal transplantation, and glaucoma surgery, and to serve as vitreous humor substitute, high molecular weight viscous HA solutions (AMVISCs and AMVISCs PLUS) are being used. Viscous HA solutions (SYNVISCs, ORTHOVISCs) are clinically used as a synovial fluid substitute to relieve pain and improve joint mobility in osteoarthritis patients [52]. Recent studies show the advantages of exogenous HA in treating vascular diseases [53].

11.2.11 Glycosaminoglycans

Glycosaminoglycans (GAGs) are polysaccharides which naturally cover the surface of all eukaryotic cells. GAGs are negatively charged polysaccharides composed of repeating disaccharides units. GAGs are often located on the surface of cells or within the ECM. They are generally covalently linked to core proteins comprising larger glycoconjugates called *proteoglycans* (*PGs*) and participate in a wide variety of biological events, which depend on their core structures, core proteins, and sulfation patterns. Variable patterns of substitution of the disaccharide subunits with *N*-sulfate, *O*-sulfate, and *N*-acetyl groups give rise to a large number of complex sequences. Heparin (HP) and heparan sulfate (HS) are structurally the most complex members of the GAG family of polysaccharides, which also includes chondroitin sulfate (CS), dermatan sulfate (DS), and keratin sulfate.

11.2.12 Heparin (HP)

HP is located in the mast cells and its exact biological function is not clear, but it is considered to be involved in allergic and inflammatory responses. It is also is well known for its anticoagulant activity; it has been used clinically as an anticoagulant for over 60 years. The release of lipoprotein lipase and hepatic lipase, inhibition of complement activation, and inhibition of angiogenesis and tumor growth, and antiviral activity are other biological activities of HP. These activities originates from its interaction with proteins, the most well studied and characterized being its interaction with antithrombin, a serine protease inhibitor that mediates the anticoagulant activity of HP. Its biological activities are advantageous in therapy, such as in modulation of angiogenesis, tumor metastasis [54, 55], and viral invasion, because HP – protein binding serves as a model for the interaction of proteins with the highly sulfated regions (NS domains) of the HS chains of cell-surface HS PGs [56].

11.2.13
Heparan Sulfate

HP PGs are recognized as ubiquitous protein ligands. Binding of proteins to HS chains may serve a variety of functional purposes, from simple immobilization or protection against proteolytic degradation to distinct modulation of biological activity. Because of such interactions HS PGs are critically involved in a variety of biological phenomena at various levels of complexity, including organogenesis in embryonic development, angiogenesis, regulation of blood coagulation and GF/cytokine action, cell adhesion, and lipid metabolism [57, 58]. HS plays essential roles in many biological processes, including blood coagulation, viral/bacterial infections, tumor growth, and embryonic development [59]. These HS/HP oligosaccharides are used to probe the structural selectivity in HS-mediated biological functions. Several works in the literature clearly show that there is a specificity directing the interactions of HS and target proteins, regarding both the fine structure of the polysaccharide chain and precise protein motifs. Thus, they can interact with a diverse range of proteins leading to biological activities as shown in Figure 11.2 [60].

Due to their vast structural diversity, HS chains are able to bind and interact with a wide variety of proteins, such as GFs, chemokines, morphogens, ECM components, and enzymes, among others. HS chains are located facing the extracellular compartment, and thus their biological roles can be related to assemble the ECM [61] to modulate the activity of enzymes and/or their inhibitors [62], to provide an extracellular gradient of GFs and chemokines [63], as well as to prevent degradation of GFs. Nevertheless, HS PGs can trigger cell response through signal transduction pathways, as well as by translocation to intracellular compartments, due to interactions of the polysaccharide chains and/or the core protein with specific ligands. HS play a role in cellular signaling as either receptors or coreceptors for

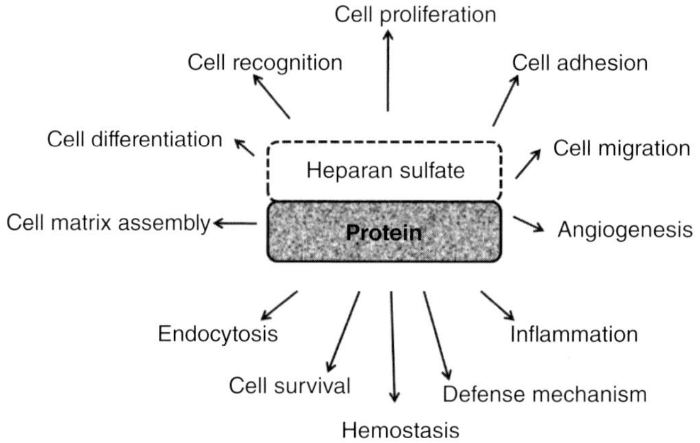

Figure 11.2 Biological activities modulated by the interaction of proteins with heparan sulfate [60].

different ligands. The activation of downstream pathways is related to phosphorylation of different cytosolic proteins either directly or by involving cytoskeleton interactions leading to gene regulation.

11.2.14 Chondroitin Sulfate

CS is a major component of aggrecan. It is found in abundance in the proteoglycans of articular cartilage. It can stimulate the metabolic response of cartilage tissue and has anti-inflammatory properties [64]. It is involved in intracellular signaling, cell recognition, and the connection of ECM components to cell-surface glycoproteins. CS disaccharides in mammals are found to be monosulfated in the 4th or 6th position of the GalNAc residue or disulfated in the 2nd and 6th positions of the GlcA and GalNAc or in the 4th and 6th positions of GalNAc residue [65]. Chondroitin sulfotransferases are responsible for these modifications. An important phase of wound healing process involves the secretion of glycosaminoglycan by fibroblast cells to form a hydrophilic matrix, which makes it suitable for remodeling. The significance of CS as natural polymer for use in biomedical applications has been shown in a recent study using rat embryonic fibroblast cells where the majority of the glycosaminoglycan chains were synthesized [66]. CS hydrogels have been extensively investigated for their role in wound dressing applications due to its biocompatibility, nonimmunogenicity, and pliability [67]. Numerous physical and chemical cross-linking techniques have been developed to prepare CS hydrogels in biomedical applications [68]. CS has been extensively investigated as a scaffolding material for cartilage tissue engineering, since it helps regulate the expression of the chondrocyte phenotype. Significance of this study includes successful cartilage regeneration through the use of a tissue engineered implant, only if the seeded cells undergo normal proliferation and phenotype development within the biodegradable scaffold together with the production of a new cartilage-specific ECM. The efficacy of using composite scaffolds composed of CS and other biopolymers, such as collagen or synthetic biodegradable polymers, as scaffolds for cartilage tissue engineering were investigated, and these studies have shown a strong correlation between the use of CS and the bioactivity of the seeded chondrocyte [69].

11.2.15 Dermatan Sulfate

DS is a macromolecule belonging to a class of natural, structurally complex, sulfated, linear polymers, namely, GAGs. DS, produced by extraction and purification from different animal tissues, has several fundamental biological activities, as well as pharmacological properties, making it an experimental therapeutic agent to modulate a variety of these biological processes [70, 71]. Biological activities of DS chains possibly involve various GFs and chemokines, and these functions are closely associated with the sulfation patterns and characteristics of the polysaccharide chains. DS may help in the development of targeted therapeutics, in particular those used for parasitic and viral infections; regenerative medicine based on the idea that minute amounts of functional poly(oligo)saccharides can be used for tissue regeneration; and antitumor drugs, in particular in tumor cell proliferation and metastasis. DS (and other GAGs) functions and possible therapeutic applications are closely related to its specific structure and properties as well as distinctive oligosaccharide sequences inside the polymer chains. DS is particularly interesting for further studies and applications because it is expressed in many tissues and it is the predominant glycan present in skin. GAG is an important cofactor in a variety of cell behaviors, in the development of the CNS, and also acts as a receptor for various pathogens [72].

11.2.16
Keratin Sulfate

Keratins are a group of cysteine-rich structural proteins formed in the epithelial cells of higher vertebrates that exhibit high mechanical strength due to a large number of disulfide bonds. These proteins, along with others, are found in hard or filamentous structures such as hair, nails, horns, hoofs, and feathers. Because of its water insolubility and the limited number of methods available for extraction and processing, keratin has attracted only minor interest in the past as a biomaterial in the field of regenerative medicine, in contrast to the attention garnered by proteins such as collagen. However, in the past decade, and particularly over the past 5 years, new methods have been described for the use of keratin or modified keratin, mainly obtained from wool, as a substrate or scaffold in cell cultivation and tissue engineering. Reichl *et al.* reported that keratin films could be a promising replacement for amniotic membrane in ophthalmology [73]. Due to the nonimmunogenic nature of keratin, proteins, and their evolutionary structural conservation across species [74, 75], it is hypothesized that keratose implants will be tolerated by the cell-mediated immune system and can incorporate with host tissues during the wound healing process. Extracts of human hair fibers were found to contain cortical keratins and, therefore, lack the ability to form disulfide crosslinks due to oxidation of free thiol groups. The absence of covalent disulfide bonds enables the hydrogel material to degrade relatively fast. Implantation in the subcutaneous layer of the mouse showed that keratose is compatible with the tissue since it integrates as evidenced by minimal fibrous capsule formation and infiltration of host cells and new blood vessels. The material was resorbed and eventually replaced with a natural collagen structure, suggesting that keratose implants can be used as temporary matrices for delivery of bioactive molecules and cells for tissue engineering and regenerative medicine applications. Highly water-stable nanoparticles of around 70nm and capable of distributing with high uptake in certain organs of mice were developed from feather keratin. Nanoparticles could provide novel veterinary diagnostics and therapeutics to boost efficiency in the identification and treatment of livestock diseases to improve protein supply and ensure safety and quality of food. Nanoparticles could penetrate easily into cells

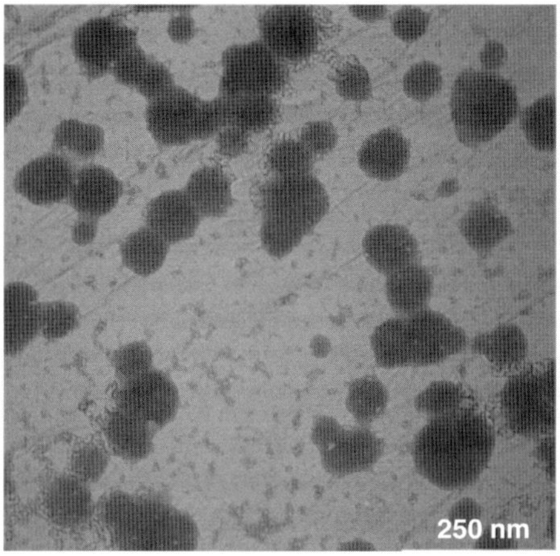

Figure 11.3 Morphologies of keratin nanoparticles in a TEM image. (Xu 2014 [76]. Reproduced with permission from American Chemical Society.)

and small capillaries, surpass detection of the immune system, and reach targeted organs because of their nanoscale sizes, as shown in Figure 11.3 [76].

Fibrous capsule is formed around implants to wall off and isolate foreign materials that cannot be eliminated by the cellular immune system. Since the keratose implant degrades relatively fast, minimal fibrous encapsulation was detected. The capsule thickness in response to keratose is less than the typical 50–200 mm range for biocompatible materials [77]. The PLGA scaffold induced a sharp increase in capsule thickness due to the delayed degradation, but once the bulk material lost its mechanical integrity (i.e., polymeric chain degradation to lactic acid and glycolic acid), the phagocytes were able to ingest the particles, leading to better host integration and decreased fibrous capsule thickness. In contrast, keratose capsule thickness plateaued directly to about 20 mm. The relatively fast resorption time, successful integration into the host system, and complete resorption of formed structures imply that the keratose extract can be used as a temporary tissue filler for injured soft tissues with a short healing phase (lasting within a few weeks) [78].

11.2.17 Dextran

Dextran is a polysaccharide which consists of basically 1,6- linked D-glucopyranose residues with a few percent of -1,2, -1,3, or -1,4-linked side chains (Figure 11.4) [79]. Due to its biocompatibility, low toxicity, relatively low cost, and simple modification, it has been widely used for biomedical applications. Clinically it has been used for more than five decades as a plasma volume expander, peripheral flow enhancer, and antithrombolytic agent as well as for the rheological improvement, for example, artificial tears [80].

Dextran shows stability under mild acidic and basic conditions and is highly water soluble. The presence of large amount of hydroxylic groups makes it

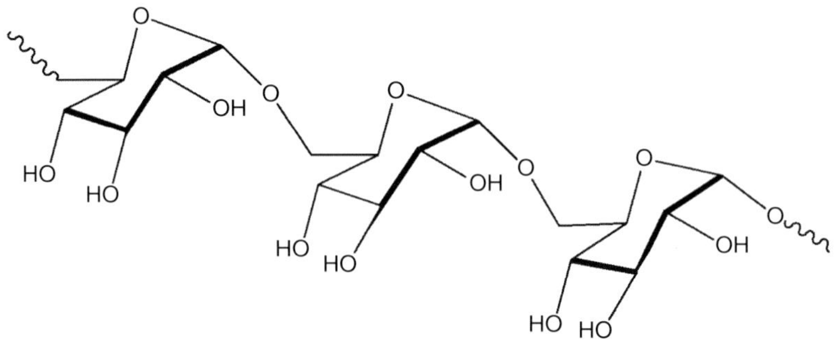

Figure 11.4 Chemical structure of dextran [79].

suitable for derivatization and subsequent chemical and physical cross-linking [81]. Compared with other polysaccharides (e.g., glycogen with −1,4 linkages) it will slowly be degraded by human enzymes and cleaved by microbial dextranases in the gastrointestinal tract. Hence it is chosen as good candidate for many biomedical applications. To increase the longevity of therapeutic agents in systemic circulation, it has been used as a macromolecular carrier for delivery of drugs and proteins. *In vivo* immunogenicity of proteins and enzymes is decreased by dextran. Molecules with Mw >40 kDa have larger half-lives and would be isolated in the liver and spleen and then hydrolyzed by endo- and exodextranases, whereas molecules with molecular weight of <40 kDa can be eliminated through renal clearance and have a half-life of 8 h [82]. Dextran has also been used in a large number of *in vivo* imaging techniques such as diagnostic magnetic resonance (DMR), photodynamic therapy (PDT), positron emission tomography (PET) imaging, and finally, magnetic resonance imaging (MRI), which may lead to promising treatments in atherosclerosis and cancer [83]. Drug delivery applications aim at delivering any drug with the correct timing in a safe and reproducible manner to a specific target in a given concentration level. Due to their significant physical properties, dextran hydrogels have been extensively explored in drug delivery applications. The moieties present in the dextran-based hydrogels are able to interact with biomolecules. Recently dextran-based hydrogels used as instructive scaffolds to promote neovascularization and skin regeneration in third-degree burn wounds. A schematic representation of the preparation of amphogels (AmB) is shown in Figure 11.5 [84]. Dextran plays an important role in reducing the intra-abdominal adhesions. Succinyl chitosan and dextran aldehyde hydrogels significantly reduce the formation of intra-abdominal adhesions without adversely affecting wound healing [85]. The antifungal agent AmB is loaded in dextran-based hydrogel, and AmB killed fungi within 2 h of contact and could be reused for at least 53 days without losing its effectiveness against *Candida albicans*.

The antifungal material used here is biocompatible *in vivo* and did not cause hemolysis in human blood. AmB inoculated with *C. albicans* and implanted in mice prevented fungal infection and also reduce fungal biofilm formation. A

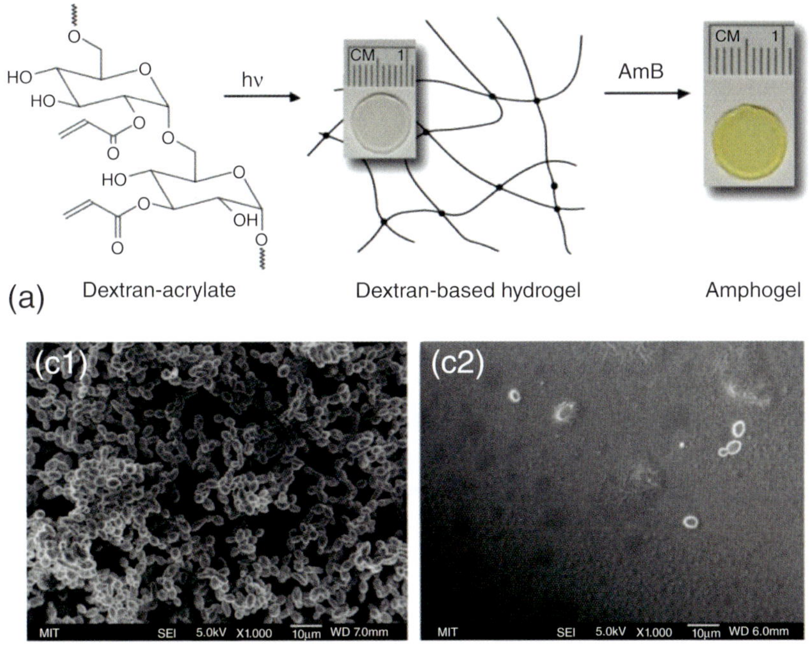

Figure 11.5 Antifungal properties of dextran-based hydrogels with or without AmB. (a) Schematic representation of the preparation of amphogels, (c) SEM images of dextran-based gels without (c1) and with (c2) AmB incubated with *Candida albicans* for 48 h. (Sun 2011 [84]. Reproduced with permission from PNAS.)

variety of medical devices, for example, catheters, as well as industrial surfaces [86] are coated with dextran and also used as an antifungal matrix. Dextran-based hydrogels may be also used as injectable in situ cross-linking networks for the delivery of amphotericin. Here AmB was first reacted with dexOx, and the resulting conjugate was cross-linked with carboxymethylcellulose (CMC) hydrazide. The gel provided *in vitro* antifungal activity for 11 days, and contact with the gel killed Candida for three weeks [87]. The gel had acceptable *in vivo* biocompatibility after implantation in the murine peritoneum.

11.2.18 Pectin

Pectin is a natural polymer constituting the cell walls of most plants, and it is extensively employed in the food industry, as a thickener or stabilizing agent. It is usually extracted from several types of fruits, by chemical or enzymatic methods. It is composed of at least three polysaccharide domains: homogalacturonan (HGA), rhamnogalacturonan-I (RG-I), and rhamnogalacturonan-II (RG-II) [88]. HGA is the major component of pectin polysaccharides and contains α-(1 → 4)-D-linked galacturonic acids (1,4-α-D-GalpA) that are partially methyl-esterified and sometimes partially acetyl-esterified. The promising features of pectin gels for biomedical applications are related to easily tunable physical properties, high water content, and their ability to homogeneously immobilize cells, genes, proteins, drugs, or GFs [89]. There are many different biomedical applications for which gels are suitable, such as drug delivery, gene delivery, tissue engineering, and wound healing [90]. Pectin has interesting properties that make it a promising candidate for drug delivery applications, such as mucoadhesiveness, the ease of dissolution in basic environments, and the ability to form gels in acid environments. Mucoadhesiveness can be exploited to target and control drug delivery in the nasal or gastric environment, while the ease of dissolution in basic environments, associated with its resistance to proteases and amylases, makes pectin suitable to release drugs in the colon. In addition, the possibility of forming gels in acid conditions enhances the contact time of drugs for gastric or ocular treatments [91, 92]. Sriamornsak *et al.* reported that the mucoadhesive potential of LM pectin was due to hydrogen bonding between pectin-free acid groups and mucin under appropriated conditions: pectin reverts from an aqueous solution to a gel when applied to mucosal surfaces. Among the applications, fentanyl (an opioid painkiller), a pectin nasal spray, was proven to improve the analgesic onset, treatment efficacy, and acceptability in treating cancer pain [93–95] where a rapid drug release is requested. Alternatively, pectin has been used in combination with peptides or with chlorpromazine hydrochloride [96] in the treatment of psychotic symptoms showing interesting absorption properties and a sustained systemic release. Nasal pectin sprays containing nicotine have also been suggested as an alternative approach for smoking cessation [97]. Pectins were considered in the preparation of capsules for sustained drug delivery and for taste masking. The ability of pectins to be resistant to proteases and amylases, which are active in the gastrointestinal tract, and to be degraded by the intestinal microflora makes them suitable for colon drugs, proteins, or polypeptide delivery [98]. However, as a drawback, pectin gels swell in aqueous media, and a small amount of drug may be released in the gastrointestinal tract. To overcome this problem, divalent ions, such as Ca^{2+} and Zn^{2+}, or other polymers, such as chitosan, ethyl cellulose, or hydroxypropyl methylcellulose (HPMC) [99–101], are used to form strong pectin gels for drug delivery in the colon. The use of water-soluble polymers, such as pectin, that form hydrogels in physiological conditions has been evaluated as a new strategy to enhance the contact time and drug penetration [92]. An alternative approach was the application of pectin systems for an *in situ* gel formation [102], where pectin is applied in a liquid form, which then gels in the eye. The gelation is mainly triggered by the pH content of the tears and by the presence of electrolytes in the tear film. Pectin appears to be able to inhibit cancer metastasis and primary tumor growth in multiple types of cancer in animals [103]. Modified pectins, possibly loaded with cytotoxic drugs to induce neoplastic cell apoptosis, hold the potential to dramatically increase the efficiency of a conventional chemotherapy. A possible approach to the treatment of genetic disorders is gene therapy. The main objective in gene therapy consists in replacing defective genes. The transfer of genetic materials to the targeted tissues can be performed with either viral or nonviral transfection vectors. Among nonviral vectors, polycationic polymers such as branched polyethylenimine (b-PEI) [104] or chitosan [105] have shown high transfection efficiency both *in vitro* and *in vivo*. However, a drawback is that the positive charge of the polycations may cause high cytotoxicity and instability in the presence of serum or ECM components. To overcome this limitation, different anionic polymers have been employed to decrease the surface charge of the polyelectrolyte complexes [106]. Pectin was found to be suitable for coating b-PEI polyplexes to form pectin-coated polyplexes with a reduced surface charge that, in turn, led to decreased transfection with a concomitant lower cytotoxicity and higher stability [107]. Pectin hydrogels were found to have a great potential for bone tissue engineering (BTE) applications, as they promote the nucleation of a mineral phase if immersed in adequate physiological solutions, with the formation of biomimetic constructs better mimicking the natural architecture of the bone. Unmodified and chemically modified pectin gel, microspheres, and coatings were studied for the 2D and 3D culture of bone cells, showing interesting properties for cell viability, metabolic activity, and differentiation [108, 109]. When pectin is added to the wound, it serves as a binding agent, protecting GFs from degradation. A wide variety of hydrocolloid pectin-based wound dressings have been patented and are currently commercially available. They are mainly composed of adhesive, absorbent polymers, pectin gelling agents, and sodium carboxymethyl cellulose (SCMC). The hydrophilic pectin particles react within the dressing with the wound fluid to form a soft gel over the wound bed, thus removing or controlling exudates in wounds. The acid environment obtained with pectin solubilization may further act as a bacterial or viral barrier. In addition, pectin hydrogels provide improved systems of loading and releasing drugs, that is, antibiotics, pain relievers, and/or tissue repair factors at the site of action (Table 11.1) [110].

Table 11.1 Pectin-containing hydrocolloid wound dressings [110].

Type of dressing	Composition	Uses
CombiDERM® (ConvaTec Ltd.)	Cellulose, pectin, Salsorb90 (acrylic polymer)	Cavity or flat shallow wounds with low to medium exudates; absorbent; conformable; suitable for "problematic" areas: heel, elbow, sacrum
DuoDERM® (ConvaTec Ltd.)	Carboxymethylcellulose, pectin, propylene glycol	
Granuflex® (ConvaTec Ltd.)	Polyurethane foam sheet coated with pectin, gelatin, and carboxymethylcellulose	
Hydrocoll® (Hartmann)	Pectin, gelatin, and carboxymethylcellulose	
GranuGel® paste (Convatec Ltd.)	Pectin, carboxymethylcellulose, propylene glycol	Useful debriding agent, conformable, may be left in place for several days.
CitruGel® (Advances medical)	Pectin, carboxymethylcellulose	

11.2.19 Gelatin

Gelatin is a natural material based on animal proteins. It is derived from collagen and consists of elongated fibrils and is mostly found in fibrous tissues such as tendon, ligament, and skin. It is also abundant in cornea, cartilage, bone, blood vessels, gut, and intervertebral discs. It is commonly used for biomedical applications due to its biodegradability and biocompatibility in physiological environments, in contact with living tissues. Collagen gel has been widely used in pharmaceutical applications as it fulfills the diverse requirements of a drug delivery system such as good biocompatibility, low antigenicity, and degradability upon implantation. Furthermore, collagen gels are one of the first natural polymers to be used as a promising matrix for drug delivery and tissue engineering. Biodegradable collagen-based systems have served as 3D scaffolds for cell culture, used to enhance survival of transfected fibroblasts, and in gene therapy. In this case, collagen scaffolds were fabricated by introducing various chemical cross-linking agents (i.e., glutaraldehyde, formaldehyde, carbodiimide) or by physical treatments (i.e., UV irradiation, freeze-drying, and heating). For various applications gelatin can be modified into PEGylated gelatin nanoparticles [111], fluoride anion-modified gelatin nanogel system for ultrasound-triggered drug release [112], antibody-modified gelatin nanoparticles as drug carrier system for uptake in lymphocytes [113], agar-modified gelatin A and gelatin B [114], gelatin thiol-modified nanoparticles for intracellular DNA delivery [115], hydrophobic hexanoyl anhydrides grafting to the amino groups of primitive gelatin [116], cationized gelatin, DNA-loaded gelatin nanoparticles [117], and modified gelatin microspheres impregnated collagen scaffold [118]. PEG-modified gelatin nanoparticles were prepared by Kaul *et al.* and are used for long-circulating intracellular delivery of DNA [111]. Daocheng *et al.* prepared adriamycin gelatin nanogel, modified with fluoride anion by the coprecipitation method with fluoride anion and sodium sulfate targeted and controlled drug release delivery system for cancer and other diseases [112]. Gelatin nanoparticles for the attachment of biotinylated anti-CD3 antibodies by avidin-biotin complex formation were used by Balthasar *et al.*, which represent for a promising carrier system for specific drug targeting to T lymphocytes [113]. Saxena *et al.* established agar-gelatin compositions and tablets made of agar, gelatin A, gelatin B, and their blends agar-gelatin A, agar-gelatin B, gelatin A, gelatin B in a 1 : 1 ratio. Salbutamol is used as the model drug [119].

11.2.20 Starch

The use of either native or modified starch in drug delivery applications is very important due to its biocompatibility, nontoxicity, biodegradability, eco-friendly, and cost-effective nature. It is a nonpolluting renewable source for sustainable supply of cheaper pharmaceutical product. Nasal delivery of drugs and oral and intramuscular delivery of vaccines are administered through starch microparticles. Bioadhesive systems based on polysaccharide microparticles have been reported to significantly enhance the systemic absorption of conventional drugs and polypeptides across the nasal mucosa, even when devoid of absorption-enhancing agents. Balmayor *et al.* suggest that starch-poly-ε-caprolactone microparticles containing dexamethasone microparticular systems seem to be quite promising for controlled-release applications especially as carriers in tissue engineering [120]. *In vitro* release behavior of diclofenac sodium from sweet potato starch microparticles was investigated by Liu *et al.*, and it exhibited controlled drug delivery properties. The encapsulation efficiencies of the microparticle, formulations were between 95.1% and 98.2%, and the mechanism of drug release from the microparticles was Fickian diffusion [121]. Silva *et al.* found that starch-based microparticles are suitable vehicles for the incorporation and release of GF, and that the incorporation and release did not affect the biological activity of the GFs. This suggests their ability to enhance the regenerating potential of tissue engineering hybrid constructs [122]. Delivery of living cells for improving bone regeneration in tissue engineering is reported by Malafaya *et al.* [123]. This study proved that starch microspheres could be prepared at room temperature to allow for the loading of labile biologically active agents. Microparticles obtained from blends of high-amylase cornstarch (HACS)/pectin were effective in targeted drug release to the colon. This improves the encapsulation efficiency and decreased the drug dissolution in the gastric condition (pH 1.2), as reported by Desai *et al.* [124]. A review article by Rydell *et al.* [125] focuses on the use of starch, a natural biocompatible and biodegradable polymer, for the production of various particulate adjuvant formulations, which can induce mucosal as well as systemic immune responses. McDermott *et al.* [126] summarized that a novel silicone polymer-grafted starch microparticle system developed for the delivery of small quantities of antigen, especially intranasally, may be useful for the induction of oral tolerance. In this study, Heritage *et al.* [127] prepared a novel microparticle fabrication technique where human serum albumin (HSA) was entrapped in starch microparticles grafted with 3-(triethoxysilyl)-propyl-terminated polydimethylsiloxane (TS-PDMS). The authors reported that the microparticles have potential as systemic and mucosal vaccine delivery vehicles. Degling *et al.* [128] found that recombinant mouse interferon-γ (mu IFN-γ) was covalently coupled with polyacryl starch microparticles, a lysosomotropic drug carrier. The microparticle-bound mu IFN was made to activate cultured macrophages for nitrite production and had an antileishmanial effect in mice. The effect of polyacryl starch microparticles on arachidonic acid metabolism in macrophage cultures and in mice was studied by Artursson *et al.* [129]. Two of the major metabolites were produced when macrophages were incubated with the microparticles. When the mice were treated with inhibitors of arachidonic acid metabolism, the microparticle-induced hepatomegaly was partly inhibited. Baillie *et al.* [130] found that when the drug sodium stibogluconate was covalently bound to polyacryl starch microparticles, it was 100 times more effective than the free form in this murine model of visceral leishmaniasis, whereas empty microparticles had no effect on liver parasites. Starch microcapsules have different applications: they can bind electrostatically to drugs [131] and can be used as coatings for food-grade enteric coatings [132], biodegradable microcapsules for oral protein administration, coating materials for encapsulating pancreatic protease [133], and macrophage uptake by polyacryl starch microparticles. Starch nanoparticles have been used in transdermal delivery [134] and as a transnasal mucoadhesive carrier [135] and anticancer drug carrier [136, 137]. Native starch is almost completely broken down by pancreatic enzymes after oral ingestion, with subsequent absorption from the small intestine into the systemic circulation. Usually, a certain proportion of starch, called *resistant starch*, escapes digestion in the small intestine and undergoes fermentation by bacteria in the colon. To inhibit or reduce the enzymatic degradation taking place in the stomach in order to allow adequate amount of the therapeutic agent to be absorbed, starch has been combined with other polymers to impart this desired property. Thiele *et al.* [138] found a new modular concept for the formation of nanoparticles from poorly soluble drugs using readily available building blocks. Stable spherical nanoparticles (NPs) were formulated mixing aqueous solutions of the anionic copolymers and of a cationic thioether of ß-cyclodextrin (ß-CD). The starch/ß-CD NPs could be loaded with hydrophobic guest molecules like 1,4-dihydroxyanthraquinone (DHA), which served as a model for the important class of anthracycline antibiotics used in cancer therapy. Kumari and Rani [139] reported that metformin-loaded chitosan- and starch-blended beads prepared by cross-linking possess suitable controlled-release properties. Biocompatible, biodegradable, stable, nontoxic, autofluorescent, and pH-responsive microcapsules were successfully prepared by Jia *et al.* [140] using dialdehyde heparin (DHP) and dialdehyde starch (DAS) as the wall components to cross-link with chitosan for the fabrication of the microcapsules. The results confirmed that the method used could be applied over a wide range of polysaccharides. Studies suggested by Zhang *et al.* [141] found that oyster peptide-loaded alginate/chitosan/starch microcapsules could be a suitable copolymeric carrier system for intestinal protein or peptide delivery in the intestine. Chowdary and Murali [142] synthesized starch–urea–borate and evaluated it for controlled-release properties in matrix tablets of diclofenac and gliclazide. The authors reported that starch–urea–borate is a better release rate-controlling polymer than HPMC and SCMC. Levy *et al.* [143] observed the presence of A novel polysaccharide cross-bridging protein comprising a cellulose-binding domain from *Clostridium cellulovorans* and a starch-binding domain from *Aspergillus niger* B1. The two genes were fused in-frame via a synthetic elastin gene to construct a cellulose/starch cross-bridging protein. Recombinant CSCP was expressed in *Escherichia coli* and successfully refolded from inclusion bodies. CSCP demonstrated cross-bridging ability in different model systems composed of insoluble or soluble starch and cellulose. Starch at submicron sizes is also finding application in tissue engineering. The general requirements for a scaffold material to be considered suitable for tissue engineering, namely, biocompatibility, appropriate mechanical properties, controlled degradation rate, and appropriate pore size and morphology, can easily be imparted on starch by modification, which have made it very useful as carriers in tissue engineering. Sachan *et al.* [144] prepared good quality microbeads by an industrially feasible microorifice ionotropic gelation method using glutinous starch from Assam Bora rice and sodium alginate backbone. Drug release properties from the prepared microdevices were excellent. Here, a novel approach of forming hydroxyapatite (HA) [145] and pure beta-tricalcium phosphate (ß-TCP)-based porous scaffolds by applying together starch consolidation with foaming method was developed. The ability of these starch-based scaffolds to release drugs suitably for osteomyelitis was confirmed *in vitro*. Duarte *et al.* [146] reported highly porous and interconnected starch-based scaffolds using supercritical immersion precipitation technique to prepare scaffolds of a polymeric blend of starch and poly(L-lactic acid) for tissue engineering purposes. In this report, Sundaram *et al.* [147] explain about hydroxyapatite (HA). It is a fundamental mineral-based biomaterial used for preparing composites for bone repair and regeneration. A gelatin–starch blend reinforced with HA nanocrystals gave biocompatible composites enhanced mechanical properties. New scaffolds based on a 50/50 (wt%) blend of cornstarch/ethylene vinyl alcohol were prepared by Salgado *et al.* [148]. After characterization, cytotoxicity evaluation, direct contact assays, cell viability assay, and Western blot analysis, the authors concluded that the starch-based scaffolds should be considered as an alternative for BTE applications in the near future. Torres *et al.* [149] reported that starches obtained from potato, sweet potato, cornstarch, and nonisolated amaranth and quinoa starch were used to produce porous biodegradable scaffolds suitable for tissue engineering. Study reports by Gomes *et al.* [150] confirm the suitability of starch-based 3D scaffolds exhibiting distinct porous structures for the proliferation and osteogenic differentiation of rat bone marrow (RBM) stromal cells in tissue engineering. Lam *et al.* [151] developed a unique blend of starch-based polymer powders (cornstarch, dextran, and gelatin) for the 3DP process. Cylindrical scaffolds of five different designs were fabricated and postprocessed to enhance the mechanical and chemical properties. Gomes *et al.* [152] proposed various alternative methodologies for the preparation of starch scaffolds. Scaffolds obtained from these using these methodologies may constitute an important alternative to the materials currently used in tissue engineering. The development of new partially biodegradable acrylic bone cements based on cornstarch/cellulose acetate blends was reported by Espigares *et al.* [153]. The developed systems show a range of properties that might allow for their application as self-curing bone cements, exhibiting several advantages with respect to other commercially available bone cements. A new simple processing route to produce starch-based porous materials was developed by Malafaya *et al.* [154], and it is based on a microwave baking methodology. This processing route was used to obtain nonloaded controls and loaded drug delivery carriers, incorporating a nonsteroid anti-inflammatory agent. Gomes *et al.* [150] describe the preliminary study on the development of a new method to produce biodegradable scaffolds from a range of cornstarch-based polymers. The scaffolds could be molded into complex shapes, and the blowing additives do not affect the noncytotoxic behavior of the starch-based materials.

11.2.21 Alginate

Alginate is composed of alternating blocks of 1,4 linked-α-L-guluronic and α-D-mannuronic acid residue. It is a water-soluble linear polysaccharide extracted from brown seaweed. Modified alginate systems for drug delivery applications includes thiolated alginate–albumin nanoparticles [155], alginate combined with CHI, alginate–poloxamer microparticles, hydrated thiolated alginate, alginate-poly(lactic-co-glycolic acid) nano/microhydrogel matrices [156], CHI-Ca-alginate microspheres [157], alginate modified by microenvironmental interaction with calcium ion, polyethylene glycol–anthracene modified alginate [158], photocross-linked heparin-alginate hydrogels [159], micelles/sodium-alginate composite gel beads [160], alginate-guar gum hydrogel, dual cross-linked alginate/*N*-α-glutaric acid CHI [161], alginate/scleroglucan/borax gels, and alginate-based mesalazine tablets for intestinal drug delivery. Hydrogel-forming polymers such as alginates and poloxamers are used as encapsulation materials by Moebus *et al.* They are used for controlled drug delivery to mucosal tissue [162]. Mucoadhesive drug delivery systems based on hydrated thiolated alginate were prepared by Davidovich-Pinhas *et al.* Dry, uncross-linked, compressed tablets made from thiolated polymers adhere better to the mucus layer compared to native polymers [163]. CHI-Ca-alginate microspheres were developed by Mennini *et al.* The prepared microspheres are used for colon delivery of celecoxib-hydroxypropyl-beta-cyclodextrin-PVP complex. Ciofani *et al.* developed alginate-based drug delivery system for neurological applications by considering neural regeneration and neuroprotection [164].

11.2.22 Guar Gum

The ground endosperm of guar beans contains mainly guar gum, which is obtained by dehusking, milling, and screening. Modifications of guar gum are graft copolymers of *N*-vinyl-2-pyrrolidone onto guar gum for sorption of $Fe^{2+}$and Cr^{6+} ions [165], partially carboxymethylated guar gum-*g*-*N*-vinyl-2-pyrrolidone [166], cross-linking of alginate guar gum with glutaraldehyde [167], carboxymethyl guar films for the formulation of transdermal therapeutic systems, partially carboxymethylated guar gum-*g*-methacrylic acid [168], complexation of cupric ion-guar gum-graft-acrylamide, phosphated cross-linked guar gum, polyester-guar gum/hydroxypropyl guar gum, and yttrium cross-linked guar gum-*g*-acrylamide gel systems. Nayak *et al.* developed a system containing swellable polymer (l-hydroxypropyl cellulose (L-HPC), xanthan gum, polyethylene oxide, or sodium alginate) together with drug tablet and erodible tablet

(L-HPC or guar gum) in a precoated capsule. The purpose of the study was to develop pulsatile capsule dosage form of valsartan for controlled delivery. This provides a useful means for timed release of valsartan and may be helpful for patients with morning surge [169]. Soppimath *et al.* prepared new spherically shaped cross-linked hydrogels of polyacrylamide-grafted guar gum by the emulsification method. These pH-sensitive microgels were loaded with diltiazem hydrochloride and nifedipine (both antihypertensive drugs), and their release studies were performed in both the simulated gastric and intestinal pH conditions [170]. Ji *et al.* prepared a pH- and enzyme-dependent colon-targeted multiunit delivery system of indomethacin by coating guar gum and Eudragit FS 30D sequentially onto drug-loaded pellets in a fluidized bed coater. It is indicated that the guar gum/Eudragit FS 30D-coated system has potential to be used to deliver drugs to the colon. Krishnaiah *et al.* investigated *in vivo* study in humans with guar gum-based matrix tablets of 5-fluorouracil (5-FU). These tablets showed delayed absorption time T, decreased C_{max}, and absorption rate constant compared with tablets that showed immediate release [171]. By graft copolymerization using methacrylic acid (MAA) with guar gum [172] or by using various polysaccharides, Mundargi *et al.* prepared tablets of metronidazole. Hydrocortisone hydrogels were prepared by Kabir *et al.* using guar gum which is cross-linked with trisodium trimetaphosphate [173]. Carboxymethyl guar gum was prepared by Murthy *et al.* It is an anionic semisynthetic guar gum for use in transdermal drug delivery systems. Terbutaline sulfate was used as a model drug [174].

11.2.23 Xanthan Gum

Xanthan gum (XG) is a polysaccharide secreted by the bacterium *Xanthomonas campestris*. It contains a cellulose backbone ß-(1 4)-D-glucopyranose glucan and backbone with side chains of (3→1)α-linked D-mannopyranose-(2→1)-ß-D-glucuronic acid-(4→1)-ß-D-mannopyranose on alternating residues [175]. Due to the hydrophilic nature, its use is limited in thickening, suspending, and emulsifying water-based systems. XG is gaining more attention for the fabrication of matrices with uniform drug release features [176, 177]. Few modifications of XG include gelatinized ST−XG hydrogel system, acrylamide-grafted XG, graft copolymerization of ethyl acrylate onto XG [178], XG combined with konjac glucomannan, XG combined with boswellia gum (3 : 1), XG combined with guar gum (10 : 20), and XG combined with locust bean gum (LG) in a 1 : 1 [179] ratio. A matrix tablet of cimetidine is prepared by Jiangyang *et al.* by combining XG with konjac glucomannan [180]. Sinha *et al.* developed a colon-specific compression-coated systems of 5-FU for the treatment of colorectal cancer using XG, boswellia gum, and HPMC as the coating materials. It was found that the ratio of XG/guar gum mixture and XG/boswellia gum mixture is 10:20 and 3:1, respectively. So the compression coating of 5-FU is a tool for delaying the release of the drug, which ensures better clinical management of the disease

[181]. The use of xanthan-grafted copolymer of acrylamide as a controlled release matrix for antihypertensive drugs such as atenolol and carvedilol was examined by Mundargi [182]. Bose *et al.* prepared sustained-release floating tablets of diltiazem HCl used XG for the treatment of angina and hypertension [183]. Modified-release tablet formulation of metoprolol succinate using HPMC and XG [184] was developed by Gohel *et al.* A constant rate delivery formulation of diclofenac sodium to release the drug in the intestine was developed by Ahmed *et al.* Matrix tablets and triple-layer matrix tablets were formulated by using LG, XG, and a mixture of LG:XG in 1 : 1 ratio as a matrix forming agent, and anionic SCMC was compressed on both the surfaces of the matrix core [179]. Venkataraju *et al.* established controlled delivery system for propranolol hydrochloride using the synergistic activity of LG and XG to avoid first-pass effect [185].

11.2.24 Gellan Gum

Gellan gum is a bacterial exopolysaccharide that is commercially prepared by aerobic submerged fermentation of *Sphingomonas elodea*. Gellan gum is a linear tetrasaccharide built up by (alpha-1 → 4)-L-rhamnopyranosyl-(alpha-1 → 3)-D-glucopyranosyl-(ß-1 → 4)-D-glucuronopyranosyl-(ß-1 → 4)-D-glucopyranosyl-(ß-1 →) with *O*(2) L-glyceryl and *O*(6) acetyl substitutes on the 3-linked glucose. Few modified forms of gellan gum include deacetylated gellan gum, methacrylated gellan gum hydrogel [186], gellan gum-poly(vinyl alcohol) hydrogel, gellan gum films with 1-ethyl-3-(3-dimethylaminopropyl)carbodiimide, Al ion cross-linked gellan hydrogel [187], and b-PEI blended with gellan gum [188]. Gellan gum blended with PEI nanocomposites was prepared by Goyal *et al.* and is used for gene delivery applications. By extruding the dispersion of cephalexin and gellan gum into a solution containing a mixture of calcium and zinc ions, gellan gum beads were prepared by Agnihotri *et al.* [189] and are used for controlled release of drug. Agnihotri *et al.* produce gellan gum-poly(vinyl alcohol) hydrogel microspheres for the controlled release of carvedilol [190]. For ophthalmic delivery of methylprednisolone [191], Sanzgiri *et al.* developed gellan-based systems. Gellan-chitosan hybrid capsules [192] encapsulated with alkaline phosphatase were developed by Fujii *et al.* [192] Oral sustained delivery of paracetamol from in situ-gelling gellan and sodium alginate formulations was prepared by Kubo *et al.* [193].

11.2.25 Zein

Excellent biocompatibility, biodegradability, and high surface contact are the significant properties of zein. Hence zein-based micro- and nanocomposites present good applications in the drug release field [194]. Acting as delivery vehicles, zein can interact more efficiently with hydrophobic and hydrophilic drug. Due to its high percentages of hydrophobic amino acid residues, zein is able to release encapsulated compounds and is insoluble in physiological conditions [195]. For oral delivery applications, zein is highly suitable, and it is found that zein degradation occurs through a number of enzymes [196]. The N-terminal region of zein interacts with cell membranes, acting as a peptide carrier for drugs across cell membranes [197]. Hydrophobic drugs present poor absorption and low bioavailability; therefore they cannot be absorbed by the body. Zein-based materials are applied extensively for the delivery of hydrophobic drugs. Zein proteins have good hydrophobic-hydrophilic property so they will act as an intermediary agent between the hydrophobic drug and the epithelial cells of the colon. This leads to an increase in the mucoadhesion of zein-based material with the epithelial cells in the gastrointestinal tract. Here zein acts as a targeted delivery and controlled release agent, where it increases hydrophobic drug permeation and absorption [198]. Li *et al.* prepared microcomposites of zein/ibuprofen (zein/IBU) using a modified electrospraying process. The DSC curve of the hydrophobic IBU shows a single endothermic peak at 77 °C which is attributed to the melting point. Zein /IBU microparticles did not show fusion peaks or phase transition, which is a clear evidence for the amorphous nature of IBU in the microcomposites and its noncrystalline nature. For the development of advanced pharmaceutical materials, this type of modification is useful [199]. Nanoparticles of zein/lutein (zein/LUT) were prepared by Hu *et al.*, and these nanoparticles are obtained from solution-enhanced dispersion by supercritical fluids (SEDS) [200]. In Hu *et al.*'s study, they encapsulated the lutein (LUT) into zein nanoparticles, and this zein coating prevents LUT from light degradation. This improves its aqueous solubility and enables specific drug delivery in the colon region. The interactions between zein/LUT enabled an amorphous state in the nanoparticles, and this interaction significantly changes the drug's physicochemical properties. Through liquid-liquid phase separation associated with the ionic gelation technique, Luo *et al.* established the nanoparticles of zein and zein/carboxymethyl CHI. Hydrophobic and bioactive compounds such as indole-3-carbinol (I3C) and 3,3′-diindolylmethane (DIM) are extracted from cruciferous vegetables that have good potential for cancer treatment. But both of them have low stability in gastric conditions and degrade when exposed to light and heat. During oligomerization under acidic conditions, I3C and DIM form a mixture of compounds known as *acid condensation products*. The nanoparticles of zein and zein/CMCS protect the labile compounds from harsh conditions and provide controlled release and targeted delivery of drug bioactive. The stability of both bioactive compounds is significantly improved after nanoparticle encapsulation. Both zein and zein/CMCS nanoparticles offer good protection against degradation in UV light. Zein/CMCS nanoparticles also offer better protection of I3C under thermal conditions against degradation and oligomerization [201].

In PBS buffer solution, the controlled release of α-tocopherol (TOC) was greatly improved by the zein nanoparticles, but chitosan coating did not affect the encapsulation efficiency. This indicates the nanoparticles of zein coated with CS can be used as a new TOC supplementation or treatment. A schematic illustration for the development of zein/CHI complex is shown in Figure 11.6 [202]. Muller *et al.*

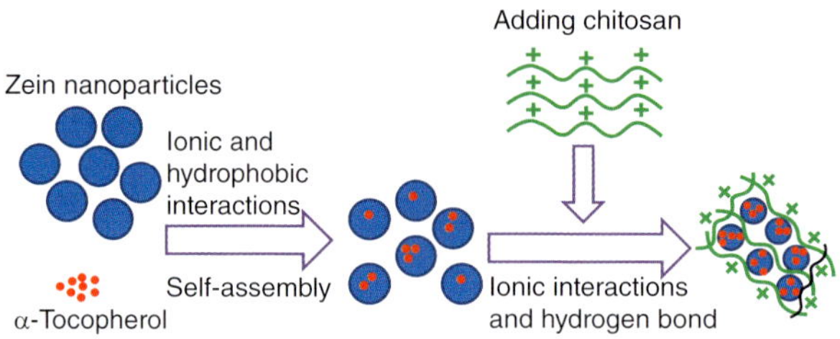

Figure 11.6 Schematic illustration of the formation of the zein/chitosan complex for encapsulation of α-tocopherol [202].

developed a carrier matrix for controlled drug release using zein and zein/CS microparticles [203]. Bobokalonov *et al.* studied the release kinetics of piroxicam drug (a therapeutic agent) from zein/pectin microparticles, and they prepared zein/pectin microspheres for drug delivery applications. Peppas' model [204] and first-order equation model [205] were used to find the kinetic parameters of piroxicam release. The rate-limiting step in the drug release from the microspheres mainly was the diffusion of piroxicam. Mehta *et al.* [206] also prepared the zein-based microspheres encapsulated with antituberculosis drugs. First-order kinetics model is followed by the controlled release of rifampicin, isoniazid, and pyrazinamide drugs, whose stability was increased by zein microparticles. To avoid direct contact of the drug with food and to enhance long-term effectiveness of antimicrobials in food, these zein microparticles are used. Spray-drying at different temperatures is used to obtain zein microcapsules. The *in vitro* study of nisin also was investigated. Nisin is a well-known bacteriocin with 34 amino acids and a molecular weight of 3510 Da. The antimicrobial activity of nisin is decreased when it is applied in foods, maybe due to its binding with food matrix components, which makes the antimicrobial unavailable to inactivate microorganisms. Hydrogen bonding helps in the interaction between nisin and zein, and even if the release of such a drug is favored only in a certain condition, the release profiles can be used as guidelines to recognize the applicability of a particular nisin delivery system in a given food product [207]. Nanofibers based on zein, poly(ethylene oxide), and CS with a good mucoadhesion property in the gastrointestinal tract were prepared by Wongsasulak *et al.* [208]. The significance of these nanofibers is related to the development of new dug carrier systems with targeted drug release in that that the gastromucoadhesion was initiated by wetting and swelling of the polymeric molecular chains of fiber, which led to a molecular interaction between the fiber and mucin molecules (protein of epithelial tissues). Wongsasulak *et al.* [209] reported the effects of encapsulation of hydrophobic drug such as TOC on the gastromucoadhesion property of electrospun fibers of zein/PEO/CS. It showed that the fiber morphology is independent on the TOC but significantly improved on the zein/PEO/CS mucoadhesive property [210]. Hordein/zein protein-based nanofibers were developed by Wang and Chen. Zein exhibited a stable assembled network structure, good stability in water, and good tensile strength with 30wt% of fiber content. Results show that fibers with a 3D porous structure could be used as carriers for the controlled release of incorporated bioactive compounds (as, e.g., riboflavin) in a PBS buffer solution. These nanofibers could be digested in a simulated intestinal fluid (SIF) for gradual release of the incorporated compounds where they are normally absorbed, are pepsin resistant, and are stable in simulated gastric fluid (SGF) [211]. Regeneration or reconstruction of hard tissues like bone and cartilage needs tissue engineering techniques. Temporary porous scaffolds surrounded by the cells are seeded and cultured *in vitro* before implantation [212]. Scaffolds provide proper environment for cell differentiation, proliferation, and the formation of new tissues [213]. Pore size, suitable porosity, and pore structure are necessary for the ingrowth of cells and the formation of new tissue. Also scaffolds should possess good biodegradability, good biocompatibility, suitable mechanical property, and a suitable degradation rate to match the new tissue formation rate. Some of the most important organic components of the ECM of the native bone has some similarity with the natural-based biopolymers. Proteins (zein, collagen, gelatin, and silk) and some polysaccharides (ST, alginate, cellulose, and CHI) are primary candidates for the design of bioactive composites for BTE applications. To improve the mechanical and biological response of scaffold materials, poly(ε-caprolactone) (PCL), HA particles [214], polyurethane (PU) [215], and so on were associated with biopolymers. The fabrication of zein/PCL porous scaffolds were studied by Wu *et al.* They obtain porous biocomposite scaffolds with a porosity of around 70% and with a well-interconnected network. The degradation rate of the scaffold could be tuned by adjusting the zein content in the composite, and results of drop-water contact angle measurement show that the zein improved hydrophilicity. So the fabricated zein/PCL biocomposite scaffolds can be used in tissue engineering strategies to regenerate bone defects [216].

The supercritical CO_2 foaming process is used for developing biodegradable porous scaffolds of PCL/thermoplastic zein (ZT) (or PCL/ZT scaffolds) in which the multiphase blend consists of water/oil, the oil phase being composed of PEG400 (special for BTE). Here the HA particles (conc. of 10 and 20 wt%) were interdispersed into PCL/ZT scaffolds. The porosity of scaffolds was controlled by varying the material formulation and foaming temperature (T_F). *In vitro* biocompatibility, biodegradation analyses, morphology, and microstructure of the scaffolds were tested. Both HA concentration and TF significantly affected the microstructural features of the scaffolds. Scaffolds with biodegradability sufficient for bone tissue engineering, mechanical properties, pore size distribution, and porosity were designed and produced by selecting TF equal to 100 °C for all of the used compositions. It is clear from the *in vitro* study that the proposed scaffolds allowed for the adhesion and colonization of preosteoblast MG63 and hMSCs cells. Salerno *et al.* prepared bimodal porous scaffolds for bone tissue engineering by combining porogen leaching and supercritical CO_2 (scCO) foaming techniques. To induce pore formation saturation, temperatures, pressures, and depressurization time were selected, and the pore structure of the foams is also optimized. As a result a macroporosity fitted for bone cell colonization and adhesion was obtained. Green chemistry process involves the formation of PCL/TZ and PCL/TZ–HA composite scaffolds. Macroporosity of the scaffolds is 20 and 400 μm. Bone tissue engineering demonstrates the potential of the colonization-induced scaffold, cell adhesion, and proliferation within 28 days. Scaffolds of PCL/ZT, ZT/HA, PCL/HA, and PCL/ZT/HA composites prepared by Salerno *et al.* [217] show that zein elevated the degradation of PCL/ZT and PCL/ZT/HA composites and improved the wettability of PCL. Tensile properties of the biomaterials decreased considerably than that of PCL scaffolds. Significant increase of the osteogenic properties of the materials results from the simultaneous addition of ZT and HA particles into PCL. This is caused by higher calcium deposit by the osteoblast cells, relative to pure PCL. The design of multiphase 3D porous scaffolds suitable for BTE needs good selection of experimental conditions. Yao *et al.* [218] and Zhang *et al.* [219] obtained nanofibers of zein/HA with a reasonable tensile strength, and also they applied these nanofibers as scaffolds for tissue repair. *In vitro* cytotoxicity and osteoblast adhesion tests showed that the mineralized zein nanofibrous membranes had a positive effect on osteoblast growth and did not induce cytotoxic action. Unique nanofibrous structural features and a coating of HA nanocrystallites can be applied during bone repair and regeneration. So the electrospun zein/HA fibrous membranes show promise for BTE applications. Physical blending of zein with polyurethane/cellulose acetate (PU/CA) was prepared, and the electrospun nanofibrous scaffolds show diameters around 400 to 700 nm. The nanoscaffolds of zein/PU/CA showed an enhanced blood clotting ability compared to PU nanofibers. Wound healing is improved by the presence of zein and CA in the nanofiber structure, which increased hydrophilicity and bioactivity; as a result, a moist environment for the wound was formed. In tissue engineering protein-based biomaterials show excellent properties in connection with other types of structures. To increase the water stability of electrospun protein scaffolds, many attempts have been made using cross-linking. Zein containing citric acid as a nontoxic cross-linker agent to improve the water stability and promote good cytocompatibility of zein fibers was prepared by Jiang *et al.* using a new method based on cross-linking electrospinning [220]. Here electrospun zein fibers containing citric acid were obtained without using toxic catalysts. Using PBS they found that the cross-linked electrospun fiber has good stability after the immersion for 15 days at 37 °C. The fibers promoted the proliferation of mouse fibroblast cells. Zein fibers without citric acid did not promote fibroblast cell proliferation; conversely electrospun zein scaffolds cross-linked with citric acid showed attachment and allowed the proliferation of fibroblast cells. Using various proteases α-zein can be hydrolyzed, and the ultrafiltrated α-zein hydrolysate reduces blood pressure. In this study Miyoshi *et al.* [221] demonstrated that when the unpurified thermolysin hydrolysate of α-zein was orally administered to spontaneously hypertensive rats, their blood pressure was reduced. Garcia *et al.* [222] and Parris *et al.* [223] developed a dry and wet bioprocess to enhance the value of proteins from deoiled corn germ using different proteases. Nearly all the ACE inhibitory peptides were in the <1 kDa fraction after both wet and dry-milled hydrolysate had been membrane fractionated. From wet- and dry-milled germ, the control of total protein extracts (before treatment with proteases) showed that neither had ACE inhibitory properties. Yamamoto *et al.* [224] presented a review on biogenic peptides and their potential uses. In this they updated different works demonstrating strong blood pressure-lowering activity for the peptide Leu-Arg-Pro, which was isolated from α-zein hydrolysate prepared with thermolysin peptide. Sweeping frequency ultrasound (SFU) as a previous treatment of zein provided augmentation of the degree of hydrolysis (DH) in a solution (pH 8 using 1MNaOH) at 50 °C containing alcalase enzyme (3500 Ug^{-1} of protein). In this study Ren *et al.* [225] concluded that the SFU treatment increased the DH and that the hydrolysate presented a higher inhibitory effect on ACE. Scanning electron micrographs and atomic force micrographs show that the ultrasonic pretreatment ruptures the fine mesh work structure of zein and causes the subsequent appearance of several microholes in zein. SFU pretreatment promotes the release of ACE inhibitory peptides from zein by altering the secondary structure and loosening the protein. The encapsulation of micronutrients such as vitamins, minerals, and nutraceuticals has increased nowadays for the development of colloidal particles in delivery applications. To improve human health through diet, the incorporation of these kinds of micronutrients in food and beverages increases their functional behavior [226]. Patel *et al.* established the development and application of zein colloidal particles for nutraceutical encapsulation [227]. In this study they used sodium caseinate as an electrostatic stabilizer by the antisolvent precipitation method for the preparation of zein colloidal particles. An average size of 20 nm and a positively charged surface were found in the colloidal particles. Sodium caseinate did not change the particle size but changed the surface charge that shifts from positive to negative. Chemical interaction between zein and sodium caseinate was not observed from FTIR analyses. Sodium caseinate acted as a stabilizer of zein colloidal particles at neutral pH, and these particles had stability at high ionic strength and the dried powder could be redispersed. Colloidal particles have the potential to be used in an all-natural biopolymer-based colloidal delivery system for encapsulating/embedding bioactive molecules in food (e.g., nutraceuticals), pharmaceutical (e.g., drug), and agricultural formulations. Because stabilization is merely due to the adsorption of protein on the particles and the antisolvent used was water, Patel *et al.* incorporated curcumin in zein colloidal particles and sodium caseinate as the stabilizer in oral delivery. Spherical zein/ curcumin particles were obtained at the size of around 100–150 nm. The increase in curcumin proportion decreased with encapsulation efficiency. The pH and UV stabilities were improved with curcumin encapsulation, mainly at physiological pH, and also they measured the photostability, pH stability, and stability in simulated gastrointestinal conditions. It was found that the colloidal particles were stable in the simulated gastrointestinal conditions. Patel *et al.* found the encapsulation of quercetin, a polyphenol that presents physiological benefits to human health, such as in antioxidant, anticancer, and antiviral activities [228].

Here they prepared colloidal particles by precipitating quercetin and zein into an antisolvent, with the presence of sodium caseinate as an electrosteric stabilizer. The average size of the spherical-shaped particles ranged from 130 to 161 nm. The presence of sodium caseinate forms the particles' surfaces, which became negatively charged, with the surface potential ranging from −30 to 41 mV. Ferric reducing antioxidant power (FRAP) method was used to measure the antioxidant activity of quercetin for determining the stability of quercetin during photodegrading assays at different pHs. The antioxidant property of quercetin encapsulated in zein colloidal particles remained almost constant during the photodegradation study, as compared to quercetin in solution. It indicates that encapsulation into zein colloidal particles enhanced quercetin's molecular stability when exposed to UV irradiation at alkaline conditions. Encapsulation of curcumin (water insoluble) and indigo carmine (water soluble) in zein colloidal particles was studied by Patel *et al.* They prepared composites and loaded different ratios of curcumin and indigo carmine and generated different shades of color in the yellow–green–blue range. The average particle size ranges from 76 to 300 nm. Soft lithography techniques were used for the fabrication of zein film with several microstructures such as channels and grids [229]. Zein is a potential candidate for microfluidic device base material due to its ease of fabrication at mild temperatures. Microfluidic device with the entire manufacturing materials is made by Leucha *et al.* The advantages of the devices are that they are disposable and environmentally friendly microchips. Reliable fabricated thin zein films with diverse microfluidic designs were obtained by standard soft lithography and stereolithography techniques. Solvent bonding and vapor deposition methods are used to obtain zein films with microfluidic channels. Zein film tends to be opaque due to protein precipitation when in contact with water. Zein films can be used as a green alternative to nondegradable PDMS and plastic material for microfluidic applications in agriculture. There is no need for expensive equipment like oxygen and plasma generator because zein film can make quick and ease bonding with different kinds of materials. Zein microfluidic devices show different permeabilities to small molecules that helps in diffusive exchange between fluid flows and bulk zein microfluidic channels. In a more complex micrototal analysis application, zein microfluidic devices with micromixing channels have the potential to be used as fluid manipulators that can be coupled with other analytical components. For the fabrication into multilayer microfluidic devices, the flexibility and the ease of the bonding process make the zein film as a good candidate. Compared to PDMS the main advantage of zein is that it is biodegradable, and this property is very important for a greener approach in the field of portable and disposable microdevices. The adsorption capacity of hydrophobic membranes and the control of the wettability of the surface are the very attractive features for biomedical applications and electronic devices [230]. Through a facile and inexpensive method, Dong *et al.* [231] established a zein-based material with a hydrophobic surface using self-assembled monolayer (SAM)-assisted evaporation-induced self-assembly (EISA). Biopolymers such as zein make biomaterials with excellent properties such as biodegradability, renewability, flexibility, good surface wettability, and good absorption potential which still remain inexpensive. Synthetic compounds have more hydrophobic surfaces but are not biodegradable and still present low mechanical flexibility and are usually expensive.

11.2.26
Curdlan

Curdlan is a neutral water-insoluble bacterial exopolysaccharide composed primarily of linear β-(1,3)-glycosidic linkages. Recently, there has been growing interest in the biomedical applications of curdlan and its derivatives particularly in the field of immunology. Curdlan and its derivatives at dosages from 10 to 20 $mg\,kg^{-1}$ body weight were found to inhibit tumors [232]. Jagodzinski *et al.* [233] and Gordon *et al.* [234] have demonstrated the anti-HIV effect of the sulfated derivative of curdlan. The immunostimulatory effects of β-glucans have long been identified to play critical roles in the host defense of the innate immune system. The dectin-1 receptor capable of recognizing β-glucans has been identified in dendritic cells, macrophages, and monocytes/neutrophils. It triggers specific cellular antimicrobial responses such as formation of reactive oxygen species and phagocytosis. Curdlan also triggers Src/Syk-dependent downstream signals in dendritic cells, neutrophils, and macrophages to activate NF-kB, mitogen-activated protein kinases, and NFAT transcription factors [235]. Curdlan, which is insoluble in water, forms a particulate that induces dectin-1-dependent reactions, such as induction of tumor necrosis factor alpha, interleukin-6, phagocytosis, and reactive oxygen species by dendritic cells and bone marrow-derived macrophages [236]. Curdlan also acts on the complement receptor-3 (CR3) [237] as well as on Toll-like receptor-2/6 and induces the activities of immune cells such as macrophages [238], monocytes, neutrophils, dendritic cells, as well as those of natural killer cells, particularly against fungal infections [239]. Consequently, curdlan is capable of modulating both innate and adaptive immune responses. Palma *et al.* [240] made "designer" microarrays from curdlan oligosaccharides. Dectin-1 binding was found to the β-1,3-linked glucose oligomers. The minimum degree of polymerization of curdlan oligomers that can be detected is 10–11. Dry tablet encapsulation of theophylline by co-spray drying of the curdlan/theophylline suspension/solution has been shown to improve the pharmacokinetics of theophylline. Curdlan was also used in the gel encapsulation of salbutamol sulfate, prednisolone, and indomethacin in the form of gel suppositories, which facilitate sustained drug diffusion and bioavailability in the lower rectum, thus avoiding the first-pass metabolic clearance by the liver when taken orally or by injection. The increasing interest in the development of polysaccharide–polynucleotide complexes as an improved therapeutic agent during the past decade led to the innovative approach of using β-(1,3)-glucans, which form hydrogen-bonded helical structures similarly to what occurs in hydrogen bonding in the polynucleotide chains of DNA to facilitate the delivery of the pharmaceutical to its intended target site. Curdlan with hydrolytic cleavage of its backbone and thus reduction of its molecular weight to make a complex with the polynucleotide polycytosine was produced as a therapeutic agent

[241]. Addition of solubilizing carbohydrate appendages also enables curdlan to bind polycytosine as an innovative pharmaceutical agent [242]. Solid lipid nanoparticles have been produced with curdlan and cacao butter. When it was added to ammonium hydroxide solution and loaded with the drug verapamil for nanoparticle drug delivery, the drug was released quickly because of its high solubility in the lipid core [243]. The cancer chemotherapy drug doxorubicin was encapsulated by curdlan with a particle size of <200 nm to prolong its stability to up to a year of frozen storage [244]. Carboxymethylated curdlan was conjugated to cholesterol to encapsulate another cancer chemotherapy drug epirubicin through self-assembly of amphiphilic copolymer by probe sonication [245].

11.2.27
Pullulan

Pullulan is a neutral linear polysaccharide consisting of α-1,6 linked maltotriose residues, and it is soluble in water. Due to its nontoxic, nonimmunogenic, and biodegradable properties, it is extensively studied for various biomedical fields. Unlike the popular polysaccharide dextran, its degradation rate in serum is low. After an incubation period of 48 h, the degradation index of pullulan is 0.7 compared to 0.05 for dextran. Varying the degrees of chemical modification regulate or decrease the degradation rate. The strong binding of pullulan to the asialoglycoprotein receptor with high affinity has been observed by Kaneo *et al.* In this study, the bound molecule is internalized to the hepatocyte via receptor-mediated endocytosis [246]. Pullulan is widely exploited for targeted drug/gene delivery to liver because it accumulates in the liver insignificantly in higher amounts than other water-soluble polymers. In the conventional monotherapy of hepatic virus C-induced liver diseases, interferon (IFN) is used. But currently the efficiency of IFN therapies is reported to be clinically inadequate. Suginoshita *et al.* attempt to target the liver by complexing the IFN with pullulan. They later concluded that pullulan is a promising candidate for IFN therapy due to the liver-targeting ability [247]. They reported that intravenous administration of the IFN-DTPA-pullulan conjugate in mice showed enhanced IFN activity than free IFN. Lately the role of polysaccharides in developing controlled drug delivery systems has increased significantly, and pullulan is gaining significant attraction toward biomedical applications. Some examples are self-assembling nanoparticles from hydrophobized pullulan, pH-sensitive derivatized pullulan nanoparticles, and anionic/amphiphilic microparticles [248]. By complexing the hydrogel nanoparticle of cholesterol-bearing pullulan, Akiyoshi *et al.* developed an insulin delivery system of the size of 20–30 nm. Insulin aggregation and enzymatic degradation were suppressed by these stable complex nanoparticles. *In vivo* the biological activity of the complexed insulin remained intact. In contrast to pullulan, carboxymethylated pullulan has low affinity for asialoglycoprotein receptors due to its negative charge [249]. The liver uptake clearance of pullulan was decreased by the more than hundredfold. The pullulan derivative was further investigated for chemotherapy applications.

Carboxymethylated pullulan is conjugated with doxorubicin, a known chemotherapy drug used for various cancer treatments, via a peptide linker. Macromolecular prodrugs are small molecular drugs which are conjugated to polysaccharides that make them inactive. For the conjugated drug to be pharmacologically active, it should be released from the prodrug. Conjugation helps reduce free drug plasma concentration and drug exposure to other susceptible tissues. The advantage of prodrugs is that they have long half-life compared with the free drug, which leads to passive accumulation of prodrugs to the tumor. Due to the leaky vasculature as well as the retention of these macromolecular conjugates that enhanced the permeability of the prodrugs to the tumor, the lymphatic drainage will decrease. Nogusa *et al.* concluded in an *in vivo* study that that the conjugated drug was more effective than the free drug [250]. They used both the conjugate and the free drug on murine carcinoma models, solid tumor (lung carcinoma and reticulosarcoma), and nonsolid tumor (P388 leukemia). Compared with free drug, the conjugate was more effective in reducing the tumor volume and increasing the survival rate, indicating that the conjugate was very effective only against solid tumors and did not have any effect on leukemia cells. Hydrophobically modified pullulan originated from self-assembled nanoparticles. pH-sensitive self-assembled nanoparticles of succinylated pullulan acetate/sulfonamide (PA/SDM) conjugates that are responsive to even minute pH variations were created by Na *et al.* [251].

The size of the nanoparticles ranges <70 nmood, which were developed for targeting solid tumors and inflammatory regions in this area. Adriamycin (doxorubicin) is used for loading and release properties of these nanoparticles. The drug release depends on PA/SDM nanoparticles. The release rare of the dug from these nanoparticles are pH dependent, and they were significantly enhanced below a pH of 6.8. The advantages of these pH-responsive PA/SDM nanoparticles for targeted anticancer drug delivery include particle aggregation and enhanced drug release rates at tumor pH. The application of pullulan in gene therapy is another area being explored. Endocytic pathway is used in gene delivery applications. Viruses are also used for gene therapy, despite being known to be immunogenic and can be hazardous. To develop nonviral vectors, cationic derivatives of natural polymers are investigated for this application. Currently pullulan is investigated for gene delivery application due to its biocompatible and nontoxicity. Hosseinkhani *et al.* prepared a pullulan–DTPA derivative in which metal-chelating residues combined with a plasmid DNA in aqueous solution containing Zn^{2+} ions to get the conjugate of pullulan derivative and plasmid DNA with Zn^{2+} coordination. Cholesterol pullulan and amino-group-modified cholesterol showed good stability but shrank and aggregated below pH 7.0. Extracellular pH (pH 6.5–7.2) is lower than normal tissues and blood. Pullulan nanogel were developed by Hasegawa *et al.* In this study the amino-group-modified cholesterol pullulan nanogel acts as a novel carrier to deliver QD into cells in comparison to conventional cationic liposome and has the disadvantage of forming aggregates once it is internalized in the cell [252]. By simply mixing nanogels of cholesterol-bearing pullulan modified with amino groups and quantum dots, nanoparticles were formed, and their size is about 38 nm. The intensity of fluorescence per cell of CHPNH2–QD nanoparticles was comparable to that of a liposome–QD complex. It also shows that with higher number of amino groups, the fluorescence can be up to 3.4 times than that of the control. Therefore the authors established that these nanoparticles could be a promising fluorescent probe for bioimaging due to chemical modification of CHP enhancing its cellular uptake and simultaneous delivering QD than the conventional cationic liposome. Carboxymethyl pullulan was developed and conjugated to HP by Na *et al.*, who also investigated its properties with regard to tissue engineering applications [253]. In tissue engineering applications, scaffolds or artificial ECM are required, since they can accommodate cells and regulate growth, leading to 3D tissue regeneration. *In vitro* it shows that the proliferation of SMCs is inhibited by the HP-conjugated pullulan. So this material can be used for the proliferation of vascular endothelial cells and to inhibit the proliferation of SMCs. Irreversible aggregation due to host-guest interaction prevents irreversible aggregation was suppressed by the selective binding of molecular chaperons to denatured proteins. This chaperon-like activity helps to catch and release the proteins. The refolded form of protein was released by the host chaperon. A water-soluble polymer such as PEO is used to increase the recovery yield of the native protein during refolding. The purpose of using this type of polymers is that they will block the exposed hydrophobic surface on the denatured proteins in such a way that it just prevents the aggregation of proteins. Folding to the native confirmation has been prevented by excessively strong binding to intermediates. Hydrophobized pullulan nanogels are developed by Nomura *et al.* These nanogels thus possess the properties of molecular chaperons [254]. In the presence of cyclodextrin, the complex proteins were effectively released from the nanogels in their refolded forms. So the authors concluded that this nanogel system is a promising technique for protein refolding. The binding and release of proteins in the active form are being explored toward tissue engineering applications. Similar to dextran, pullulan is largely explored as a potential blood-plasma substitute. The significant property for plasma expanders is its high water solubility, which made pullulan a great example. These blood plasma expanders operates through colloidal osmotic pressure induced by the macromolecules. So in order to attain this property, pullulan should have a molecular weight of about 60 kDa. Low molecular weight pullulan gets rapidly excluded from the organism resulting in a secondary hemorrhagic shock, while higher molecular weight pullulan increased venous pressure. For this purpose pullulan should be in a therapeutic molecular range. Anionically modified pullulan via γ-irradiation was used as the base for blood-plasma substitute by Shingel *et al.* [255]. The resistance of pullulan to degradative action amylase is increased by the presence of carboxyl and carbonyl groups.

11.2.28 **Casein**

Casein films have been shown to exhibit high tensile strength making them suitable candidates for coatings for tablets. There have been no reports investigating the use of this highly acceptable biopolymer for tablet coating processes until Abu Diak *et al.* [256] evaluated casein as a film former for tablet coating with the aid of different water-soluble and insoluble plasticizers. In this study, diltiazem HCl core tablets were coated with casein using a pan coater, and the efficacy of four different plasticizing agents (glycerol, triethyl citrate, dibutyl sebacate, and oleic acid) in producing a continuous tablet coat was evaluated. Interestingly, as only those films formed using oleic acid were capable of producing a continuous and acceptable coat, casein can be considered as a potential film former for the coating of pharmaceutical dosage forms. Macheras *et al.* [257] have observed increases in bioavailability of drug–milk preparations relative to the pure drug. Subsequent binding studies in casein solutions showed increases in drug solubility, which could not be explained by normal protein binding. Watanabe *et al.* [258] observed that the release rate of phenytoin from a solid mass containing sodium caseinate and microcrystalline cellulose decreased gradually in comparison with its release from intact phenytoin powder. They related that decrease to the adsorption of sodium caseinate protein on the hydrophobic surface of phenytoin crystal. Caseins possess a number of favorable characteristics suitable for the development of hydrogel biomaterials, such as high hydrophilicity; good biocompatibility, particularly in oral delivery applications; lack of toxicity; and availability of reactive sites for chemical modification. Genipin is found in traditional Chinese medicine and is extracted from the gardenia fruit. It is an effective naturally occurring cross-linking agent that can react with amino acids or proteins [259]. Many researchers have investigated the cytotoxicity, feasibility, and biocompatibility of genipin for tissue fixation and found that genipin was 10 000 times less cytotoxic than the commonly used glutaraldehyde solution. Novel casein-based hydrogel for the controlled release of BSA has been prepared for the first time using genipin to cross-link casein protein in an aqueous system [260]. The mechanical strength of the cross-linked casein hydrogel could be tuned depending on the amount of genipin. At pH 1.2, the swelling ratio of the hydrogel and the amount of BSA released were relatively low. However, a higher amount of swelling and BSA release were observed at pH 7.4. The release behavior could be related to cross-linking and swelling degrees of the hydrogel networks formed by various amounts of genipin. It is suggested that the genipin-cross-linked casein hydrogels might be a suitable polymeric carrier for protein drug delivery in the intestine, as shown in Figure 11.7. [261]

Various chemical or physical cross-linking methods have been used for the gelation of aqueous casein systems. Among them, enzyme-induced cross-linking has been found to be an attractive route. Transglutaminase (TGase) catalyzes covalent inter molecular cross-linking through an acyl-transfer reaction, between the g-carboxyamide group of a peptide-bound glutamine residue (acyl donor) and the primary amino group of an amine (acyl acceptor) [262]. Song *et al.* used microbial transglutaminase (MTGase) to assist the gelation of an aqueous casein system for controlled drug release. Increasing the amount of MTGase resulted in a decrease in gelation time and an enhancement of hydrogel strength.

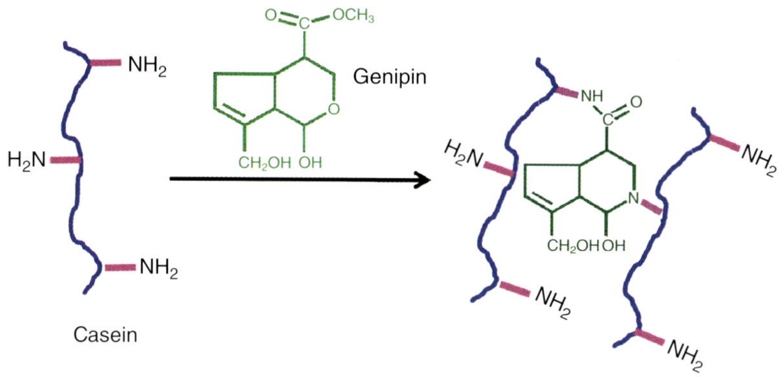

Figure 11.7 Possible cross-linking mechanism for the reaction of casein with genipin in an aqueous system [261].

Compared with the casein hydrogel without the added MTGase, the enzyme-induced casein hydrogel is characterized by a more complex network structure with higher fractal dimension. By means of this enzyme-assisted gelation, as a model drug, vitamin B12 was incorporated into the casein hydrogel matrix under mild conditions. This hydrogel was found to have potential use as a new matrix for the entrapment and controlled release of vitamin B12 [263]. Casein has been used to prepare biodegradable microspheres by an emulsification technique. The microspheres obtained by this technique do not show any floating properties. However, casein foaming properties cause the incorporation of air bubbles that act as air reservoirs in the floating systems. Fluorescein sodium (FluNa)-loaded casein–gelatin floating beads have been prepared by an emulsification extraction method and cross-linked with D,L-glyceraldehyde. Emulsifying properties of casein caused air bubble incorporation and formation of large holes in the beads. The high porosity of the matrix influences bead properties such as drug loading, drug release, and floatation. These effects are significant when compared to those with low-porosity beads that are artificially prepared without cavities. The percentage of casein in the matrix increased drug loading of both low-porosity and high-porosity matrices, with the loading of high-porosity matrices being lower than that of low-porosity ones. The drug release rate increase in high-porosity matrix, in comparison with beads without cavities, is due to the rapid diffusion of the drug through water-filled pores. The study shows that cavities act as an air reservoir and enables the beads to float. Therefore, casein seems to be a material suitable for the inexpensive formation of air reservoirs for floating systems. Casein microspheres may be advantageous to be used as an alternative to albumin as a matrix for microsphere drug carriers. Casein microspheres are relatively inexpensive; they have better amphiphilicity and good dispersibility in aqueous systems, and they form uniform spherical structures. Particle amphiphilicity is important for post-synthesis drug loading as well as for easy wetting and rapid reconstitution in aqueous solutions. Casein microspheres have been prepared through a number of techniques. In emulsification–chemical cross-linking, cross-linked casein microspheres were successfully used as parenteral biodegradable carriers for sustained delivery of drugs via intramuscular, intraperitoneal, and direct intratumoral injection, or intra-arterially for embolization in solid tumor deposits. Enzymatically cross-linked casein micelles (CM) can be transformed from associating colloids with microgel particles, which can provide very interesting and promising controlled-release drug delivery systems [264], coacervation, and electrostatic complexation in aqueous systems. Casein-based nanovehicles were used for drug and nutraceutical delivery applications varying from nanosized micelles to enzymatically cross-linked nanogel particles, or nanoparticles prepared by graft copolymerization, heat gelation, or polyelectrolyte ionic complexation. Milk CM represent a natural nano delivery system. They are part of the milk transport system in which nutrients are passed from the mother to a suckling offspring as a primary source of amino acids and calcium phosphates essential for neonates. The micelles are very stable in processing and retain their basic structural identity during the processing of milk into various products [265]. CM have received much attention in many fields such as food, cosmetics, and medicine. In general, caseins can be thought of as block copolymers consisting of blocks with high levels of hydrophobic or hydrophilic amino acid residues. Semo *et al.* [265] have demonstrated the possibility to encapsulate the fat-soluble vitamin D2 as a model hydrophobic nutraceutical compound within CM, using the natural self-assembly tendency of bovine caseins. The complexation of the poorly soluble chemopreventive agent curcumin with the natural nanostructure of bovine CM, and its application in drug delivery to cancer cells were investigated. The interaction of CM with gold nanoparticles (GNPs) was studied. It was believed that CM–GNP conjugates are desirable nanobiotechnology materials for future applications in genomics, proteomics, biomedical, and bioanalytical areas. Beta-casein (β-CN) micelles have also been studied as nanovehicles for hydrophobic bioactives. The pronounced self-associating behavior into micelles makes casein a promising candidate for drug delivery applications. The micelles can potentially encapsulate and stabilize bioactive compounds, particularly drugs and therapeutic compounds of hydrophobic as well as amphiphilic character [266]. A drug delivery system comprising a model hydrophobic anticancer drug, mitoxantrone (MX), entrapped within β-CN-based nanoparticles was introduced [267]. β-CN nanoparticles may serve as effective oral delivery nanovehicles for solubilization and stabilization of hydrophobic drugs. Mandelbaum and Danino [268] focused their research on encapsulation of celecoxib and budesonide, both having low bioavailability, into nanostructured β-CN assemblies. Zhu and Li [269] prepared poly(methyl methacrylate) (PMMA)/casein core–shell nanoparticles via a graft copolymerization of methyl methacrylate (MMA) with CM induced by a small amount of copper ions. Thus, this process is considered commercially viable and could be used as a drug delivery vehicle. Pan *et al.* [270] grafted dextran to casein to increase its hydrophilicity through the Maillard reaction, which is a nontoxic reaction that happens naturally during the processing, cooking, and storage of foods [271]. Nanoparticles encapsulating extremely insoluble β-carotene were fabricated via self-assembly of casein-*graft*-dextran copolymer. The amphiphilic character of the particles provides a possibility for practical applications of the particles to deliver unstable and hydrophobic nutrients and drugs. Nanogel casein particles were prepared by cross-linking the CM with the enzyme TGase [272]. Casein nanogel particles were more stable to heat-induced coagulation but less stable to acid-induced coagulation than native CM. Casein nanogel particles offer applications not only in traditional dairy products but also in applications where the integrity and biocompatibility of the nanogel particle are important such as their use in drug delivery applications. Heat-induced protein denaturation causes proteins to lose their compact structure, to expose their hydrophobic residues to the surface, and to exchange their disulfide bonds, resulting in intermolecular interactions [273, 274]. Pan *et al.* [275] studied the self-assembly of β-CN and lysozyme, having isoelectric points of pH 5.0 and 10.7, respectively, to form polydisperse electrostatic complex nanoparticles. The nanoparticles formed due to interactions between these biomacromolecules may find a potential application in encapsulation and controlled release of drugs, nutraceuticals, and other bioactive compounds. Major challenges of milk proteins include identification of specific targets and targeting mechanisms for oral delivery of anticancer drugs and advancing nanotechnology for food and drug applications. In the field of nutraceuticals, these include protecting oxidation-sensitive hydrophobic and hydrophilic nutraceuticals in their long shelf life and exploring the digestive or systemic fate of vehicles developed and their bioactive cargo and applying this knowledge to the design of smarter, more effective targeted vehicles for both nutraceuticals and drugs. The main technological challenges in this respect are to control digestibility, to program the release of the bioactive payload to occur at the desired target location along the gastrointestinal tract, and to promote its bioavailability [276].

11.2.29 Silk

The most important and ancient insect-derived protein materials used by humans are silk. Silkworm silk and spider silk are the different sources of silk that have been studied. Dragline spider silk is the toughest of all types [277]. In tissue engineering studies, silk and silklike polypeptides (SLPs) have been used extensively. Naturally derived silk fibroin from silkworms is a readily available source of these proteins. It has been processed to form hydrogels, films, and electrospun nanofibers, as well as porous scaffolds. Perrone *et al.* recently investigated that the tough silk fibroin can be processed into devices such as biodegradable screws and plates useful for craniofacial bone-fixing applications [278]. Spider silks have also been used in applications that require durable materials [279, 280]. Dragline spider silk harvested from *Nephila* spp. was used to fabricate woven scaffolds as artificial skin, able to support fibroblasts and keratinocytes. The combination of crystalline, flexible, and amorphous domains in the protein makes spider silk the toughest among silks. However, the limitations of natural silk from spiders and silkworms are that the harvesting of mechanically robust silk spidroin is impractical and they lack intrinsic bioactivity and cannot be genetically modified like recombinant proteins. Researchers using recombinantly expressed SLPs have focused on the spider silk-derived consensus sequences from spiders such as *Nephila clavipes* and *Araneus diadematus* [281]. The mechanical robustness of native spider silks has been used to improve SLPs to fabricate tough structures such as fibers, films, and coatings. Such structures would be useful to replace skeletal tissues and skin as well as for many nonbiological uses [282]. The bioapplications of SLP have mainly focused on exploring the biocompatibility of the proteins and on ways to impart bioactivity and synthesizing different forms of scaffolds rather than using the strongest versions of SLP fibers. For example, porous scaffolds fabricated using *N. clavipes* MaSp1 sequence-derived SLP expressed in *E. coli* have been shown to not only be biocompatible but also show vascularization and tissue in growth during subcutaneous implantation in BALB/c mice [283]. Moisenovich *et al.* observed that the porous scaffolds show bone healing capabilities after defect repair with these scaffolds compared to the control in Wistar rats. *N. clavipes*-derived sequence is used to synthesize SLPs with various functionalities including RGD-functionalized SLPs to improve cell adhesion, silaffin-derived R5 sequence to mineralize silica [284], and dentin matrix protein 1 sequence to mineralize calcium phosphate by Kaplan and coworkers [285]. An alternative type of SLP used to develop cell-interactive substrates is the *Euprosthenops australis*-derived 4RepCT. 4RepCT has been used to prepare films, foams, fibers, and meshes that were tested for interactions with human primary fibroblasts [286]. Widhe *et al.* show that all the substrates were compatible with the fibroblasts and sustained similar cell properties such as collagen formation even after 14 days of culture. Lewicka *et al.* observed that 4RepCT films are compatible with neural stem cell culture and are comparable to plates coated with poly-L-ornithine and fibronectin from bovine plasma [287]. Recently, 4RepCT films fused with cell adhesion motifs such as RGD, IKVAV, and YIGSR were shown to promote better cell adhesion than controls especially for Schwann cells on IKVAV functional 4RepCT compared with laminin-coated control [288]. Furthermore, 4RepCT fusions with different biomolecule-binding domains such as IgG binding, biotin binding, and albumin binding have also been prepared [289]. Site-specific immobilization of different biomolecules can be a powerful method to impart ECM-like activity to SLP or any other PBP used for cell interaction and tissue engineering. Silk and silk fibroins from silkworms are used heavily for drug delivery applications. Silk fibroin has been processed into films, fibers, hydrogels, and coatings [290]. Delivery of biomolecules has been obtained using SLP sequences derived from two sources: major ampule proteins ADF4 and MaSp1 from *A. diadematus* and *N. clavipes*, respectively. Among the different structures, the most commonly fabricated one is nanoparticle delivery agents. Low molecular weight hydrophobic drug molecules can easily diffuse into these nanoparticles, and hydrophobic interactions with the β-sheet-rich core trap the molecules within the particles [291]. Furthermore, eADF4(C16) has an isoelectric point of pH 3.48, which makes it a negatively charged polypeptide at a high pH; thus, positively charged drugs show a higher encapsulation efficiency at physiological pH than those with a negative charge. The charge on the eADF4(C16) peptides also allows for pH-responsive drug delivery; for example, >80% of the loaded drug (ethacridine lactate) was released in 1 day at pH2, whereas only 10% was released in the same time at pH 7 and above. The drug-loaded nanoparticles can also be enzymatically degraded by trypsin and elastase, making the particles useful for cell activity-mediated drug release. Hofer *et al.* [292] used similar particles composed of eADF4(C16) for lysozyme delivery. The positively charged lysozyme was easily loaded in the eADF4(C16) nanoparticles, and the *in vitro* release tests showed a pH- and ionic strength-dependent protein release. The researchers also showed that SLP nanoparticles can be lyophilized for long-term storage without any damage. On the other hand, *N. clavipes* MaSp1 protein-derived sequence has been used to design self-assembling nanoparticles useful for gene delivery. Numata *et al.* [293] synthesized a triblock SLP containing six repeats of the MaSp1 consensus, poly(L-lysine) with 30 lysine residues, and either a tumor lymphatics-targeting domain or cell death-inducing domain. The triblock polypeptides self-assemble to form nanoparticles in the presence of negatively charged genes. Particles with tumor lymphatics-homing peptide showed better transfection efficiency, resulting in their use in a mouse model for *in vivo* gene delivery. In addition, the particles also have a tunable enzymatic degradation rate dependent on its β-sheet content that can be regulated by methanol treatment of the particles. Other scaffold structures made of SLP being developed for drug delivery are films. Similarly to the SLP nanoparticles for gene delivery, films can also have tunable degradation and drug release by changing film crystallinity. A standard method used to increase the β-sheet content of silk structures is via dehydration using nonsolvents such as methanol [294]. Spiess *et al.* [295] observed that due to changes in SLP crystallinity and packing, the mechanical properties of the films would simultaneously affect the release rates of loaded drugs. Tuning the release rate of drugs from SLP films is to mix the polypeptide with a synthetic polymer as shown by Hardy *et al.* [296]. The films cast with a combination of eADF4(C16) and polycaprolactone or pellethane show degradation and drug release that is dependent on the amount of synthetic polymer; lower polymer results in faster degradation and drug release, and vice versa.

11.3 Conclusion

Currently natural biodegradable polymers are very significant in terms of their applications in fields with respect to environmental protection and physical health. The demand for natural biopolymers includes a wide range of biomedical applications such as wound dressing membranes, scaffolds for tissue engineering, resorbable surgical sutures, matrices for the controlled release of drugs, and resorbable devices such as bone cements, pins, screws, and plates. Natural polymers have many advantages over synthetic polymers because of many reasons such as their natural resources, being inexpensive, and having the capability of chemical modification.

Abbreviations

b-PEI	branched polyethylenimine
ß-TCP	beta-tricalcium phosphate
BTE	bone tissue engineering
BSA	bovine serum albumin
β-CN	beta-casein
CM	casein micelles
CaP	calcium phosphate
CHI	chitosan
CA	cellulose acetate
DIM	3,3′-diindolylmethane
DHA	1,4-dihydroxyanthraquinone
DS	dermatan sulfate
DMR	diagnostic magnetic resonance
DH	degree of hydrolysis
DHP	dialdehyde heparin
DAS	dialdehyde starch
ELP	elastin-like polypeptides
ECM	extracellular matrix
EISA	evaporation-induced self-assembly
FRET	Förster resonance energy transfer
FRAP	ferric reducing antioxidant power
GNPs	gold nanoparticles
GBR	guided bone regeneration
GAGs	glycosaminoglycans
GF	growth factor
HP	heparin
HS	heparan sulfate
HGA	homogalacturonan
HACS	high-amylase cornstarch
HSA	human serum albumin
HA	hydroxyapatite
ITT	inverse temperature transition
IBU	ibuprofen
IFN	interferon
LUT	lutein
MAA	methacrylic acid
MTGase	microbial transglutaminase
MX	mitoxantrone
MMA	methyl methacrylate
MRI	magnetic resonance imaging

NPs	nanoparticles
PGs	proteoglycans
PET	positron emission tomography
PDT	photodynamic therapy
(pAAm-*g*-GG)	polyacrylamide-grafted guar gum
PCL	poly(ε-caprolactone)
PU	polyurethane
PDMS	poly(dimethylsiloxane)
PMMA	poly(methyl methacrylate)
RBM	rat bone marrow
ST	starch
SGF	simulated gastric fluid
SIF	simulated intestinal fluid
SFU	sweeping frequency ultrasound
SAM	self-assembled monolayer
SMCs	smooth muscle cells
SLPs	silklike polypeptides
TOC	α-tocopherol
TF	foaming temperature
TGase	transglutaminase
ZT	thermoplastic zein

References

1. Liu, J. *et al.* (2015) A review of bioactive plant polysaccharides: biological activities, functionalization, and biomedical applications. *Bioact. Carbohydr. Dietary Fibre*, **5**, 31–61.
2. Sharma, K. *et al.* (2011) Natural biodegradable polymers as matrices in transdermal drug delivery. *Int. J. Drug Dev. Res.*, **3** (2), 85–103.
3. Chifiriuc, M.C. *et al.* (2013) Biomedical applications of natural polymers for drug delivery. *Curr. Org. Chem.*, **18**, 152–164.
4. Athanasiou, K.A., Shah, A.R., Hernandez, R.J., and Le Baron, R.G. (2001) Basic science of articular cartilage repair. *Clin. Sports Med.*, **20**, 223–247.
5. Madihally, S.V. and Matthew, H.W.T. (1999) Porous chitosan scaffolds for tissue engineering. *Biomaterials*, **20**, 1133–1142.
6. Park, S.Y., Lee, B.I., Jung, S.T., and Park, J.H. (2001) Biopolymer composite films based on k-carrageenan and chitosan. *Mater. Res. Bull.*, **36**, 511–519.
7. Shi, C., Zhu, Y., Ran, X., Wang, M., Su, Y., and Cheng, T. (2006) Therapeutic potential of chitosan and its derivatives in regenerative medicine. *J. Surg. Res.*, **133**, 185–192.
8. Seeherman, H., Li, R., and Wozney, J. (2003) A review of preclinical program development for evaluating injectable carriers for osteogenic factor. *J. Bone Joint Surg. Am.*, **85A**, 96–108.
9. Chesnutt, B.M., Viano, A.M., Yuan, Y., Yang, Y., Guda, T., Appleford, M.R., Ong, J.L., Haggard, W.O., and Bumgardner, J.D. (2009) Design and characterization of a novel chitosan/nanocrystalline calcium phosphate composite scaffold for bone regeneration. *J. Biomed. Mater. Res. Part A*, **88A**, 491–502.
10. Thein-Han, W.W. and Misra, R.D.K. (2009) Biomimetic chitosan– nanohydroxyapatite composite scaffolds for bone tissue engineering. *Acta Biomater.*, **5**, 1182–1197.

11. Lee, J.Y., Kim, K.H., Shin, S.Y., Rhyu, I.C., Lee, Y.M., Park, Y.J., Chung, C.P., and Lee, S.J. (2006) Enhanced bone formation by transforming growth factor- β1-releasing collagen/chitosan microgranules. *J. Biomed. Mater. Res.*, 7, 530–539.
12. Zhao, H. and Ma, L. (2008) Fabrication and properties of mineralized collagen-chitosan/hydroxyapatite scaffold. *Polym. Adv. Technol.*, **19**, 1590–1596.
13. Lee, E.J., Shin, D.S., Kim, H.E., Kim, H.W., Koh, Y.H., and Jang, J.H. (2009) Membrane of hybrid chitosan–silica xerogel for guided bone regeneration. *Biomaterials*, **30**, 743–750.
14. Zhou, H., Qian, J., Wang, J., Yao, W., Liu, C., Chen, J., and Cao, X. (2009) Enhanced bioactivity of bone morphogenetic protein-2 with low dose of 2-N, 6-Osulfated chitosan in vitro and in vivo. *Biomaterials*, **30**, 1715–1724.
15. D'Ayala, G., De Rosa, A., Laurienzo, P., and Malinconico, M. (2007) Development of a new calcium sulphate-based composite using alginate and chemically modified chitosan for bone regeneration. *J. Biomed. Res.*, **81**, 811–820.
16. Bhattacharya, M., Malinen, M.M., Lauren, P., Lou, Y.-R., Kuisma, S.W., Kanninen, L., Lille, M., Corlu, A., GuGuen-Guillouzo, C., Ikkala, O., Laukkanen, A., Urtti, A., and Yliperttula, M. (2012) Nanofibrillar cellulose hydrogel promotes three-dimensional liver cell culture. *J. Controlled Release*, **164**, 291–298.
17. Valoa, H., Arolab, S., Laaksonenb, P., Torkkelic, M., Peltonena, L., Linderb, M.B., Serimaac, R., Kugad, S., Hirvonena, J., and Laaksonena, T. (2013) Drug release from nanoparticles embedded in four different nanofibrillar cellulose aerogels. *Eur. J. Pharm. Sci.*, **50**, 69–77.
18. Meinel, L., Hofmann, S., Karageorgiou, C., Kirker-Head, C., Cool, M. *et al.* (2005) The inflammatory responses to silk fibers in vitro and in vivo. *Biomaterials*, **26**, 147–155.
19. Haarer, J.C., Inskeep, B.D., and Dee, K.C. (2006) Proteins and amino acid-derived polymers, in *An Introduction to Biomaterials* (eds S.A. Guelcher and J.O. Hollinger), CRC, Taylor & Francis, Boca Raton, FL, pp. 121–138.
20. Nair, L.S. and Laurencin, C.T. (2007) Biodegradable polymers as biomaterials. *Prog. Polym. Sci.*, **32**, 762–798.
21. Pachence, J.M. (2007) Biodegradable polymers, in *Principles of Tissue Engineering*, 3rd edn, Burlington, MA, Academic Press.
22. Altman, G.H., Diaz, F., Jakuba, C., Calabro, T., Horan, R.L., and Chen, J. (2003) Silk based biomaterials. *Biomaterials*, **24**, 410–416.
23. Chevallay, B. and Herbage, D. (2000) Collagen-based biomaterials as 3D scaffold for cell cultures: applications for tissue engineering and gene therapy. *Med. Biol. Eng. Comput.*, **38**, 211–218.
24. Wang, Y., Yang, C., Chen, X., and Zhao, N. (2006) Biomimetic formation of hydroxyapatite/collagen matrix composite. *Adv. Eng. Mater.*, **8**, 97–100.
25. Hsu, F.Y., Chueh, S.C., and Wang, Y.J. (1999) Microspheres of hydroxyapatite/reconstituted collagen as supports for osteoblast cell growth. *Biomaterials*, **20**, 1931–1936.
26. Dos Santos, I., Mazères, S., Freche, M., Lacout, J., and Sautereau, A. (2008) FRET: a tool to study the interaction between apatite and collagen? *Mater. Lett.*, **62**, 4377–4379.
27. Rodrigues, C.V., Serricella, P., Linhares, A.B.R., Guerdes, R.M., Borojevic, R., Rossi, M.A., Duarte, M.E.L., and Farina, M. (2003) Characterization of a bovine collagen-hydroxyapatite composite scaffold for bone tissue engineering. *Biomaterials*, **24**, 4987–4997.
28. Brodie, J.C., Goldie, E., Connel, G., Merry, J., and Grant, M.H. (2005) Osteoblast interactions with calcium phosphate ceramics modified by coating with type I collage. *J. Biomed. Mater. Res.*, **73**, 409–421.
29. Zou, C., Weng, W., Deng, X., Cheng, K., Liu, X., Du, P., Shen, G., and Han, G. (2005) Preparation and characterization of porous b-tricalcium phosphate/collagen composites with an integrated structure. *Biomaterials*, **26**, 5276–5284.

30. Schneiders, W., Reinstorf, A., Pompe, W., Grass, R., Biewener, A., Holch, M., Zwipp, H., and Rammelt, S. (2007) Effect of modification of hydroxyapatite/collagen composites with sodium citrate, phosphoserine, phosphoserine/RGD-peptide and calcium carbonate on bone remodeling. *Bone*, **40**, 1048–1059.
31. Tamimi, F., Kumarasami, B., Doillon, C., Gbureck, U., Le Nihouannen, D., Cabarcos, E.L., and Barralet, J.E. (2008) Brushite–collagen composites for bone regeneration. *Acta Biomater.*, **4**, 1315–1321.
32. Barralet, J.E., Gbureck, U., and Grover, L.M. (2004) Ionic modification of calcium phosphate cement viscosity. Part II: hypodermic injection and strength improvement of brushite cement. *Biomaterials*, **25**, 2197–2203.
33. Rahman, A.M., Mubarak, A.K., and Tareq, S.M. (2010) Preparation and characterization of polyethylene oxide (PEO)/gelatin blend for biomedical application: Effect of gamma radiation. *J. Appl. Polym. Sci.*, **117** (4), 2075–2082.
34. Mithieux, S.M., Rasko, J.E.J., and Weiss, A.S. (2004) Synthetic elastin hydrogels derived from massive elastic assemblies of self-organized human protein monomers. *Biomaterials*, **25**, 4921–4927.
35. Woodhouse, K.A., Klement, P., Chen, V., Gorbet, M.B., Keeley, F.W. *et al.* (2004) Investigation of recombinant human elastin polypeptides as non-thrombogenic coatings. *Biomaterials*, **25**, 4543–4553.
36. McMillan, R.A. and Conticello, V.P. (2000) Synthesis and characterization of elastin-mimetic protein gels derived from a well-defined polypeptide precursor. *Macromolecules*, **33**, 4809–4821.
37. Mithieux, S.M., Rasko, J.E.J., and Weiss, A.S. (2004) Synthetic elastin hydrogels derived from massive elastic assemblies of self- organized human protein monomers. *Biomaterials*, **25**, 4921–4927.
38. Nath, N. and Chilkoti, A. (2001) Interfacial phase transition of an environmentally responsive elastin biopolymer adsorbed on functionalized gold nanoparticles studied by colloidal surface plasmon resonance. *J. Am. Chem. Soc.*, **123**, 8197–8202.
39. Chilkoti, A., Christensen, T., and Mackay, J.A. (2006) Stimulus responsive elastin biopolymers: applications in medicine and biotechnology. *Curr. Opin. Chem. Biol.*, **10**, 652–657.
40. Betre, H., Ong, S.R., Guilak, F., Chilkoti, A., Fermor, B., and Setton, L.A. (2006) Chondrocytic differentiation of human adipose-derived adult stem cells in elastin-like polypeptide. *Biomaterials*, **27**, 91–99.
41. Liu, J.C., Heilshorn, S.C., and Tirrell, D.A. (2004) Comparative cell response to artificial extracellular matrix proteins containing the RGD and CS5 cell-binding domains. *Biomacromolecules*, **5**, 497–504.
42. Prinsen, B.H. and de Sain-van der Velden, M.G. (2004) Albumin turnover: experimental approach and its application in health and renal diseases. *Clin. Chim. Acta*, **347** (1–2), 1–14.
43. Chuang, V.T., Kragh-Hansen, U., and Otagiri, M. (2002) Pharmaceutical strategies utilizing recombinant human serum albumin. *Pharm. Res.*, **19** (5), 569–577.
44. Uchida, M., Ito, A., Furukawa, K.S., Nakamura, K., Onimura, Y., Oyane, A. *et al.* (2005) Reduced platelet adhesion to titanium metal coated with apatite, albumin–apatite composite, or laminin– apatite composite. *Biomaterials*, **26**, 6924–6931.
45. Grassl, E. and Tranquillo, R.T. (2006) Fibrillar fibrin gels, in *Scaffolds in Tissue Engineering* (eds X.P. Ma and J. Elisseeff), CRC, Taylor & Francis, Boca Raton, FL, pp. 61–70.
46. Wong, C., Inman, E., Spaethe, R., and Helgerson, S. (2003) Fibrin-based biomaterials to deliver human growth factors. *Thromb. Haemost.*, **89**, 573.
47. Mana, M., Cole, M., Cox, S., and Tawil, B. (2006) Human U937 monocyte behavior and protein expression on various formulations of three-dimensional

fibrin clots. *Wound Repair Regen.*, **14**, 72–80.
48. Al-Assaf, S., Navaratnam, S., Parsons, B.J., and Phillips, G.O. (2003) The chain scission of hyaluronan by peroxynitrite. *Arch. Biochem. Biophys.*, **411**, 73–82.
49. Brekke, J.H. and Thacker, K. (2006) Hyaluronan as a biomaterial, in *An Introduction to Biomaterials* (eds S.A. Guelcher and J.O. Hollinger), CRC, Taylor & Francis, Boco Raton, FL, pp. 219–248.
50. Hunt, D.R., Joanovic, S.A., Wikesjo, U.M.E., Wozney, J.M., and Bernard, D.W. (2001) Hyaluronan supports recombinant human bone morphogenetic protein-2 induced bone reconstruction of advanced alveolar ridge defects in dogs. A pilot study. *J. Periodontol.*, **72**, 651–657.
51. Eppley, B.L. and Dadvand, B. (2006) Injectable soft-tissue fillers: clinical overview. *Plast. Reconstr. Surg.*, **118**, 98e–106e.
52. Kato, Y., Nakamura, S., and Nishimura, M. (2006) Beneficial actions of hyaluronan (HA) on arthritic joints: effects of molecular weight of HA on elasticity of cartilage matrix. *Biorheology*, **43**, 347–354.
53. Volpi, N. (2006) Therapeutic applications of glycosaminoglycans. *Curr. Med. Chem.*, **13**, 1799–1810.
54. Parrish, C.R., Freeman, C., and Hulett, M.D. (2001) Heparanase: a key enzyme involved in cell invasion. *Biochim. Biophys. Acta*, **1471**, M99.
55. Borsig, L., Wong, R., Feramisco, J., Nadeau, D.R., Varki, N.M., and Varki, A. (2001) Synergistic effects of L- and P-selectin in facilitating tumor metastasis can involve non-mucin ligands and implicate leukocytes as enhancers of metastasis. *Proc. Natl. Acad. Sci. U.S.A.*, **98**, 3352.
56. Sasisekharan, S. and Venkataraman, G. (2000) Heparin and heparan sulfate: biosynthesis, structure and function. *Curr. Opin. Chem. Biol.*, **4**, 626.
57. Salmivirta, M., Lidholt, K., and Lindahl, U. (1996) Heparan sulfate: a piece of information. *FASEB J.*, **10**, 1270–1279.
58. Rosenberg, R.D., Shworak, N.W., Liu, J., Schwartz, J.J., and Zhang, L. (1997) Heparan sulfate proteoglycans of the cardiovascular system. Specific structures emerge but how is synthesis regulated? *J. Clin. Invest.*, **99**, 2062–2070.
59. Bishop, J., Schuksz, M., and Esko, J.D. (2007) Heparan sulphate proteoglycans fine-tune mammalian physiology. *Nature*, **446**, 1030.
60. Dreyfuss, J.L., Regatieri, C.V., Jarrouge, T.R., Cavalheiro, R.P., Sabmpaio, L.O., and Nader, H.B. (2009) Heparan sulfate proteoglycans: structure, protein interactions and cell signalling. *Ann. Braz. Acad. Sci.*, **81** (3), 409–429.
61. Peretti, T., Waisberg, J., Mader, A.M., DE Matos, L.L., DA Costa, R.B., Conceicao, G.M., Lopes, A.C., Nader, H.B., and Pinhal, M.A. (2008) Heparanase-2, syndecan-1, and extracellular matrix remodeling in colorectal carcinoma. *Eur. J. Gastroenterol. Hepatol.*, **20**, 756–765.
62. Raman, R., Sasisekharan, V., and Sasisekharan, R. (2005) Structural insights into biological roles of protein-glycosaminoglycan interactions. *Chem. Biol.*, **12**, 267–277.
63. Grunert, M., Nurcombe, V., and Cool, S.M. (2008) Stem cell fate decisions: the role of heparan sulfate in the control of autocrine and paracrine signals. *Curr. Stem Cell Res. Ther.*, **3**, 1–8.
64. Chan, P.S., Caron, J.P., Rosa, G.J., and Orth, M.W. (2005) Glucosamine and chondroitin sulfate regulate gene expression and synthesis of nitric oxide and prostaglandin E(2) in articular cartilage explants. *Osteoarthr. Cartil.*, **13**, 387–394.
65. Sugahara, K., Mikami, T., Uyama, T., Mizuguchi, S., Nomura, K., and Kitagawa, H. (2003) Recent advances in the structural biology of chondroitin sulfate and dermatan sulfate. *Curr. Opin. Struct. Biol.*, **13**, 612–620.
66. Kosir, M.A., Quinn, C.C.V., Wang, W., and Tromp, G. (2000) Matrix glycosaminoglycans in the growth phase of Fibroblasts: more of the story in wound healing. *J. Surg. Res.*, **92**, 45–52.
67. Gilbert, M.E., Kirker, K.R., Gray, S.D., Ward, P.D., Szakacs, J.G., Prestwich, G.D. *et al.* (2004) Chondroitin sulfate

hydrogel and wound healing in rabbit maxillary sinus mucosa. *Laryngoscope*, **114** (8), 1406–1409.

68. Kirker, K.R., Luo, Y., Nielson, J.H., Shelby, J., and Prestwich, G.D. (2002) Glycosaminoglycan hydrogel films as bio-interactive dressings for wound healing. *Biomaterials*, **17**, 3661–3671.
69. van Susante, J.L., Pieper, J., Buma, P., van Kuppevelt, T.H., Beuningen, H.V., van der Kraan, P.M. *et al.* (2001) Linkage of chondroitin-sulfate to type I collagen scaffolds stimulates the bioactivity of seeded chondrocytes in vitro. *Biomaterials*, **22**, 2359–2369.
70. Trowbridge, J.M. and Gallo, R.L. (2002) Dermatan sulfate: new functions from an old glycosaminoglycan. *Glycobiology*, **12**, 117R–125R.
71. Volpi, N. and Maccari, F. (2009) Structural characterization and antithrombin activity of dermatan sulfate purified from marine clam Scapharca inaequivalvis. *Glycobiology*, **19** (4), 356–367.
72. Volpi, N. (2010) Dermatan sulfate: recent structural and activity data. *Carbohydr. Polym.*, **82**, 233–239.
73. Reichl, S., Borrelli, M., and Geerling, G. (2011) Keratin films for ocular surface reconstruction. *Biomaterials*, **32**, 3375–3386.
74. Fuchs, E. (1995) Keratins and the skin. *Annu. Rev. Cell Dev. Biol.*, **11**, 123–153.
75. Kirfel, J., Magin, T.M., and Reichelt, J. (2003) Keratins: a structural scaffold with emerging functions. *Cell. Mol. Life Sci.*, **60** (1), 56–71.
76. Xu, H., Shi, Z., Reddy, N., and Yang, Y. (2014) Intrinsically water-stable keratin nanoparticles and their in vivo biodistribution for targeted delivery. *J. Agric. Food Chem.*, **62**, 9145–9150.
77. Morais, J.M., Papadimitrakopoulos, F., and Burgess, D.J. (2010) Biomaterials/tissue interactions: possible solutions to overcome foreign body response. *AAPS J.*, **12** (2), 188–196.
78. de Guzman, R.C., Merrill, M.R., Richter, J.R., Hamzi, R.I., Greengauz-Roberts, O.K., and Van Dyke, M.E. (2011) Mechanical and biological properties of keratose biomaterials. *Biomaterials*, **32**, 8205–8217.
79. Gil, M.H. (2014) *Carbohydrates Applications in Medicine*, Research Signpost, pp. 31–53. ISBN: 978-81-308-0523-8
80. Mehvar, R. (2000) Dextrans for targeted and sustained delivery of therapeutic and imaging agents. *J. Controlled Release*, **69**, 1.
81. Tomme, S.R.V. and Hennink, W.E. (2007) Biodegradable dextran hydrogels for protein delivery applications. *Expert Rev. Med. Devices*, **4**, 147.
82. Khalikova, E., Susi, P., and Korpela, T. (2005) Microbial dextran-hydrolyzing enzymes: fundamentals and applications. *Microbiol. Mol. Biol. Rev.*, **69**, 306.
83. Tassa, C., Shaw, S.Y., and Weissleder, R. (2011) Dextran-coated iron oxide nanoparticles: a versatile platform for targeted molecular imaging, molecular diagnostics, and therapy. *Acc. Chem. Res.*, **44**, 842.
84. Sun, G. *et al.* (2011) Dextran hydrogel scaffolds enhance angiogenic responses and promote complete skin regeneration during burn wound healing. *Proc. Natl. Acad. Sci. U.S.A.*, **108**, 20976.
85. Lauder, C.I., Garcea, G., Strickland, A., and Maddern, G.J. (2011) Use of a modified chitosan-dextran gel to prevent peritoneal adhesions in a rat model. *J. Surg. Res.*, **171**, 877.
86. Zumbuehl, A. *et al.* (2007) Antifungal hydrogels. *Proc. Natl. Acad. Sci. U.S.A.*, **104**, 12994.
87. Hudson, S.P., Langer, R., Fink, G.R., and Kohane, D.S. (2009) Injectable in situ cross-linking for local antifungal therapy. *Biomaterials*, **31**, 1444.
88. Yapo, B.M. (2011) Pectic substances: from simple pectic polysaccharides to complex pectins—A new hypothetical model. *Carbohydr. Polym.*, **86**, 373–385.
89. Munarin, F., Petrini, P., Tanzi, M.C., Barbosa, M.A., and Granja, P.L. (2012) Biofunctional chemically modified pectin for cell delivery. *Soft Matter*, **8**, 4731–4739.
90. Tan, H. and Marra, K.G. (2010) Injectable, biodegradable hydrogels for tissue engineering applications. *Materials*, **3**, 1746–1767.

91. Sriamornsak, P., Wattanakorn, N., and Takeuchi, H. (2010) Study on the mucoadhesion mechanism of pectin by atomic force microscopy and mucin-particle method. *Carbohydr. Polym.*, **79**, 54–59.
92. Ludwig, A. (2005) The use of mucoadhesive polymers in ocular drug delivery. *Adv. Drug Delivery Rev.*, **57**, 1595–1639.
93. Taylor, D., Galan, V., Weinstein, S.M., Reyes, E., Pupo-Araya, A.R., and Rauck, R. (2010) Fentanyl pectin nasal spray in breakthrough cancer pain. *J. Support. Oncol.*, **8**, 184–190.
94. Portenoy, R.K., Burton, A.W., Gabrail, N., and Taylor, D. (2010) A multicenter, placebo-controlled, double-blind, multiple-crossover study of Fentanyl Pectin Nasal Spray (FPNS) in the treatment of breakthrough cancer pain. *Pain*, **151**, 617–624.
95. Fisher, A., Watling, M., Smith, A., and Knight, A. (2010) Pharmacokinetics and relative bioavailability of fentanyl pectin nasal spray 100 – 800 μg in healthy volunteers. *Int. J. Clin. Pharmacol. Ther.*, **48**, 860–867.
96. Luppi, B., Bigucci, F., Abruzzo, A., Corace, G., Cerchiara, T., and Zecchi, V. (2010) Freeze-dried chitosan/pectin nasal inserts for antipsychotic drug delivery. *Eur. J. Pharm. Biopharm.*, **75**, 381–387.
97. Illum, L. (1999) Nasal drug delivery composition containing nicotine. US Patent 5935604.
98. Paharia, A., Yadav, A.K., Rai, G., Jain, S.K., Pancholi, S.S., and Agrawal, G.P. (2007) Eudragit-coated pectin microspheres of 5-fluorouracil for colon targeting. *AAPS Pharm- SciTech*, **8**, 87–93.
99. Dhalleine, C., Assifaoui, A., Moulari, B., Pellequer, Y., Cayot, P., Lamprecht, A., and Chambin, O. (2011) Zinc-pectinate beads as an in vivo self-assembling system for pulsatile drug delivery. *Int. J. Pharm.*, **414**, 28–34.
100. Perera, G., Barthelmes, J., and Bernkop-Schnürch, A. (2010) Novel pectin-4-aminothiophenole conjugate microparticles for colon-specific drug delivery. *J. Controlled Release*, **145**, 240–246.
101. Das, S., Chaudhury, A., and Ng, K.Y. (2011) Preparation and evaluation of zinc–pectin–chitosan composite particles for drug delivery to the colon: role of chitosan in modifying *in vitro* and *in vivo* drug release. *Int. J. Pharm.*, **406**, 11–20.
102. Ni, Y. and Yates, K.M. (2004) In situ gel formation of pectin. US Patent 6777000.
103. Glinsky, V.V. and Raz, A. (2009) Modified citrus pectin anti-metastatic properties: one bullet, multiple targets. *Carbohydr. Res.*, **344**, 1788–1791.
104. Wightman, L., Kircheis, R., Rössler, V., Carotta, S., Ruzicka, R., Kursa, M., and Wagner, E. (2001) Different behavior of branched and linear polyethylenimine for gene delivery in vitro and in vivo. *J. Gene Med.*, **3**, 362–372.
105. Köping-Höggard, M., Tubulekas, I., Guan, H., Edwards, K., Nilsson, M., and Varum, K.M. (2001) Chitosan as a nonviral gene delivery system. Structure–property relationships and characteristics compared with polyethylenimine in vitro and after lung administration in vivo. *Gene Ther.*, **8**, 1108–1121.
106. Guo, W. and Lee, R.J. (2000) Efficient gene delivery using anionic liposome-complexed polyplexes (LPDII). *Biosci. Rep.*, **20**, 419–432.
107. Asnaghi, A.M., Candiani, G., Farè, S., Fiore, G.B., Petrini, P., Raimondi, M.T., Soncini, M., and Mantero, S. (2011) Trends in biomedical engineering: focus on Regenerative Medicine. *J. Appl. Biomater. Biomech.*, **9**, 73–86.
108. Coimbra, P., Ferreira, P., de Sousa, H.C., Batista, P., Rodrigues, M.A., Correia, I.J., and Gil, M.H. (2011) Preparation and chemical and biological characterization of a pectin/chitosan polyelectrolyte complex scaffold for possible bone tissue engineering applications. *Int. J. Biol. Macromol.*, **48**, 112–118.
109. Munarin, F., Guerreiro, S.S., Grellier, M.A., Tanzi, M.C., Barbosa, M.A., Petrini, P., and Granja, P.L. (2011) Pectin-based injectable biomaterials

for bone tissue engineering. *Biomacromolecules*, **12**, 568–577.

110. Munarin, F., Tanzi, M.C., and Petrini, P. (2012) Advances in biomedical applications of pectin gels. *Int. J. Biol. Macromol.*, **51**, 681–689.
111. Kaul, G. and Amiji, M. (2002) Long-circulating poly(ethylene glycol)-modified gelatin nanoparticles for intracellular delivery. *Pharm. Res.*, **19**, 1061–1067.
112. Wu, D. and Wan, M. (2008) A novel fluoride anion modified gelatine nanogel system for ultrasound-triggered drug release. *J. Pharm. Pharm. Sci.*, **11**, 32–45.
113. Balthasar, S., Michaelis, K., Dinauer, N. *et al.* (2005) Preparation and characterisation of antibody modified gelatin nanoparticles as drug carrier system for uptake in lymphocytes. *Biomaterials*, **26**, 2723–2732.
114. Saxena, A., Tahir, A., Kaloti, M., and Ali, J. (2011) Effect of agar-gelatin compositions on the release of salbutamol tablets. *Int. J. Pharm. Investig.*, **4**, 93–98.
115. Kommareddy, S. and Amiji, M. (2005) Preparation and evaluation of thiol-modified gelatin nanoparticles for intracellular DNA delivery in response to glutathione. *Int. J. Pharm. Investig.*, **16**, 1423–1432.
116. Li, W., Liu, D., and Chen, S. (2005) Amphiphilically-modified gelatine nanoparticles: self-assembly behavior, controlled biodegradability, and rapid cellular uptake for intracellular drug delivery. *Biomaterials*, **16**, 1423–1432.
117. Kommareddy, S. and Amiji, M. (2002) Cell transfection and analysis using DNA-loaded gelatin nanoparticles. *Pharm. Res.*, **19**, 1061–1067.
118. Adhirajan, N., Shanmugasundaram, N., Shanmuganathan, S., and Babu, M. (2009) Functionally modified gelatin microspheres impregnated collagen scaffold as novel wound dressing to attenuate the proteases and bacterial growth. *Pharm. Res.*, **36**, 235–245.
119. Saxena, A., Tahir, A., Kaloti, M., and Ali, J. (2011) Effect of agar-gelatin compositions on the release of salbutamol tablets. *Int. J. Pharm. Invest.*, **1** (2), 93–98.
120. Balmayor, E.R., Tuzlakoglu, K., Azevedo, H.S., and Reis, R.L. (2009) Preparation and characterization of starch-poly-[epsilon]-caprolactone microparticles incorporating bioactive agents for drug delivery and tissue engineering applications. *Acta Biomater.*, **5** (4), 1035–1045.
121. Liu, C.-S., Desai, K.G.H., Meng, X.-H., and Chen, X.-G. (2007) Sweet potato starch microparticles as controlled drug release carriers: preparation and in vitro drug release. *Drying Technol.*, **25** (4–6), 689–693.
122. Silva, G.A., Coutinho, C.O., Ducheyne, P., Shapiro, I.M., and Reis, R.L. (2007) Starch-based microparticles as vehicles for the delivery of active platelet-derived growth factor. *Tissue Eng.*, **13** (6), 1259–1268.
123. Malafaya, P.B., Stappers, F., and Reis, R.L. (2006) Starch-based microspheres produced by emulsion crosslinking with a potential media dependent responsive behavior to be used as drug delivery carriers. *J. Mater. Sci.: Mater. Med.*, **17**, 371–377.
124. Desai, K.G.H. (2005) Preparation and characteristics of high-amylose corn starch/pectin blend microparticles: a technical note. *AAPS Pharm. Sci. Technol.*, **6** (2), E202–E208.
125. Rydell, N., Stertman, L., and Sjöholm, I. (2005) Starch microparticles as vaccine adjuvant. *Expert Opin. Drug Delivery*, **2** (5), 807–828.
126. McDermott, M.R., Heritage, P.L., Bartzoka, V., and Brook, M.A. (1998) Polymer-grafted starch microparticles for oral and nasal immunization. *Immunol. Cell Biol.*, **76** (3), 256–262.
127. Heritage, P.L., Loomes, L.M., Jianxiong, J., Brook, M.A., Underdown, B.J., and McDermott, M.R. (1996) Novel polymer-grafted starch microparticles for mucosal delivery of vaccines. *Immunology*, **88** (1), 162–168.
128. Degling, L., Stjärnkvist, P., and Sjöholm, I. (1993) Interferon- in starch microparticles: nitric oxide-generating activity in vitro and antileishmanial effect in mice. *Pharm. Res.*, **10** (6), 783–790.

129. Artursson, P., Ericsson, J.L.E., and Sjöholm, I. (1988) Inflammatory response to polyacryl starch microparticles, role of arachidonic acid metabolites. *Int. J. Pharm.*, **46** (1–2), 149–157.
130. Baillie, A.J., Coombs, G.H., Dolan, T.F., Hunter, C.A., Laakso, T., Sjöholm, I. *et al.* (2012) Biodegradable microspheres: polyacryl starch microparticles as a delivery system for the antileishmanial drug, sodium stibogluconate. *J. Pharm. Pharmacol.*, **39** (10), 832–835.
131. Fundueanu, G., Constantin, M., Ascenzi, P., and Simionescu, B. (2010) An intelligent multicompartmental system based on thermo-sensitive starch microspheres for temperature-controlled release of drugs. *Biomed. Microdevices*, **12** (4), 693–704.
132. Dimantov, A., Greenberg, M., Kesselman, E., and Shimoni, E. (2004) Study of high amylase corn starch as food grade enteric coating in a microcapsule model system. *Innovative Food Sci. Emerg. Technol.*, **5** (1), 93–100.
133. Lin, C.W. and Lee, T.G. (1993) A note on the microencapsulation of pancreatic protease for protection against gastric digestion. *Anim. Sci.*, **56** (03), 413–417.
134. Santander-Ortega, M.J., Stauner, T., Loretz, B., Ortega-Vinuesa, J.L., Bastos-González, D., Wenz, G. *et al.* (2010) Nanoparticles made from novel starch derivatives for transdermal drug delivery. *J. Controlled Release*, **141** (1), 85–92.
135. Jain, A.K., Khar, R.K., Ahmed, F.J., and Diwan, P.V. (2008) Effective insulin delivery using starch nanoparticles as a potential trans-nasal mucoadhesive carrier. *Eur. J. Pharm. Biopharm.*, **69** (2), 426–435.
136. Yu, D., Xiao, S., Tong, C., Chen, L., and Liu, X. (2007) Dialdehyde starch nanoparticles: preparation and application in drug carrier. *Chin. Sci. Bull.*, **52** (21), 2913–2918.
137. Xiao, S., Tong, C., Liu, X., Yu, D., Liu, Q., Xue, C. *et al.* (2006) Preparation of folate conjugated starch nanoparticles and its application to tumor-targeted drug delivery vector. *Chin. Sci. Bull.*, **51** (14), 1693–1697.
138. Thiele, C., Auerbach, D., Jung, G., Qiong, L., Schneider, M., and Wenz, G. (2011) Nanoparticles of anionic starch and cationic cyclodextrin derivatives for the targeted delivery of drugs. *Polym. Chem.*, **2** (1), 209–215.
139. Kumari, K. and Rani, U. (2011) Controlled release of metformin hydrochloride through crosslinked blends of chitosan-starch. *Pelagia Res. Lib. Adv. Appl. Sci. Res.*, **2** (2), 48–54.
140. Jia, Y., Jinbo, J., Cui, Y., Yang, Y., Gao, L., and Li, J. (2011) pH-responsive polysaccharide microcapsules through covalent bonding assembly. *Chem. Commun.*, **47**, 1175–1177.
141. Zhang, L., Liu, Y., Wu, Z., and Chen, H. (2009) Preparation and characterization of coacervate microcapsules for the delivery of antimicrobial oyster peptides. *Drug Dev. Ind. Pharm.*, **35** (3), 369–378.
142. Chowdary, K.P.R. and Murali, K.M.N. (2008) Synthesis and evaluation of starch–urea–borate as rate controlling matrix for controlled release. *Int. J. Pharm. Sci. Nanotechnol.*, **1** (2), 167–170.
143. Levy, I., Paldi, T., and Shoseyov, O. (2004) Engineering a bifunctional starch–cellulose cross-bridge protein. *Biomaterials*, **25**, 1841–1849.
144. Sachan, N.K., Ghosh, S.K., and Bhattacharya, A. (2010) Evaluation of glutinous rice starch based matrix microbeads using scanning electron microscopy. *J. Chem. Pharm. Res.*, **2** (3), 433–452.
145. Kundu, B., Lemos, A., Soundrapandian, C., Sen, P., Datta, S., Ferreira, J. *et al.* (2010) Development of porous HAp and -TCP scaffolds by starch consolidation with foaming method and drug-chitosan bilayered scaffold based drug delivery system. *J. Mater. Sci. - Mater. Med.*, **21** (11), 2955–2969.
146. Duarte, A.R.C., Mano, J.F., and Reis, R.L. (2009) Preparation of starch-based scaffolds for tissue engineering by supercritical immersion precipitation. *J. Supercrit. Fluids*, **49** (2), 279–285.
147. Sundaram, J., Durance, T.D., and Wang, R. (2008) Porous scaffold of

gelatin-starch with nanohydroxyapatite composite processed via novel microwave vacuum drying. *Acta Biomater.*, **4** (4), 932–942.

148. Salgado, A.J., Coutinho, O.P., and Reis, R.L. (2004) Novel starch-based scaffolds for bone tissue engineering: cytotoxicity, cell culture, and protein expression. *Tissue Eng.*, **10** (3–4), 465–474.
149. Torres, F.G., Boccaccini, A.R., and Troncoso, O.P. (2007) Microwave processing of starch-based porous structures for tissue engineering scaffolds. *J. Appl. Polym. Sci.*, **103** (2), 1332–1339.
150. Gomes, M.E., Ribeiro, A.S., Malafaya, P.B., Reis, R.L., and Cunha, A.M. (2001) A new approach based on injection moulding to produce biodegradable starch-based polymeric scaffolds: morphology, mechanical and degradation behaviour. *Biomaterials*, **22** (9), 883–889.
151. Lam, C.X.F., Mo, X.M., Teoh, S.H., and Hutmacher, D.W. (2002) Scaffold development using 3D printing with a starch-based polymer. *Mater. Sci. Eng., C*, **20** (1–2), 49–56.
152. Gomes, M.E., Godinho, J.S., Tchalamov, D., Cunha, A.M., and Reis, R.L. (2002) Alternative tissue engineering scaffolds based on starch: processing methodologies, morphology, degradation and mechanical properties. *Mater. Sci. Eng., C*, **20** (1–2), 19–26.
153. Espigares, I., Elvira, C., Mano, J.F., Vázquez, B., San Román, J., and Reis, R.L. (2002) New partially degradable and bioactive acrylic bone cements based on starch blends and ceramic fillers. *Biomaterials*, **23** (8), 1883–1895.
154. Malafaya, P.B., Elvira, C., Gallardo, A., San Román, J., and Reis, R.L. (2001) Porous starch-based drug delivery systems processed by a microwave route. *J. Biomater. Sci., Polym. Ed.*, **12**, 1227–1241.
155. Martinez, A., Iglesias, I., Lozanob, R., Teijon, J., and Blanco, M. (2011) Synthesis and characterization of thiolated alginate-albumin nanoparticles stabilized by disulfide bonds. Evaluation as drug delivery systems. *Carbohydr. Polym.*, **83**, 1311–1321.
156. El-Sherbiny, I., Abdel-Mogib, M., Elsayed, A., and Hugh, D. (2011) Synthetic biodegradable pH-responsive alginate-poly (lactic-co-glycolic acid) nano/micro hydrogel matrices for oral delivery of silymarin. *Carbohydr. Polym.*, **83**, 1345–1354.
157. Mennini, N., Furlanetto, S., Cirri, M., and Mura, P. (2012) Quality by design approach for developing chitosan-Ca-alginate microspheres for colon delivery of celecoxib-hydroxypropyl-b-cyclodextrin-PVP complex. *Eur. J. Pharm. Biopharm.*, **80** (1), 67–75.
158. Wells, L. and Sheardown, H. (2011) Photosensitive controlled release with glycol–anthracene modified alginate. *Eur. J. Pharm. Biopharm.*, **79** (2), 304–313.
159. Jeon, O., Powell, C., Solorio, L., Krebs, M., and Alsberg, E. (2011) Affinity-based growth factor delivery using biodegradable, photocrosslinked heparin-alginate hydrogels. *J. Controlled Release*, **154**, 258–266.
160. Huang, X., Xiao, Y., and Lang, M. (2011) Micelles/sodium-alginate composite gel beads: a new matrix for oral drug delivery of indomethacin. *Carbohydr. Polym.*, **87** (1), 790–798.
161. Gong, R., Li, C., Zhu, S., Zhang, Y., Du, Y., and Jiang, J. (2011) A novel pH-sensitive hydrogel based on dual crosslinked alginate/N- -glutaric acid chitosan for oral delivery. *J. Controlled Release*, **85**, 869–874.
162. Moebus, K., Siepmann, J., and Bodmeier, R. (2009) Alginate–poloxamer microparticles for controlled drug delivery to mucosal tissue. *Eur. J. Pharm. Biopharm.*, **72**, 42–53.
163. Davidovich-Pinhas, M., Harari, O., and Bianco-Peled, H. (2009) Evaluating the mucoadhesive properties of drug delivery systems based on hydrated thiolated alginate. *J. Controlled Release*, **136**, 38–44.
164. Ciofani, G., Raffa, V., Pizzorusso, T., Menciassi, A., and Dario, P. (2008) Characterization of an alginate-based drug delivery system for neurological applications. *Med. Eng. Phys.*, **7**, 848–855.

165. Sharma, R.L. (2011) Synthesis and characterization of graft copolymers of N-Vinyl-2-Pyrrolidone onto guar gum for sorption of Fe^{2+} and Cr^{6+}ions. *Carbohydr. Polym.*, **83**, 1929–1936.
166. Mishra, M.M., Yadav, M., Mishra, D., and Behari, K. (2011) Synthesis of graft copolymer (CmgOH-g-NVP) and study of physicochemical properties: characterization and application. *Carbohydr. Polym.*, **83**, 1749–1756.
167. Rana, V., Rai, P., Tiwary, A., Singh, R., Kennedy, J., and Knill, C. (2011) Modified gums: approaches and applications in drug delivery. *Carbohydr. Polym.*, **83**, 1031–1047.
168. Yadav, M., Mishra, D.K., and Behari, K. (2011) Synthesis of partially hydrolyzed graft copolymer (H-partially carboxymethylated guar gum-g-methacrylic acid): a superabsorbing material. *Carbohydr. Polym.*, **85**, 29–36.
169. Nayak, U., Shavi, G., Nayak, Y., Averinen, R., Mutalik, S., Reddy, S., Das Gupta, P., and Udupa, N. (2009) Chronotherapeutic drug delivery for early morning surge in blood pressure: a programmable delivery system. *J. Controlled Release*, **136**, 125–131.
170. Soppimath, K.S., Kulkarni, A.R., and Aminabhavi, T.M. (2001) Chemically modified polyacrylamide-g-guar gum-based crosslinked anionic microgels as pH-sensitive drug delivery q systems: preparation and characterization. *J. Controlled Release*, **75**, 331–345.
171. Krishnaiah, Y.S.R., Satyanarayana, V., Kumar, D., Karthikeyan, R.S., and Bhaskar, P. (2003) In vivo pharmacokinetics in human volunteers: oral administered guar gum-based colon-targeted 5-fluorouracil tablets. *Eur. J. Pharm. Sci.*, **19**, 355–362.
172. Mundargi, R.C., Patil, S.A., Agnihotri, S.A., and Aminabhavi, T.M. (2007) Development of polysaccharide-based colon targeted drug delivery systems for the treatment of amoebiasis. *Drug Dev. Ind. Pharm.*, **33**, 255–264.
173. Kabir, I.G., Yagen, B., Penhasi, A., and Rubinstein, A. (2000) Phosphated-physicochemical characterization. *J. Controlled Release*, **63**, 121–127.
174. Murthy, S., Hiremath, S., and Paranjothy, K. (2007) Evaluation of carboxymethyl guar films for the formulation of transdermal therapeutic systems. *Drug Dev. Ind. Pharm.*, **33**, 255–264.
175. Bhardwaj, T.R., Kanwar, M., Lal, R., and Gupta, A. (2000) Natural gums and modified natural gums as sustained-release carriers. *Drug Dev. Ind. Pharm.*, **26**, 1025–1038.
176. Alvarez-Mancenido, F., Landin, M., and Martinez, P.R. (2008) Konjac glucomannan/xanthan gum enzyme sensitive binary mixtures for colonic drug delivery. *Eur. J. Pharm. Biopharm.*, **69**, 573–581.
177. Shalviri, A., Liu, Q., Mohammad, J., and Wu, X. (2010) Novel modified starch–xanthan gum hydrogels for controlled drug delivery: synthesis and characterization. *Carbohydr. Polym.*, **79**, 898–907.
178. Pandey, S. and Mishra, S. (2011) Graft copolymerization of ethylacrylate onto xanthan gum using potassium perdisulfide as an initiator. *Int. J. Biol. Macromol.*, **49**, 527–535.
179. Ahmed, M.L. and Rao, Y.M. (2010) Formulation & characterization of matrix & triple layer matrix tablets for orally controlled drug delivery. *Int. J. Pharm. Pharm. Sci.*, **2**, 137–143.
180. Jiangyang, F., Wang, K., Liu, M., and He, Z. (2008) In vitro evaluations of konjac glucomannan and xanthan gum mixture as the sustained release material of matrix tablet. *Carbohydr. Polym.*, **73**, 241–247.
181. Sinha, V.R., Singh, A., Singh, S., and Binge, J.R. (2007) Compression coated systems for colonic delivery of 5-fluorouracil. *J. Pharm. Pharmacol.*, **59**, 359–365.
182. Mundargi, R., Patil, S., and Aminabhavi, T. (2007) Evaluation of acrylamide-grafted-xanthan gum copolymer matrix tablets for oral controlled delivery of antihypertensive drugs. *Carbohydr. Polym.*, **69**, 130–141.
183. Bose, P., Reddy, P., Ravi, V., Sarita, D., and Pramod, K.T. (2011) Formulation and evaluation of sustained release floating tablets of diltiazem HCl using

xanthan gum. *Res. J. Pharm. Biol. Chem. Sci.*, **2**, 319–328.

184. Gohel, M., Parikh, R., Nagori, S., and Jena, D. (2009) Fabrication of modified release tablet formulation of metoprolol succinate using hydroxypropyl methylcellulose and xanthan gum. *AAPS PharmSciTech*, **10**, 62–68.
185. Venkataraju, M., Gowda, D., Rajesh, K., and Shivakumar, H. (2007) Xanthan and locust bean gum (from Ceratonia siliqua) matrix tablets for oral controlled delivery of propranolol hydrochloride. *Asian J. Pharm. Sci.*, **2**, 239–248.
186. Coutinho, D.F., Sant, S.V., Shin, H. *et al.* (2010) Modified gellan gum hydrogels with tunable physical and mechanical properties. *Biomaterials*, **31** (29), 7494–7502.
187. Maiti, S., Ranjit, S., Mondol, R., Ray, S., and Sa, B. (2011) Al+3 ion crosslinked and acetalated gellan hydrogel network beads for prolonged release of glipizide. *Carbohydr. Polym.*, **85**, 164–172.
188. Goyal, R., Tripathi, S.K., Tyagi, S. *et al.* (2011) Gellan gum blended PEI nanocomposites as gene delivery agents: evidences from in vitro and in vivo studies. *Eur. J. Pharm. Biopharm.*, **79**, 3–14.
189. Agnihotri, S.A., Jawalkar, S.S., and Aminabhavi, T.M. (2006) Controlled release of cephalexin through gellan gum beads: effect of formulation parameters on entrapment efficiency, size, and drug release. *Eur. J. Pharm. Biopharm.*, **63**, 249–261.
190. Sanzgiri, Y.D., Maschi, S., Crescenzi, V., Callegaro, L., Topp, E.M., and Stella, V.J. (1993) Gellan-based systems for ophthalmic sustained delivery of methylprednisolone. *J. Controlled Release*, **26**, 195–201.
191. Agnihotri, S.A. and Aminabhavi, T.M. (2005) Development of novel interpenetrating network gellan gum poly(vinyl alcohol) hydrogel microspheres for the controlled release of carvedilol. *Drug Dev. Ind. Pharm.*, **31**, 491–503.
192. Fujii, T., Ogiwara, D., Ohkawa, K., and Yamamoto, H. (2005) Alkaline phosphatase encapsulated in gellan–chitosan hybrid capsules. *Macromol. Biosci.*, **5**, 394–400.
193. Kubo, W., Miyazaki, S., and Attwood, D. (2003) Oral sustained delivery of paracetamol from in situ-gelling gellan and sodium alginate formulations. *Int. J. Pharm.*, **258**, 55–64.
194. Jiang, Y.-N., Mo, H.-Y., and Yu, D.-G. (2012) Electrospun drug-loaded core-sheath PVP/zein nanofibers for biphasic drug release. *Int. J. Pharm.*, **438**, 232–239.
195. Hurtado-Lopez, P. and Murdan, S. (2006) Zein microspheres as drug/antigen carriers: a study of their degradation and erosion, in the presence and absence of enzymes. *J. Microencapsul.*, **23**, 303–314.
196. Gong, S.-J., Sun, S.-X., Sun, Q.-S., Wang, J.-Y., Liu, X.-M., and Liu, G.-Y. (2011) Tablets based on compressed zein microspheres for sustained oral administration: design, pharmacokinetics, and clinical study. *J. Biomater. Appl.*, **26**, 195–208.
197. Fernandez-Carneado, J., Kogan, M.J., Castel, S., and Giralt, E. (2004) Potential peptide carriers: amphipathic proline-rich peptides derived from the N-terminal domain of gamma-zein. *Angew. Chem. Int. Ed.*, **43**, 1811–1814.
198. Regier, M.C., Taylor, J.D., Borcyk, T., Yang, Y., and Pannier, A.K. (2012) Fabrication and characterization of DNA-loaded zein nanospheres. *J. Nanobiotechnol.*, **10**, 44.
199. Li, W., Yu, D.-G., Chen, K., Wang, G., and Williams, G.R. (2013) Smooth preparation of ibuprofen/zein microcomposites using an epoxy-coated electrospraying head. *Mater. Lett.*, **93**, 125–128.
200. Hu, D., Lin, C., Liu, L., Li, S., and Zhao, Y. (2012) Preparation, characterization, and in vitro release investigation of lutein/zein nanoparticles via solution enhanced dispersion by supercritical fluids. *J. Food Eng.*, **109**, 545–552.
201. Luo, Y., Wang, T.T.Y., Teng, Z., Chen, P., Sun, J., and Wang, Q. (2013) Encapsulation of indole-3-carbinol and 3,3'-diindolylmethane in zein/carboxymethyl chitosan nanoparticles with controlled

release property and improved stability. *Food Chem.*, **139**, 224–230.
202. Muniz, E.C. *et al* (2014) Recent advances in food packing, pharmaceutical and biomedical applications of zein and zein based materials. *Int. J. Mol. Sci.*, **15**, 22438–22470.
203. Mueller, V., Piai, J.F., Fajardo, A.R., Favaro, S.L., Rubira, A.F., and Muniz, E.C. (2011) Preparation and characterization of zein and zein-chitosan microspheres with great prospective of application in controlled drug release. *J. Nanomater.*, **2011**, 1–6, doi: 10.1155/2011/928728.
204. Korsmeyer, R.W., Gurny, R., Doelker, E., Buri, P., and Peppas, N.A. (1983) Mechanisms of solute release from porous hydrophilic polymers. *Int. J. Pharm.*, **15**, 25–35.
205. Bobokalonov, J.T., Kasimova, G.F., Muhidinov, Z.K., Jonmurodov, A.S., Khalikov, D.K., and Liu, L. (2012) Kinetics of piroxicam release from low-methylated pectin/zein hydrogel microspheres. *Pharm. Chem. J.*, **46**, 50–53.
206. Mehta, S.K., Kaur, G., and Verma, A. (2011) Fabrication of plant protein microspheres for encapsulation, stabilization and in vitro release of multiple anti-tuberculosis drugs. *Colloids Surf., A*, **375**, 219–230.
207. Xiao, D. and Zhong, Q. (2011) In vitro release kinetics of nisin as affected by Tween 20 and glycerol co-encapsulated in spray-dried zein capsules. *J. Food Eng.*, **106**, 65–73.
208. Wongsasulak, S., Puttipaiboon, N., and Yoovidhya, T. (2013) Fabrication, gastromucoadhesivity, swelling, and degradation of zein-chitosan composite ultrafine fibers. *J. Food Sci.*, **78**, N926–N935.
209. Wongsasulak, S., Pathumban, S., and Yoovidhya, T. (2014) Effect of entrapped alpha-tocopherol on mucoadhesivity and evaluation of the release, degradation, and swelling characteristics of zein-chitosan composite electrospun fibers. *J. Food Eng.*, **120**, 110–117.
210. Anderson, T.J. and Lamsal, B.P. (2011) Development of new method for extraction of alpha-zein from corn gluten meal using different solvents. *Cereal Chem.*, **88**, 356–362.
211. Wang, Y. and Chen, L. (2012) Fabrication and characterization of novel assembled prolamin protein nanofabrics with improved stability, mechanical property and release profiles. *J. Mater. Chem.*, **22**, 21592–21601.
212. Nitta, S.K. and Numata, K. (2013) Biopolymer-based nanoparticles for drug/gene delivery and tissue engineering. *Int. J. Mol. Sci.*, **14**, 1629–1654.
213. Wang, H.-J., Gong, S.-J., Lin, Z.-X., Fu, J.-X., Xue, S.-T., Huang, J.-C., and Wang, J.-Y. (2007) In vivo biocompatibility and mechanical properties of porous zein scaffolds. *Biomaterials*, **28**, 3952–3964.
214. Zhang, M., Liu, Y., Jia, Y., Han, H., and Sun, D. (2014) Preparation and evaluation of electrospun zein/HA fibers based on two methods of adding HA nanoparticles. *J. Bionic Eng.*, **11**, 115–124.
215. Unnithan, A.R., Gnanasekaran, G., Sathishkumar, Y., Lee, Y.S., and Kim, C.S. (2014) Electrospun antibacterial polyurethane-cellulose acetate-zein composite mats for wound dressing. *Carbohydr. Polym.*, **102**, 884–892.
216. Wu, F., Wei, J., Liu, C., O'Neill, B., and Ngothai, Y. (2012) Fabrication and properties of porous scaffold of zein/PCL biocomposite for bone tissue engineering. *Composites Part B*, **43**, 2192–2197.
217. Salerno, A., Zeppetelli, S., Oliviero, M., Battista, E., di Maio, E., Iannace, S., and Netti, P.A. (2012) Microstructure, degradation and in vitro MG63 cells interactions of a new poly(epsilon-caprolactone), zein, and hydroxyapatite composite for bone tissue engineering. *J. Bioact. Compat. Polym.*, **27**, 210–226.
218. Yao, C., Li, Y., and Wu, F. (2013) Zein nanofibrous membranes as templates for biomineralization of hydroxyapatite crystallites. *Polym. Compos.*, **34**, 1163–1171.
219. Zhang, M., Liu, Y., Jia, Y., Han, H., and Sun, D. (2014) Preparation and evaluation of electrospun zein/HA fibers based on two methods of adding

HA nanoparticles. *J. Bionic Eng.*, **11**, 115–124.

220. Jiang, Q., Reddy, N., and Yang, Y. (2010) Cytocompatible cross-linking of electrospun zein fibers for the development of water-stable tissue engineering scaffolds. *Acta Biomater.*, **6**, 4042–4051.

221. Miyoshi, S., Kaneko, T., Yoshizawa, Y., Fukui, F., Tanaka, H., and Maruyama, S. (1991) Hypotensive activity of enzymatic alpha-zein hydrolysate. *Agric. Biol. Chem.*, **55**, 1407–1408.

222. Garcia, M.C., Puchalska, P., Esteve, C., and Marina, M.L. (2013) Vegetable foods: a cheap source of proteins and peptides with antihypertensive, antioxidant, and other less occurrence bioactivities. *Talanta*, **106**, 328–349.

223. Parris, N., Moreau, R.A., Johnston, D.B., Dickey, L.C., and Aluko, R.E. (2008) Angiotensin I converting enzyme-inhibitory peptides from commercial wet- and dry-milled corn germ. *J. Agric. Food Chem.*, **56**, 2620–2623.

224. Yamamoto, N., Ejiri, M., and Mizuno, S. (2003) Biogenic peptides and their potential use. *Curr. Pharm. Des.*, **9**, 1345–1355.

225. Ren, X., Ma, H., Mao, S., and Zhou, H. (2014) Effects of sweeping frequency ultrasound treatment on enzymatic preparations of ACE-inhibitory peptides from zein. *Eur. Food Res. Technol.*, **238**, 435–442.

226. Joye, I.J., Davidov-Pardo, G., and McClements, D.J. (2014) Nanotechnology for increased micronutrient bioavailability. *Trends Food Sci. Technol.*, **40** (2), 168–182.

227. Patel, A.R. and Velikov, K.P. (2014) Zein as a source of functional colloidal nano- and microstructures. *Curr. Opin. Colloid Interface Sci.*, **19**, 450–458.

228. Zheng, Y., Haworth, I.S., Zuo, Z., Chow, M.S.S., and Chow, A.H.L. (2005) Physicochemical and structural characterization of quercetin-beta-cyclodextrin complexes. *J. Pharm. Sci.*, **94**, 1079–1089.

229. Luecha, J., Hsiao, A., Brodsky, S., Liu, G.L., and Kokini, J.L. (2011) Green microfluidic devices made of corn proteins. *Lab Chip*, **11**, 3419–3425.

230. Liu, J., Huang, W., Xing, Y., Li, R., and Dai, J. (2011) Preparation of durable superhydrophobic surface by sol-gel method with water glass and citric acid. *J. Sol-Gel Sci. Technol.*, **58**, 18–23.

231. Dong, F., Padua, G.W., and Wang, Y. (2013) Controlled formation of hydrophobic surfaces by self-assembly of an amphiphilic natural protein from aqueous solutions. *Soft Matter*, **9**, 5933–5941.

232. Sasaki, T., Abiko, N., Sugino, Y., and Nitta, K. (1978) Dependence on chain length of anti-tumor activity of (1,3)-β-D-glucan from Alcaligenes faecalis var. myxogenes, IFO 13140, and its acid-degraded products. *Canccer Res.*, **38**, 379–383.

233. Jagodzinski, P.P., Wiaderkiewicz, R., Kurzawski, G., Kloczewiak, M., Nakkashima, H., Hyjek, E., Yamamoto, N., Uryu, T., Kaneko, Y., Posner, M.R., and Kozbor, D. (1994) Mechanism of the inhibitory effect of curdlan sulfate on HIV-1 infection in vitro. *Virology*, **202**, 735–745.

234. Gordon, M., Guralnik, M., Kaneko, Y., Mimura, T., Goodgame, J., and Lang, W. (1995) Further clinical-studies of curdlan sulfate (Crds): an anti- HIV agent. *J. Med.*, **26**, 97–131.

235. Kerrigan, A.M. and Brown, G.D. (2010) Syk-coupled C-type lectin receptors that mediate cellular activation via single tyrosine based activation motifs. *Immunol. Rev.*, **234**, 335–352.

236. Goodridge, H.S., Reyes, C.N., Becker, C.A., Katsumoto, T.R., Ma, J., Wolf, A.J., Bose, N., Chan, A.S.H., Magee, A.S., Danielson, W.A., and Vasilakos, U.D.M. (2011) Activation of the innate immune receptor Dectin-1 upon formation of a 'phagocytic synapse'. *Nature*, **472**, 471–475.

237. Kumar, H., Kumagai, Y., Tsuchida, T., Koenig, P.A., Satoh, T., Guo, Z.J., Jang, M.H., Saitoh, T., Akira, S., and Kawai, T. (2009) Involvement of the NLRP3 inflammasome in innate and humoral adaptive immune responses to fungal β-glucan. *J. Immunol.*, **183**, 8061–8067.

238. Kataoka, K., Muta, T., Yamazaki, S., and Takeshige, K. (2002) Activation

of macrophages by linear (1→3)-β-D-glucans implications for the recognition of fungi by innate immunity. *J. Biol. Chem.*, **277**, 36825–36831.

239. Minari, J., Mochizuki, S., Matsuzaki, T., Adachi, Y., Ohno, N., and Sakurai, K. (2011) Enhanced cytokine secretion from primary macrophages due to Dectin-1 mediated uptake of CpG DNA/beta-1,3-glucan complex. *Bioconjugate Chem.*, **22**, 9–15.

240. Palma, A.S., Feizi, T., Zhang, Y., Stoll, M.S., Lawson, A.M., Diaz-Rodriguez, E., Campanero-Rhodes, M.A., Costa, J., Gordon, S., Brown, G.D., and Chai, W. (2006) Ligands for the beta-glucan receptor, Dectin-1, assigned using "designer" microarrays of oligosaccharide probes (neoglycolipids) generated from glucan polysaccharides. *J. Biol. Chem.*, **281**, 5771–5779.

241. Koumoto, K., Kimura, T., Kobayashi, H., Sakurai, K., and Shinkai, S. (2011) Chemical modification of curdlan to induce an interaction with poly(C). *Chem. Lett.*, **9**, 908–909.

242. Hasegawa, T., Numata, M., Okumura, S., Kimura, T., Sakurai, K., and Shinkai, S. (2007) Carbohydrate appended curdlan as a new family of glycoclusters with binding properties both for a polynucleotide and lectins. *Org. Biomol. Chem.*, **5**, 2404–2412.

243. Kim, B.D., Na, K., and Choi, H.K. (2005) Preparation and characterization of solid lipid nanoparticles (SLN) made of cacao butter and curdlan. *Eur. J. Pharm. Sci.*, **24**, 199–205.

244. Subedi, R.K., Kang, K.W., and Choi, H. (2009) Preparation and characterization of solid lipid nanoparticles loaded with doxorubicin. *Eur. J. Pharm. Sci.*, **37**, 508–513.

245. Li, L., Gao, F., Tang, H., Bai, Y., Li, R., Li, X., Liu, L., Wang, Y., and Zhang, Q. (2010) Self-assembled nanoparticles of cholerterol-conjugated carboxymethyl curdlan as a novel carrier of epirubicin. *Nanotechnology*, **21**, 265601.

246. Kaneo, Y., Tanaka, T., Nakano, T., and Yamaguchi, Y. (2001) Evidence for receptor-mediated hepatic uptake of pullulan in rats. *J. Controlled Release*, **70** (3), 365–373.

247. Suginoshita, Y. *et al.* (2002) Liver targeting of human interferon-β with pullulan based on metal coordination. *J. Controlled Release*, **83**, 75–88.

248. Na, K., Seong-Lee, E., and Bae, Y.H. (2003) Adriamycin loaded pullulan acetate/sulfonamide conjugate nanoparticles responding to tumor pH: pH-dependent cell interaction, internalization and cytotoxicity in vitro. *J. Controlled Release*, **87** (1-3), 3–13.

249. Nogusa, H., Yamamoto, K., Yano, T., Kajiki, M., Hamana, H., and Okuno, S. (2000) Distribution characteristics of carboxymethylpullulan–peptide-doxorubicin conjugates in tumour–bearing rats: different sequence of peptide spacers and doxorubicin contents. *Biol. Pharm. Bull.*, **23** (5), 621–626.

250. Nogusa, H., Hamana, H., Uchida, N., Maekawa, R., and Yoshioka, T. (2000) Improved in vivo antitumor efficacy and reduced systemic toxicity of carboxymethyl pullulan-peptide-doxorubicin conjugate. *Jpn. J. Cancer Res.*, **91** (12), 1333–1338.

251. Na, K. and Bae, Y.H. (2002) Self-assembled hydrogel nanoparticles responsive to tumor extracellular pH from pullulan derivative/sulfonamide conjugate: characterization, aggregation, and adriamycin release in vitro. *Pharm. Res.*, **19** (5), 681–687.

252. Hasegawa, U., Nomura, S.M., Kaul, S.C., Hirano, T., and Akiyoshi, K. (2005) Nanogel-quantum dot hybrid nanoparticles for live cell imaging. *Biochem. Biophys. Res. Commun.*, **331**, 917–921.

253. Na, K., Shin, D., Yun, K., Park, K.-H., and Lee, K.C. (2003) Conjugation of heparin into carboxylated pullulan derivatives as an extracellular matrix for endothelial cell culture. *Biotechnol. Lett*, **25**, 381–385.

254. Nomura, Y., Ikeda, M., Nozomi, M., Yamaguchi, N., Aoyama, Y., and Akiyoshi, K. (2003) Protein refolding assisted by self-assembled nanogels as novel artificial molecular chaperone. *FEBS Lett.*, **553**, 271–276.

255. Shingel, K.I. and Petrov, P.T. (2002) Behavior of γ-ray-irradiated pullulan in aqueous solutions of cationic (cetyltrimethylammonium hydroxide) and anionic (sodium dodecyl sulfate) surfactants. *Colloid Polym. Sci.*, **280**, 176–182.
256. Abu Diak, O., Bani-Jaber, A., Amro, B., Jones, D., and Andrews, G.P. (2007) The manufacture and characterization of casein films as novel tablet coatings. *Food Bioprod. Process.*, **85**, 284–290.
257. Macheras, P., Ismailos, G., and Reppas, C. (1991) Bioavailability study of a freeze-dried sodium phenytoin-milk formulation. *Biopharm. Drug Dispos.*, **12**, 687–695.
258. Watanabe, A., Hanawa, T., Sugihara, M., and Yamamoto, K. (1994) Release profiles of phenytoin from new oral dosage form for the elderly. *Chem. Pharm. Bull.*, **42**, 1642–1645.
259. Yuan, Y., Chesnutt, B.M., Utturkar, G., Haggard, W.O., Yang, Y., Ong, J.L., and Bumgardner, J.D. (2007) The effect of cross-linking of chitosan microspheres with genipin on protein release. *Carbohydr. Polym.*, **68**, 561–567.
260. Song, F., Zhang, L.-M., Yang, C., and Yan, L. (2009) Genipin-crosslinked casein hydrogels for controlled drug delivery. *Int. J. Pharm.*, **373**, 41–47.
261. Elzoghby, A.O., Samy, W.M., and Elgindy, N.A. (2013) Novel spray-dried genipin-crosslinked casein nanoparticles for prolonged release of alfuzosin hydrochloride. *Pharm. Res.*, **30**, 512–522.
262. Song, F., Zhang, L.-M., Shi, J.-F., and Li, N.-N. (2010) Novel casein hydrogels: formation, structure and controlled drug release. *Colloids Surf., B*, **79**, 142–148.
263. Bulgarelli, E., Forni, F., and Bernabei, M.T. (2000) Effect of matrix composition and process conditions on casein–gelatin beads floating properties. *Int. J. Pharm.*, **198**, 157–165.
264. Huppertz, T., Smiddy, M.A., and de Kruif, C.G. (2007) Biocompatible micro-gel particles from cross-linked casein micelles. *Biomacromolecules*, **8**, 1300–1305.
265. Semo, E., Kesselman, E., Danino, D., and Livney, Y.D. (2007) Casein micelle as a natural nanocapsular vehicle for nutraceuticals. *Food Hydrocolloids*, **21**, 936–942.
266. Portnaya, I., Ben-Shoshan, E., Cogan, U., Khalfin, R., Fass, D., Ramon, O., and Danino, D. (2008) Self-assembly of bovine β-casein below the isoelectric pH. *J. Agric. Food Chem.*, **56**, 2192–2198.
267. Shapira, A., Markman, G., Assaraf, Y.G., and Livney, Y.D. (2010) β-casein–based nanovehicles for oral delivery of chemotherapeutic drugs: drug-protein interactions and mitoxantrone loading capacity. *Nanomedicine*, **6**, 547–555.
268. Mandelbaum, A. and Danino, D. (2009) Nanostructured β-Casein Assemblies for the Delivery of Anti-Inflammatory Drugs, http://ism.technion.ac.il/Docs/2009/Posters-Bio/Mandelbaum.pdf (accessed 22 June 2016).
269. Zhu, J. and Li, P. (2003) Synthesis and characterization of poly(methyl methacrylate)/casein nanoparticles with a well-defined core-shell structure. *J. Polym. Sci., Part A: Polym. Chem.*, **41**, 3346–3353.
270. Pan, X., Yao, P., and Jiang, M. (2007) Simultaneous nanoparticle formation and encapsulation driven by hydrophobic interaction of casein-graft-dextran and β-carotene. *J. Colloid Interface Sci.*, **315**, 456–463.
271. Pan, X.Y., Mu, M.F., Hu, B., Yao, P., and Jiang, M. (2006) Acidic solution properties of β-casein-graft dextran copolymer prepared through maillard reaction. *Biopolymers*, **81**, 29.
272. Huppertz, T. and de Kruif, C.G. (2008) Structure and stability of nanogel particles prepared by internal cross-linking of casein micelles. *Int. Dairy J.*, **18**, 556–565.
273. Dreis, S., Rothweiler, F., Michaelis, M., Cinatl, J. Jr., Kreuter, J., and Langer, K. (2007) Preparation, characterisation and maintenance of drug efficacy of doxorubicin-loaded human serum albumin (HSA) nanoparticles. *Int. J. Pharm.*, **341**, 207–214.
274. Wartlick, H., Spänkuch-Schmitt, B., Strebhardt, K., Kreuter, J., and

Langer, K. (2004) Tumour cell delivery of antisense oligonucleotides by human serum albumin nanoparticles. *J. Controlled Release*, **96**, 483–495.

275. Pan, X., Yu, S., Yao, P., and Shao, Z. (2007) Self-assembly of β-casein and lysozyme. *J. Colloid Interface Sci.*, **316**, 405–412.

276. Livney, Y.D. (2010) Milk proteins as vehicles for bioactives. *Curr. Opin. Colloid Interface Sci.*, **15**, 73–83.

277. Omenetto, F.G. and Kaplan, D.L. (2010) New opportunities for an ancient material. *Science*, **329**, 528–531.

278. Perrone, G.S., Leisk, G.G., Lo, T.J., Moreau, J.E., Haas, D.S., Papenburg, B.J., Golden, E.B., Partlow, B.P., Fox, S.E., Ibrahim, A.M.S. *et al.* (2014) The use of silk-based devices for fracture fixation. *Nat. Commun.*, **5**, 3385.

279. Gellynck, K., Verdonk, P.C.M., Nimmen, E., Almqvist, K.F., Gheysens, T., Schoukens, G., Langenhove, L., Kiekens, P., Mertens, J., and Verbruggen, G. (2008) Silkworm and spider silk scaffolds for chondrocyte support. *J. Mater. Sci. Mater. Med.*, **19**, 3399–3409.

280. Wendt, H., Hillmer, A., Reimers, K., Kuhbier, J.W., Schäfer-Nolte, F., Allmeling, C., Kasper, C., and Vogt, P.M. (2011) Artificial skin—culturing of different skin cell lines for generating an artificial skin substitute on cross-weaved spider silk fibres. *PLoS One*, **6**, e21833.

281. Lazaris, A. (2002) Spider silk fibers spun from soluble recombinant silk produced in mammalian cells. *Science*, **295**, 472–476.

282. Vendrely, C. and Scheibel, T. (2007) Biotechnological production of spidersilk proteins enables new applications. *Macromol. Biosci.*, **7**, 401–409.

283. Moisenovich, M.M., Pustovalova, O., Shackelford, J., Vasiljeva, T.V., Druzhinina, T.V., Kamenchuk, Y.A., Guzeev, V.V., Sokolova, O.S., Bogush, V.G., Debabov, V.G. *et al.* (2012) Tissue regeneration in vivo within recombinant spidroin 1 scaffolds. *Biomaterials*, **33**, 3887–3898.

284. Wong Po Foo, C., Patwardhan, S.V., Belton, D.J., Kitchel, B., Anastasiades, D., Huang, J., Naik, R.R., Perry, C.C., and Kaplan, D.L. (2006) Novel nanocomposites from spider silk-silica fusion (chimeric) proteins. *Proc. Natl. Acad. Sci. U.S.A.*, **103**, 9428–9433.

285. Huang, J., Wong, C., George, A., and Kaplan, D.L. (2007) The effect of genetically engineered spider silk-dentin matrix protein 1 chimeric protein on hydroxyapatite nucleation. *Biomaterials*, **28**, 2358–2367.

286. Widhe, M., Bysell, H., Nystedt, S., Schenning, I., Malmsten, M., Johansson, J., Rising, A., and Hedhammar, M. (2010) Recombinant spider silk as matrices for cell culture. *Biomaterials*, **31**, 9575–9585.

287. Lewicka, M., Hermanson, O., and Rising, A.U. (2012) Recombinant spider silk matrices for neural stem cell culture. *Biomaterials*, **33**, 7712–7717.

288. Widhe, M., Johansson, U., Hillerdahl, C.-O., and Hedhammar, M. (2013) Recombinant spider silk with cell binding motifs for specific adherence of cells. *Biomaterials*, **34**, 8223–8234.

289. Jansson, R., Thatikonda, N., Lindberg, D., Rising, A., Johansson, J., Nygren, P.-Å., and Hedhammar, M. (2014) Recombinant spider silk genetically functionalized with affinity domains. *Biomacromolecules*, **15**, 1696–1706.

290. Numata, K. and Kaplan, D. (2010) Silk-based delivery systems of bioactive molecules. *Adv. Drug Delivery Rev.*, **62**, 1497–1508.

291. Lammel, A., Schwab, M., Hofer, M., Winter, G., and Scheibel, T. (2011) Recombinant spider silk particles as drug delivery vehicles. *Biomaterials*, **32**, 2233–2240.

292. Hofer, M., Winter, G., and Myschik, J. (2012) Recombinant spider silk particles for controlled delivery of protein drugs. *Biomaterials*, **33**, 1554–1562.

293. Numata, K., Hamasaki, J., Subramanian, B., and Kaplan, D.L. (2010) Gene delivery mediated by recombinant silk proteins containing cationic and cell binding motifs. *J. Controlled Release*, **146**, 136–143.

294. Numata, K. and Kaplan, D.L. (2010) Silk-based gene carriers with cell

membrane destabilizing peptides. *Biomacromolecules*, **11**, 3189–3195.

295. Spiess, K., Ene, R., Keenan, C.D., Senker, J., Kremer, F., and Scheibel, T. (2011) Impact of initial solvent on thermal stability and mechanical properties of recombinant spider silk films. *J. Mater. Chem.*, **21**, 13594–13604.

296. Hardy, J.G., Leal-Egaña, A., and Scheibel, T.R. (2013) Engineered spider silk protein-based composites for drug delivery. *Macromol. Biosci.*, **13**, 1431–1437.

12
Synthetic Biodegradable Polymers for Medical and Clinical Applications

Raju Francis, Nidhin Joy, and Anjaly Sivadas

12.1
Introduction

Biodegradation of a polymer is defined as the deterioration of its physical and chemical properties and the decrease of its molecular mass down to the formation of CO_2, H_2O, CH_4, and other low-molecular weight products under the influence of microorganisms in both aerobic and anaerobic conditions [1].

In modern medicine polymeric biomaterials have a specific role because they are broken down after their served function, and therefore they are preferred in clinical applications. In order to fit functional demand, materials with the desired physical, chemical, biological, biomechanical, and degradation properties must be selected. Fortunately, a wide range of synthetic degradable polymers have been investigated and developed to meet new challenges in the biomedical field.

Biomedical applications of synthetic biodegradable polymer:

1) Tissue engineering
2) Drug delivery and control release
3) Bioseparation and diagnosis
4) Medical devices
   Drug-eluting stents
   Orthopedic devices
   Disposable medical devices
   Other medical devices
5) Gene delivery
   Poly(L-lysine)-based systems
   Polyphosphoester-based systems
   Polyethylenimine (PEI)-based systems
   Poly(β-amino ester)s-based systems
   Other degradable polymers-based systems

Properties of synthetic biodegradable polymer materials offer more advantages than natural materials: freedom from concerns of immunogenicity, predictable

Biomedical Applications of Polymeric Materials and Composites, First Edition.
Edited by Raju Francis and Sakthi Kumar.

uniformity, and reliability of the source of raw material because polymer materials with fundamental building block units have simple and well-known structures and properties. Synthetic materials have many advantages, which include their use as scaffolds. These polymers can be tailored to exhibit a wide range of mechanical properties and degradation rates and to also serve as a more reliable source of raw materials with the ability to evoke an immune response in the body. Furthermore, polymers can be designed with chemical functional groups that can induce tissue in growth.

Coulembier *et al.* explain the many specific requirements of biodegradable polymers that are used in drug delivery systems [2]. The selection of biopolymers that are natural or synthetic depends on these requirements:

1) Biocompatibility of both polymer and its degradation products
2) Mechanical strength sufficient to meet the needs of specific applications
3) Solubility in various solvents
4) Processibility using available equipment
5) Economically acceptable shelf life
6) Chemical, structural, and application versatility
7) Degradability with degradation kinetics matching a biological process such as wound healing
8) EMEA or FDA, US approval for a polymer, additives, and its degradation products

Attempts to find tissue-engineered solutions to cure orthopedic injuries/diseases have made the development of new polymers essential. The new polymer demands that the scaffold is capable of providing mechanical support and gradually degrades to biocompatible products. More demanding requirements are the ability to incorporate cells, growth factors, and so on and to provide osteoconductive and osteoinductive environments. Star biopolymers have more enhanced properties compared to linear polymers. There has been more focus on poly(L-lactic acid) (PLLA) and poly(ε-caprolactone), due to their availability and ease of use. Thermal, physical, and self-assembly properties can all be tuned by altering the polymer composition, the number and length of the polymer arms, and the polymer tacticity. Biodegradable polymers can be classified into natural polymers, synthetic polymers, and modified copolymers (Figure 12.1). Various biodegradable polymers are described with respect to their composition, structure, properties, and applicability.

The aim of this chapter is to briefly discuss the major classes of biodegradable polymers and their potential in various biomedical applications. This work focuses on the potential applications, biocompatibility, and biodegradation of these polymers to help the reader to further explore the use of polymers or precursors with similar characteristics for developing new polymer compositions in the biomedical field. Continued investigation of new polymer compositions, methods of polymerization, and catalysts is critical to meet the changing and varied demands of polymer properties for medical devices, drug–device combinations, and tissue-engineered scaffolds.

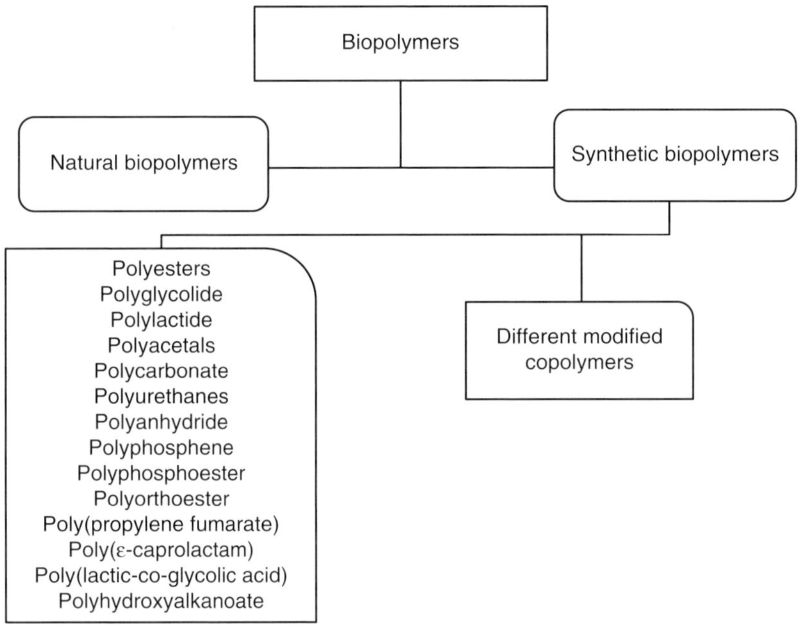

Figure 12.1 Classification of biodegradable polymer.

12.2 Polyesters/Poly(α-hydroxy acids)

Among the families of synthetic polymers, the polyesters have been attractive for these applications because of their ease of degradation by hydrolysis of ester linkage and the ability of the degraded products to be resorbed through the metabolic pathways. Polyesters have also been considered for the development of tissue engineering applications. Although a number of polyesters are commercially available and all are theoretically degradable, the hydrolytically stable nature of the ester bond implies that only polyesters with reasonably short aliphatic chains can be used as degradable polymers for biomedical applications. Although these polymers are often mildly hydrophobic, ester bond stability causes them to undergo bulk erosion. Poly(α-hydroxy acids) are considered as one of the most widely and most primitive researched class of biodegradable polymers. They can be produced from a collection of monomers, for example, glycolide, caprolactone, and lactide [3–6]. The chemical properties of these polymers allow hydrolytic degradation through de-esterification. The degraded monomeric components of each polymer are removed by natural pathways. The human body already contains a highly regulated mechanism that completely removes monomeric components of lactic and glycolic acids [7, 8]. The limitation of this polymer in biomedical fields is that the degradation products reduce the local pH value, which, in turn, may accelerate the polyester's degradation rates. Another disadvantage is that the mechanical properties of the porous scaffolds made from polyesters are relatively weak, which limits their use for bone tissue engineering.

12.3
Poly(glycolide)

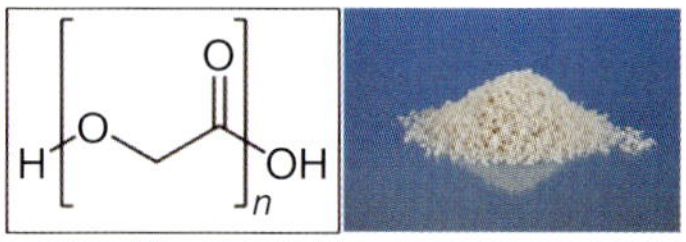

Poly(glycolide) (PGA) or polyglycolic acid was the first biodegradable polymer synthesized in 1971 [9]. A vast majority of the biodegradable polymers studied belong to the polyester family, which includes polyglycolides and polylactides (PLAs). It is the simplest linear, aliphatic polyester and also a biodegradable, synthetic, and thermoplastic polymer. The glass transition and melting temperatures of PGA are 36 and 225 °C, respectively. Because of high crystallinity (46–50%), PGA is not soluble in most organic solvents. In the biomedical field, polyglycolide and its copolymers were broadly utilized as a material for the synthesis of absorbable sutures and being assessed thoroughly at this time. Degradation of polyglycolide into its monomer glycolic acid takes place in two steps. Degradation mainly takes place at the ester bonds. PGA is used in bone tissue engineering and medical application owing to its degradation properties.

The immobilization of biological ligands (such as biotin and peptides) onto polyglycolide is complicated by the absence of functional groups on the polymer backbone. By attaching (+)-biotinyl-3,6,9-trioxaundecanediamine to the surface of PGA sutures, which immobilizes the ligand through an amide bond between amine (ligands) and carboxylic acid groups (surface-hydrolyzed PGA sutures), Lee *et al.* demonstrated a new method for overcoming this problem [10]. This strategy can be applied to surface modifications of other bioaliphatic polyesters, which would improve the active targeting of drugs based on ligand-attached, polymeric drug delivery systems.

Due to its good mechanical properties, PGA has been investigated for application in bone internal fixation devices. However, its degradation rate is very high, which in the end would limit the mechanical properties and biomedical applications for PGA.

12.4
Polylactide

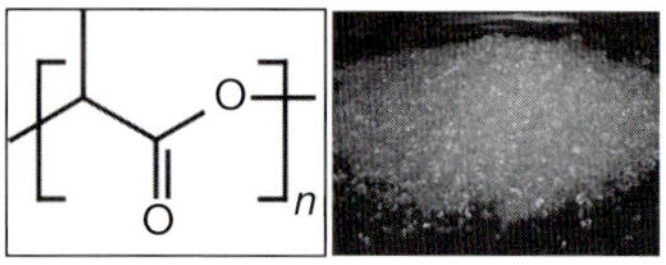

Polylactide possesses chiral molecules. PLAs come in four forms: PLLA, PDLA, PDLLA – a racemic mixture of PLLA and PDLA, and meso-poly(lactic acid).

Poly(lactic acid) is synthesized by the cyclic dimer of lactic acid (LA) that mainly exists as two optical isomers: D- and L-lactate, the latter being the naturally occurring isomer; and D,L-lactide is the synthetic blend of D-lactide and L-lactide. The semicrystalline homopolymer L-lactide has high tensile strength, elongation, good mechanical strength, degradation, biocompatibility, and modulus, all of which make it more suitable for load-bearing applications such as sutures, scaffolds for tissue engineering, drug carriers, and orthopedic fixation. The additional methyl group in PLA causes the polymer to be much more hydrophobic and stable against hydrolysis than PGA. PLLA systems have only limited application due to their slow degradation time. Radiation technique was used for solving this limitation [11, 12]. Radiation creates radicals in the ester alpha carbon, which upon rearrangement shortens the polymer backbone through the removal of an ester bond and the release of carbon dioxide. Recombination of carbon radicals induces branching and cross-linking causing a decrease in crystallinity. Shortening of the polymer and a decrease in crystallinity work in concert with fine-tuning of PLLA degradation behavior; even heavily irradiated PLLA is not completely absorbed until months after being delivered *in vivo*. This holds promise for use in birth control delivery devices. PLLA has been extensively used in bone fixator and tissue engineering applications ranging from scaffolds for bone, cartilage, tendon, neural, and vascular regeneration. PLA can be dissolved in various organic solvents, such as chloroform, methylene chloride, methanol, ethanol, benzene, acetone, and dimethylformamide.

Compared to linear polymers, star polymers exhibit lower melting temperatures (*T*m), glass transition temperatures (*T*g), and crystallization temperatures (*T*c) [13–19]. Star-shaped PLAs have lower hydrodynamic volumes and higher viscosity than linear polymers. The two main factors affecting the properties of star PLAs are the nature of the core and the selection of catalyst. The hydrolytic degradation stability of polymer significantly affects the terminal end group of star arms. The hydrolytic degradation of star-shaped PLAs is a key factor to note when using these materials in controlled release drug delivery systems [20]. PLA star polymers have been investigated for their potential effectiveness as drug delivery vectors and self-assembled micelles, because they can encapsulate dyes, drugs, big, and small molecules.

12.5 Poly(lactic-co-glycolic) Acid

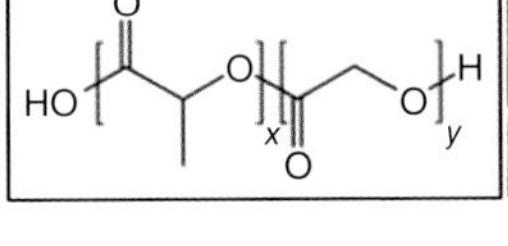

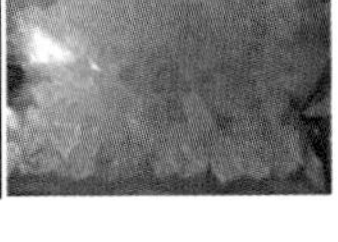

Poly(lactic-co-glycolic) acid (PLGA) is a biocompatible, nontoxic, and noninflammatory polymer formed by the combination of lactic and glycolic acid monomers. Copolymers of glycolide such as PLGA have attracted considerable interest as a base material for biomedical applications due to their

(i) biocompatibility, (ii) tailored biodegradation rate, (iii) approval for clinical use in humans, and (iv) potential to modify surface properties [21]. PLGA has been used in a wide variety of forms, such as films, porous scaffolds, hydrogels, or microspheres. Due to the biological safety and tunable degradation properties of PLGA, it is favored in bone tissue engineering. The mechanical properties and biodegradation rate of PLGA can be manipulated to some extent by controlling the molecular weight and the unit ratio of the copolymer. Due to its low mechanical strength, PLGA cannot be used in load-bearing applications.

12.6 Poly(ε-caprolactone)

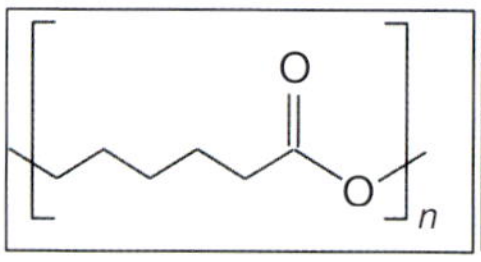

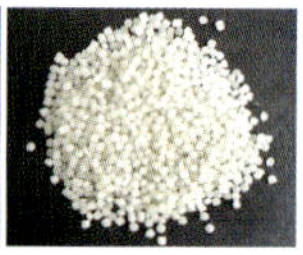

Polycaprolactone (PCL) is a semicrystalline polyester with great organic solvent solubility and low tensile strength, but very high elongation at breakage, low *in vivo* degradation rate, high thermal stability, high decomposition temperature, and high drug permeability. PCL has found favor as a long-term implant delivery device and elastic biomaterial, in drug delivery applications and tissue engineering applications. PCL and PCL composites have been used as tissue engineering scaffolds for the regeneration of bone, ligament, cartilage, skin, nerve, and vascular tissues. With regard to bone engineering, PCL can be categorized as a promising biocompatible and biodegradable polymer. However, due to the slow degradation limits, its application in bone engineering is not favored [22–24].

12.7 Polyurethanes

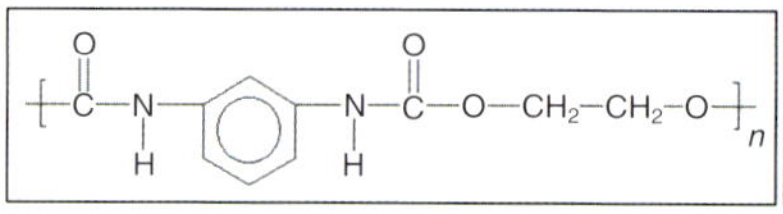

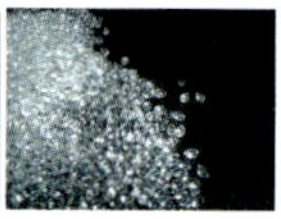

Polyurethanes (PU) are synthetic elastomers that have been evaluated for a variety of medical implants; they have excellent mechanical properties, are biostable and moldable, and have good biocompatibility that helps enhance their medical applications such as scaffolds for tissue engineering. For improving the *in vivo* stability, silicon-based PU were developed. They are used in the fabrication of medical implants such as cardiac pacemakers and vascular grafts. PU can also be designed to have chemical linkages that are degradable in the biological environment such as in both *in vitro* and *in vivo* studies; however, a major problem has been the toxicity of degradation products. PU has ester bonds with geminal amide bonds synthesized by polycondensation of diisocyanates with alcohols and amines [25]. PU are composed of hard and soft segments that can undergo microphase separation provided these polymers have high mechanical properties. PU have been used extensively in prostheses such as cardiac-assist devices, small vascular shunts, and tracheal tubes.

12.8 Polyanhydrides

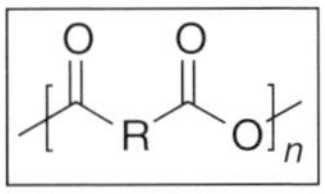

Polyanhydrides (PAs) are a class of surface-eroding biopolymers that contain two carbonyl groups bound together by an ether bond. Poly(sebacic anhydride) is an example of aliphatic homo-PAs, but it has limited applications due to their rapid degradation. PAs are synthesized by dehydration of the diacid, and dicarboxylic acid monomers are converted to the mixed anhydride of acetic acid [26]. High molecular weight polymers are prepared by melt polycondensation of prepolymers. PAs have been used for the delivery of chemotherapeutics, antibiotics, vaccines, and proteins. PAs have limited mechanical properties that control their use in orthopedics. Tyrosine-based polycarbonates are degradable polymers used in load-bearing applications. PAs degrade by hydrolysis of the anhydride linkage. PAs degrade by surface erosion, and their main applications are in controlled drug delivery systems and have been used clinically.

12.9 Polyphosphazenes

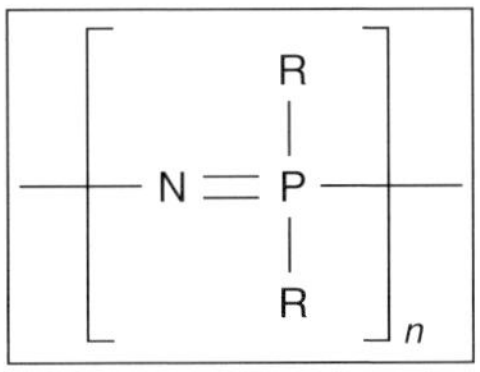

The polyphosphazenes consist of several hundred different polymers; their backbone is completely inorganic consisting of phosphorous and nitrogen bonded linearly through alternating single and double bonds. Most of the polyphosphazenes are biostable, and incorporation of specific side groups such as amino acid esters, glucosyl, glyceryl, lactate, or imidazolyl units renders it biodegradable. Physical properties and degradation rates of polymers are also greatly affected by the selection of the side group. Different polyphosphazenes are made by macromolecular substitution reactions of poly(dichlorophosphazene) reactive polymeric intermediates. The choice of side groups and the processibility of polyphosphazenes have allowed them to form particles, micelles, and gels. Polyphosphazenes have significant promise in tissue engineering applications, drug delivery, chemotherapeutics, growth factors, DNA, proteins, and vaccines. Immune-activating polyphosphazenes have great potential as adjuvants, nonspecific boosting substances, and rapid-degrading polyphosphazenes and are used in drug delivery applications, while the more hydrophobic side group-substituted polyphosphazenes are used in tissue engineering applications.

12.10 Polyhydroxyalkanoates

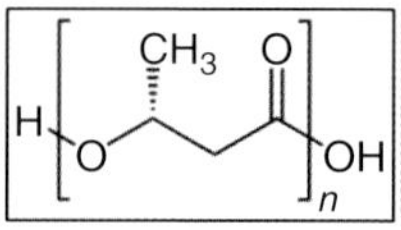

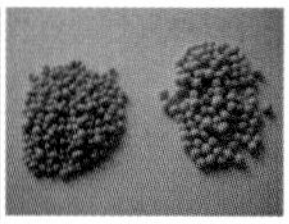

Polyhydroxyalkanoates are biodegradable polyesters that can be synthesized by both (natural) bacterial and synthetic routes. Poly(3-hydroxybutyrate) (PHB), a semicrystalline isotactic polymer, which belongs to this family undergoes surface erosion due to the hydrophobicity of its backbone and its crystallinity. PHB is an excellent candidate for use in tissue engineering applications due to its processibility, biocompatibility, and degradability [27–29]. The main disadvantage of PHB is the limited use in controlled drug delivery due to its stability.

12.11 Polyorthoesters

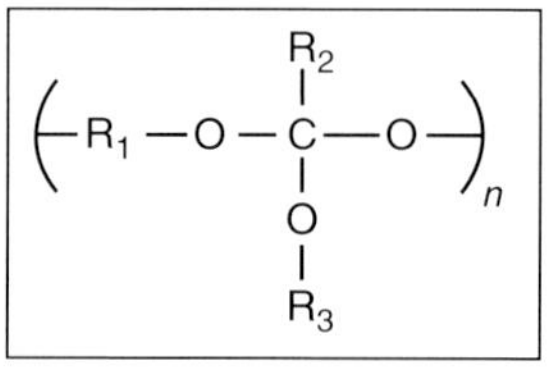

Poly(ortho esters) (POEs) are hydrophobic, surface-eroding polymers, which were developed for drug delivery application and have three geminal ether bonds suitable for orthopedic (load-bearing) applications. Addition of lactide segments in the polymeric structure enhances its tunable degradation times to hundreds of days. POE enhances the bone growth compared to other polymers, but its weak mechanical property limits its application.

12.12 Poly(propylene fumarate)

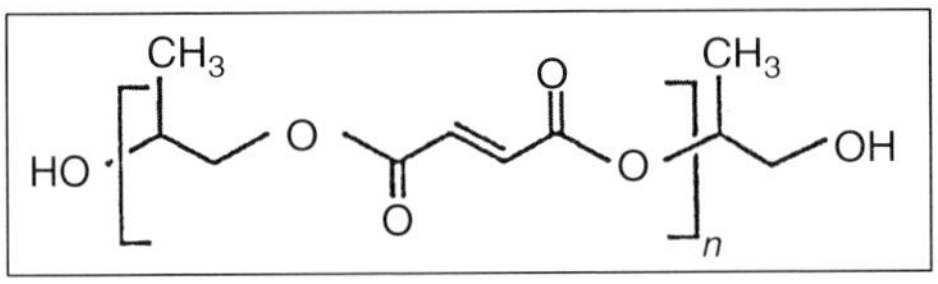

Poly(propylene fumarate) (PPF) is a high-strength biopolymeric material due to the cross-linking of unsaturated bonds in its backbone. The liquid phase of PPF is changed by the addition of a cross-linker; therefore, it is favored in biomedical applications such as bone filling. The degradation rate of PPF depends on the molecular weight, cross-linker, and cross-linking density [30]. Combination of ceramics with PPF helps in osteogenic tissue engineering due to the construction of stronger, more bioactive scaffolds.

12.13 Polyacetals

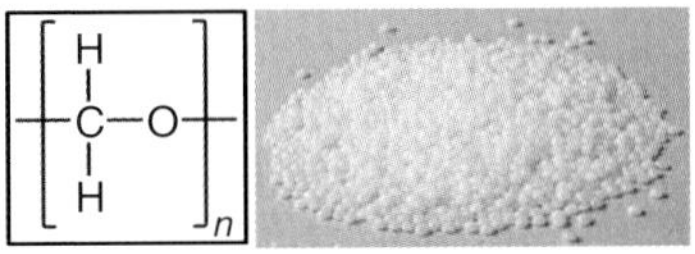

Polyacetals are degradable polymers in which two ether bonds are connected to the geminal carbon molecule and exhibit surface-eroding properties. Polyacetals and polyketals are the two subgroups of polyacetals used in the biomedical field because their acid-catalyzed degradation products possess no carboxylic acids [31, 32]. Low stability of polyacetals limits their application in many areas. To create osteogenic biomaterials for bone tissue engineering scaffolds from polyacetals, cyclic polyacetal monomers with two ester acrylate end groups have been synthesized, which can then be cross-linked [33–35].

12.14 Polycarbonates

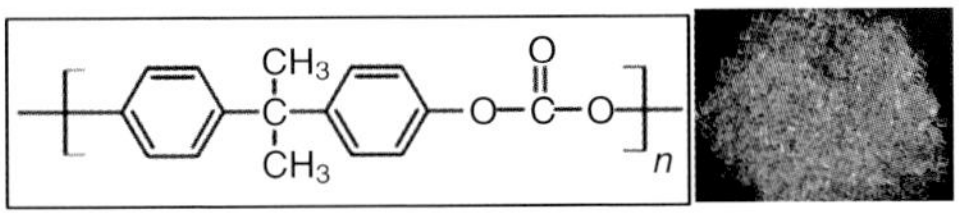

Polycarbonates are linear polymers that have two hydrolytically stable germinal ether bonds and a carbonyl bond. Poly(trimethylene carbonate) (PTMC) is an elastomeric aliphatic polycarbonate with great flexibility and slow degradation, but poor mechanical strength. PTMC is used in the delivery of angiogenic agents and antibiotics in the form of microparticles, discs, and gels. 1,3-Propanediol is a non-acidic biocompatible degradation product of PTMC. α,ω-Dihydroxy telechelic PTMC, HO-PTMC-OH, is a linear dihydroxytelechelic PTMC readily usable as biomaterials. HO-PTMC-OH is synthesized from the controlled "immortal" ring-opening polymerization (ROP) of trimethylene carbonate under mild conditions, using a catalyst precursor [36].

Other polycarbonates are tyrosine-derived polycarbonates and poly (desaminotyrosyl-tyrosine alkyl ester carbonates) (PDTEs). Tyrosine-derived polycarbonates are used as fixators and tissue engineering scaffolds. PDTEs have been studied for their potential in tissue engineering of bone, vasculature, and muscle due to their good physical properties like slow degradation and minimal mass loss [37].

Zhang *et al.* report a facile and efficient method to synthesize linear atactic poly(1,2-glycerol carbonate) using copolymerization of benzyl glycidyl ether with CO_2 using Co-salen complexes [38]. This atactic poly(1,2-glycerol carbonate) showed a remarkable increase in degradation rate compared to poly(1,3-glycerol carbonate). These chiral polycarbonates, from simple and abundant starting materials, expand the repertoire of readily degradable polymers that are available for biomedical applications.

12.15 Polyphosphoesters

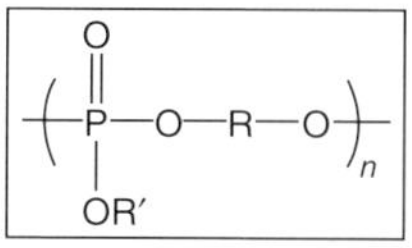

Polyphosphoesters form another class of flexible biomaterials similar to biomacromolecules and are composed of phosphorous-incorporated monomers synthesized by ROP, polyaddition, and polycondensation. These polymers consist of phosphates with two R groups: one in the backbone and the other in the side group [39]. Polyphosphoesters, similar to biomacromolecules, undergo relatively rapid hydrolytic cleavage of the phosphate bonds in the backbone leading to the production of bioresorbable or excretable phosphates, alcohols, and diols. The different forms of polymer such as particles, micelles, films, and gels have been used in various applications like scaffolds in bone tissue engineering. Polyphosphonates and polyphosphates are two different classes of polyphosphoesters. Polyphosphonates have alkyl or aryl R groups, and polyphosphates have alkoxy or aryloxy R groups in their phosphates. Physical properties and degradation rates of polyphosphoesters depend on the selection of R groups.

12.16 Synthesis and Application of Different Modified Synthetic Biopolymer

Well-defined mid-disulfide-functionalized amphiphilic comb-like copolymers with alternating poly(ethylene glycol) (PEG) and poly(ε-caprolactone) side chains were synthesized by a combination of RAFT process and ROP [40]. As compared with linear PEG-*b*-PCL copolymers with similar chain length and weight content of PCL segment, comb-like copolymers comprising PEG and PCL pendant chains usually exhibited decreased crystallization temperature, maximal melting temperature, and high degree of crystallinity, indicating that macromolecular architecture plays an important role in affecting the physicochemical properties of copolymers with similar chemical compositions. The disulfide-linked comb-like copolymer aggregates could rapidly release the encapsulated drug when triggered by 10 mM DL-dithiothreitol and have potential as controlled delivery vehicles due to their excellent storage stability, satisfactory DLC, and rapid drug release in response to reductive environment. Cytotoxicity studies revealed that copolymer aggregates were nontoxic and biocompatible.

Biopolymer-based materials have evinced increasing attention from the packaging industry due to concerns expressed in recent years from both environmental and economic perspectives on the hazards of use of traditional petroleum-based polymers. The extensive use of these traditional synthetic polymers has already resulted in serious ecological problems. Recently, biopolymers have been increasingly found in applications such as food, pharmaceutical, and consumer goods packaging, since they are either totally or partially from renewable resources and have the potential to be biodegradable and/or compostable.

Nitric oxide (NO) is a naturally occurring signaling agent that is responsible for maintaining the functional performance of blood vessel cells in the body and other vascular functions that include modulating hemostasis, regulating vascular tone, and promoting revascularization [41–44]. Overall, compelling evidence suggests that biodegradable materials release NO at tunable levels.

NO-releasing biodegradable polymers have been synthesized by derivatizing poly(lactic-co-glycolic-co-hydroxymethyl propionic acid) (PLGH) polymers with structurally unique thiol functionalities followed by nitrosation to yield pendant S-nitrosothiol moieties [45].The nature of the thiol group was found to greatly influence the overall properties of the polymer, including NO storage as well as the total amount and kinetics of NO release. Stabilization of the S-nitrosated species via cyclic intermediates prevents the rapid and uncontrollable initial decay of the NO donor and results in a clinically relevant level of release. Because of the very short half-life of the NO moiety, it was concluded that the degradation profile of these polymers tends to follow the same pattern as that of the nonnitrosated parent thiol polymers. The degree of cell lysis of a polymer sample suggested that there is no observed cytotoxicity. The functional utility of these materials is demonstrated in that these nontoxic polymers release NO under physiological conditions, have degradation profiles that are appropriate for tissue scaffolds, and can be prepared as electrospun nanofibers, commonly used in tissue and bone regeneration applications.

Prasanna *et al.* developed environment-friendly cathodes using biopolymer chitosan with enhanced electrochemical behavior for use in lithium-ion batteries [46]. Chitosan is compared to the conventional binder, polyvinylidene fluoride (PVDF). Dispersion of the active material, $LiFePO_4$, and conductive agent, Super P carbon black, was tested using a viscosity analysis. Electrochemical impedance spectroscopy (EIS) analysis showed that the $LiFePO_4$ electrode with the chitosan binder had high ionic conductivity and a smaller increase in charge transfer resistance based on time compared to the $LiFePO_4$ electrode with the PVDF binder (Figure 12.2).

Strain-stiffening behavior common to biopolymer networks is difficult to reproduce in synthetic networks. Physically associating synthetic polymer networks can be an exception to this rule and can demonstrate strain-stiffening behavior at relatively low values of strain. Erk *et al.* synthesized synthetic and biopolymer Poly(methyl methacrylate)–poly(*n*-butyl acrylate)–poly-(methyl methacrylate) triblock copolymers for solving this problem [47]. These polymer networks could be useful model systems for biological materials due to (i) the observed similarity in strain-stiffening behavior, which can be quantified and related to network structure, and (ii) the tunable structure of the physically associating network, which can be manipulated to yield a desired response.

Hemorrhage (severe blood loss) from traumatic injury is a leading cause of death for soldiers in combat as well as for young civilians. Dowling *et al.* demonstrated that a sprayable polymer-based foam can be effective for treating bleeding from

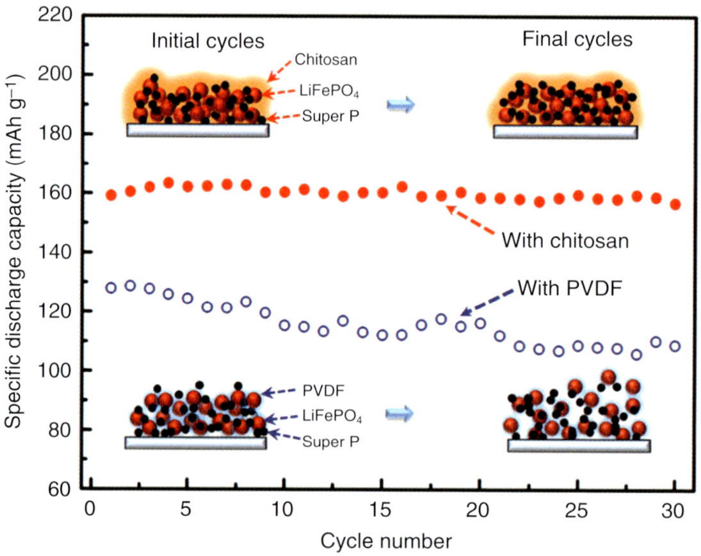

Figure 12.2 Cycling performance of $LiFePO_4$ electrodes prepared using different binders, at 0.1 °C between 2.7 and 4.3 V at room temperature. (Prasanna 2015 [46]. Reproduced with permission from American Chemical Society.)

a soft tissue without the need for compression [48]. When the foam is sprayed into an open cavity created by an injury, it expands and forms a self-supporting barrier that counteracts the expulsion of blood from the cavity. The active material in this foam is the amphiphilic biopolymer, hydrophobically modified chitosan (hmC), which physically connects blood cells into clusters via hydrophobic interaction. Hemostasis was achieved within minutes after application of the hmC foams. The total blood loss was 90% lower with the hmC foam relative to controls (Figure 12.3).

Gualandi *et al.* synthesized a new class of multiblock copolyesters by reactive blending using butylene succinate and triethylene succinate with the same chemical composition but different block lengths – $P(BS_{18}TES_{18})$, $P(BS_9TES_9)$, $P(BS_4TES_4)$, and $P(BS_2TES_2)$. Different types of characterization show that polymer crystallinity, thermal and mechanical properties, wettability, and degradation rate can be controlled by changing the block length. Stiffness of copolymers depends on the crystallinity degree, a tunable range of degradation rates, and surface hydrophilicity [49]. These copolyesters are not cytotoxic, and protein adsorption capability and ability to support cell growth can be controlled by surface hydrophilicity. These characterizations are performed by using fluorescein isothiocyanate (FITC), a model molecule. Depending on comonomer distribution, the polyesters are capable of releasing FITC in a tailorable manner.

β-Calcium metaphosphate (CMP), $Ca(PO_3)_2$, is a kind of bioactive ceramic having high biological compatibility to evoke specific biological responses and safety in living tissues [50, 51]. It can produce a strong bond between the tissue and materials, but due to its brittleness and stiffness, it cannot be used in fracture fixation. For improving the strength, fracture resistance, bone-bonding ability, and biocompatibility, β-CMP is combined with PLLA by a two-step

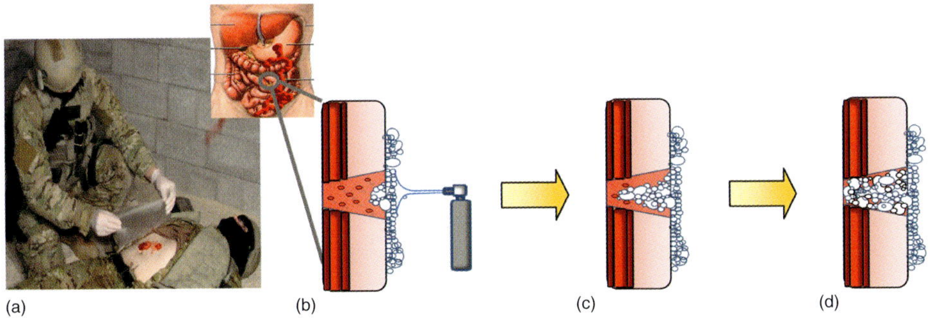

Figure 12.3 Concept of a hemostatic foam to treat noncompressible hemorrhage. (a) Hemorrhage occurring from a wound in the torso region cannot be treated by applying compression of a bandage. (b) Hemostatic foam can be sprayed into the wound cavity. (c) The foam expands into the cavity and forms a solid barrier that counteracts the expulsion of blood. Active ingredients in the foam can also interact with the blood, promoting blood clotting or gelation. (d) The net result is that hemostasis is rapidly achieved, and the bleeding is thereby contained. (Dowling 2015 [48]. Reproduced with permission from American Chemical Society.)

compression-molding method that consists of a low-temperature (50 °C) molding step and a high-temperature (200 °C) molding step [52]. The resultant product is biodegradable and has high mechanical strength.

Polylysine (PLL) is an interesting polymer in gene therapy since it is synthesized from a naturally occurring, noncytotoxic monomer with polyamino acid as its polymer. Terminal amines in its side group have an ability to protonate at physiological pH, which enhances its application in gene therapy techniques [53–64]. The molecular weight of PLL has a major outcome on cell toxicity, transfection efficiency, and biodistribution [65]. Park and Healy synthesized terpolymers of poly(lysine-*g*-(lactide-*b*-ethylene glycol)) through an ROP and functional end-group grafting, which are capable of self-assembling with plasmid DNA [66]. Minimizing the amount of PLL in terpolymer, which is necessary for complete plasmid condensation, may improve transfection efficiency and reduce overall cytotoxicity. Terplex DNA delivery system using PLL has the advantage of being a nonviral gene delivery carrier, good biocompatibility, and high transfection efficiency [67]. Currently, several endogenous lipids incorporated PLL to serve as effective DNA carriers. Carriers with high molecular weight and lipid methylene content increased cellular uptake, generating significant gene expression with relatively low toxicity on bone marrow stromal cells. Myristic, palmitic, and stearic acid-substituted polymers were most effective in DNA delivery [68].

Zeng *et al.* evaluated the cellular uptake profiles and intracellular trafficking of polymer micelles built from the hyperbranched polyester Boltorn, fitted with PEG and fluorescent groups in MDA-MB-468 breast cancer cells [69]. Results showed that the uptake of these nanoparticles correlated positively with both time and concentration, and that the uptake of the nanoparticles was energy dependent (Figure 12.4).

Poly(β-amino ester)s are more suitable for gene delivery because they contain degradable linkages, exhibit ease in synthesis, do not produce byproducts, and so on; they can be synthesized by Michael addition of primary amines to diacrylate esters [70–75]. Poly(4-hydroxy-l-proline ester) was the first biodegradable poly(β-amino ester) used as a gene carrier. Poly(β-amino ester)s synthesized from 2-(pyridyldithio)ethylamine are degradable and contain pyridyldithio functionalities in the side chains that show high specificity toward thiol ligands [76]. This poly(β-amino ester) has low cellular toxicity and may serve as a modular platform for polymer-mediated gene delivery.

Lim *et al.* synthesized poly[α-(4-aminobutyl)-L-glycolic acid], a biodegradable cationic polymer that has ester linkage because polyesters usually show biodegradability [77]. The overall positive charge of the polymer promotes the formation of stable complexes with DNA. Transfection efficiency of the polymer–DNA complex is higher, which possibly arises from the nontoxicity and degradability of the polymer. The polymer is nontoxic, and its final degradation product is a degraded monomer, L-oxylysine.

Around 140 degradable poly(β-amino esters) were prepared by parallel synthesis via the conjugate addition of 20 primary or secondary amine monomers to seven different diacrylate monomers. Akinc *et al.* investigated the ability of each

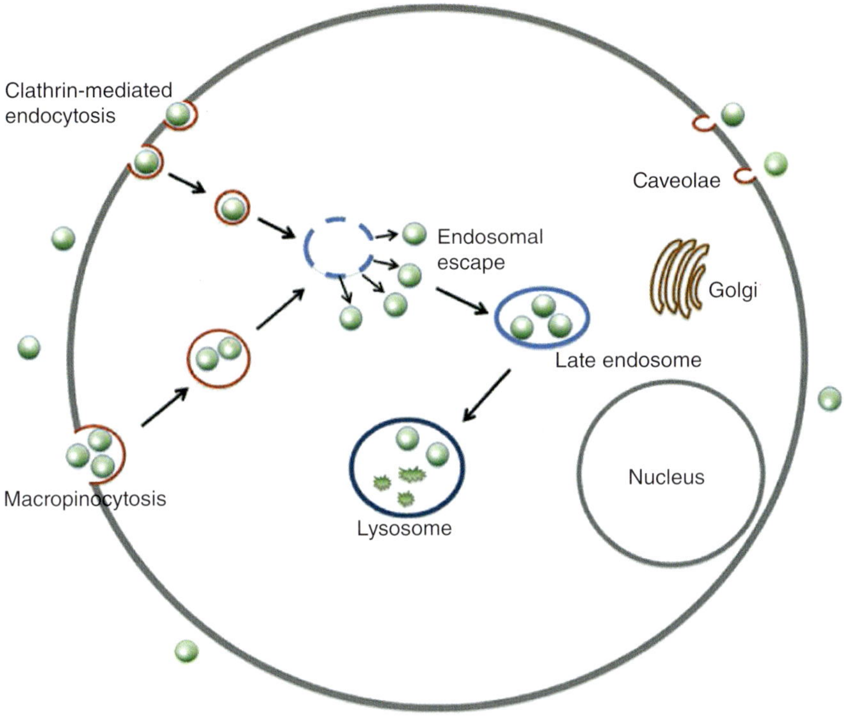

Figure 12.4 Endocytic uptake and intracellular trafficking of hyperbranched copolymer-based micelles in cells. (Zeng 2012 [69]. Reproduced with permission from American Chemical Society.)

DNA-complexing polymer to overcome important cellular barriers to gene transfer [78]. Effective diameter and zeta potential measurements indicated that small particle size and positive surface charge led to higher internalization rates.

The delivery of genetic material to cells offers the potential to treat many genetic diseases. PEI has been used for both *in vitro* and *in vivo* gene-delivery applications [79–83]. Cationic polymers, specifically PEI, are promising gene delivery vectors due to their inherent ability to condense genetic material and successfully affect its transfection. However, PEI and many other cationic polymers also exhibit high cytotoxicity [84]. To overcome the cytotoxicity of PEI, different modifications were carried out using degradable polymers that could retain the high transfection efficiency of PEI. High molecular weight PEI is used in nonviral gene therapy, but its methylene backbone ($-CH_2CH_2N_x-$) and high charge density can result in poor biodegradability and high toxicity to cells [85]. Xiong *et al.* hypothesized that optimizing the polymer length and charge density of PEI may result in decreased toxicity, and higher transfection efficiency, and *in vivo* biocompatibility. Secondary amino groups of branched PEI were linked with cholesteryl chloroformate to form a water-soluble lipopolymer [86]. In this system, the primary amino group was used for conjugation,

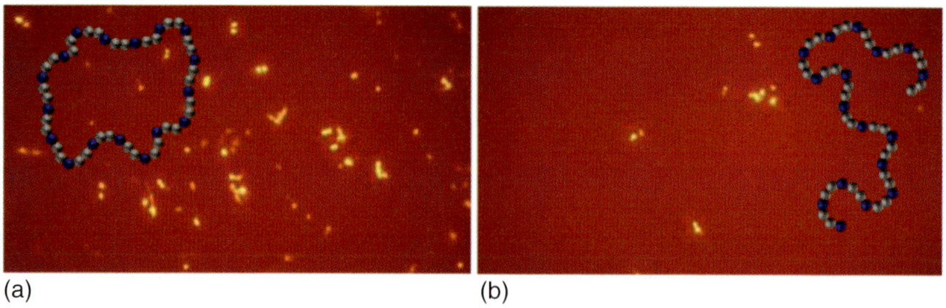

Figure 12.5 PEI in red fluorescent protein (RFP). (a) Cyclic PEI RFP expression and (b) linear PEI RFP expression. (Xiong 2007 [85]. Reproduced with permission from Elsevier.)

as it has a significant role in DNA condensation. Each PEI grafted with one cholesterol molecule provides enough space for the steric interactions of primary amines with the DNA. The interaction between polymer and DNA was carried out by band retardation studies and circular dichroism spectroscopy (Figure 12.5).

Water-soluble complex copolymers were obtained by the reaction between hyperbranched PEI and hydrophobic poly(*g*-benzyl L-glutamate) (PBLG) segment [87]. Experiments show that PBLG at the chain ends of PEI can effectively condense DNA into particles. Cytotoxicity studies by MTT colorimetric assays suggested that the copolymer had much lower toxicity than PEI. Transfection efficiency of the copolymer was considerably improved in HeLa cells, Vero cells, and 293T cells as compared to its corresponding homopolymer.

A series of cationic polymers, multiarmed poly(aspartate-graft-oligoethylenimine) (MP-*g*-OEI) copolymers, were synthesized by grafting different types of oligoethylenimine (OEI) to a multiarmed poly(L-aspartic acid) backbone [88]. These MP-*g*-OEI copolymers exhibited good capacity for condensing nucleic acids (pDNA or siRNA) into nanosized particles with positive surface charges. MP-*g*-OEI copolymers have improved gene transfection activity and lower cytotoxicity. These results suggest that MP-*g*-OEI copolymers may be potential nonviral gene carriers for the delivery of nucleic acids in gene therapy.

12.17 Conclusion

The major classes of polymers are briefly discussed here with regard to synthesis, properties, biodegradability, known degradation modes, and products. Synthetic biopolymers include polyesters, polyamides, polyureas, poly(amide-enamine)s, PAs, and so on. Many of the currently available natural biodegradable polymers do not fulfill all of these requirements, and significant chemical changes to their structure may be required if they are to be expressed for such applications. These show the significance of synthetic biopolymers.

Abbreviations

BS	butylene succinate
CMP	calcium metaphosphate
EMEA	European Medicine Evaluation Agency
FDA	Food and Drug Administration
FITC	fluorescein isothiocyanate
PAs	polyanhydrides
PCL	polycaprolactone
PDLA	poly(D-lactic acid)
PDLLA	poly(D,L-lactic acid)
PEG	poly(ethylene glycol)
PEI	polyethylenimine
PGA	poly(glycolide)
PHB	poly(3-hydroxybutyrate)
PLA	polylactide
PLL	polylysine
PLLA	poly(L-lactic acid)
PLGA	poly(lactic-co-glycolic) acid
PPF	poly(propylene fumarate)
PTMC	poly(trimethylene carbonate)
PU	polyurethanes
PVDF	polyvinylidene fluoride
ROP	ring-opening polymerization
TES	triethylene succinate

References

1. Decriaud, A.C., Maurel, V.B., and Silvestre, F. (1998) in *Block-copolymers – Polyelectrolytes – Biodegradation, Advanced Polymer Science*, vol. 135 (ed. A.C. Albertsson), Springer, Berlin, pp. 207–226.
2. Coulembier, O., Dege, P., Hedrick, J.L., and Dubois, P. (2006) From controlled ring-opening polymerization to biodegradable aliphatic polyester: especially poly(β-malic acid) derivatives. *Prog. Polym. Sci.*, **31**, 723–747.
3. Jagur-Grodzinski, J. (1999) Biomedical application of functional polymers. *React. Funct. Polym.*, **39**, 99–138.
4. Kohn, J.R.L. (1996) in *Biomaterials Science: an Introduction to Materials in Medicine* (eds B.D. Hoffman and A.S. Schoen), Academic Press, New York, pp. 64–72.
5. Mano, J.F., Sousa, R.A., Boesel, L.F., Neves, N.M., and Reis, R.L. (2004) Bioinert, biodegradable and injectable polymeric matrix composites for hard tissue replacement: state of the art and recent developments. *Compos. Sci. Technol.*, **64**, 789–817.
6. Seal, B.L., Otero, T.C., and Panitch, A. (2001) Polymeric biomaterials for tissue and organ regeneration. *Mater. Sci. Eng., R*, **34**, 147–230.
7. Godbey, W.T. and Atala, A. (2002) In vitro systems for tissue engineering. *Ann. N.Y. Acad. Sci.*, **961**, 10–26.
8. Rezwan, K., Chen, Q.Z., Blaker, J.J., and Boccaccini, A.R. (2006) Biodegradable and bioactive porous polymer/inorganic composite scaffolds for bone tissue engineering. *Biomaterials*, **27**, 3413–3431.

9. Frazza, E.J. and Schmitt, E.E. (1971) A new absorbable suture. *J. Biomed. Mater. Res.*, **5**, 43–58.
10. Lee, K.B., Yoon, K.R., Woo, S.I., and Choi, I.S. (2003) Surface modification of poly(glycolic acid) (PGA) for biomedical applications. *J. Pharm. Sci.*, **92** (5), 933–937.
11. Loo, J.S.C., Oooi, C.P., and Boey, F.Y.C. (2005) Degradation of poly(lactide-co-glycolide) (PLGA) and poly(L-lactide) (PLLA) by electron beam radiation. *Biomaterials*, **26**, 1359–1367.
12. Loo, S.C.J., Tan, H.T., Ooi, C.P., and Boey, Y.C.F. (2006) Hydrolytic degradation of irradiated and non-irradiated PLLA. *Acta Biomater.*, **2**, 287–296.
13. Stanford, M.J. and Dove, A.P. (2010) Stereocontrolled ring-opening polymerisation of lactide. *Chem. Soc. Rev.*, **39**, 486–494.
14. Labet, M. and Thielmans, W. (2009) Synthesis of polycaprolactone: a review. *Chem. Soc. Rev.*, **38**, 3484–3504.
15. Gunatillake, P., Mayadunne, R., and Adhitari, R. (2006) Recent developments in biodegradable synthetic polymers. *Biotechnol. Annu. Rev.*, **12**, 301–347.
16. Astruc, D., Boisselier, E., and Ornelas, C. (2010) Dendrimers designed for functions: from physical, photophysical, and supramolecular properties to applications in sensing, catalysis, molecular electronics, photonics, and nanomedicine. *Chem. Rev.*, **110**, 1857–1959.
17. Voit, B.I. (2003) Hyperbranched polymers: a chance and a challenge. *C.R. Chim.*, **6**, 821–832.
18. Zhu, K.J., Song, B., and Yang, S. (1989) Super microcapsules' (SMC). I. Preparation and characterization of star polymethylene oxide (PEO) polylactide (PLA) copolymers. *J. Polym. Sci., Part A: Polym. Chem.*, **27**, 2151–2159.
19. Kim, E.S., Kim, B.C., and Kim, S.H. (2004) Structural effect of linear and star-shaped poly(L-lactic acid) on physical properties. *J. Polym. Sci., Part B: Polym. Phys.*, **42**, 939–946.
20. Cameron, D.J.A. and Shaver, M.P. (2011) Aliphatic polyester polymer stars: synthesis, properties and applications in biomedicine and nanotechnology. *Chem. Soc. Rev.*, **40**, 1761–1776.
21. Gentile, P., Chiono, V., Carmagnola, I., and Hatton, P.V. (2014) An overview of poly(lactic-co-glycolic) acid (PLGA)-based biomaterials for bone tissue engineering. *Int. J. Mol. Sci.*, **15**, 3640–3659.
22. Pitt, C.G., Gratzel, M.M., and Kimmel, G.L. (1981) Aliphatic polyesters. 2. The degradation of poly(DL-lactide), poly(e-caprolactone) and their copolymers in vivo. *Biomaterials*, **2**, 215–220.
23. Porter, J.R., Henson, A., and Popat, K.C. (2009) Biodegradable poly(3- caprolactone) nanowires for bone tissue engineering applications. *Biomaterials*, **30**, 780–788.
24. Mondrinos, M.J., Dembzynski, R., Lu, L., Byrapogu, V.K.C., Wootton, D.M., Lelkes, P.I., and Zhou, J. (2006) Porogen-based solid freeform fabrication of polycaprolactone-calcium phosphate scaffolds for tissue engineering. *Biomaterials*, **27**, 4399–4408.
25. Guelcher, S.A. (2008) Biodegradable polyurethanes: synthesis and applications in regenerative medicine. *Tissue Eng. Part B*, **14**, 3–17.
26. Kipper, M.J., Wilson, J.H., Wannemuehler, M.J., and Narasimhan, B. (2006) Single dose vaccine based on biodegradable polyanhydride microspheres can modulate immune response mechanism. *J. Biomed. Mater. Res. Part A*, **76**, 798–810.
27. Bernd, H.E., Kunze, C., Freier, T., Sternberg, K., Kramer, S., Behrend, D., Prall, F., Donat, M., and Kramp, B. (2009) Poly(3-hydroxybutyrate) (PHB) patches for covering anterior skull base defects – an animal study with minipigs. *Acta Otolaryngol.*, **129**, 1010–1017.
28. Gredes, T., Spassov, A., Mai, R., Mack, H., Loster, B.W., Mazurkiewicz-Janik, M., Kubein-Meesenburg, D., Fanghanel, J., and Gedrange, T. (2009) Changes in insulin like growth factors, myostatin and vascular endothelial growth factor in rat *musculus latissimus dorsi* by poly-3-hydroxybutyrate implants. *J. Physiol. Pharmacol.*, **60**, 77–81.
29. Ahmed, T., Marcal, H., Lawless, M., Wanandy, N.S., Chiu, A., and

Foster, L.J.R. (2010) Polyhydroxybutyrate and its copolymer with polyhydroxyvalerate as biomaterials: influence on progression of stem cell cycle. *Biomacromolecules*, **11**, 2707–2715.

30. He, S., Timmer, M.D., Yaszemski, M.J., Yasko, A.W., Engel, P.S., and Mikos, A.G. (2001) Synthesis of biodegradable poly(propylene fumarate) networks with poly(propylene fumarate)–diacrylate macromers as crosslinking agents and characterization of their degradation products. *Polymer*, **42**, 1251–1260.
31. Weiner, A.A., Moore, M.C., Walker, A.H., and Shastri, V.P. (2008) Modulation of protein release from photocrosslinked networks by gelatin microparticles. *Int. J. Pharm.*, **360**, 107–114.
32. Lee, S., Yang, S.C., Heffernan, M.J., Taylor, W.R., and Murthy, N. (2007) Polyketal microparticles: a new delivery vehicle for superoxide dismutase. *Bioconjugate Chem.*, **18** (1), 4–7.
33. Moreau, J.L., Kesselman, D., and Fisher, J.P. (2007) Synthesis and properties of cyclic acetal biomaterials. *J. Biomed. Mater. Res.*, **81**, 594–602.
34. Betz, M.W., Modi, P.C., Caccamese, J.F., Coletti, D.P., Sauk, J.J., and Fisher, J.P. (2008) Cyclic acetal hydrogel system for bone marrow stromal cell encapsulation and osteodifferentiation. *J. Biomed. Mater. Res. Part A*, **86**, 662–670.
35. Falco, E.E., Roth, J.S., and Fisher, J.P. (2008) EH networks as a scaffold for skeletal muscle regeneration in abdominal wall hernia repair. *J. Surg. Res.*, **149**, 76–83.
36. Helou, M., Miserque, O., Brusson, J.-M., Carpentier, J.-F., and Guillaume, S.M. (2009) Highly effective and green catalytic approach toward a,v-dihydroxy-telechelic poly(trimethylenecarbonate). *Macromol. Rapid Commun.*, **30**, 2128–2135.
37. Tangpasuthadol, V., Pendharkar, S.M., Peterson, R.C., and Kohn, J. (2000) Hydrolytic degradation of tyrosine-derived polycarbonates, a class of new biomaterials. Part II: 3-yr study of polymeric devices. *Biomaterials*, **21**, 2379–2387.
38. Zhang, H. and Grinstaff, M.W. (2013) Synthesis of atactic and isotactic poly(1,2-glycerol carbonate)s: degradable polymers for biomedical and pharmaceutical applications. *J. Am. Chem. Soc.*, **135**, 6806–6809.
39. Ulery, B.D., Nair, L.S., and Laurencin, C.T. (2011) Biomedical applications of biodegradable polymers. *J. Polym. Sci., Part B: Polym. Phys.*, **49**, 832–864.
40. Li, S., Ye, C., Zhao, G., Zhang, M., and Zhao, Y. (2012) Synthesis and properties of monocleavable amphiphilic comblike copolymers with alternating PEG and PCL grafts. *J. Polym. Sci., Part A: Polym. Chem.*, **50**, 3135–3148.
41. Furchgott, R.F. (1999) Endothelium-derived relaxing factor: discovery, early studies, and identification as nitric oxide (nobel lecture). *Angew. Chem. Int. Ed.*, **38**, 1870.
42. Ignarro, L.J., Buga, G.M., Wood, K.S., Byrns, R.E., and Chaudhuri, G. (1987) Endothelium-derived relaxing factor produced and released from artery and vein is nitric oxide. *Proc. Natl. Acad. Sci. U.S.A.*, **84**, 9265.
43. Luque Contreras, D., Vargas Robles, H., Romo, E., Rios, A., and Escalante, B. (2006) The role of nitric oxide in the post-ischemic revascularization process. *Pharmacol. Ther.*, **112**, 553.
44. Gallo, O., Fini-Storchi, I., Vergari, W.A., Masini, E., Morbidelli, L., Ziche, M., and Franchi, A. (1998) Role of nitric oxide in angiogenesis and tumor progression in head and neck cancer. *J. Natl. Cancer Inst.*, **90**, 587–596.
45. Damodaran, V.B., Joslin, J.M., Wold, K.A., Lantvita, S.M., and Reynolds, M.M. (2012) S-nitrosated biodegradable polymers for biomedical applications: synthesis, characterization and impact of thiol structure on the physicochemical properties. *J. Mater. Chem.*, **22**, 5990–6001.
46. Prasanna, K., Subburaj, T., Jo, Y.N., Lee, W.J., and Lee, C.W. (2015) Environment-friendly cathodes using biopolymer chitosan with enhanced electrochemical behavior for use in lithium ion batteries. *ACS Appl. Mater. Interfaces*, **7**, 7884–7890.

47. Erk, K.A., Henderson, K.J., and Shull, K.R. (2010) Strain stiffening in synthetic and biopolymer networks. *Biomacromolecules*, **11**, 1358–1363.
48. Dowling, M.B., MacIntire, I.C., White, J.C., Narayan, M., Duggan, M.J., King, D.R., and Raghavan, S.R. (2015) Sprayable foams based on an amphiphilic biopolymer for control of hemorrhage without compression. *ACS Biomater. Sci. Eng.*, **1**, 440–447.
49. Gualandi, C., Soccio, M., Saino, E., Focarete, M.L., Lotti, N., Munari, A., Moronig, L., and Visai, L. (2012) Easily synthesized novel biodegradable copolyesters with adjustable properties for biomedical applications. *Soft Matter*, **8**, 5466–5476.
50. Jung, Y., Kim, S.S., Kim, Y.H., Kim, S.H., Kim, B.S., Kim, S., Choi, C.Y., and Kim, S.H. (2005) A poly (lactic acid)/calcium metaphosphate composite for bone tissue engineering. *Biomaterials*, **26**, 6314–6322.
51. Jaw, K.-S. (2006) The effects on the devitrification mechanism for a certain composition of CaO/P_2O_5 glass with additives of HAp, TCP, and β-CaP_2O_6 whisker. *J. Therm. Anal.*, **83**, 151–156.
52. Liao, L., Lin, C., Chen, A.-Z., Xi-Ming, P., Kang, Y.-Q., Yao, Y.-D., Liao, X.-M., Huang, Z.-b., and Yin, G.-F. (2007) Preparation and characteristics of novel poly-L-lactide/β-calcium metaphosphate fracture fixation composite rods. *J. Mater. Res.*, **22**, 3324–3329.
53. Zauner, W., Ogris, M., and Wagner, E. (1998) Polylysine-based transfection systems utilizing receptor-mediated delivery. *Adv. Drug Delivery Rev.*, **30**, 97–113.
54. Schatzlein, A.G. (2001) Non-viral vectors in cancer gene therapy: principles and progress. *Anti-Cancer Drugs*, **12**, 275–304.
55. Kwoh, D.Y., Coffin, C.C., Lollo, C.P., Jovenal, J., Banaszczyk, M.G., Mullen, P., Phillips, A., Amini, A., Fabrycki, J., and Bartholomew, R.M. (1999) Stabilization of poly-L-lysine/DNA polyplexes for in vivo gene delivery to the liver. *Biochim. Biophys. Acta, Gene Struct. Expression*, **1444**, 171–190.
56. Jeong, J.H. and Park, T.G. (2002) Poly (L-lysine)-g-poly (D,L-lactic-co-glycolic acid)micelles for low cytotoxic biodegradable gene delivery carriers. *J. Controlled Release*, **82**, 159–166.
57. Wolfert, M.A., Schacht, E.H., Toncheva, V., Ulbrich, K., Nazarova, O., and Seymour, L.W. (1996) Characterization of vectors for gene therapy formed by self-assembly of DNA with synthetic block co-polymers. *Hum. Gene Ther.*, **7**, 2123–2133.
58. Park, S. and Healy, K.E. (2004) Compositional regulation of poly (lysine-*g*-(lactide-*b*-ethylene glycol))–DNA complexation and stability. *J. Controlled Release*, **95**, 639–651.
59. Bikram, M., Ahn, C.H., Chae, S.Y., Lee, M., Yockman, J.W., and Kim, S.W. (2004) Biodegradable poly(ethylene glycol)-*co*-poly(L-lysine)-*g*-histidine multiblock copolymers for nonviral gene delivery. *Macromolecules*, **37**, 1903–1916.
60. Bikram, M., Lee, M., Chang, C.W., Janat-Amsbury, M.M., Kern, S.E., and Kim, S.W. (2005) Long-circulating DNA-complexed biodegradable multiblock copolymers for gene delivery: degradation profiles and evidence of dysopsonization. *J. Controlled Release*, **103**, 221–233.
61. Hashida, M., Takemura, S., Nishikawa, M., and Takakura, Y. (1998) Targeted delivery of plasmid DNA complexed with galactosylated poly (l-lysine). *J. Controlled Release*, **53**, 301–310.
62. Shimizu, N., Chen, J., Gamou, S., and Takayanagi, A. (1996) Immunogene approach toward cancer therapy using erythrocyte growth factor receptor-mediated gene delivery. *Cancer Gene Ther.*, **3**, 113–120.
63. Kang, H.C., Kim, S., Lee, M., and Bae, Y.H. (2005) Polymeric gene carrier for insulin secreting cells: poly (l-lysine)-g-sulfonylurea for receptor mediated transfection. *J. Controlled Release*, **105**, 164–176.
64. Mislick, K.A., Baldeschwieler, J.D., Kayyem, J.F., and Meade, T.J. (1995) Transfection of folate-polylysine DNA complexes: evidence for lysosomal delivery. *Bioconjugate Chem.*, **6**, 512–515.

65. Ward, C.M., Read, M.L., and Seymour, L.W. (2001) Systemic circulation of poly(L-lysine)/DNA vectors is influenced by polycation molecular weight and type of DNA: differential circulation in mice and rats and the implications for human gene therapy. *Blood*, **97**, 2221–2229.
66. Park, S. and Healy, K.E. (2003) Nanoparticulate DNA packaging using terpolymers of poly(lysine-*g*-(lactide-*b*-ethylene glycol)). *Bioconjugate Chem.*, **14**, 311–319.
67. Kim, J.S., Maruyama, A., Akaike, T., and Kim, S.W. (1998) Terplex DNA delivery system as a gene carrier. *Pharm. Res.*, **15**, 116–121.
68. Incani, V., Lin, X., Lavasanifar, A., and Uludag, H. (2009) Relationship between the extent of lipid substitution on poly (L-lysine) and the DNA delivery efficiency. *ACS Appl. Mater. Interfaces*, **1**, 841–848.
69. Zeng, X., Zhang, Y., and Nystrom, A.M. (2012) Endocytic uptake and intracellular trafficking of bis-MPA-based hyperbranched copolymer micelles in breast cancer cells. *Biomacromolecules*, **13**, 3814–3822.
70. Lynn, D.M. and Langer, R. (2000) Degradable poly (β-amino esters): synthesis,characterization, and self-assembly with plasmid DNA. *J. Am. Chem. Soc.*, **122**, 10761–10768.
71. Lynn, D.M., Anderson, D.G., Putnam, D., and Langer, R. (2001) Accelerated discovery of synthetic transfection vectors: parallel synthesis and screening of a degradable polymer library. *J. Am. Chem. Soc.*, **123**, 8155–8156.
72. Lim, Y., Choi, Y.H., and Park, J. (1999) A self-destroying polycationic polymer: biodegradable poly (4-hydroxy-l-proline ester). *J. Am. Chem. Soc.*, **121**, 5633–5639.
73. Koh, J.J., Ko, K.S., Lee, M., Han, S., Park, J.S., and Kim, S.W. (2000) Degradable polymeric carrier for the delivery of IL-10 plasmid DNA to prevent autoimmune insulitis of NOD mice. *Gene Ther.*, **7**, 2099–2104.
74. Christensen, L.V., Chang, C.W., Kim, W.J., Kim, S.W., Zhong, Z., Lin, C., Engbersen, J.F.J., and Feijen, J. (2006) Reducible poly(amido ethylenimine)s designed for triggered intracellular gene delivery. *Bioconjugate Chem.*, **17**, 1233–1240.
75. Anderson, D.G., Peng, W., Akinc, A., Hossain, N., Kohn, A., Padera, R., Langer, R., and Sawicki, J.A. (2004) A polymer library approach to suicide gene therapy for cancer. *Proc. Natl. Acad. Sci. U.S.A.*, **101**, 16028–16033.
76. Zugates, G.T., Anderson, D.G., Little, S.R., Lawhorn, I.E.B., and Langer, R. (2006) Synthesis of poly (β-amino ester) s with thiol-reactive side chains for DNA delivery. *J. Am. Chem. Soc.*, **128**, 12726–12734.
77. Lim, Y.B., Han, S.O., Kong, H.U., Lee, Y., Park, J.S., Jeong, B., and Kim, S.W. (2000) Biodegradable polyester, poly [α-(4-aminobutyl)-L-glycolic acid], as a non-toxic gene carrier. *Pharm. Res.*, **17**, 811–816.
78. Akinc, A., Lynn, D.M., Anderson, D.G., and Langer, R. (2003) Parallel synthesis and biophysical characterization of a degradable polymer library for gene delivery. *J. Am. Chem. Soc.*, **125**, 5316–5323.
79. Bragonzi, A., Boletta, A., Biffi, A., Muggia, A., Sersale, G., Cheng, S.H., Bordignon, C., Assael, B.M., and Conese, M. (1999) Comparison between cationic polymers and lipids in mediating systemic gene delivery to the lungs. *Gene Ther.*, **6**, 1995–2004.
80. Jeong, G.J., Byun, H.M., Kim, J.M., Yoon, H., Choi, H.G., Kim, W.K., Kim, S.J., and OhYK (2007) Biodistribution and tissue expression kinetics of plasmid DNA complexed with polyethylenimines of different molecular weight and structure. *J. Controlled Release*, **118**, 118–125.
81. Boeckle, S., von Gersdorff, K., van der Piepen, S., Culmsee, C., Wagner, E., and Ogris, M. (2004) Purification of polyethylenimine polyplexes highlights the role of free polycations in gene transfer. *J. Gene Med.*, **6**, 1102–1111.
82. Thomas, M., Ge, Q., Lu, J.J., Chen, J., and Klibanov, A. (2005) Cross-linked small polyethylenimines: while still nontoxic, deliver DNA efficiently to mammalian cells in vitro and in vivo. *Pharm. Res.*, **22**, 373–380.

83. Godbey, W.T., Wu, K.K., and Mikos, A.G. (2001) Poly(ethylenimine)-mediated gene delivery affects endothelial cell function and viability. *Biomaterials*, **22**, 471–480.

84. Cortez, M.A., Godbey, W.T., Fang, Y., Payne, M.E., Cafferty, B.J., Kosakowska, K.A., and Grayson, M. (2015) The synthesis of cyclic poly(ethylene imine) and exact linear analogues: an evaluation of gene delivery comparing polymer architectures. *J. Am. Chem. Soc.*, **137**, 6541–6549.

85. Xiong, M.P., Laird Forrest, M., Ton, G., Zhao, A., Davies, N.M., and Kwon, G.S. (2007) Poly(aspartate-*g*-PEI800), a polyethylenimine analogue of low toxicity and high transfection efficiency for gene delivery. *Biomaterials*, **28**, 4889–4900.

86. Wang, D., Narang, A.S., Kotb, M., Gaber, A.O., Miller, D.D., Kim, S.W., and Mahato, R.I. (2002) Novel branched poly(ethylenimine)-cholesterol water-soluble lipopolymers for gene delivery. *Biomacromolecules*, **3**, 1197–1207.

87. Tian, H., Xiong, W., Wei, J., Wang, Y., Chen, X., Jing, X., and Zhu, Q. (2007) Gene transfection of hyperbranched PEI grafted by hydrophobic amino acid segment PBLG. *Biomaterials*, **28**, 2899–2907.

88. Chen, L., Tian, H., Chen, J., Chen, X., Huang, Y., and Jing, X. (2009) Multi-armed poly(L-glutamic acid)-graft-oligoethylenimine copolymers as efficient nonviral gene delivery vectors. *J. Gene Med.*, **12**, 64–76.

Index

Biomedical Applications of Polymeric Materials and Composites, First Edition.
Edited by Raju Francis and Sakthi Kumar.

r

s